CONTROVERSIES IN SHOULDER INSTABILITY

CONTROVERSIES IN SHOULDER INSTABILITY

Editors

Christopher C. Dodson, MD
Sports Medicine Service
The Rothman Institute
Associate Professor of Orthopaedic Surgery
Thomas Jefferson University
Philadelphia, Pennsylvania

David M. Dines, MD
Senior Attending
Sports Medicine and Shoulder Service
Hospital for Special Surgery

Clinical Professor of Orthopedic Surgery
Weill Cornell Medical College of Cornell University
New York, New York

Joshua S. Dines, MD
Sports Medicine and Shoulder Service
Hospital for Special Surgery

Assistant Professor of Orthopedic Surgery
Weill Cornell Medical College
New York, New York

Gilles Walch, MD
Hôpital Privé J Mermoz
Centre Orthopédique Santy
Lyon, France

Gerald R. Williams, Jr, MD
Professor of Orthopaedic Surgery
Chief, Division of Shoulder and Elbow Surgery
The Rothman Institute
Thomas Jefferson University
Philadelphia, Pennsylvania

. Wolters Kluwer | Lippincott Williams & Wilkins
Health
Philadelphia · Baltimore · New York · London
Buenos Aires · Hong Kong · Sydney · Tokyo

Acquisitions Editor: Brian Brown
Product Manager: Dave Murphy
Production Project Manager: Marian Bellus
Manufacturing Manager: Beth Welsh
Marketing Manager: Daniel Dressler
Design Manager: Joan Wendt
Composition: Aptara, Inc.

Library of Congress Cataloging-in-Publication data available on request from the publisher.

DISCLAIMER

Care has been taken to confirm the accuracy of the information presented and to describe generally accepted practices. However, the authors, editors, and publisher are not responsible for errors or omissions or for any consequences from application of the information in this book and make no warranty, expressed or implied, with respect to the currency, completeness, or accuracy of the contents of the publication. Application of this information in a particular situation remains the professional responsibility of the practitioner; the clinical treatments described and recommended may not be considered absolute and universal recommendations.

The authors, editors, and publisher have exerted every effort to ensure that drug selection and dosage set forth in this text are in accordance with the current recommendations and practice at the time of publication. However, in view of ongoing research, changes in government regulations, and the constant flow of information relating to drug therapy and drug reactions, the reader is urged to check the package insert for each drug for any change in indications and dosage and for added warnings and precautions. This is particularly important when the recommended agent is a new or infrequently employed drug.

Some drugs and medical devices presented in this publication have Food and Drug Administration (FDA) clearance for limited use in restricted research settings. It is the responsibility of the health care provider to ascertain the FDA status of each drug or device planned for use in his or her clinical practice.

To purchase additional copies of this book, call our customer service department at (800) 638-3030 or fax orders to (301) 223-2320. International customers should call (301) 223-2300.

Visit Lippincott Williams & Wilkins on the Internet: at LWW.com. Lippincott Williams & Wilkins customer service representatives are available from 8:30 am to 6 pm, EST.

10 9 8 7 6 5 4 3 2 1

Dedication

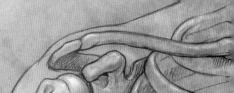

To my wife, Cara, and my children, Connor, Avery, and Lauren, for their endless love, patience, and support. You remind me every day of what is most important in my life.

To my parents, Cloyd and Patricia Dodson, for their years of sacrifice, love, and encouragement.

To my friend and mentor, David Altchek, MD, who has been instrumental in my development as a shoulder surgeon.

To my co-editors for their years of friendship and camaraderie; this collaboration with you has truly been an honor for me.

—Christopher C. Dodson, MD

To my wife and children for their love and support which makes this book and all aspects of my professional career worthwhile.

To my students, residents, and fellows over all these years who by their energy and will to learn stimulate me to be the best educator and clinician that I can be.

—David M. Dines, MD

This book is the result of friendships both here and abroad, and it is an honor to have been part of it. Furthermore, it couldn't have happened without the constant love and support of my family, especially my—expecting—wife, Kathryn, and Humphrey.

—Joshua S. Dines, MD

It's a tremendous honor to be part of this dream team as a co-editor. I dedicate this work to the friendship developed with my colleagues from America. This friendship of 20 years has made my career fascinating and most enjoyable. Nicole, my wife, and my three children made it possible and I thank them for their understanding and support.

—Gilles Walch, MD

I would like to dedicate this book to all of my patients (past, present, and future) who have trusted me with their care, my teachers (especially Dr. Charles Rockwood) who have helped shape my thoughts and professional life, my colleagues and friends who have shared their wisdom along the way (especially my co-editors), and my family (especially my wife, Robin, and my children, Mark and Alexis) without whose love, patience, and support none of this would have been possible.

—Gerald R. Williams, Jr, MD

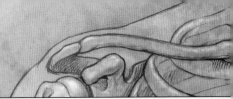

Contributors

Joseph A. Abboud, MD
Associate Professor
Director of Research, Shoulder
    and Elbow Division
Rothman Institute
Shoulder and Elbow Surgery
Thomas Jefferson University
    Hospitals
Philadelphia, Pennsylvania

Jeffrey S. Abrams, MD
Attending Surgeon
University Medical Center at
    Princeton
Department of Surgery
Princeton, New Jersey
Clinical Professor Seton Hall
    University
Department of Surgery
Orange, New Jersey

Answorth A. Allen, MD
Sports Medicine and Shoulder Service
Hospital for Special Surgery
New York, New York

Bashar Alolabi, MD
Fellow
Department of Orthopaedic Surgery
Cleveland Clinic Foundation
Cleveland, Ohio

David W. Altchek, MD
Attending Orthopaedic Surgeon
Department of Orthopaedic
    Surgery
Hospital for Special Surgery
Co-Chief, Sports Medicine and
    Shoulder Service
Hospital for Special Surgery
Professor of Clinical Orthopedic
    Surgery
Weill Cornell Medical College
New York, New York

Michael E. Angeline, MD
Attending Orthopaedic Surgeon
Department of Orthopaedic Surgery
Mercy Health System
Janesville, Wisconsin

Evan Argintar, MD
University Southern California
Department of Orthopedics
Santa Monica, California

Michael B. Banffy, MD
Beach Cities Orthopedics and Sports
    Medicine
Manhattan Beach, California

Asheesh Bedi, MD
Medsport
Department of Orthopaedic Surgery
University of Michigan
Ann Arbor, Michigan

Pascal Boileau, MD
Professor and Chairman
Department of Orthopaedic Surgery
    and Sports Traumatology
Hôpital de L'Archet 2, University
    of Nice-Sophia-Antipolis
Nice, France

Aaron J. Bois, MD, MSc, FRCSC
Department of Orthopaedic Surgery
Orthopaedic and Rheumatologic
    Institute
Cleveland Clinic
Cleveland, Ohio

James P. Bradley, MD
Head Team Physician, Pittsburgh
    Steelers
Clinical Professor
University of Pittsburgh Medical
    Center
Department of Orthopaedic Surgery
Burke and Bradley Orthopaedics
Pittsburgh, Pennsylvania

Robert T. Burks, MD
Professor
Orthopaedic Surgery and Sports
    Medicine
University of Utah
Salt Lake City, Utah

Curtis Bush, MD
Orthopedic Specialty Associates
Fort Worth, Texas

Jon-Michael E. Caldwell, BS
Center for Shoulder, Elbow and
    Sports Medicine
Columbia University Medical
    Center
New York, New York

Kirk A. Campbell, MD
Department of Orthopaedic Surgery
Division of Sports Medicine
New York University Hospital for
    Joint Diseases
New York, New York

Kaitlin M. Carroll, BS
Beach Cities Orthopedics and Sports
    Medicine
Manhattan Beach, California

Ryan T. Cassilly, MD
Center for Shoulder, Elbow and
    Sports Medicine
Columbia University Medical Center
New York, New York

Edward S. Chang, MD
Department of Orthopaedic Surgery
Thomas Jefferson University
Philadelphia, Pennsylvania

Michael G. Ciccotti, MD
Professor of Orthopaedic Surgery
Chief, Division of Sports Medicine
Director, Sports Medicine
    Fellowship and Research
Rothman Institute, Thomas
    Jefferson University
Head Team Physician
Philadelphia Phillies and
    St. Joseph's University
Philadelphia, Pennsylvania

Steven Cohen, MD
Associate Professor
Department of Orthopaedic Surgery
Thomas Jefferson University
Philadelphia, Pennsylvania
Director of Sports Medicine
    Research
Rothman Institute
Philadelphia, Pennsylvania

Edward V. Craig, MD
Sports Medicine and Shoulder Service
Hospital for Special Surgery
New York, New York

Demetris Delos, MD
Sports Medicine and Shoulder Service
Hospital for Special Surgery
New York, New York

Patrick J. Denard, MD
Southern Oregon Orthopedics
Medford, Oregon

David M. Dines, MD
Senior Attending
Sports Medicine and Shoulder Service
Hospital for Special Surgery
New York, New York

Joshua S. Dines, MD
Sports Medicine and Shoulder
  Service
Hospital for Special Surgery
New York, New York

Christopher C. Dodson, MD
Sports Medicine Service
Rothman Institute
Associate Professor of Orthopaedic
  Surgery
Thomas Jefferson University
Philadelphia, Pennsylvania

Jeffrey R. Dugas, MD
Orthopaedic Surgeon
Andrews Sports Medicine &
  Orthopaedic Center
Fellowship Director
American Sports Medicine Institute
Birmingham, Alabama

T. Bradley Edwards, MD
Fondren Orthopedic Group
Texas Orthopedic Hospital
Houston, Texas

Neal S. ElAttrache, MD
Kerlan-Jobe Orthopaedic Clinic
Los Angeles, California

Rachel M. Frank, MD
Resident
Department of Orthopaedic Surgery
Rush University Medical Center
Chicago, Illinois

Mark A. Frankle, MD
Florida Orthopaedic Institute (FOI)
Foundation for Orthopaedic
  Research and Education (FORE)
Temple Terrace, Florida

Jeffrey Gagliano, MD
North Denver Orthopedic Specialists
Thornton, Colorado

Itai Gans, BS
Division of Orthopaedic Surgery
The Children's Hospital of
  Philadelphia
Philadelphia, Pennsylvania

Grant Garrigues, MD
Duke University Medical Center
Durham, North Carolina

Elizabeth Gausden, MD
Sports Medicine and Shoulder
  Service
Hospital for Special Surgery
New York, New York

Albert O. Gee, MD
Department of Orthopaedics and
  Sports Medicine
University of Washington
Seattle, Washington

Antonios Giannakos, MD
Head of Shoulder and Elbow
  Surgery
Asklepios Klinik St. Georg
Hamburg, Germany

Michael J. Griesser, MD
Sports Health Center, Cleveland
  Clinic Foundation
Garfield Heights, Ohio

Lawrence V. Gulotta, MD
Assistant Attending Orthopedic
  Surgeon
Shoulder Surgery and Sports
  Medicine
Hospital for Special Surgery
New York, New York

Stephen C. Hamilton, MD
Steadman Hawkins Clinic of the
  Carolinas
Greenville Hospital System
Greenville, South Carolina

Thomas C. Harris, MS
Massachusetts General Hospital
Boston, Massachusetts

Richard J. Hawkins, MD
Steadman Hawkins Clinic of the
  Carolinas
Greenville Hospital System
Greenville, South Carolina

Waqas M. Hussain, MD
Department of Orthopaedic Surgery
Orthopaedic and Rheumatologic
  Institute
Cleveland Clinic
Cleveland, Ohio

Kristofer J. Jones, MD
Fellow
Sports Medicine and Shoulder
  Service
Department of Orthopaedic Surgery
Hospital for Special Surgery
New York, New York

Richard W. Kang, MS, MD
Hospital for Special Surgery
New York, New York

Kenneth A. Kearns, MD
Orlin & Cohen Orthopedic
  Associates
Rockville Centre, New York

Anne M. Kelly, MD
Sports Medicine and Shoulder
  Service
Hospital for Special Surgery
New York, New York

M. Michael Khair, MD
Resident in Orthopaedic Surgery
Hospital for Special Surgery
New York, New York

Sumant G. Krishnan, MD
The Shoulder Center
Baylor University Medical Center
Dallas, Texas

John E. Kuhn, MD
Associate Professor
Chief of Shoulder Surgery
Vanderbilt University Medical
  Center
Nashville, Tennessee

Laurent Lafosse, MD
Chairman
Clinique Générale d'Annecy
Chairman of Alps Surgery Institute
Annecy, France

Tom Lawrence, MSc, MD, FRCS (Tr & Orth)
Consultant Shoulder and Elbow
    Surgeon
University Hospital Coventry and
    Warwickshire
Coventry, United Kingdom

Mark D. Lazarus, MD
Associate Professor
The Rothman Institute
Department of Orthopaedic Surgery
Thomas Jefferson University
    Medical School
Philadelphia, Pennsylvania

Jason D. Lehman, BA
Medical Student
Research Assistant
Hospital for Special Surgery
New York, New York

James P. Leonard, MD
Midwest Orthopaedic Consultants
Orland Park, Illinois

Bryson P. Lesniak, MD
Department of Orthopaedic Surgery
University of Miami School of
    Medicine
Miami, Florida

William N. Levine, MD
Vice Chairman and Professor
Department of Orthopaedic Surgery
Co-Director
Center for Shoulder, Elbow and
    Sports Medicine
NYP/Columbia University Medical
    Center
New York, New York

Xinning Li, MD
Massachusetts General Hospital
    Shoulder Service
Massachusetts General Hospital
Boston, Massachusetts

Eddie Y. Lo, MD
The Shoulder Center
Baylor University Medical Center
Dallas, Texas

Bryan J. Loeffler, MD
OrthoCarolina
Hand and Upper Extremity Surgery
Shoulder and Elbow Surgery
Charlotte, North Carolina

Travis G. Maak, MD
Assistant Professor
Orthopaedic Surgery and Sports
    Medicine
University of Utah
Salt Lake City, Utah

Moira M. McCarthy, MD
Sports Medicine and Shoulder Service
Hospital for Special Surgery
New York, New York

Walter B. McClelland, Jr, MD
Peachtree Orthopaedic Clinic
Atlanta, Georgia

Frank McCormick, MD
Fellow, Section of Sports Medicine
Department of Orthopaedic Surgery
Rush University Medical Center
Chicago, Illinois

Brett W. McCoy, MD
Department of Orthopaedic Surgery
Orthopaedic and Rheumatologic
    Institute
Cleveland Clinic
Cleveland, Ohio

John McNeil, BA
Department of Orthopaedics
Naval Medical Center San Diego
San Diego, California

Matthew Mendez-Zfass, MD
Department of Orthopaedic Surgery
University of Miami School of Medicine
Miami, Florida

Andrew L. Merritt, MD
Hospital for Special Surgery
New York, New York

Anthony Miniaci, MD, FRCSC
Sports Health Center, Cleveland
    Clinic Foundation
Garfield Heights, Ohio
Department of Biomedical
    Engineering
Lerner Research Institute
Cleveland Clinic
Cleveland, Ohio

Anand M. Murthi, MD
Department of Orthopaedic
    Surgery and Sports Medicine
MedStar Union Memorial Hospital
Baltimore, Maryland

Thomas Obermeyer, MD
Fellow
Department of Orthopaedic
    Surgery
Mount Sinai Medical Center
New York, New York

Michael J. O'Brien, MD
Department of Orthopaedics
Tulane University School of
    Medicine
New Orleans, Louisiana

Stephen J. O'Brien, MD, MBA
Sports Medicine and Shoulder
    Service
Hospital for Special Surgery
New York, New York

Thomas O'Hagan, MD
Sports Medicine Fellow
Department of Orthopaedic
    Surgery
Thomas Jefferson University
Rothman Institute
Philadelphia, Pennsylvania

Ioannis P. Pappou, MD, PhD
Florida Orthopaedic Institute
    (FOI)
Foundation for Orthopaedic
    Research and Education (FORE)
Temple Terrace, Florida

Brad Parsons, MD
Assistant Professor
Department of Orthopaedic
    Surgery
Mount Sinai Medical Center
New York, New York

CDR Matthew T. Provencher,
MD, MC, USN
Professor of Orthopaedics, USUHS
Director, Orthopaedic Shoulder,
    Knee and Sports Surgery
Department of Orthopaedic
    Surgery
Naval Medical Center San Diego
San Diego, California

Patric Raiss, MD
Clinic for Orthopaedic and Trauma
  Surgery
University of Heidelberg
Heidelberg, Germany

Centre Orthopédique Santy
Lyon, France

Miguel A. Ramirez, MD
Department of Orthopaedic Surgery
  and Sports Medicine
MedStar Union Memorial Hospital
Baltimore, Maryland

Matthew L. Ramsey, MD
Rothman Institute
Philadelphia, Pennsylvania

Eric T. Ricchetti, MD
Department of Orthopaedic Surgery
Cleveland Clinic
Cleveland, Ohio

Clay Riley, MD
Martin Knee and Sports Medicine
  Center
Arkansas Surgical Hospital
Little Rock, Arkansas

Scott A. Rodeo, MD
Sports Medicine and Shoulder Service
Hospital for Special Surgery
New York, New York

Anthony Romeo, MD
Department of Orthopaedic Surgery
Section of Shoulder and Elbow
  Surgery
Division of Sports Medicine
Rush University Medical Center
Chicago, Illinois

Gabriel J. Rulewicz, MD
North Mississippi Sports Medicine
  and Orthopaedic Clinic
Tupelo, Mississippi

Richard K.N. Ryu, MD
Senior Surgeon
The Ryu Hurvitz Orthopedic Clinic
Santa Barbara, California

Felix H. Savoie, III, MD
Department of Orthopaedics
Tulane University School of Medicine
New Orleans, Louisiana

Daniel G. Schwartz, MD
Shoulder and Elbow Surgery
Florida Orthopaedic Institute
Tampa, Florida

Nicholas R. Slenker, MD
Kerlan-Jobe Orthopaedic Clinic
Los Angeles, California

Nicole Sliva, BA
Sports Medicine and Shoulder
  Service
Hospital for Special Surgery
New York, New York

Christopher J. Smithers, MD
Nuffield Orthopaedic Centre
Oxford, Oxfordshire, United
  Kingdom

John Sperling, MD
Professor Orthopaedic Surgery
Mayo Clinic
Rochester, Minnesota

Eric J. Strauss, MD
Department of Orthopaedic
  Surgery
Division of Sports Medicine
New York University Hospital for
  Joint Diseases
New York, New York

Sabrina Strickland, MD
Hospital for Special Surgery
New York, New York

Hiroyuki Sugaya, MD
Director, Shoulder & Elbow Service
Funabashi Orthopaedic Sports
  Medicine Center
Chiba, Japan

Misty Suri, MD
Orthopedic Surgery and Sports
  Medicine
Ochsner Health System

Team Physician
New Orleans Saints
Jefferson, Louisiana

Samuel A. Taylor, MD
Sports Medicine and Shoulder
  Service
Hospital for Special Surgery
New York, New York

Sam G. Tejwani, MD
Southern California Permanente
  Medical Group
Kaiser Permanente
Department of Orthopaedic
  Surgery
Division of Sports Medicine
Fontana, California

Matthew J. Teusink, MD
Florida Orthopaedic Institute (FOI)
Foundation for Orthopaedic
  Research and Education (FORE)
Temple Terrace, Florida

Charles-Edouard Thélu, MD
Department of Orthopaedic
  Surgery and Sports Traumatology
Hôpital de L'Archet 2, University of
  Nice-Sophia-Antipolis
Nice, France

Matthew M. Thompson, MD
Sports Medicine and Shoulder
  Service
Hospital for Special Surgery
Senior Clinical Associate in
  Orthopaedic Surgery
Weill Cornell Medical College
New York, New York

James E. Tibone, MD
Department of Orthopedics
University Southern California
Los Angeles, California

John M. Tokish, MD
Director, Orthopedic Residency
Tripler Army Medical
Honolulu, Hawaii

Bradford Tucker, MD
The Rothman Institute
Thomas Jefferson University
Philadelphia, Pennsylvania

Ekaterina Urch, MD
Hospital for Special Surgery
New York, New York

Corinne VanBeek, MD
Fellow, Shoulder and Elbow
  Surgery
Thomas Jefferson University
Philadelphia, Pennsylvania

Nikhil N. Verma, MD
Department of Orthopaedic Surgery
Section of Shoulder and Elbow
  Surgery
Division of Sports Medicine
Rush University Medical Center
Chicago, Illinois

Gilles Walch, MD
Hôpital Privé J Mermoz
Centre Orthopédique Santy
Lyon, France

Jon J.P. Warner, MD
Chief of the Shoulder Service
Professor of Orthopaedic Surgery
Massachusetts General Hospital
  Shoulder Service
Massachusetts General Hospital
Boston, Massachusetts

Russell F. Warren, MD
Professor of Orthopedics, Weil
  Cornell
Professor of Orthopedics, Hospital
  for Special Surgery
Surgeon in Chief Emeritus, Hospital
  for Special Surgery
New York, New York

Lawrence Wells, MD
Division of Orthopaedic Surgery
The Children's Hospital of
  Philadelphia
Philadelphia, Pennsylvania

Matthew J. White, MD
Orthopedic Surgeon
Physicians' Clinic of Iowa
Cedar Rapids, Iowa

Gerald R. Williams, Jr, MD
Professor of Orthopaedic Surgery
Chief, Division of Shoulder and
  Elbow Surgery
The Rothman Institute
Thomas Jefferson University
Philadelphia, Pennsylvania

Phillip N. Williams, MD
Hospital for Special Surgery
New York, New York

Paul Yannopoulos, BA
Research Assistant
Massachusetts General Hospital
  Shoulder Service
Massachusetts General Hospital
Boston, Massachusetts

Foreword

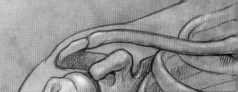

Controversies in Shoulder Instability, as edited by noted shoulder surgeons, Drs. Williams, Walch, Dines, Dines, and Dodson, is a timely text on the treatment of the unstable shoulder. The surgical treatment of the unstable shoulder is clearly in an evolutionary phase.

Just when we thought that we had all the answers many, many controversies have arisen—the role of arthroscopic stabilization, the management of bony deficiency, and revision surgery to name a few. These authors have done a fabulous job assembling a knowledgeable group of authors to help us begin to make some sense out of these complex topics.

I hope you will enjoy this text and learn as much as I have.

David W. Altchek, MD
Hospital for Special Surgery
Co-Chief Sports Medicine & Shoulder Service
New York, New York

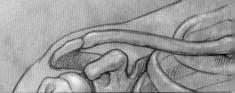

Acknowledgment

*T*he authors would like to say a special thank you to Robyn Alvarez, David Murphy Jr. and Indu Jawwad for their dedication and assistance in the compilation of this text.

Preface

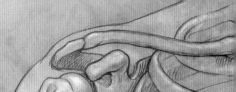

While the treatment of shoulder instability was first reported in Roman times, the subject of glenohumeral instability has remained controversial and complicated for all orthopedic surgeons for centuries. Instability stands as one of the major causes of shoulder disability; and, in spite of significant research on the topic, there remains significant controversy regarding its etiology, pathophysiology, and treatment.

While classification systems for instability have been well defined, many issues have become more confused in recent years. Despite improvements in surgical techniques, the role of open and arthroscopic treatments continues to be debated. More controversy surrounds the ideal treatment for first time dislocators, and how to best treat instability after arthroplasty continues to evoke discussion.

In an attempt to cover the topic of glenohumeral instability in a most comprehensive and contemporary manner, we have assembled an all-star, international group of shoulder surgeons across several generations. Each author was selected for his or her recognized expertise in a specific area of instability. Each chapter and section was created to give the reader the most up-to-date information on that topic. The book encompasses every aspect of shoulder instability including pathophysiology, diagnosis, treatment of acute trauma, rehabilitation, and all types of surgical techniques including their associated complications and treatment. To make these issues even more contemporary, we have included point–counterpoint debate chapters to bring these issues to life for the reader.

I wish to thank my co-editors and all of the authors for their diligence and effort in making each chapter a stand-alone reference work on their topic. Through their efforts, the reader will be given a most up-to-date and comprehensive understanding of shoulder instability and successful treatment concepts.

David M. Dines, MD

Contents

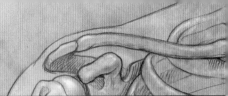

CONTROVERSIES IN
SHOULDER INSTABILITY

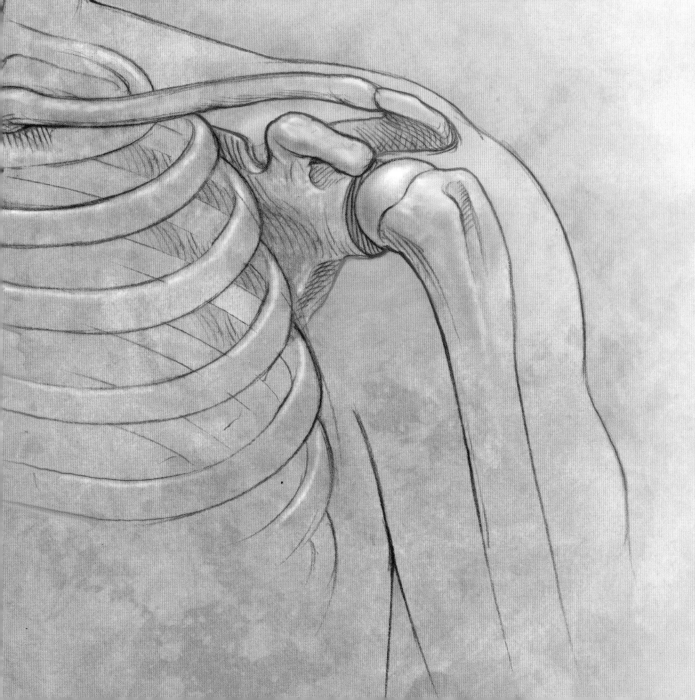

GENERAL PRINCIPLES OF SHOULDER INSTABILITY

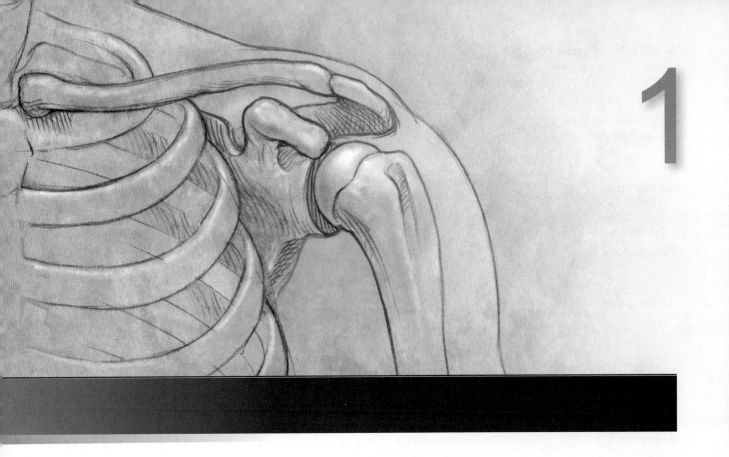

Gross and Arthroscopic Anatomy of the Glenohumeral Joint

M. Michael Khair / Jason D. Lehman /
Lawrence V. Gulotta

Introduction

The glenohumeral joint is a multiaxial ball-and-socket synovial joint formed by the humeral head and the glenoid surface of the scapula (Fig. 1-1). This articulation provides remarkable range of motion at the expense of a compromise in biomechanical stability. Generally, descriptions of the anatomy of the glenohumeral articulation, with an emphasis on shoulder stability, focus on static and dynamic anatomic restraints. A thorough understanding of the gross anatomy of the glenohumeral joint, emphasizing the static and dynamic factors, is fundamental to treating shoulder instability.

Static Factors: Bony Restraints

With the arm relaxed in an adducted position, the scapula faces 30 degrees anteriorly on the posterior chest wall and tilts 20 degrees forward relative to the sagittal plane and 3 degrees upward relative to the transverse plane (1). Projecting laterally from the scapular body is the glenoid, which functions as the socket of the glenohumeral

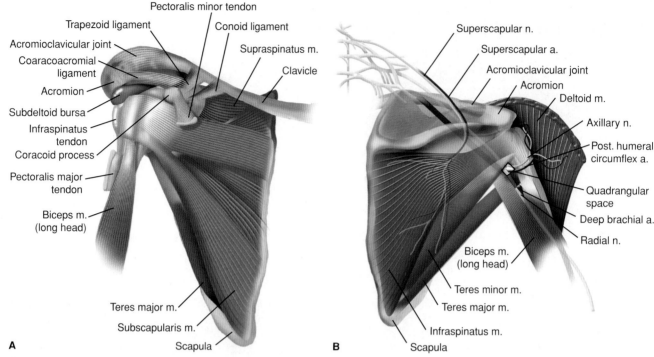

▲ **FIGURE 1-1:** Gross anatomy of the glenohumeral joint.

joint. Glenoid anatomy varies widely among individuals. In a study by Saha (2) it was found that glenoid surfaces were retroverted in approximately 75% of persons with an average of 7 degrees, and anteverted between 2 and 10 degrees in the other 25% of persons. A more recent study of 344 cadaveric scapulae revealed an average of 1.23 degrees of retroversion with a range of 9.5 degrees anteversion to 10.5 degrees retroversion (3). In terms of inclination, Churchill et al. found an average superior tilt of approximately 4.2 degrees with a range of 15.8 degrees superior inclination to 7 degrees inferior inclination.

The surface of the glenoid, or the glenoid fossa, is "pear-shaped" and often likened to an inverted comma. Its superior portion is narrow and its inferior portion is broad. The average vertical dimension of the glenoid is 39 mm, and the average transverse dimension ranges from 23 mm at the midpoint of the upper half to 29 mm at the midpoint of the lower half (4). Thus, the ratio of the transverse dimension of the lower half of the glenoid to that of the upper half is approximately 1:0.8 (4). The concave surface of the glenoid is covered by a hyaline cartilage surface that is thickest at the periphery and becomes thinner centrally.

In contrast, the humeral head is a large, spherical structure with a surface area three times greater than that of the glenoid (5). The articular surface of the head constitutes approximately one-third of a sphere and is angled between 130 and 150 degrees in relation to the humeral shaft (6). The actual size of the head is widely variable but in the study by Boileau and Walch (7), the average diameter of the humeral head was determined to be 43.2 mm with an average articular cartilage thick-

ness of 15.2 mm. The head is retroverted with respect to the transepicondylar axis of the distal humerus an average of 30 degrees with a range of 10 to 55 degrees (8). The central portion of the articular surface is spherical, but the dimensions become slightly elliptical on the periphery (4).

Given the nature of glenoid and humeral head anatomy, it is given that there is a significant surface area mismatch between the glenoid and the humeral head such that only 25% to 30% of the humeral head is in contact with the glenoid at any shoulder position (9). Despite this difference in surface area, there is remarkable congruence between the glenoid and the articulating humeral head (10). While perfect congruence (equal to 0) occurs in only 9% of individuals (11), a study by Soslowsky et al. (5) of 32 shoulders showed close to 90% of individuals had congruence within 2 mm, and all were congruent within 3 mm.

STATIC FACTORS: SOFT TISSUE RESTRAINTS

Adding further static stability to the glenohumeral joint is the glenoid labrum, a rim of fibrous tissue that surrounds the glenoid (Fig. 1-2). The labrum attaches to the glenoid articular cartilage through a fibrocartilaginous transition zone (12), and its inner surface is covered with synovium. The labrum serves to deepen the glenoid cavity by up to 50% or 9 mm in the superior–inferior plane and 5 mm in the anterior–posterior plane (13). In addition to increasing the depth of the socket the labrum

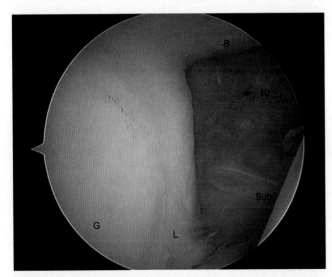

▲ **FIGURE 1-2:** Basic arthroscopic view of the glenohumeral joint from a posterior viewing portal (B, biceps; G, glenoid; L, anterior labrum; RI, rotator interval; Sub, subscapularis).

also serves to increase the surface area contact with the humeral head (14,15). The labrum also serves an attachment site for several structures involved in shoulder stability. As the tendon of the long head of the biceps brachii courses to insert in the supraglenoid tubercle, its fibers are often continuous with the superior labrum.

The inferior portion of the glenoid labrum serves as an attachment site for the inferior glenohumeral ligament. By deepening the glenoid cavity, the labrum decreases resistance to translation by up to 20% (16).

The glenohumeral joint capsule originates at the glenoid neck and extends laterally to the anatomical neck of the humerus and onto the shaft of the humerus. It often extends superiorly to the coracoid process and on either side of the scapular body via the anterior and posterior recesses, but there is substantial variation among individuals (17). Although less than 5 mm thick (18), the capsule confers substantial stability to the glenohumeral joint by limiting translation and rotation through the ligamentous structures contained within it. In addition to the glenohumeral ligaments detailed below, the capsule is strengthened anteriorly by the attachment of the subscapularis tendon, and posteriorly by the attachments of the teres minor and infraspinatus tendons (19,20). The capsule is lined by synovial membrane and contains on average between 28 and 35 mL of fluid (17). Synovial fluid contributes to shoulder stability through negative intra-articular pressure (21) and adhesion–cohesion forces (22).

The ligamentous structures of the glenohumeral joint serve primarily to stabilize the joint at extremes of motion (Fig. 1-3). The functions of each ligament vary

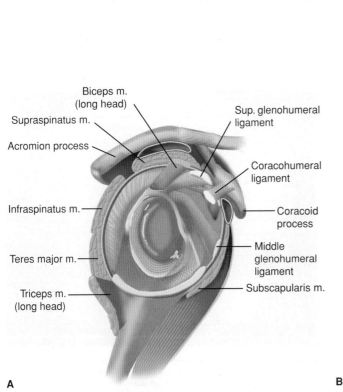

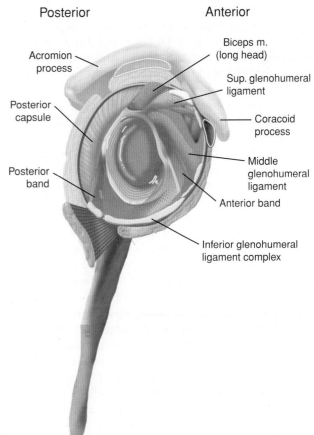

A   **B**

▲ **FIGURE 1-3:** Ligamentous anatomy of the glenohumeral joint.

depending on the anatomic position of the ligament, the position of the upper extremity, and the directions of forces placed on the joint. In addition, considerable anatomic variation exists in these structures, further contributing to differences in function by individual.

The coracohumeral ligament (CHL) is a broad (1 to 2 cm) fibrous structure that originates from the lateral aspect of the base of the coracoid process and extends inferiorly and laterally to attach to the lesser and greater tuberosities of the humerus where it converges with the insertions of the supraspinatus and subscapularis muscles. There remains some controversy as to the specific function of the CHL, but it is believed to serve as an important restraint to external rotation of the adducted arm (23). A recent study has suggested that the corocoacromial ligament (CAL) may influence the function of the CHL through a structural connection between the two called the falx (24). The authors suggest disruption of the CAL can hinder the stabilizing functions of the CHL and allow for increased translation in the anterior and inferior directions. Others have questioned the clinical significance of this increase due to smaller increases in translation in a muscularly intact shoulder (25).

Although the size of the superior glenohumeral ligament (SGHL) varies greatly, it is present in some form in over 90% of cases (26). It is attached proximally to the supraglenoid tubercle and superior labrum, then courses parallel to the CHL before inserting just superior to the lesser tuberosity along with the CHL. A recent cadaveric study suggests that the SGHL comprises two distinct groups of fibers: Oblique and direct (27). The direct fibers arise from the glenoid labrum and run parallel to the tendon of the long head of the biceps brachii before inserting into either the lesser tubercle or bridge over the bicipital groove to form the superior part of the transverse humeral ligament. The oblique fibers arise from the supraglenoid tubercle and insert below the CHL. Again, there are differences in opinion as to the main function of the SGHL. Despite these differences in opinion, the current consensus appears to be that both the SGHL and CHL work together to constrain the humeral head on the glenoid. They accomplish this by limiting inferior translation and external rotation when the arm is adducted. In addition, they appear to limit posterior translation when the arm is adducted, internally rotated and forward flexed. More research needs to be done before the exact contribution of these two ligamentous structures is completely known.

The middle glenohumeral ligament (MGHL) shows the greatest individual variation of all the glenohumeral ligaments. The classic anatomic study by DePalma et al. (26) mentioned above found an SGHL in over 90% of cases, and a well-formed MGHL in only 70%. The MGHL was poorly defined in 17% of cases, and completely absent in the other 13% of cases. A similar study done more recently found the MGHL to be absent in over 25%

of cases (28). A series of 108 MR arthrograms in asymptomatic patients found an SGHL and IGHL in 99% of cases, but an MGHL in only 79% of cases (29). When present, several morphologic forms exist. The ligament can appear linear and sheet-like or rounded and cord-like. It originates from the anterosuperior surface of the labrum or glenoid and inserts just medial to the lesser tuberosity of the humerus beneath the subscapularis tendon to which it is attached (30). One important variant of the MGHL is called the Buford complex, in which a cord-like version of the ligament exists in the absence of a well-defined anterosuperior labrum (31). Although recognized in only 1% to 2% of cases (29,31), this is important to the clinician as it is often misdiagnosed as a tear of the anterior labrum (32–34). The MGHL may serve as a secondary stabilizer of inferior translation with the arm in adduction (35), but its most prominent role is to limit both anterior and posterior translations of the humeral head with the arm in abduction and external rotation. When prominent (cord like) it can play an important role in preventing anterior translation, especially in the presence of a damaged anterior portion of the inferior glenohumeral ligament (36).

Of all the glenohumeral ligaments, the most important contributor to glenohumeral stability is the inferior glenohumeral ligament. It was first described in 1948 (26) before Turkel et al. (30) further elaborated on the different parts of the ligament by describing a superior band as well as anterior and posterior axillary pouches. The use of arthroscopy allowed O'Brien et al. (37) to further define the structure as the inferior glenohumeral ligament complex (IGHLC) consisting of three components: An anterior band, a posterior band, and the axillary pouch situated in between the bands (Fig. 1-4). The anterior and posterior bands of the IGHLC take origin

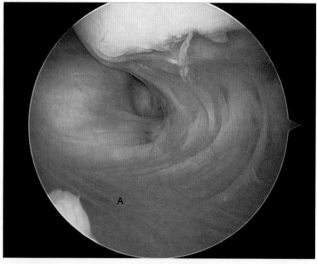

▲ **FIGURE 1-4:** Arthroscopic view of the axillary pouch, and the capsular attachment to the humerus (A, axillary pouch of the capsule).

from the labrum or the periosteum of the glenoid neck. The generally thicker anterior band arises from the 2-o'clock to 4-o'clock position (when viewing the right shoulder), and the thinner posterior band from the 7-o'clock to 9-o'clock position (37). They run circumferentially around the glenohumeral joint before attaching to the humerus just below the articular margin of the head. Two different humeral attachments have been described—the "split type" and "broad type" (38). The split type has a capsular bifurcation with loose connective tissue between internal and external folds, while the broad type has no separate folds.

The unique geometry of the IGHLC allows for it to play both a large and diverse role in the stabilization of the glenohumeral joint. O'Brien et al. (37) described the region between the anterior and posterior bands as acting like a hammock in its support of the humeral head. When the arm is abducted, the complex shifts beneath the humeral head to limit inferior translation. If the abducted arm is then externally rotated, the anterior band shifts to cover the humeral head anteriorly and resist anterior translation. When the abducted arm shifts to internal rotation; however, the posterior band resists posterior translation. This reciprocal load sharing has obvious clinical implications for the overhead athlete. A study using a biomechanical cadaveric model also found the IGHLC to be the most important restraint to external rotation in both the neutral and abducted positions (23).

DYNAMIC FACTORS: THE ROTATOR CUFF

The rotator cuff is composed of four muscles: The supraspinatus, infraspinatus, teres minor, and, subscapularis. Each of these musculotendinous units originates on the body of the scapula and terminates on the tuberosities of the humerus effectively enveloping the humeral head.

The supraspinatus originates on the suprascapular fossa and inserts into the greater tuberosity of the proximal humerus (39) (Fig. 1-5). It receives its primary innervation from the suprascapular nerve which originates from the upper trunk of the brachial plexus. The supraspinatus is fundamental to glenohumeral compression during active shoulder motion and also aids in abduction of the shoulder (13). The muscle sits between the humeral head and the acromial arch. It is protected by bursae on both sides.

The subscapularis muscle originates along the costal surface of the scapula and inserts on the lesser tuberosity of the proximal humerus. The subscapularis is considered the largest and most powerful of the four rotator cuff muscles. It has dual innervation from the upper and lower subscapular nerves which are both derived from the posterior cord of the brachial plexus. The subscapularis is known to be the main internal rotator of the

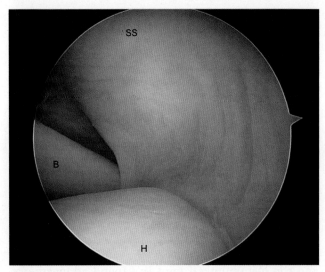

▲ FIGURE 1-5: Arthroscopic view of the supraspinatus (SS, supraspinatus; B, biceps; H, humeral head).

shoulder. However, it also contributes a great deal to arm abduction, humeral head depression, and functions to limit anterior translation of the humeral head.

The infraspinatus and teres minor muscles make up the posterior rotator cuff. They originate on the infraspinatus fossa and the dorsolateral border of the scapula and both insert into the greater tuberosity. The infraspinatus is innervated by the suprascapular nerve and the teres minor is innervated by the axillary nerve. Both muscles function to externally rotate the humerus as well as stabilize the glenohumeral joint in concert with the supraspinatus and subscapularis.

While there continues to be debate over some of the functions of the rotator cuff, there is an abundance of data to support the role of the rotator cuff muscles in dynamic stabilization of the shoulder. The four muscles of the rotator cuff work in concert to achieve humeral depression, rotation, adduction, and compression. It has been shown that the four rotator cuff muscles are perfectly aligned to effectively compress the humeral head into the glenoid at all shoulder positions (24). In addition, the direct connection between the rotator cuff muscles and capsuloligamentous structures in the shoulder allows for ligament dynamization which helps to stabilize the shoulder through the midrange of shoulder rotation where the ligaments and capsule can be more lax.

BURSAE AND RECESSES

There are several bursae present in the shoulder region, and the two most important clinically are the subacromial bursa and subscapular bursa. The subacromial bursa lies between the deltoid muscle and the shoulder capsule and serves to facilitate the motion of the muscles of the rotator cuff beneath the overlying acromion and acromioclavicular joints. While important in several pathologic conditions, it does not under normal circumstances communicate with the glenohumeral joint. The subscapularis bursa, on the other hand, communicates freely with the glenohumeral joint. It is located just inferior to the coracoid process between the neck of the scapula and the subscapularis tendon and it serves to protect the subscapularis tendon as it passes above the neck of the scapula and below the coracoid process. The top of the bursa is linked to the coracoid process by a fibrous attachment called the suspensory ligament, and in close to one-third of cases it connects with the subcoracoid bursa to form one large bursa (40). Several synovial recesses in the anterior shoulder capsule permit communication between the subscapularis bursa and the glenohumeral joint in varying arrangements. DePalma et al. (26) categorized these variations into six commonly found types: (type 1) one synovial recess above the MGHL, (type 2) one synovial recess below the MGHL, (type 3) one recess above and one recess below the MGHL, (type 4) one large recess with an absent MGHL, (type 5) the MGHL appears as two small synovial folds, and (type 6) there are no synovial recesses present but all the ligaments are well defined.

VASCULAR SUPPLY TO THE GLENOHUMERAL JOINT

The blood supply of the glenohumeral joint is derived from the subclavian (and later axillary) artery and its branches (Fig. 1-6). The subclavian arises from the brachiocephalic trunk on the right side and the aortic arch on the left. As it courses the superior border of the first rib and before crossing behind the anterior scalene muscle, it branches into the thyrocervical trunk. In addition to the ascending cervical, inferior thyroid, and transverse cervical arteries, the thyrocervical trunk also divides into the suprascapular artery, which supplies blood to the shoulder region. As it crosses the first rib and passes beneath the clavicle, the subclavian artery becomes the axillary artery. The axillary artery is divided into three parts based on its location relative to the pectoralis minor muscle. As it continues laterally through the axilla posterior to the pectoralis minor, the axillary artery gives off six branches, each originating from the anteroinferior surface of the vessel. Four of these branches are important to the vascular supply of the glenohumeral joint (from medial to lateral): The thoracoacromial artery, subscapular artery, anterior circumflex artery, and posterior circumflex artery. The thoracoacromial artery further divides into four branches: The clavicular, acromial, deltoid, and pectoral branches. The subscapular artery divides into the circumflex scapular artery and thoracodorsal artery. The anterior and posterior circumflex humeral arteries course around the neck of the humerus before anastomosing and giving off other small branches to supply the humerus and surrounding musculature. Each of these arteries combines to form a vascular network that supplies the glenohumeral joint and surrounding structures with a rich blood supply.

There are three major contributing vessels to the blood supply of the glenoid labrum: The suprascapular artery, circumflex scapular branch of the subscapular

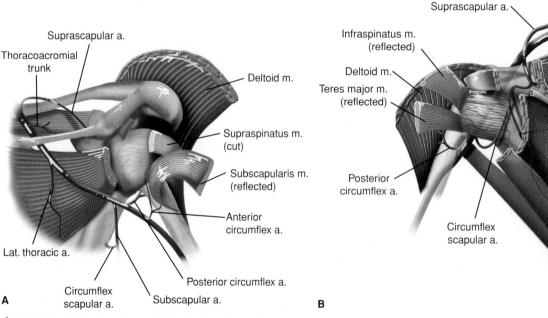

A

Suprascapular a.
Thoracoacromial trunk
Deltoid m.
Supraspinatus m. (cut)
Subscapularis m. (reflected)
Anterior circumflex a.
Lat. thoracic a.
Circumflex scapular a.
Subscapular a.
Posterior circumflex a.

B

Suprascapular a.
Infraspinatus m. (reflected)
Deltoid m.
Teres major m. (reflected)
Posterior circumflex a.
Circumflex scapular a.

▲ **FIGURE 1-6:** Vascular supply to the glenohumeral joint.

artery, and the posterior circumflex humeral artery. Branches from these vessels supply the glenoid labrum throughout its peripheral attachment in a predominantly radial pattern although circumferentially oriented vessels also exist (12). These vessels surround the entire periphery of the labrum but penetration into the labral tissue is limited to the peripheral attachment of the labrum, and the superior and anterior portions are less vascularized than the posterior and inferior portions (12).

Andary and Petersen (41) performed a study on 24 cadaveric shoulders to elaborate the vascular supply of the shoulder capsule and glenohumeral ligaments. They found the capsule was supplied by four arteries: The suprascapular artery, circumflex scapular branch of the subscapular artery, anterior circumflex humeral artery, and the posterior circumflex artery. These arteries enter from either the medial (scapular) side of the capsule or the lateral (humeral) side before arborizing toward the center of the capsule. The suprascapular and circumflex scapular arteries enter the capsule medially, and the anterior and posterior circumflex humeral vessels enter laterally. In addition to these vessels, the capsule also receives branches of arteries that arise from the tendons and muscles of the overlying rotator cuff. The anterior and inferior aspects of the capsule are more vascularized than the thinner posterior section, but all portions receive a consistent blood supply. It appears the dominant vessels of the shoulders run horizontally, a finding that might be important in designing surgical approaches to access the glenohumeral joint (41).

The vascular branches that supply the glenoid appear to also supply the periosteum of the scapular neck and glenoid (12). The anterior and posterior circumflex humeral arteries supply the humeral head. The anterior circumflex humeral artery arises from the third part of the axillary artery just below the inferior border of the pectoralis major, and courses beneath the coracobrachialis and short head of the biceps to reach the humerus. Its major branch, the anterolateral branch (or arcuate artery), passes beneath the tendon of the long head of the biceps, and enters the humeral head at the lateral and superior aspects of the intertubercular groove. This branch is the most important artery of the humeral head, supplying almost the entire epiphysis (42). The posterior circumflex artery also arises from the third part of the axillary artery. It courses posteriorly through the quadrangular space and supplies the posterior aspect of the greater tuberosity and the posteroinferior part of the humeral head (42). The anterior and posterior circumflex arteries anastomose with each other in addition to other arteries in the region, but complete vascularization of the humeral head is only possible through the anterolateral branch of the anterior circumflex artery (the arcuate artery).

INNERVATION OF THE GLENOHUMERAL JOINT

Nerve branches originating from the C5, C6, and C7 nerve roots innervate the shoulder region, with variable contribution from the C4 nerve root. The major contributors to the glenohumeral joint are the axillary, suprascapular, subscapular, and musculocutaneous nerves with additional contributions from branches of the posterior cord of the brachial plexus (17). The superior portion of the joint is supplied mainly by branches of the suprascapular nerve. The axillary nerve, musculocutaneous nerve, and branches from the lateral anterior thoracic nerve can also contribute to this region. The anterior portion is supplied by the axillary and suprascapular nerves with variable contributions from the musculocutaneous nerve. The subscapular nerve and branches from the posterior cord of the brachial plexus can also supply the anterior region. Posteriorly, the upper region of the capsule is supplied by the suprascapular nerve and the lower portion by the axillary nerve. The inferior region is supplied by the axillary nerve anteriorly, and by a combination of the axillary nerve and branches from the suprascapular nerve posteriorly.

References

1. O'Brien S, Arnoczky S, Warren R, et al. Developmental anatomy of the shoulder and anatomy of the glenohumeral joint. In: Rockwood CA, Matsen, FA, eds. *The Shoulder.* Philadelphia, PA: WB Saunders; 1990:1–33.
2. Saha AK. Dynamic stability of the glenohumeral joint. *Acta Orthop Scand.* 1971;42:491–505.
3. Churchill RS, Brems JJ, Kotschi H. Glenoid size, inclination, and version: An anatomic study. *J Shoulder Elbow Surg.* 2001;10:327–332.
4. Iannotti JP, Gabriel JP, Schneck SL, et al. The normal glenohumeral relationships: An anatomical study of one hundred and forty shoulders. *J Bone Joint Surg Am.* 1992;74:491–500.
5. Soslowsky L, Flatow E, Bigliani LU, et al. Articular geometry of the glenohumeral joint. *Clin Orthop Relat Res.* 1992;285:181–190.
6. Sarrafian SK. Gross and functional anatomy of the shoulder. *Clin Orthop Rel Res.* 1983;173:11–19.
7. Boileau P, Walch G. The three-dimensional geometry of the proximal humerus: Implications for surgical technique and prosthetic design. *J Bone Joint Surg Br.* 1997;79B:857–865.
8. Pearl ML, Volk AG. Coronal plane geometry of the proximal humerus relevant to prosthetic arthroplasty. *J Shoulder Elbow Surg.* 1996;5:320–326.
9. Saha A. *Theory of Shoulder Mechanism: Descriptive and Applied.* Springfield, IL: Charles C Thomas; 1961.
10. Iannotti JP, Williams GR. Total shoulder arthroplasty. *Orthop Clin North Am.* 1998;29:377–391.

11. Friedman RJ. Biomechanics and design of shoulder arthroplasties. In: Friedman RJ, ed. *Arthroplasty of the Shoulder.* New York, NY: Thieme Medical Publishers, Inc.; 1994:27–40.

12. Cooper D, Arnoczky S, O'Brien S, et al. Anatomy, histology, and vascularity of the glenoid labrum: An anatomical study. *J Bone Joint Surg Am.* 1992;74:46–52.

13. Howell SM, Galinat BJ. The glenoid-labral socket: A constrained articular surface. *Clin Orthop Relat Res.* 1989;243:122–125.

14. Bigliani LU, Kelkar R, Flatow EL, et al. Glenohumeral stability: Biomechanical properties of passive and active stabilizers. *Clin Orthop Relat Res.* 1996;330:13–30.

15. Lippitt S, Matsen F. Mechanisms of glenohumeral joint stability. *Clin Orthop Relat Res.* 1993;291:20–28.

16. Itoi E, Hsu HS, An KN. Biochemical investigation of the glenohumeral joint. *J Shoulder Elbow Surg.* 1996;5: 407–424.

17. O'Brien SJ, Voos JE, Neviaser AS, et al. Developmental anatomy of the shoulder and anatomy of the glenohumeral joint. In: Rockwood CA, Matsen FA, eds. *The Shoulder.* 4th ed. Philadelphia, PA: Saunders Elsevier; 2009:1–31.

18. Ciccone WJ II, Hunt TJ, Lieber R, et al. Multiquadrant digital analysis of shoulder capsule thickness. *Arthroscopy.* 2000;16:457–461.

19. Ovesen J, Nielsen S. Anterior and posterior shoulder instability: A cadaver study. *Acta Orthop Scand.* 1986;57: 324–327.

20. Ovesen J, Nielsen S. Posterior instability of the shoulder: A cadaver study. *Acta Orthop Scand.* 1986;57:436–439.

21. Itoi E, Motzkin NE, Browne AO, et al. Intraarticular pressure of the shoulder. *Arthroscopy.* 1993;9:406–413.

22. Matsen FI, Thomas S, Rockwood CJ. Anterior glenohumeral instability. In: Rockwood C, Matsen F, eds. *The Shoulder.* Philadelphia, PA: WB Saunders; 1990:526–622.

23. Kuhn JE, Huston LJ, Soslowsky LJ, et al. External rotation of the glenohumeral joint: Ligament restraints and muscle effects in the neutral and abducted positions. *J Shoulder Elbow Surg.* 2005;14:39S–48S.

24. Lee TQ, Black AD, Tibone JE, et al. Release of the coracoacromial ligament can lead to glenohumeral laxity: A biomechanical study. *J Shoulder Elbow Surg.* 2001;10:68–72.

25. Wellman M, Petersen W, Thore Z, et al. Effect of coracoacromial ligament resection on glenohumeral stability under active muscle loading in an in vitro model. *Arthroscopy.* 2008;11:1258–1264.

26. DePalma AF, Gallery G, Bennett GA. Shoulder joint: Variational anatomy and degenerative regions of the shoulder joint. *Instr Course Lect.* 1949;6:225–281.

27. Kask K, Poldoja E, Lont T, et al. Anatomy of the superior glenohumeral ligament. *J Shoulder Elbow Surg.* 2010;19:908–916.

28. O'Brien SJ, Warren RF, Schwarts E. Anterior shoulder instability. *Orthop Clin North Am.* 1987;18:395–408.

29. Park YH, Lee JY, Moon SH, et al. MR arthrography of the labral capsular ligamentous complex in the shoulder: Imaging variations and pitfalls. *AJR Am J Roentgenol.* 2000;175:667–672.

30. Turkel SJ, Panio MW, Marshall JL, et al. Stabilizing mechanisms preventing anterior dislocation of the glenohumeral joint. *J Bone Joint Surg Am.* 1981;63:1208–1217.

31. Williams MM, Snyder SJ, Buford D. The Buford complex – the "cord-like" middle glenohumeral ligament and absent anterosuperior labrum complex: A normal anatomical capsulolabral variant. *Arthroscopy.* 1994;10:241–247.

32. Tirman PFJ, Feller JF, Palmer WE, et al. The Buford complex – a variation of normal shoulder anatomy: MR arthrographic imaging features. *AJR Am J Roentgenol.* 1996;166:869–873.

33. Yeh LR, Kwak S, Kim YS, et al. Anterior labroligamentous structures of the glenohumeral joint: Correlation of MR arthrography and anatomic dissection in cadavers. *AJR Am J Roentgenol.* 1998;171:1229–1236.

34. Snyder SJ. Diagnostic arthroscopy: Normal anatomy and variations. In: Snyder SJ, ed. *Shoulder Arthroscopy.* New York, NY: McGraw-Hill; 1994:179–214.

35. Warner J, Deng X, Warren R, et al. Static capsuloligamentous restraints to superior-inferior translation of the glenohumeral joint. *Am J Sports Med.* 1992;20:675–685.

36. Schwartz E, Warren RF, O'Brien SJ, et al. Posterior shoulder instability. *Orthop Clin North Am.* 1987;18:409–419.

37. O'Brien SJ, Neves MC, Arnoczky SP, et al. The anatomy and histology of the inferior glenohumeral ligament complex of the shoulder. *Am J Sports Med.* 1990;18:449–456.

38. Sugalski MT, Wiater JM, Levine WN, et al. An anatomic study of the humeral insertion of the inferior glenohumeral capsule. *J Shoulder Elbow Surg.* 2005;14:91–95.

39. Volk AG, Vangsness CT Jr. An anatomic study of the supraspinatus muscle and tendon. *Clin Orthop Relat Res.* 2001;384:280–285.

40. Colas F, Nevoux J, Gagey O. The subscapular and subcoracoid bursae: Descriptive and functional anatomy. *J Shoulder Elbow Surg.* 2004;13:454–458.

41. Andary JL, Petersen SA. The vascular anatomy of the glenohumeral capsule and ligaments: An anatomic study. *J Bone Joint Surg Am.* 2002;84:2258–2265.

42. Gerber C, Schneeberger AG, Vinh TS. The arterial vascularization of the humeral head. An anatomical study. *J Bone Joint Surg Am.* 1990;72A:1486–1494.

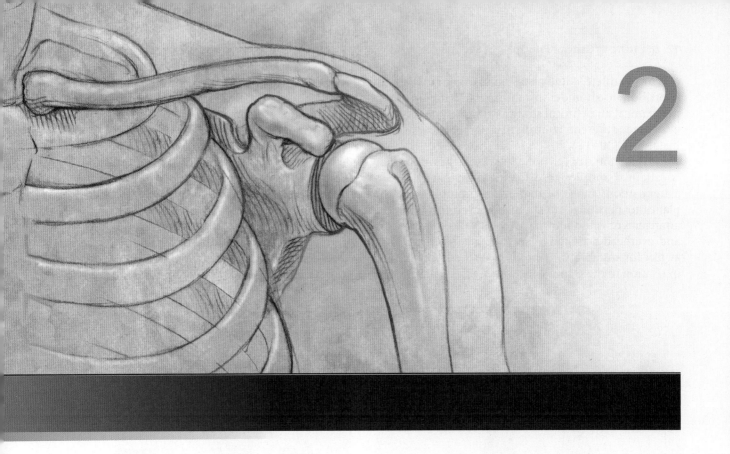

2

PATHOPHYSIOLOGY AND BIOMECHANICS OF GLENOHUMERAL INSTABILITY

Xinning Li / Paul Yannopoulos / Jon J.P. Warner

INTRODUCTION

Hippocrates was the first to investigate the pathophysiology of the unstable shoulder (anterior instability and treatment) over 1,000 years ago (1). Early investigations attributed instability to traumatic events or congenital shoulder abnormalities (2). The capsuloligamentous complex of the glenohumeral joint was first described in 1829 as consisting of the superior, middle, and inferior glenohumeral ligaments (3). Subsequent studies in the early 1900s by Perthes (4) and Thomas (5) suggested that the capsule and glenohumeral ligaments played a role in shoulder stability. In 1923, Bankart (6,7) described the detachment of the anterior inferior capsule from the glenoid as the "essential" lesion in anterior glenohumeral instability. The modern-day term "Bankart lesion" is used to describe an avulsion of the anteroinferior glenoid labrum from its attachment to the inferior glenohumeral ligament complex (IGHLC). Subsequently, Turkel et al. (8) performed the classic biomechanical cadaver study to describe the contribution of the superior, middle, and inferior glenohumeral ligaments to shoulder stability at various degrees of shoulder abduction. Subsequently, Neer hypothesized that repetitive microtrauma to the shoulder capsule, as in the case of a high-demand

11

overhead athlete, could also lead to overstretching and contribute to shoulder instability (9). Numerous biomechanical and clinical studies in the last decade have evaluated different contributing factors to shoulder instability (10–16).

The shoulder (glenohumeral joint) is minimally constrained and designed for mobility that allows for a tremendous range of motion in multiple anatomic planes to maximize function. However, this anatomic arrangement while allowing necessary motion for sports and overhead activities, places the glenohumeral joint at risk for instability. Translation of the humeral head in relation to the glenoid during activities of daily living or athletics is prevented by both the static and dynamic stabilizing mechanisms. Important static stabilizers include the articular anatomy of a joint with matched concavity and convexity of the ball-in-socket, as well as the glenoid labrum which broadens and deepens the socket depth. The vacuum seal of the closed joint capsule results in negative intra-articular pressure which may enhance the stabilizing effect of the capsular ligamentous structures. Dynamic stabilizers include the rotator cuff musculature, biceps tendon, scapulothoracic and humeral motions, and the deltoid muscle. The balance between the static and dynamic stabilizers determines the stability of the shoulder joint. An imbalance among

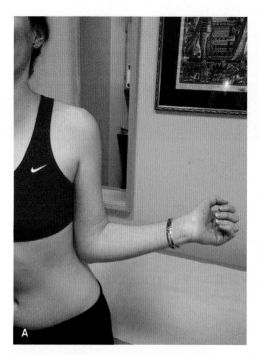
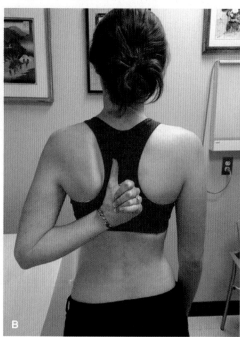
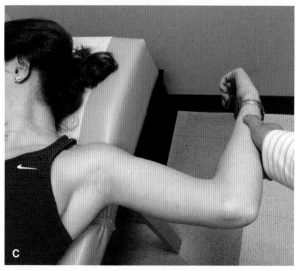
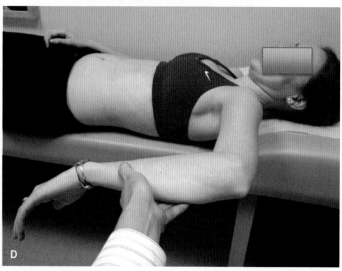

▲ **FIGURE 2-1:** A patient with clinical laxity increased range of motion in both external and internal rotations but without any symptoms of instability. External rotation at neutral measured 95 degrees **(A)**, internal rotation to T5 **(B)**, external rotation and internal rotation with the arm abducted at 90 degrees measured 100 degrees **(C)**, and 90 degrees **(D)**, respectively.

these stabilizing factors may result in instability occurring in the anterior, posterior, inferior directions or it may be multidirectional in nature (17–19). There is a spectrum of instability ranging from transient subluxation, dislocation that is self-reduced to locked dislocation requiring general anesthesia and muscle relaxation for reduction. In addition to the above dynamic and static factors, proprioception also plays a significant role in the pathoetiology of shoulder instability (20). Proprioception is the perception of motion of the joint and it is an important mechanism by which the muscles receive a message to contract and guard against instability. A failure of proprioceptive feedback may contribute to instability.

Finally, it is essential to distinguish between "laxity" and "instability." Some patients may be lax without actual instability (Fig. 2-1) and some individuals may be tight with episodes of instability. Laxity is the looseness of a joint necessary for normal shoulder motion and is often painless. It is variable between individuals. Instability is a sudden displacement of the humeral head out of the socket during shoulder motion and it is a pathologic event that is typically painful. Clinical manifestations of instability are the result of a combination of factors with both static and dynamic failure of stabilizing structures; therefore, it is essential to understand normal biomechanics if a surgeon is to formulate a logical approach to treatment on an individual patient basis. This chapter will clarify the static and dynamic contributions to stability of the shoulder joint complex and thus provide a framework for understanding surgical solutions for instability of the shoulder.

SPECTRUM AND DIRECTION OF INSTABILITY

Instability and laxity are two separate terms describing two different entities of glenohumeral translation. Laxity is defined as asymptomatic translation of the humeral head on the glenoid surface that is seen in normal shoulders and it is a requirement for normal joint motion; however, the amount of translation may differ between individuals secondary to the status of the soft tissue about the shoulder. Instability is a clinical diagnosis manifested as excessive translation of the humeral head on the glenoid surface during active shoulder rotation or motion that is associated with symptoms, usually pain or apprehension (21–25).

A spectrum of instability also exists ranging from subluxation to complete dislocation requiring sedation and muscle relaxation for successful reduction. Subluxation is defined as symptomatic translation of the humeral head out of the glenoid socket but not to the point of actual dislocation. A dislocation is complete separation of the articular surfaces, which can also range from spontaneous self-reduction termed "transient luxation" to a fixed dislocation requiring sedation and muscle relaxation for reduction of the humeral head back into the glenoid (26). Owens et al. (26) defined "transient luxation" as complete dislocation that spontaneously self reduces. Most patients who experienced a "transient luxation" will present with both a Bankart lesion and a Hill-Sachs lesion on MRI.

The primary direction of instability can be anterior, posterior, inferior, or multidirectional. Often, patients presenting with anterior instability will also have associated injury to the posterior capsule and may have excessive posterior translation when examined under anesthesia. This phenomenon is explained by the "circle concept" and by the "load and sharing concept" of glenohumeral instability (Fig. 2-2) (27). Multidirectional instability (MDI) means symptomatic instability in more than one direction (28). Typically this produces symptoms in an anterior direction in combination with the inferior direction. Less commonly, it may be posteriorly associated with inferior direction of instability. While patients with MDI are rare and may present with a Bankart lesion and a Hill-Sachs lesion, the hallmark of this condition is a redundant inferior axillary pouch and deficient rotator interval (28–30).

History and physical examination help indicate the direction of instability and examination under anesthesia confirms the diagnosis. Typically, apprehension is elicited in the abduction–external rotation position in patients with anterior instability and in the adduction–internal rotation in patients with posterior instability. A significant symptomatic inferior translation on clinical examination in addition to either anterior or posterior symptoms is the hallmark of MDI (31–36). Biomechanically, Warner et al. (22) proved the primary restraint to inferior translation of

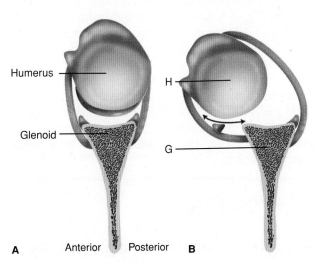

Humerus

Glenoid

H

G

A Anterior Posterior B

▲ **FIGURE 2-2:** **A:** Normal glenohumeral joint with capsulolabral complex. **B:** Anterior dislocation of the humeral head (H) in relations to the glenoid (G) results in injury to both sides of the joint and capsulolabral complex.

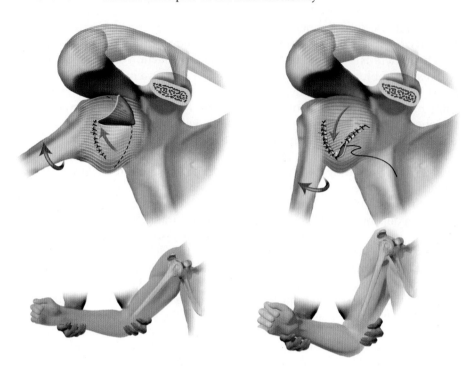

◀ **FIGURE 2-3:** Selective capsular shift in patients with both a Bankart lesion and inferior instability. The Bankart is repaired anatomically and the capsule is tightened with the arm in 30 degrees of abduction and 30 degrees of external rotation to prevent loss in range of motion.

the adducted shoulder is the superior glenohumeral ligament (SGHL). With progressive abduction of the arm, the anterior and posterior glenohumeral ligaments become the main static stabilizers in resisting inferior translation. Anterior portion was the primary restraint with the arm in 45 degrees of abduction and the posterior portion was the primary restraint with the arm in 90 degrees of abduction. Furthermore, Warner et al. (22) also showed that venting of the shoulder capsule resulted in significant inferior translation of the humeral head. Thus the so-called "sulcus sign" is the result of intra-articular vacuum effect and capsular laxity. In patients who present with both Bankart lesion and laxity, selective capsular repair with the arm in the 30 degrees of abduction and 30 degrees of external rotation (Fig. 2-3) have been recommended in the literature (37). Gerber et al. (38) have also demonstrated that total anterior capsular plication and posterior plication will significantly limit external rotation (>30 degrees) and internal rotation (>30 degrees), respectively. Inferior plication will limit shoulder range of motion in abduction, flexion, and rotation. Therefore, it is essential to diagnose the direction of instability or laxity and select the optimal location for capsular plication in order to maximize patient outcome.

STATIC STABILIZERS

Articular Geometry and Concavity

The glenohumeral joint comprises a large spherical humeral head that articulates with the smaller glenoid surface. Historically, the articular geometry was believed

to contribute minimally to the overall stability of the glenohumeral joint. This conclusion was drawn from two observations. The first is the small area of the glenoid surface relative to the large humeral head; and the second is the relative mismatch of the bony curvature of the glenoid to the humeral head (39,40). The shape of the glenoid is smaller superiorly and larger inferiorly, much like a "pear." Average vertical and transverse dimensions are 35 and 25 mm, respectively, whereas the vertical and transverse humeral head articular surface average 48 and 45 mm, respectively (41). Thus, the above measurements produce a significant surface area and radius of curvature mismatch between the joint surfaces of the glenoid and the humeral head. Furthermore, unlike the hip joint, the glenoid does not enclose the humeral head and only up to 25% to 30% of the humeral head is in contact with the glenoid at various shoulder range of motion (42,43). Although the subchondral bone on the glenoid side is flatter than the humeral head, recent studies have demonstrated that the articular surface of the glenoid is actually highly congruent to the articular surface of the humeral head. Kelkar et al. (44) reported the average radii of curvature of the humeral head and glenoid articular surfaces were 25.5 ± 1.5 mm and 27.2 ± 1.6 mm, respectively. The articular surface of the glenoid is thin in the central bare area (1.2 mm average) and thick at the periphery (3.8 mm average). In contrast, the cartilage on the humeral head is thin in the peripheral region (0.6 mm average) and thick in the central region (2 mm average) (17,42,43). Thus, the mismatch in the articular cartilage in the glenoid and humeral head increases the conformity of the overall glenohumeral joint to within

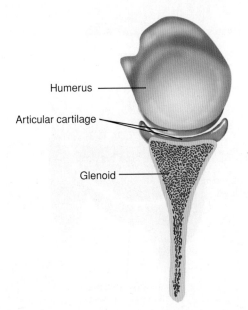

Humerus

Articular cartilage

Glenoid

▲ **FIGURE 2-4:** Illustration demonstrating the conformity of the articular cartilage surfaces of the glenoid with cartilage of the humeral head despite the relative flat osseous glenoid.

3 mm (Fig. 2-4). Furthermore, the glenoid concavity is deepened by the labrum that is attached circumferentially around the glenoid on the outer rim (45). Biomechanical studies have demonstrated that joint conformity contributes more in controlling translations during active motions, whereas capsular constraints become more important during passive motions (46).

In terms of humeral version, there is minimal evidence that abnormal version will contribute significantly to glenohumeral instability (2).

Glenoid Labrum

The labrum is a fibrocartilaginous bumper that forms a circumferential ring around the glenoid and serves as an anchoring point for the capsuloligamentous structures. Attachment to the articular cartilage occurs via a narrow fibrocartilaginous transition zone but it is otherwise fibrous throughout the entire structure (45). It is loosely attached superiorly above the equator and significant anatomic variability exists in this particular region between individuals (47). In contrast, the anterior inferior labrum is intimately attached to the glenoid rim and any detachment would indicate an abnormality (Fig. 2-5) (19). Vascular supply occurs in the peripheral attachment to the joint capsule (47). The essential contribution of the labrum to glenohumeral stability is by deepening the anterior to posterior depth of the glenoid socket from 2.5 to 5 mm and increasing the glenoid concavity to 9 mm in the superior to inferior plane. A loss of the labrum will decrease the overall depth of the socket by up to 50% in all directions (48). The stabilizing effect of the labrum is similar to a "chock block" that is used to prevent a wheel on a car or plane from rolling downhill (48). Furthermore, the glenoid labrum also increases the surface area for humeral head articulation and increases the excursion distance required for glenohumeral instability (49,50).

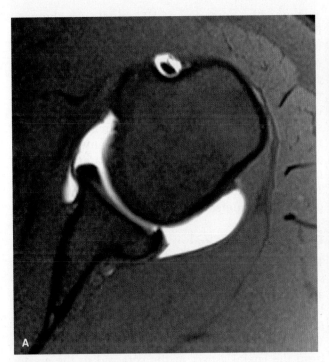

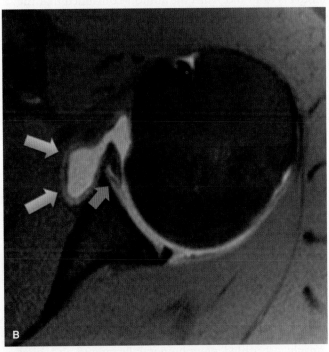

▲ **FIGURE 2-5:** Axial T2-weighted MRI images of a normal patient **(A)** and a patient with a Bankart lesion (*orange arrow*) and associated anterior capsule stretch injury (*blue arrows*) secondary to the dislocation event **(B)**.

Biomechanical studies have shown that the concavity-compression effect of the labrum is the most effective stabilizing mechanism in resisting tangential forces. With the labrum intact, the humeral head will resist tangential forces of up to 60% of the compressive load. The degree of compression stabilization also varied according to the circumferential location of the glenoid, where the greatest magnitude was observed both superiorly and inferiorly. This effect may be attributed to the greater glenoid labrum depths in those two particular areas (49). The average contribution of the labrum to glenohumeral stability through the concavity compression is around 10%. This contribution also varies according to both arm position and direction of force with increased stability seen in the adducted position and inferior direction, respectively (51,52). Rodosky et al. (53) showed that with detachment of the superior glenoid labrum, resistance to torsion is decreased and more strain is placed on the inferior glenohumeral ligament (IGHL) which can contribute to dynamic anterior instability.

Another theory on the stabilizing effect of the labrum is its contribution to the intra-articular negative pressure of the shoulder. Habermeyer et al. (54) have compared the glenohumeral joint to a piston surrounded by a valve. The labrum works as a valve block that seals the joint from atmospheric pressure. Traction of the arm in a stable shoulder with intact labrum resulted in negative pressure that correlated to the amount of forces exerted. In contrast, in the unstable shoulder with detachment of the anterior inferior labrum, the above phenomenon does not exist, thus the piston and valve model is not valid. Thus the authors concluded that the absence of negative joint pressure disturbs joint mechanics and also the receptors that control motor feedback to protect the shoulder dynamically from dislocating forces. However, in contrast to the above study, restoring the "bumper" effect after Bankart repair to recreate the glenoid labrum has not been shown in a cadaver model to increase glenohumeral translational stability when compared to fixation at the glenoid rim (55).

Capsule and Glenohumeral Ligaments

The shoulder capsule has about twice the surface area of the humeral head and allows for shoulder range of motion (17). The anterior capsule is thicker than the posterior capsule. Ciccone et al. (56) found that the anterior shoulder capsule averaged 2.42 mm, inferior capsule averaged 2.8 mm, and posterior capsule averaged at 2.2 mm thick. The range in the study was 1.32 to 4.47 mm and with significant thinning laterally from the glenoid to the humerus. These distinct thickenings in the anterior capsule are called glenohumeral ligaments and play an important role in shoulder stability. Early cadaver studies have evaluated the role and function of these lig-

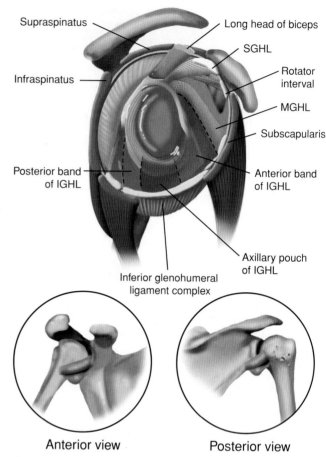

▲ **FIGURE 2-6:** Anatomic drawing of the superior, middle, and inferior glenohumeral ligaments. Both the intracapsular and extracapsular views are represented.

aments, which comprises SGHL, middle glenohumeral ligament (MGHL), and IGHL that is further separated into anterior and posterior components (Fig. 2-6). With rotation of the arm, specific ligaments tighten while others loosen. In the midranges of motion (everyday activities), the capsule and glenohumeral ligaments are in a lax state; therefore, does not contribute significantly to shoulder stability. However, at the extremes of range of motion, different glenohumeral ligaments will tighten according to the specific position of the arm and control humeral head translation to provide stability (17,19). The following subsections will discuss the contributions of each glenohumeral ligament to shoulder stability.

Rotator Interval

The "rotator interval" is a region that is between the superior border of the subscapularis tendon and the anterior border of the supraspinatus tendon. The two ligaments found within the rotator interval are the SGHL and the coracohumeral ligament (CHL) (57). The CHL is a dense fibrous structure that extends from the lateral aspect of the coracoid to the greater and lesser tuberosity of the humerus just adjacent to the bicipital groove (58). Portions of the CHL form a tunnel for the biceps tendon and blends inferiorly with the SGHL. Some investigators have demonstrated the CHL as a thin capsular fold without any ligamentous form (59), while others have suggested that the CHL may represent an accessory insertion of the pectoralis minor tendon (41). The SGHL originates from the supraglenoid tubercle anteroinferior to the origin of the long head of the biceps tendon and inserts onto the humerus on the proximal tip of the lesser tuberosity. Significant variations in the size and shape of the SGHL exist between individuals. In contrast to the CHL, Cooper et al. (59) demonstrated that the SGHL is a ligamentous structure with collagen bundles organized in a longitudinal direction. Both CHL and SGHL run parallel to each other in the rotator interval to limit inferior translation and external rotation in the adducted arm position or posterior translation with the arm in flexion, adduction, and internal rotation (17,19). Furthermore, deficiency or injury to the rotator interval may result in MDI, while contracture in this region may limit external rotation and forward flexion (60–62). Lee et al. (30) reported that in patients with MDI, the rotator interval width and depth were significantly greater than in normal patients on MRI. Furthermore, the capsular dimensions at the inferior and posteroinferior regions were larger as well. However, in contrast to the above findings, Provencher et al. (63) did not find a difference in the rotator interval distance between normal patients and instability patients. Furthermore, Mologne et al. (64) reported that with closure of the rotator interval in a cadaver model benefited or decreased anterior instability; however, posterior instability did not improve.

Middle Glenohumeral Ligament

The MGHL has the greatest variations among individuals and is absent in up to 30% of cases and poorly defined in another 10% (22,65,66). It typically originates from the superior glenoid just inferior to the SGHL between the 1-o'clock and 3-o'clock positions and blends in with the subscapularis tendon as its insertion approximately 2 cm medial to the lesser tuberosity (8,67). There are two variations to the MGHL that include a sheet-like structure that is confluent with the anterior band of the IGHL or a cord-like structure with a foraminal separation from the IGHL called a "Buford" complex (68,69). The MGHL primarily limits anterior humeral head translation with the arm abducted to 45 degrees and externally rotated. When the arm is in the adducted position, the MGHL functions to limit external rotation and inferior translation (8,17,70).

Inferior Glenohumeral Ligament

The IGHLC is a hammock-like structure that originates from the anterior inferior glenoid rim and labrum to insert below the MGHL on the inferior margin of the humeral articular surface and anatomic neck (Fig. 2-7).

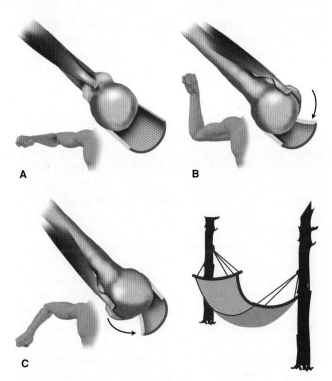

▲ **FIGURE 2-7:** The inferior glenohumeral ligament complex provide support to the humeral head like a hammock **(A)**. Reciprocal tightening in external rotation **(B)** and internal rotation **(C)** provides barrier to prevent anterior and posterior instability, respectively.

The IGHLC is divided into three main components: A thick anterior band, a thinner posterior band, and the interposed axillary pouch between the two bands (65). Cadaver studies have found that the anterior band of the IGHLC averages 2.8 mm while the posterior portion of the IGHLC averages 1.7 mm in thickness. However, the authors could not identify a distinct posterior band (71). Recent studies also support that the posterior band of the IGHLC is less consistent than both the anterior band and the axillary pouch (72). The IGHLC function to support the humeral head and prevent translation when the arm is in the abducted position (73). Global stability requires function of all three components of the IGHLC. With abduction and external rotation of the arm, the entire complex becomes taut and moves beneath the humeral head to prevent anterior translation. However, with internal rotation and abduction, the IGHLC functions to limit posterior translation (17,19). When the arm is in the 90-degree abduction and extension (30 degrees), the anterior band of the IGHLC prevents excessive anterior and posterior translation. Conversely, with the arm in the 90-degree abduction and flexion (30 degrees) position, the posterior band of the IGHLC prevents excessive anterior and posterior translation (74).

Tensile testing of the anterior band of the IGHLC in the position of clinical apprehension (abduction and external rotation) revealed that 66% of the specimens failed at the glenoid insertion while 34% failed at the midsubstance and humeral insertion.

Failure at the glenoid insertion region can be grouped into two separate pathologies. In one scenario, the failure occurred with the labrum completely avulsed from the glenoid bone (63%) and the other failure mode occurred at the ligament–labral junction with the labrum remained attached to the glenoid (37%). Before failure, all regions of the IGHLC experienced significant amount of strain (75). The ultimate load to failure of the anterior band (213 to 353 N) was not significantly different between the three modes of failure (glenoid, midsubstance, or humeral site). However, the amount of elongation was found to be greater at the glenoid and humeral insertion sites than specimens with midsubstance failures. Thus the yield strain at the glenoid and humeral region was larger than the midsubstance area prior to failure; however, permanent stretching of the anterior band IGHLC could never exceed a length greater than 4% strain (67,75). Several other studies have also investigated the strain of the IGHLC before failure and reported higher values of 9% to 11% (71,72). This difference may be attributed to the differences in the cadavers, modes of measurement, and equipment. Failure mode is also age dependent; in younger patients the disruption of the anterior band of the IGHLC typically occurs at the glenoid site while older individuals tend to fail at the midsubstance. Furthermore, the ultimate load of failure is significantly higher in the younger age group (76).

DYNAMIC STABILIZERS

Rotator Cuff Musculature and Biceps Tendon

The rotator cuff musculature comprises supraspinatus, infraspinatus, teres minor, and subscapularis muscles. Contribution of the rotator cuff muscle group to glenohumeral stability occurs through three distinct mechanisms (39,77–79) that include: (1) joint compression, (2) coordinated contraction of the cuff muscle to guide the humeral head onto the center of the glenoid, and (3) dynamization of the glenohumeral ligament with shoulder range of motion through the cuff attachments (65). The rotator cuff muscles are well positioned to provide a coordinated compressive joint load to stabilize the shoulder throughout the different ranges of motion. Lippitt et al. (49) first described the effect of "concavity compression" in which compression of the humeral head into the glenoid cavity stabilizes it against translating forces (Fig. 2-8). With the labrum intact, the humeral head resisted tangential forces of up to 60% of the compressive load before instability. The greatest stabilizing effect was seen in the superior and inferior directions (52) while the least stable direction is anterior (51), which may be attributed to the glenoid depth in these regions respectively. Furthermore, resection of

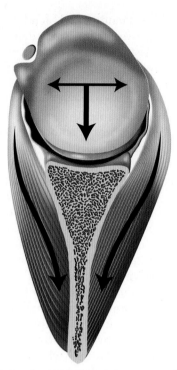

▲ **FIGURE 2-8:** Co-contraction of the rotator cuff musculature results in compression of the humeral head onto the glenoid surface to improve dynamic stability of the glenohumeral joint.

the labrum decreased the effectiveness of the compression stabilization effect by approximately 20%. This value has been debated in literature, with a more recent study demonstrating the average contribution of the labrum to glenohumeral stability through the concavity compression is only 10%. Stability was also greater in the hanging arm position compared to arm abduction–external rotation under the concavity-compression mechanism (51). These findings indicate that the effect of concavity compression may be an important stabilizer of the glenohumeral joint in the midranges of motion when the capsuloligamentous structures are lax. When the arm is in the extremes of motion, the capsuloligament structures are stretched to enhance their contribution to stability.

Co-contraction of the cuff muscles with the long head of the biceps tendon enhances the conformity fit of the humeral head onto the glenoid and further stabilizes the glenohumeral joint (80–83). The stabilizing effect of the rotator cuff on glenohumeral dynamic stability has been well demonstrated in the literature. Kronberg et al. (84) revealed altered rotator cuff and deltoid EMG activity in patients with generalized ligamentous laxity and instability when compared to normal individuals. Warner et al. (85) further demonstrated rotator cuff muscle strength differences in patients with shoulder instability compared to normal. McMahon et al. (86) has also shown significantly reduced EMG activity in the supraspinatus muscle from 30 to 60 degrees of abduction in patients with anterior shoulder instability. In a dynamic shoulder model,

50% reduction in the rotator cuff forces resulted in increased anterior displacement by 46% and posterior displacement by 31%. However, a decrease in the rotator cuff strength did not significantly influence inferior instability (79).

Many investigators have studied the contribution of the biceps tendon to glenohumeral stability. The origin of the long head of the biceps tendon arose directly from both the supraglenoid tubercle and the superior glenoid labrum. Most of the bicep attachment on the labrum is posterior in orientation (87). Itoi et al. (80) evaluated the stabilizing effect of the biceps tendon in a cadaver model and found that both the long and short head of the biceps have similar roles in preventing anterior shoulder instability with the arm in abduction and external rotation. Their role is further increased as the intrinsic shoulder stability decreases (capsule tear or Bankart lesion). Furthermore, the biceps becomes more important than the subscapularis in anterior stability as the stability from the capsuloligamentous structures decreases (81). Several other studies have also found that the magnitude of the joint compression stabilizing effect exceeds that of the static capsuloligamentous factors (49,52).

Deltoid Musculature

The deltoid muscle comprises three portions; anterior, middle, and posterior. It is a large triangular shaped bulky muscle which contributes to approximately 20% of all shoulder muscles (88). Morrey et al. (89) proposed the four essential muscle dynamic stabilizing effects contributing to shoulder stability. This includes: (1) passive tension from the muscle bulk, (2) muscle contraction that results in compression of the humeral head on the articular surface, (3) joint motion that tightens the passive ligaments of the shoulder, and (4) the barrier effect of the contracted muscle. Using a dynamic stability index, Lee and An (90) demonstrated the middle and posterior deltoid provided more stability by generating more compressive forces and lower shear forces than the anterior deltoid. Furthermore, the deltoid muscle produces more compressive force when the arm is elevated than in the neutral position. With the arm in external rotation, the insertion of the deltoid moves more posteriorly in relation to the glenohumeral joint, thus contraction at this position will produce a posteriorly directed compressive force and tensioning to reduce anterior instability. Kido et al. (91) also showed that with the capsule intact, anterior displacement is significantly reduced by application of load to the middle deltoid. However, with a simulated Bankart lesion, loading of each muscle portion significantly reduces anterior displacement. Thus the authors concluded that the stabilizing function of the deltoid becomes more essential as the shoulder becomes unstable.

Proprioception in Glenohumeral Stability

Placement of the upper extremity and hand in space for daily function is dependent on the perception of the shoulder joint position in space and motion. Capsule and ligaments function in joint stabilization by providing neurologic feedback that directly mediates joint position sensibility and muscle reflex stabilization. This sensory modality is called proprioception and mediated by receptors in the muscular and cutaneous structures of the shoulder joint. Specialized nerve endings and proprioceptive mechanoreceptors (Pacinian corpuscles, Ruffini endings, Golgi tendon endings, etc.) have been shown to exist in the capsule and ligaments (92,93). Stimulation of these mechanoreceptors result in muscle contraction around the joint that result in compressional forces which functions as an adaptive control for joint stabilization to sudden movements in acceleration or deceleration (20). It has been hypothesized that the receptors in the joint capsule responds to extremes in range of motion or deep pressure that may occur as a result of glenohumeral translation (94–96). Both Warner et al. (20) and Lephart et al. (97) have shown that the proprioception of the shoulder joint was disrupted in patients with glenohumeral instability compared to the asymptomatic shoulders. However, these differences were eliminated after surgical reconstruction. Laudner et al. (98) have also shown that shoulder proprioception at 75 degrees of external rotation decreases as the anterior glenohumeral laxity increases. After surgical reconstruction for shoulder instability, the joint position sense improved significantly in the position of abduction, flexion, and rotation from preoperative testing at greater than 5 years of follow-up. Interesting, the joint position in the contralateral shoulder also improved at final follow-up (99). Zuckerman et al. (100) also performed a similar study and reported that patients after open anterior stabilization procedure had 50% improvement of proprioceptive ability at the 6 months postsurgery time which improved to 100% or similar to the contralateral shoulder at the 1-year mark. Sullivan et al. (101) showed that patients after thermal or open capsulorrhaphy for anterior instability had significant better joint position sense than patients that had arthroscopic capsulorrhaphy. The authors attributed this finding to possible capsular retensioning and muscular scarring after the open and thermal capsulorrhaphy, respectively. Overall, the literature suggests that patients with recurrent shoulder instability will have a perceivable deficit in glenohumeral proprioception, which can be restored to normal after surgical repair or reconstruction. Capsuloligamentous structures may contribute to stability by providing the afferent feedback to reflexive muscle contraction of the rotator cuff, biceps, or deltoid. This reflexive contraction may serve as a protective mechanism via compressional forces against instability due to excessive glenohumeral translation or rotation.

S U M M A R Y

Successful management of shoulder instability requires knowledge of all factors responsible for stability and all of the potential factors that may contribute to instability. Both static and dynamic factors contribute to shoulder stability. Static factors include articular conformity of the glenohumeral joint and the negative intra-articular pressure. However, in the midranges of motion where the glenohumeral ligaments are lax, dynamic joint compression via rotator cuff muscle is responsible for joint stabilization. With the arm in the abducted and externally rotated position, the anterior portion of the IGHL is tensioned and provides a barrier to resist anterior instability. The rotator interval plays an additional role in limiting inferior translation of the humeral head when the arm in the adducted position. Co-contraction of rotator cuff musculature with the biceps tendon provides compression forces while enhancing the centering of the humeral head onto the glenoid to provide dynamic forces to stabilize the shoulder joint. Furthermore, both the deltoid muscle and proprioception also plays a dynamic role in shoulder stability. Abnormal version of either the glenoid or the humeral head has not been shown in the literature to contribute in glenohumeral instability. The spectrum of clinical instability can range from subluxation to transient luxation to dislocation. Most patients with a dislocation event will present with an injury to the anteroinferior capsulolabral complex or a "Bankart" lesion. In symptomatic patients, anatomic repair of the Bankart lesion is recommended. Some patients may also present with capsular laxity in combination to a Bankart lesion; therefore, a capsular shift may also be indicated in addition to a Bankart repair. It is essential to perform the capsular shift with the arm in specific positions (abduction of 30 degrees and external rotation of 30 degrees) to prevent overtightening and clinical loss in range of motion.

References

1. Adams FL. *The Genuine Work of Hippocrates.* New York, NY: William Wood; 1886.
2. Wang VM, Flatow EL. Pathomechanics of acquired shoulder instability: A basic science perspective. *J Shoulder Elbow Surg.* 2005;14(1 suppl S):2S–11S.
3. Field LD. Discovery of a new ligament of the shoulder. *Lancet.* 1997;1671–1672.
4. Perthes G. Operationen bei habitueller schulterluxation. *Deutsch Ztschr Chir.* 1906;85:199–227.
5. Thomas TT. Habitual or recurrent anterior dislocation of the shoulder; etiology and pathology. *Am J Med Sci.* 1909;137:229–246.
6. Bankart AS, Cantab MC. Recurrent or habitual dislocation of the shoulder-joint. 1923. *Clin Orthop Relat Res.* 1993;(291):3–6.
7. Bankart AS. Recurrent or habitual dislocation of the shoulder-joint. *Br Med J.* 1923;2(3285):1132–1133.
8. Turkel SJ, Panio MW, Marshall JL, et al. Stabilizing mechanisms preventing anterior dislocation of the glenohumeral joint. *J Bone Joint Surg Am.* 1981;63(8):1208–1217.
9. Neer CS 2nd. Dislocations. In: Reines L, ed. *Shoulder Reconstruction.* Philadelphia, PA: Saunders; 1990.
10. Ahmed I, Ashton F, Robinson CM. Arthroscopic Bankart repair and capsular shift for recurrent anterior shoulder instability: Functional outcomes and identification of risk factors for recurrence. *J Bone Joint Surg Am.* 2012; 94(14):1308–1315.
11. Milano G, Grasso A, Russo A, et al. Analysis of risk factors for glenoid bone defect in anterior shoulder instability. *Am J Sports Med.* 2011;39(9):1870–1876.
12. Provencher MT, Arciero RA, Burkhart SS, et al. Key factors in primary and revision surgery for shoulder instability. *Instr Course Lect.* 2010;59:227–244.
13. Boileau P, Villalba M, Hery JY, et al. Risk factors for recurrence of shoulder instability after arthroscopic Bankart repair. *J Bone Joint Surg Am.* 2006;88(8): 1755–1763.
14. Sener M, Yagdi S, Karapinar H. [Factors associated with failure in the surgical treatment of shoulder instability]. *Acta Orthop Traumatol Turc.* 2005;39(suppl):1134–1138.
15. Meehan RE, Petersen SA. Results and factors affecting outcome of revision surgery for shoulder instability. *J Shoulder Elbow Surg.* 2005;14(1):31–37.
16. Jahnke AH Jr, Hawkins RJ. Instability after shoulder arthroplasty: Causative factors and treatment options. *Semin Arthroplasty.* 1995;6(4):289–286.
17. McCluskey GM, Getz BA. Pathophysiology of anterior shoulder instability. *J Athl Train.* 2000;35(3):268–272.
18. Itoi E. Pathophysiology and treatment of atraumatic instability of the shoulder. *J Orthop Sci.* 2004;9(2):208–213.
19. Levine WN, Flatow EL. The pathophysiology of shoulder instability. *Am J Sports Med.* 2000;28(6):910–917.
20. Warner JJ, Lephart S, Fu FH. Role of proprioception in pathoetiology of shoulder instability. *Clin Orthop Relat Res.* 1996;(330):35–39.
21. Gibb TD, Sidles JA, Harryman DT 2nd, et al. The effect of capsular venting on glenohumeral laxity. *Clin Orthop Relat Res.* 1991;(268):120–127.
22. Warner JJ, Deng XH, Warren RF, et al. Static capsuloligamentous restraints to superior-inferior translation of the glenohumeral joint. *Am J Sports Med.* 1992;20(6):675–685.
23. Bryce CD, Davison AC, Okita N, et al. A biomechanical study of posterior glenoid bone loss and humeral head translation. *J Shoulder Elbow Surg.* 2010;19(7):994–1002.
24. Harryman DT 2nd, Sidles JA, Clark JM, et al. Translation of the humeral head on the glenoid with passive glenohumeral motion. *J Bone Joint Surg Am.* 1990;72(9): 1334–1343.

25. Harryman DT 2nd, Sidles JA, Harris SL, et al. Laxity of the normal glenohumeral joint: A quantitative in vivo assessment. *J Shoulder Elbow Surg.* 1992;1(2):66–76.

26. Owens BD, Nelson BJ, Duffey ML, et al. Pathoanatomy of first-time, traumatic, anterior glenohumeral subluxation events. *J Bone Joint Surg Am.* 2010;92(7):1605–1611.

27. Ovesen J, Nielsen S. Anterior and posterior shoulder instability. A cadaver study. *Acta Orthop Scand.* 1986;57(4):324–37.

28. Neer CS 2nd, Foster CR. Inferior capsular shift for involuntary inferior and multidirectional instability of the shoulder. A preliminary report. *J Bone Joint Surg Am.* 1980;62(6):897–908.

29. Neer CS 2nd, Foster CR. Inferior capsular shift for involuntary inferior and multidirectional instability of the shoulder: A preliminary report. 1980. *J Bone Joint Surg Am.* 2001;83-A(10):1586.

30. Lee HJ, Kim NR, Moon SG, et al. Multidirectional instability of the shoulder: Rotator interval dimension and capsular laxity evaluation using MR arthrography. *Skeletal Radiol.* 2013;42(2):231–238.

31. Abrams JS, Savoie FH 3rd, Tauro JC, et al. Recent advances in the evaluation and treatment of shoulder instability: Anterior, posterior, and multidirectional. *Arthroscopy.* 2002;18(9 suppl 2):1–13.

32. Gaskill TR, Taylor DC, Millett PJ. Management of multidirectional instability of the shoulder. *J Am Acad Orthop Surg.* 2011;19(12):758–767.

33. Provencher MT, Romeo AA. Posterior and multidirectional instability of the shoulder: Challenges associated with diagnosis and management. *Instr Course Lect.* 2008;57:133–152.

34. Millett PJ, Clavert P, Warner JJ. Arthroscopic management of anterior, posterior, and multidirectional shoulder instability: Pearls and pitfalls. *Arthroscopy.* 2003;19(suppl):186–193.

35. Paxinos A, Walton J, Tzannes A, et al. Advances in the management of traumatic anterior and atraumatic multidirectional shoulder instability. *Sports Med.* 2001;31(11):819–828.

36. Schenk TJ, Brems JJ. Multidirectional instability of the shoulder: Pathophysiology, diagnosis, and management. *J Am Acad Orthop Surg.* 1998;6(1):65–72.

37. Warner JJ, Johnson D, Miller M, et al. Technique for selecting capsular tightness in repair of anterior-inferior shoulder instability. *J Shoulder Elbow Surg.* 1995;4(5):352–364.

38. Gerber C, Werner CM, Macy JC, et al. Effect of selective capsulorrhaphy on the passive range of motion of the glenohumeral joint. *J Bone Joint Surg Am.* 2003;85-A(1):48–55.

39. Saha AK. Dynamic stability of the glenohumeral joint. *Acta Orthop Scand.* 1971;42(6):491–505.

40. Bowen MK, Deng XH, Hannafin JA, et al. An analysis of the patterns of glenohumeral joint contact and their relationships to the glenoid bare area. *Trans Orthop Res Soc.* 1992;496.

41. O'Brien SJ, Arnoczky SP, Warren RF, et al. Developmental anatomy of the shoulder and anatomy of the glenohumeral joint. In: Rockwood CA Jr, Matsen FA 3rd, eds. *The Shoulder.* Philadelphia, PA: W.B. Saunders; 1990.

42. Soslowsky LJ, Flatow EL, Bigliani LU, et al. Articular geometry of the glenohumeral joint. *Clin Orthop Relat Res.* 1992;(285):181–190.

43. Soslowsky LJ, Glatow EL, Bigliani LU, et al. Quantitation of in situ contact areas at the glenohumeral joint: A biomechanical study. *J Orthop Res.* 1992;10(4):524–534.

44. Kelkar R, Wang VM, Flatow EL, et al. Glenohumeral mechanics: A study of articular geometry, contact, and kinematics. *J Shoulder Elbow Surg.* 2001;10(1):73–84.

45. Howell SM, Galinat BJ. The glenoid-labral socket. A constrained articular surface. *Clin Orthop Relat Res.* 1989;(243):122–125.

46. Karduna AR, Williams GR, Williams JL, et al. Kinematics of the glenohumeral joint: Influences of muscle forces, ligamentous constraints, and articular geometry. *J Orthop Res.* 1996;14(6):986–993.

47. Cooper DE, Arnoczky SP, O'Brien SJ, et al. Anatomy, histology, and vascularity of the glenoid labrum. An anatomical study. *J Bone Joint Surg Am.* 1992;74(1):46–52.

48. Howell SM, Galinat BJ, Renzi AJ, et al. Normal and abnormal mechanics of the glenohumeral joint in the horizontal plane. *J Bone Joint Surg Am.* 1988;70(2):227–232.

49. Lippitt SB, Vanderhooft JE, Harris SL, et al. Glenohumeral stability from concavity-compression: A quantitative analysis. *J Shoulder Elbow Surg.* 1993;2(1):27–35.

50. Metcalf MH, Pon JD, Harryman DT 2nd, et al. Capsulolabral augmentation increases glenohumeral stability in the cadaver shoulder. *J Shoulder Elbow Surg.* 2001;10(6):532–538.

51. Halder AM, Kuhl SG, Zobitz ME, et al. Effects of the glenoid labrum and glenohumeral abduction on stability of the shoulder joint through concavity-compression: An in vitro study. *J Bone Joint Surg Am.* 2001;83-A(7):1062–1069.

52. Warner JJ, Bowen MK, Deng X, et al. Effect of joint compression on inferior stability of the glenohumeral joint. *J Shoulder Elbow Surg.* 1999;8(1):31–36.

53. Rodosky MW, Harner CD, Fu FH. The role of the long head of the biceps muscle and superior glenoid labrum in anterior stability of the shoulder. *Am J Sports Med.* 1994;22(1):121–130.

54. Habermeyer P, Schuller U, Wiedemann E. The intra-articular pressure of the shoulder: An experimental study on the role of the glenoid labrum in stabilizing the joint. *Arthroscopy.* 1992;8(2):166–172.

55. Yamamoto N, Muraki T, Sperling JW, et al. Does the "bumper" created during Bankart repair contribute to shoulder stability? *J Shoulder Elbow Surg.* 2013;22(6):828–834.

56. Ciccone WJ 2nd, Hunt TJ, Lieber R, et al. Multiquadrant digital analysis of shoulder capsular thickness. *Arthroscopy.* 2000;16(5):457–461.

57. Cain PR, Mutschler TA, Fu FH, et al. Anterior stability of the glenohumeral joint. A dynamic model. *Am J Sports Med.* 1987;15(2):144–148.

58. Jost B, Koch PP, Gerber C. Anatomy and functional aspects of the rotator interval. *J Shoulder Elbow Surg.* 2000;9(4):336–341.

59. Cooper DE, O'Brien SJ, Arnoczky SP, et al. The structure and function of the coracohumeral ligament: An

anatomic and microscopic study. *J Shoulder Elbow Surg.* 1993;2(2):70–77.

60. Nobuhara K, Ikeda H. Rotator interval lesion. *Clin Orthop Relat Res.* 1987;(223):44–50.
61. Ikeda H. ["Rotator interval" lesion. Part 2: Biomechanical study]. *Nihon Seikeigeka Gakkai Zasshi.* 1986;60(12):1275–1281.
62. Ikeda H. ["Rotator interval" lesion. Part 1: Clinical study]. *Nihon Seikeigeka Gakkai Zasshi.* 1986;60(12):1261–1273.
63. Provencher MT, Dewing CB, Bell SJ, et al. An analysis of the rotator interval in patients with anterior, posterior, and multidirectional shoulder instability. *Arthroscopy.* 2008;24(8):921–929.
64. Mologne TS, Zhao K, Hongo M, et al. The addition of rotator interval closure after arthroscopic repair of either anterior or posterior shoulder instability: Effect on glenohumeral translation and range of motion. *Am J Sports Med.* 2008;36(6):1123–1131.
65. Warner JJ, Caborn DN, Berger R, et al. Dynamic capsuloligamentous anatomy of the glenohumeral joint. *J Shoulder Elbow Surg.* 1993;2(3):115–133.
66. DePalma AF, Callery G, Bennett GA. Variational anatomy and the degenerative lesions of the shoulder joint. In: *American Academy of Orthopaedic Surgeons Instructional Course Lectures.* Vol XVI; 1949:255–281.
67. Burkart AC, Debski RE. Anatomy and function of the glenohumeral ligaments in anterior shoulder instability. *Clin Orthop Relat Res.* 2002;(400):32–39.
68. Tirman PF, Feller JF, Palmer WE, et al. The Buford complex – a variation of normal shoulder anatomy: MR arthrographic imaging features. *AJR Am J Roentgenol.* 1996;166(4):869–873.
69. Williams MM, Snyder SJ, Buford D Jr. The Buford complex – the "cord-like" middle glenohumeral ligament and absent anterosuperior labrum complex: A normal anatomic capsulolabral variant. *Arthroscopy.* 1994;10(3):241–247.
70. O'Connell PW, Nuber GW, Mileski RA, et al. The contribution of the glenohumeral ligaments to anterior stability of the shoulder joint. *Am J Sports Med.* 1990;18(6):579–584.
71. Bigliani LU, Pollock RG, Soslowsky LJ, et al. Tensile properties of the inferior glenohumeral ligament. *J Orthop Res.* 1992;10(2):187–197.
72. Ticker JB, Bigliani LU, Soslowsky LJ, et al. Inferior glenohumeral ligament: Geometric and strain-rate dependent properties. *J Shoulder Elbow Surg.* 1996;5(4):269–279.
73. O'Brien SJ, Neves MC, Arnoczky SP, et al. The anatomy and histology of the inferior glenohumeral ligament complex of the shoulder. *Am J Sports Med.* 1990;18(5):449–456.
74. O'Brien SJ, Schwartz RS, Warren RF, et al. Capsular restraints to anterior-posterior motion of the abducted shoulder: A biomechanical study. *J Shoulder Elbow Surg.* 1995;4(4):298–308.
75. McMahon PJ, Tibone JE, Cawley PW, et al. The anterior band of the inferior glenohumeral ligament: Biomechanical properties from tensile testing in the position of apprehension. *J Shoulder Elbow Surg.* 1998;7(5):467–471.

76. Lee TQ, Dettling J, Sandusky MD, et al. Age related biomechanical properties of the glenoid-anterior band of the inferior glenohumeral ligament-humerus complex. *Clin Biomech (Bristol, Avon).* 1999;14(7):471–476.
77. Thompson WO, Debski RE, Boardman ND 3rd, et al. A biomechanical analysis of rotator cuff deficiency in a cadaveric model. *Am J Sports Med.* 1996;24(3):286–292.
78. Xue Q, Huang G. Dynamic stability of glenohumeral joint during scapular plane elevation. *Chin Med J (Engl).* 1998;111(5):447–449.
79. Wuelker N, Korell M, Thren K. Dynamic glenohumeral joint stability. *J Shoulder Elbow Surg.* 1998;7(1):43–52.
80. Itoi E, Kuechle DK, Newman SR, et al. Stabilising function of the biceps in stable and unstable shoulders. *J Bone Joint Surg Br.* 1993;75(4):546–550.
81. Itoi E, Newman SR, Kuechle DK, et al. Dynamic anterior stabilisers of the shoulder with the arm in abduction. *J Bone Joint Surg Br.* 1994;76(5):834–836.
82. Pagnani MJ, Deng XH, Warren RF, et al. Role of the long head of the biceps brachii in glenohumeral stability: A biomechanical study in cadavera. *J Shoulder Elbow Surg.* 1996;5(4):255–262.
83. Warner JJ, McMahon PJ. The role of the long head of the biceps brachii in superior stability of the glenohumeral joint. *J Bone Joint Surg Am.* 1995;77(3):366–372.
84. Kronberg M, Brostrom LA, Nemeth G. Differences in shoulder muscle activity between patients with generalized joint laxity and normal controls. *Clin Orthop Relat Res.* 1991;(269):181–192.
85. Warner JJ, Micheli LJ, Arslanian LE, et al. Patterns of flexibility, laxity, and strength in normal shoulders and shoulders with instability and impingement. *Am J Sports Med.* 1990;18(4):366–375.
86. McMahon PJ, Jobe FW, Pink MM, et al. Comparative electromyographic analysis of shoulder muscles during planar motions: Anterior glenohumeral instability versus normal. *J Shoulder Elbow Surg.* 1996;5(2 pt 1):118–123.
87. Vangsness CT Jr, Jorgenson SS, Watson T, et al. The origin of the long head of the biceps from the scapula and glenoid labrum. An anatomical study of 100 shoulders. *J Bone Joint Surg Br.* 1994;76(6):951–954.
88. Bassett RW, Browne AO, Morrey BF, et al. Glenohumeral muscle force and moment mechanics in a position of shoulder instability. *J Biomech.* 1990;23(5):405–415.
89. Morrey BF, Itoi E, An KN. Biomechanics of the shoulder. In: Rockwood CA Jr, Matsen FA 3rd, eds. *The Shoulder.* Philadelphia, PA: W.B. Saunders; 1998.
90. Lee SB, An KN. Dynamic glenohumeral stability provided by three heads of the deltoid muscle. *Clin Orthop Relat Res.* 2002;(400):40–47.
91. Kido T, Itoi E, Lee SB, et al. Dynamic stabilizing function of the deltoid muscle in shoulders with anterior instability. *Am J Sports Med.* 2003;31(3):399–403.
92. Hagert E, Lee J, Ladd AL. Innervation patterns of thumb trapeziometacarpal joint ligaments. *J Hand Surg Am.* 2012;37(4):706–714.
93. Vangsness CT Jr, Ennis M, Taylor JG, et al. Neural anatomy of the glenohumeral ligaments, labrum, and subacromial bursa. *Arthroscopy.* 1995;11(2):180–184.

94. Grigg P, Hoffman AH. Properties of Ruffini afferents revealed by stress analysis of isolated sections of cat knee capsule. *J Neurophysiol.* 1982;47(1):41–54.

95. Grigg P, Hoffman AH. Calibrating joint capsule mechanoreceptors as in vivo soft tissue load cells. *J Biomech.* 1989;22(8–9):781–785.

96. Clark FJ, Burgess PR. Slowly adapting receptors in cat knee joint: Can they signal joint angle? *J Neurophysiol.* 1975;38(6):1448–1463.

97. Lephart SM, Warner JJ, Borsa PA, et al. Proprioception of the shoulder joint in healthy, unstable, and surgically repaired shoulders. *J Shoulder Elbow Surg.* 1994;3(6):371–380.

98. Laudner KG, Meister K, Kajiyama S, et al. The relationship between anterior glenohumeral laxity and proprioception in collegiate baseball players. *Clin J Sport Med.* 2012;22(6):478–482.

99. Potzl W, Thorwesten L, Gotze C, et al. Proprioception of the shoulder joint after surgical repair for Instability: A long-term follow-up study. *Am J Sports Med.* 2004; 32(2):425–430.

100. Zuckerman JD, Gallagher MA, Cuomo F, et al. The effect of instability and subsequent anterior shoulder repair on proprioceptive ability. *J Shoulder Elbow Surg.* 2003;12(2):105–109.

101. Sullivan JA, Hoffman MA, Harter RA. Shoulder joint position sense after thermal, open, and arthroscopic capsulorrhaphy for recurrent anterior instability. *J Shoulder Elbow Surg.* 2008;17(3):389–394.

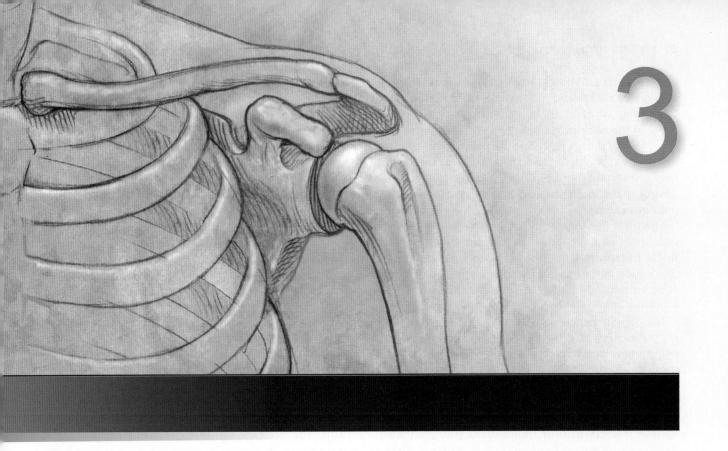

Workup of the Patient Presenting with Instability

Ryan T. Cassilly / Jon-Michael E. Caldwell /
William N. Levine

Shoulder instability is a frequently encountered diagnosis in orthopedic practices, both among athletes and the general population. Instability may present as an acute traumatic dislocation or as a chronic form of unidirectional or multidirectional instability. Recurrent subluxation and/or dislocation requires surgical intervention for definitive management in many cases. An accurate clinical diagnosis is imperative, as the complexity of shoulder anatomy lends itself to multiple forms of pathology. A thorough workup, including history, physical examination with provocative dynamic maneuvers for instability, and appropriate imaging, must be undertaken to make the appropriate diagnosis, which will ultimately drive treatment options.

PATIENT PRESENTATION

Glenohumeral instability encompasses a variety of clinical presentations and patterns of instability. Patients may present with nonspecific complaints including pain, a decrease in athletic performance, a sensation of instability, or less commonly radicular-type symptoms. Patients may recall or even demonstrate specific inciting activities or positions and modify their behavior or develop compensatory behaviors to avoid such activities (1). Symptoms may involve one or both shoulders and may be uni- or multidirectional. Presenting complaints in pediatric patients parallel those in the adult population (2).

Several details regarding the nature of the patient's instability should be ascertained from the history. Patients should be questioned regarding the degree, direction, chronology, cause, frequency, and volition of their symptoms (3). The degree and direction of instability can range from subluxation to complete dislocation in one or more directions. The most common traumatic instability pattern is an anterior glenohumeral dislocation resulting from a force applied to an externally rotated and abducted shoulder, which results in unidirectional anterior instability. These patients may either present acutely or after spontaneous reduction.

Patients with an acute posterior dislocation usually will present with a history of high-energy trauma, electrical shock, or seizure. Posterior dislocations and subsequent unidirectional posterior instability have been reported to be up to 20 times less common than anterior dislocations (3). The patient's age at first dislocation is an important prognostic indicator, as younger patients have been shown in multiple studies to have a higher risk for recurrence (4–6), up to 90% if younger than 20 years (7). Continued participation in contact sports has also been shown to have a high propensity for redislocation after the initial injury (5). While patients older than 40 years have a lower rate of recurrence of 10%, they are more prone to suffer tears of the rotator cuff (7).

The chronicity of instability can be described as either acute or chronic and the frequency of dislocations or subluxations should be noted. Patients with chronic instability may have had a single initial traumatic dislocation that has progressed to recurrent episodes of instability. Some patients, particularly overhead athletes such as those who participate in swimming and gymnastics, may also complain of multidirectional instability (MDI), which was originally described as anterior and posterior instability with involuntary inferior subluxation (8), but may simply involve two or more planes (1,9,10). In throwing athletes, it is important to determine the relationship between instability symptoms and changes in performance ability, throwing mechanics, or frequency of practice.

It is important to consider if the patient is voluntarily dislocating the shoulder or has associated psychiatric comorbidities, as these patients are thought to respond less favorably to both nonoperative and surgical interventions (11). However, care should be taken to distinguish patients who are able to demonstrate positional instability from those who willfully dislocate, as the latter may have favorable operative outcomes.

Concomitant medical conditions, such as epilepsy or collagen disorders such as Ehlers-Danlos, may also play a role in the etiology of the patient's insta-

bility and should be noted. The physician must also obtain a history of all previous treatments for instability, such as closed reductions for dislocation, use of physical therapy, periods of immobilization, or operative intervention.

PHYSICAL EXAMINATION

A careful history and physical examination can yield a diagnosis of shoulder instability in the majority of cases. General inspection should include evaluation of previous surgical scars (and any healing abnormalities which may suggest a collagen disorder), asymmetry, atrophy, arm position, and any gross deformity. In the acute anterior dislocation, patients will present with loss of normal shoulder contour, as well as an anterior fullness to the shoulder where the humeral head has displaced. Patients with acute posterior dislocation will usually present with the arm adducted and internally rotated. Those with a chronic posterior dislocation will lack external rotation when compared to the contralateral arm. The muscles and bony anatomy should then be palpated with particular attention to underlying muscle tone and any tenderness. The presence of soreness over the posterior capsule suggests anterior subluxation, while compensation for MDI often causes tenderness along the medial border of the scapula (3).

The stability of the humerus on the glenoid is maintained through a balance between the dynamic and static stabilizers (12). The humeral head is stabilized and centered on the glenoid by the coordinated forces of the rotator cuff musculature, with the capsule, coracohumeral ligament, and glenohumeral ligaments providing static restraint. Examination of supraspinatus, infraspinatus, teres minor, and subscapularis strength is important to assess the dynamic stabilization of the shoulder. Active and passive range of motion must be evaluated for every patient presenting with shoulder complaints including forward elevation, abduction, external rotation at 0 and 90 degrees of abduction, and internal rotation at 0 and 90 degrees of shoulder abduction. This will allow for the assessment of further pathology, as well as decrease or increase in range of motion from capsular contraction or laxity, respectively. Posterosuperior rotator cuff tears are a known complication of shoulder dislocation in patients older than 40 years, and correlate with the rising number of dislocations (13). As such, comprehensive assessment of cuff integrity should be included in the instability physical examination. Particular attention should be paid to the supraspinatus and infraspinatus fossae, which may demonstrate atrophy following a rotator cuff tear. However, full thickness rotator cuff tears are uncommon in the younger patient population with acute traumatic dislocations, as well as in the throwing shoulder.

Muscle wasting, paresthesias, reflex changes, or sensory or motor deficits may all be present in a patient with instability. A careful neurologic examination should be performed including the cervical spine and extremity, both proximal and distal to the shoulder for confounding pathology. In the setting of acute traumatic shoulder dislocation, one should ensure a thorough examination of the entire brachial plexus, with particular attention paid to axillary nerve function, both motor and sensory, prior to and after closed reduction maneuvers.

Ligamentous Laxity

When examining the patient, it is important to differentiate laxity from instability. Objective measures of shoulder laxity must also take into account the patient's symptoms. Only when laxity causes symptoms should it be considered pathologic for instability. Throwing athletes, for example, will typically have increased external rotation with corresponding decreased internal rotation (14). When present, this should not be considered pathologic as it is an adaptation to the repetitive throwing motion (15).

All patients should be assessed for generalized ligamentous hyperlaxity. While there is an absence of accepted definitions for hyperlaxity, it has been described by evaluating for elbow hyperextension, metacarpal–phalangeal joint hyperextension (Fig. 3-1), positive thumb-to-forearm test (Fig. 3-2) (the patient is able to contact the ipsilateral forearm with the thumb), and genu recurvatum. The prognosis and response of patients with concurrent hyperlaxity and shoulder instability to surgical intervention remains unclear, though these patients are thought to respond well to both nonoperative and operative treatments (16). Various physical examination techniques, as described below, have been used as a means to evaluate the patient for glenohumeral laxity or its subsequent pathology, and elicit symptoms that may indicate instability.

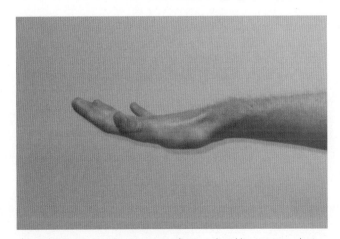

▲ **FIGURE 3-1:** Examination of generalized ligamentous laxity with MCP hyperextension. (Figure courtesy of Columbia Center for Shoulder, Elbow and Sports Medicine.)

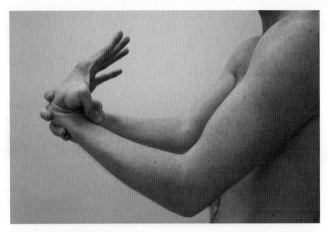

▲ **FIGURE 3-2:** Examination of generalized ligamentous laxity with thumb-to-forearm test. (Figure courtesy of Columbia Center for Shoulder, Elbow and Sports Medicine.)

Sulcus Test

The sulcus test, first described by Neer and Welsh (17), examines first for unidirectional inferior instability, but also the integrity of the rotator interval, which plays a role in MDI. The patient is placed upright in a seated position on the examination table with the shoulder in 0 degrees of abduction and neutral rotation (Fig. 3-3). Inferior longitudinal traction is placed on the humerus, forming a depression between the humerus and the lateral border of the acromion. The magnitude of translation is measured as Grade I (<1 cm), Grade II (1 to 2 cm), and Grade III (>2 cm). Both shoulders can be tested simultaneously and assessed for symmetry (Fig. 3-4). The examination is then repeated with the shoulder placed in external rotation. If the rotator interval is competent, the sulcus will decrease with external rotation.

Load and Shift

The load and shift is used to examine anterior and posterior laxity of the shoulder (18). The patient is placed upright in a seated position on the examination table (Fig. 3-5). The arm is supported in 20 degrees of abduction, 20 degrees of forward flexion, and neutral rotation. With the physician standing behind the patient, one hand stabilizes the scapula, while the other hand grasps the proximal humerus. A compressive load is placed on the humerus to center it within the glenoid, and an anteriorly directed force is used to translate the humeral head. The test is then repeated with a posterior directed force. The magnitude of translation is measured as Grade I (to glenoid rim), Grade II (over glenoid rim with spontaneous reduction), or Grade III (over glenoid rim without reduction; i.e., dislocation). This test may also be performed while the patient is supine with the shoulder at the edge of the examination table, using both of the physician's hands to stabilize and shift the humerus (Fig. 3-6).

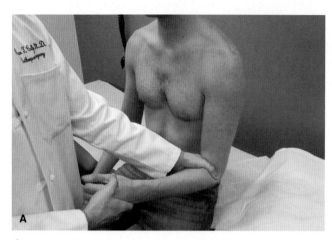
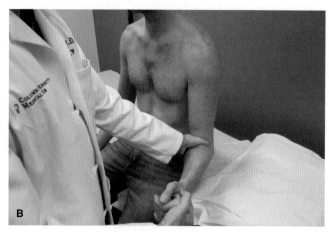

▲ **FIGURE 3-3:** Assessing inferior instability and rotator interval integrity via the sulcus test, performed in **(A)** internal and **(B)** external rotation. (Figure courtesy of Columbia Center for Shoulder, Elbow and Sports Medicine.)

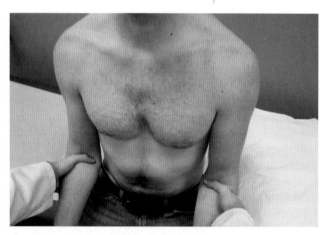

▲ **FIGURE 3-4:** The sulcus test may be performed sitting using the contralateral extremity for comparison. (Figure courtesy of Columbia Center for Shoulder, Elbow and Sports Medicine.)

Active Compression Test

The active compression test as described by O'Brien et al. (19) may be used to evaluate for labral pathology, which may have resulted during episodes of instability. The patient is placed upright in a seated or standing position with the shoulder in 90 degrees of forward flexion, 15 degrees of adduction, elbow in full extension, and the arm internally rotated with the thumb pointing down (Fig. 3-7). A uniform downward force is applied to the arm, with the patient resisting. The examination is then repeated with the arm in supination with the palm facing upward. If the patient experiences pain "deep" within the joint with the first maneuver that is alleviated with supination, the test is considered positive for pathology within the glenoid labrum. This test can also be used for acromioclavicular joint (ACJ) pathology if the patient experiences pain superficially over the AC joint. O'Brien found the examination to be 100% sensitive and 98.5%

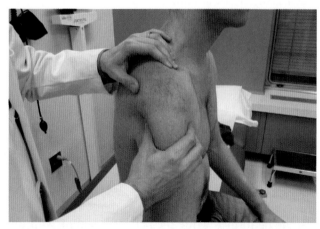

▲ **FIGURE 3-5:** The load and shift test assesses for anterior and posterior instability, using one hand to stabilize the scapula. (Figure courtesy of Columbia Center for Shoulder, Elbow and Sports Medicine.)

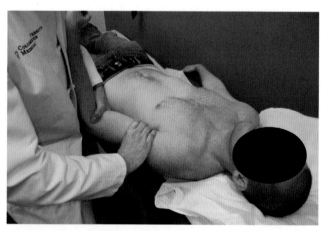

▲ **FIGURE 3-6:** The load and shift test may also be performed supine. (Figure courtesy of Columbia Center for Shoulder, Elbow and Sports Medicine.)

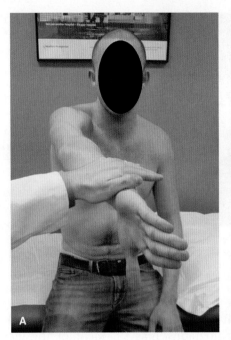 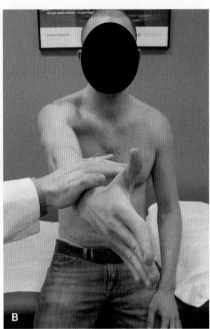

▶ **FIGURE 3-7:** Examination of labral pathology with the active compression test performed with shoulder **(A)** internal rotation and **(B)** external rotation. (Figure courtesy of Columbia Center for Shoulder, Elbow and Sports Medicine.)

specific for labral pathology, although recent meta-analysis has found this test to be 67% sensitive with 37% specific for detecting labral pathology (20).

Apprehension Test

The apprehension test evaluates the patient for symptoms of anterior instability. It is performed with the patient supine on the examination table with the shoulder in 90 degrees of abduction, neutral rotation, and the elbow in 90 degrees of flexion (Fig. 3-8). The shoulder is then slowly maximally externally rotated by the physician with a simultaneous anterior directed force, and is considered positive if the patient senses a feeling of apprehension from impending instability. Jobe et al. (21) found that when the apprehension test was per-

formed with maximal external rotation, it was a valuable diagnostic tool to differentiate between anterior instability and rotator cuff impingement. The sensitivity and specificity of the apprehension test have been found to be 53% to 72% and 96% to 99%, respectively (22,23). In terms of stratifying patients following an acute traumatic dislocation, Safran found that at 2 years, 71% of individuals with positive apprehension test 6 weeks after dislocation had suffered a recurrent dislocation, with a positive predictive value of 71%, suggesting that the examination can be used to stratify patients into a high and low risk category for future instability.

Relocation Test

The relocation test is a variation of the apprehension test that further evaluates for anterior instability. The arm is returned to neutral position, and the physician's hand applies a posteriorly directed force to the humeral head to stabilize it within the glenoid (Fig. 3-9). The shoulder is again slowly maximally externally rotated. If the symptoms of instability felt by the patient during the apprehension test are alleviated with the stabilizing force, the test is considered positive. The relocation test has been found to be 44% to 82% sensitive and 54% to 92% specific for anterior instability, and Farber et al. (22) concluded that apprehension was a better indication of instability than pain alone (24).

IMAGING

The findings of the physical examination guide the selection of an appropriate imaging modality to

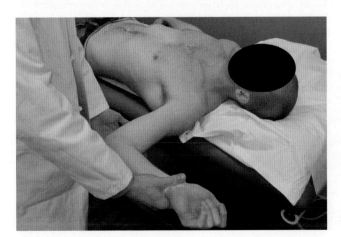

▲ **FIGURE 3-8:** Assessing for subjective sense of impending anterior instability with the apprehension test. (Figure courtesy of Columbia Center for Shoulder, Elbow and Sports Medicine.)

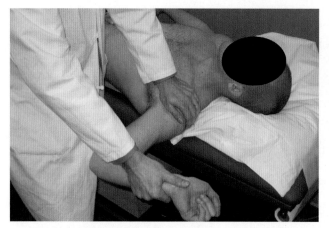

▲ **FIGURE 3-9:** The subjective sense of instability with the apprehension test should improve with a posterior directed humerus-stabilizing force in the relocation test. (Figure courtesy of Columbia Center for Shoulder, Elbow and Sports Medicine.)

continue the workup of the patient with glenohumeral instability, and may include radiographs, magnetic resonance imaging (MRI), MR arthrography, computed tomography (CT scan), or CT arthrogram. All patients should initially undergo radiographic imaging, including a true anterior-posterior (AP) of the shoulder joint with the humerus in internal, neutral, and external rotation. Equally as important are the orthogonal scapular-Y and axillary views. True AP images are acquired perpendicular to the plane of the glenoid fossa, typically with 30 to 45 degrees of rotation of the body toward the cassette. Specialized views

such as the West Point view or Stryker notch view may be indicated for further evaluation of the humerus or glenoid, respectively. In the patient presenting with an acute dislocation, it is imperative to obtain postreduction films to evaluate for appropriate reduction as well as the presence of fractures of the glenoid or proximal humerus.

X-ray Pathology

Bony Bankart

The most common structural lesion during traumatic dislocation, known as the essential lesion of instability, or Bankart lesion, results from detachment of the anterior–inferior labrum and glenohumeral ligament from the glenoid (25), and can be found in over 90% of patients (26). This may purely consist of a disruption of the fibrocartilaginous tissue, which will only be visualized on MRI, but may be notable on radiographs if there is an associated bony avulsion fragment of the glenoid, the so-called "bony Bankart" lesion (Fig. 3-10). A glenoid defect greater than 20% of the length of the glenoid has been shown to significantly increase instability (27). Although described as the essential lesion, consensus is that a Bankart lesion alone is insufficient to allow the humeral head to dislocate (28).

Hill-Sachs

A Hill-Sachs lesion is the resultant compression fracture of the posterolateral humeral head due to impaction

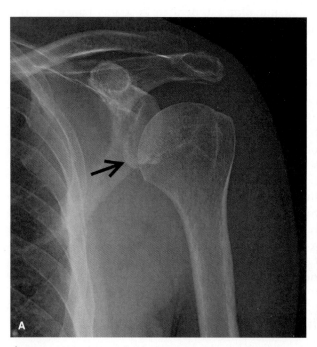
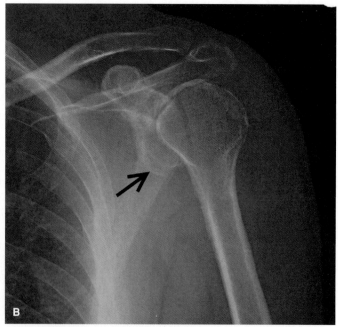

▲ **FIGURE 3-10:** Left shoulder neutral rotation **(A)** and internal rotation **(B)** radiographs demonstrating "bony Bankart" lesion of the anteroinferior glenoid rim (*arrows*). (Figure courtesy of Columbia Center for Shoulder, Elbow and Sports Medicine.)

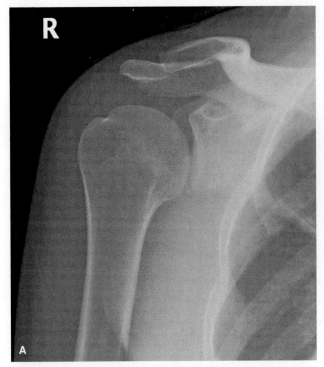

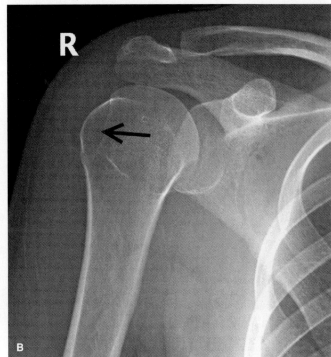

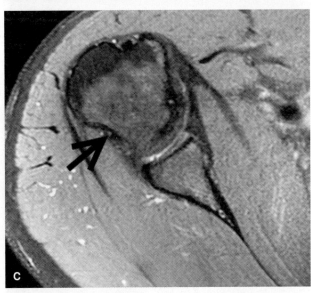

▲ **FIGURE 3-11:** Right shoulder external rotation **(A)** and internal rotation **(B)** radiographs demonstrating Hill-Sachs lesion (arrows), better visualized on the internal rotation view. Axial MRI **(C)** confirms the lesion with associated humeral head edema. (Figure courtesy of Columbia Center for Shoulder, Elbow and Sports Medicine.)

against the anterior glenoid rim during an anterior dislocation (29). It is best seen on the internal rotation AP shoulder radiograph, as this places the posterolateral aspect of the humeral head in profile (Fig. 3-11). Over 90% of patients will show evidence of the lesion after their first traumatic dislocation (26). A posterior glenohumeral dislocation will create a similar characteristic lesion, the reverse Hill-Sachs, on the anteromedial humeral head.

CT Scan Pathology

CT scan can be used to evaluate for underlying bony morphology of the unstable shoulder, including adequacy of reductions for glenohumeral fracture–dislocations of the proximal humerus and measurement of the size of Hill-Sachs (Fig. 3-12) and bony Bankart lesions (Fig. 3-13). With chronic instability in particular, the integrity of the glenoid rim should be evaluated for attritional loss (Fig. 3-14) which will lead to further progression instability (30). CT scan used in conjunction with arthrography may be used to evaluate the integrity of the glenoid labrum and rotator cuff. Such characteristics will guide the ultimate treatment options.

MRI Pathology

The workup of patients with glenohumeral instability has been greatly facilitated with MRI and MRI arthrography,

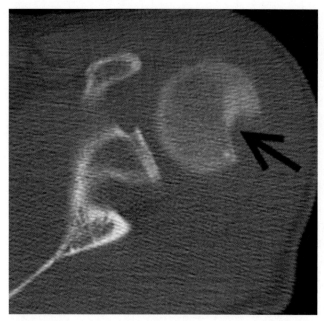

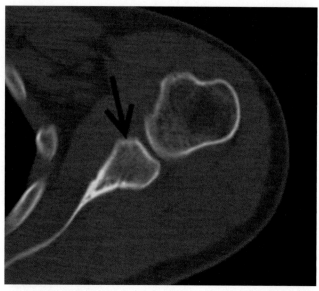

▲ **FIGURE 3-12:** Left shoulder axial CT image demonstrating Hill-Sachs lesion (*arrow*). (Figure courtesy of Columbia Center for Shoulder, Elbow and Sports Medicine.)

▲ **FIGURE 3-14:** Left shoulder CT axial image demonstrating anterior–inferior glenoid attrition from recurrent instability (*arrows*). (Figure courtesy of Columbia Center for Shoulder, Elbow and Sports Medicine.)

from which a wealth of information regarding pathology and ultimately treatment options can be gained. This is especially true when evaluating whether a soft tissue reconstruction will be sufficient or whether bony augmentation will be necessary depending on concurrent bony pathology. Intra-articular gadolinium contrast can be particularly helpful with assessment of the glenoid labrum such as posttraumatic Bankart lesions (Fig. 3-15).

Characteristic Lesions

ALPSA. ALPSA lesions (Anterior Labroligamentous Periosteal Sleeve Avulsion) are the result of chronic instability that causes displacement of the anterior labroligamentous complex (31) (Fig. 3-16). Over time there is medialization and scarring of the labroligamentous complex and periosteum to the medial glenoid neck, and has been shown to be more

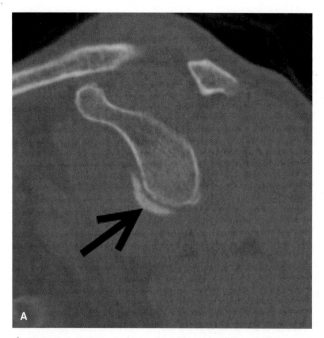

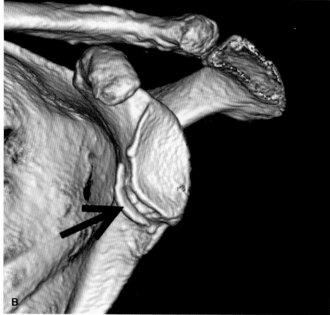

▲ **FIGURE 3-13:** Left shoulder CT sagital **(A)** and 3D reconstruction **(B)** images demonstrating "bony Bankart" lesion of the anteroinferior glenoid rim (*arrows*). (Figure courtesy of Columbia Center for Shoulder, Elbow and Sports Medicine.)

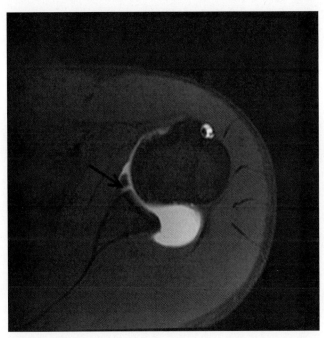

▲ **FIGURE 3-15:** Left shoulder MRI arthrogram axial image demonstrating Bankart lesion, avulsion of the anteroinferior glenoid labrum (*arrow*). Notice the intra-articular dye turning the corner between the torn labrum and the glenoid. (Figure courtesy of Columbia Center for Shoulder, Elbow and Sports Medicine.)

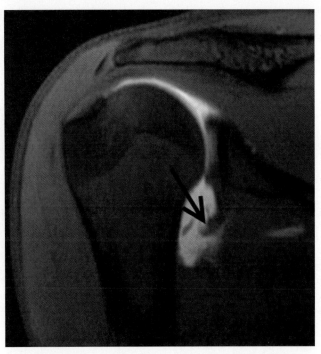

▲ **FIGURE 3-17:** MRI arthrogram demonstrating humeral avulsion of the glenohumeral ligament (HAGL). (Figure courtesy of Columbia Center for Shoulder, Elbow and Sports Medicine.)

prevalent in patients with chronic instability than patients with isolated traumatic dislocations (32).

HAGL. Disruption of the glenohumeral capsuloligamentous complex is not isolated to the glenoid rim. As seen on MRI, the capsule may avulse off of the humeral attachment, leading to the so-called HAGL lesion (Humeral Avulsion of the Glenohumeral Ligament) (Fig. 3-17). This can be noted approximately 10% of the time, as the majority avulse from the glenoid attachment.

GLAD. GLAD lesions (Glenolabral Articular Disruption) consist of a depression of the articular cartilage on the glenoid fossa from impaction injury of the humeral head, and are best appreciated on MRI (Fig. 3-18). This lesion has been shown to cause a significant amount of posttraumatic anterior shoulder pain (33).

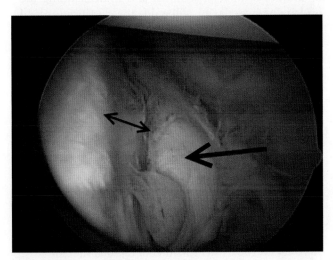

▲ **FIGURE 3-16:** MRI T2-weighted axial image demonstrating Anterior Labroligamentous Periosteal Sleeve Avulsion (ALPSA). Double arrow indicates the medial scapular neck where the labrum should be. The large arrow indicates the medially healed labrum (ALPSA lesion). (Figure courtesy of Columbia Center for Shoulder, Elbow and Sports Medicine.)

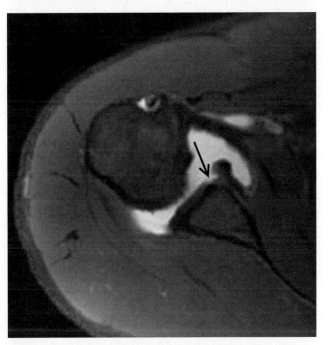

▲ **FIGURE 3-18:** Right shoulder MR arthrogram axial image demonstrating glenolabral articular disruption (GLAD). (Figure courtesy of Columbia Center for Shoulder, Elbow and Sports Medicine.)

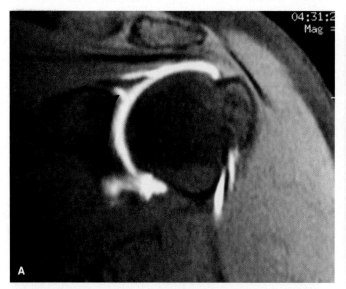 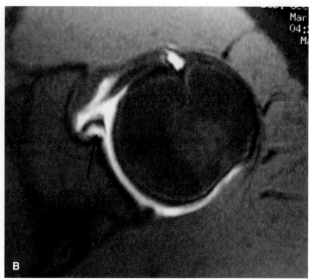

▲ **FIGURE 3-19:** Right shoulder MRI T2-weighted coronal **(A)** and axial **(B)** imaging demonstrating superior labral, anterior to posterior (SLAP) tear (*arrow*). (Figure courtesy of Columbia Center for Shoulder, Elbow and Sports Medicine.)

SLAP. SLAP lesions (Superior Labrum Anterior to Posterior) that involve only fraying of the labrum are typically related to degenerative changes. However disruption of the superior labrum from the glenoid or tears within the labrum may be indicative of a trau-matic etiology related to traction injuries or repetitive trauma in overhead athletes, and may confer a degree of instability to the glenohumeral joint (Fig. 3-19). Posterior instability typically leads to fraying of the labrum as opposed to an overt tear.

S U M M A R Y

Diagnosis of the patient with shoulder instability relies on the interplay between symptoms, physical examination findings, and corresponding pathology noted on imaging studies. It should again be stressed that shoulder laxity, in and of itself, does not imply underlying pathology and may be inherent or an adaptation to overhead use in athletes. Clinical laxity with associated symptoms is the hallmark of glenohumeral instability, and may be reproduced though provocative physical examination maneuvers as described above. Determining whether the patient is presenting with unidirectional or multidirectional instability, and understanding the underlying hyperlaxity, will guide the classification and treatment for the unstable shoulder.

References

1. Gaskill TR, Taylor DC, Millett PJ. Management of multi-directional instability of the shoulder. *J Am Acad Orthop Surg.* 2011;19(12):758–767.
2. Lawton RL, Choudhury S, Mansat P, et al. Pediatric shoulder instability: Presentation, findings, treatment, and outcomes. *J Pediatr Orthop.* 2002;22(1):52–61.
3. Robinson CM, Seah M, Akhtar MA. The epidemiology, risk of recurrence, and functional outcome after an acute traumatic posterior dislocation of the shoulder. *J Bone Joint Surg Am.* 2011;93(17):1605–1613.
4. Robinson CM, Howes J, Murdoch H, et al. Functional outcome and risk of recurrent instability after primary traumatic anterior shoulder dislocation in young patients. *J Bone Joint Surg Am.* 2006;88(11): 2326–2336.
5. Sachs RA, Lin D, Stone ML, et al. Can the need for future surgery for acute traumatic anterior shoulder dislocation be predicted? *J Bone Joint Surg Am.* 2007; 89(8):1665–1674.
6. Owens BD, Dawson L, Burks R, et al. Incidence of shoulder dislocation in the United States military: Demographic considerations from a high-risk population. *J Bone Joint Surg Am.* 2009;91(4):791–796.
7. McLaughlin HL, Cavallaro WU. Primary anterior dislocation of the shoulder. *Am J Surg.* 1950;80(6):615–621; passim.
8. Neer CS 2nd, Foster CR. Inferior capsular shift for involuntary inferior and multidirectional instability of the shoulder. A preliminary report. *J Bone Joint Surg Am.* 1980;62(6):897–908.
9. Pollock RG, Owens JM, Flatow EL, et al. Operative results of the inferior capsular shift procedure for

multidirectional instability of the shoulder. *J Bone Joint Surg Am.* 2000;82-A(7):919–928.

10. Neer CS 2nd. Involuntary inferior and multidirectional instability of the shoulder: Etiology, recognition, and treatment. *Instr Course Lect.* 1985;34:232–238.

11. Rowe CR, Pierce DS, Clark JG. Voluntary dislocation of the shoulder. A preliminary report on a clinical, electromyographic, and psychiatric study of twenty-six patients. *J Bone Joint Surg Am.* 1973;55(3):445–460.

12. Soslowsky LJ, Flatow EL, Bigliani LU, et al. Articular geometry of the glenohumeral joint. *Clin Orthop Relat Res.* 1992;(285):181–190.

13. Porcellini G, Paladini P, Campi F, et al. Shoulder instability and related rotator cuff tears: Arthroscopic findings and treatment in patients aged 40 to 60 years. *Arthroscopy.* 2006;22(3):270–276.

14. Bigliani LU, Codd TP, Connor PM, et al. Shoulder motion and laxity in the professional baseball player. *Am J Sports Med.* 1997;25(5):609–613.

15. Ireland M. *Instructional Course Lectures: Sports Medicine.* Rosemont, IL: American Academy of Orthopaedic Surgeons; 2005.

16. Johnson SM, Robinson CM. Shoulder instability in patients with joint hyperlaxity. *J Bone Joint Surg Am.* 2010;92(6):1545–1557.

17. Neer CS 2nd, Welsh RP. The shoulder in sports. *Orthop Clin North Am.* 1977;8(3):583–591.

18. Silliman JF, Hawkins RJ. Classification and physical diagnosis of instability of the shoulder. *Clin Orthop Relat Res.* 1993;(291):7–19.

19. O'Brien SJ, Pagnani MJ, Fealy S, et al. The active compression test: A new and effective test for diagnosing labral tears and acromioclavicular joint abnormality. *Am J Sports Med.* 1998;26(5):610–613.

20. Hegedus EJ, Goode AP, Cook CE, et al. Which physical examination tests provide clinicians with the most value when examining the shoulder? Update of a systematic review with meta-analysis of individual tests. *Br J Sports Med.* 2012;46(14):964–978.

21. Jobe FW, Kvitne RS, Giangarra CE. Shoulder pain in the overhand or throwing athlete. The relationship of anterior instability and rotator cuff impingement. *Orthop Rev.* 1989;18(9):963–975.

22. Farber AJ, Castillo R, Clough M, et al. Clinical assessment of three common tests for traumatic anterior shoulder instability. *J Bone Joint Surg Am.* 2006;88(7):1467–1474.

23. Lo IK, Nonweiler B, Woolfrey M, et al. An evaluation of the apprehension, relocation, and surprise tests for anterior shoulder instability. *Am J Sports Med.* 2004;32(2):301–307.

24. Oh JH, Kim JY, Kim WS, et al. The evaluation of various physical examinations for the diagnosis of type II superior labrum anterior and posterior lesion. *Am J Sports Med.* 2008;36(2):353–359.

25. Bankart AS. The pathology and treatment of recurrent dislocation of the shoulder joint. *Br J Surg.* 1938;26:23–29.

26. Owens BD, Nelson BJ, Duffey ML, et al. Pathoanatomy of first-time, traumatic, anterior glenohumeral subluxation events. *J Bone Joint Surg Am.* 2010;92(7):1605–1611.

27. Itoi E, Lee SB, Berglund LJ, et al. The effect of a glenoid defect on anteroinferior stability of the shoulder after Bankart repair: A cadaveric study. *J Bone Joint Surg Am.* 2000;82(1):35–46.

28. Levine WN, Flatow EL. The pathophysiology of shoulder instability. *Am J Sports Med.* 2000;28(6):910–917.

29. Hill H, Sachs M. The grooved defect of the humeral head: A frequently unrecognized complication of dislocations of the shoulder joint. *Radiology.* 1940;35(6):690–700.

30. Dumont GD, Russell RD, Robertson WJ. Anterior shoulder instability: A review of pathoanatomy, diagnosis and treatment. *Curr Rev Musculoskelet Med.* 2011;4(4):200–207.

31. Neviaser TJ. The anterior labroligamentous periosteal sleeve avulsion lesion: A cause of anterior instability of the shoulder. *Arthroscopy.* 1993;9(1):17–21.

32. Spatschil A, Landsiedl F, Anderl W, et al. Posttraumatic anterior-inferior instability of the shoulder: Arthroscopic findings and clinical correlations. *Arch Orthop Trauma Surg.* 2006;126(4):217–222.

33. Neviaser TJ. The GLAD lesion: Another cause of anterior shoulder pain. *Arthroscopy.* 1993;9(1):22–23.

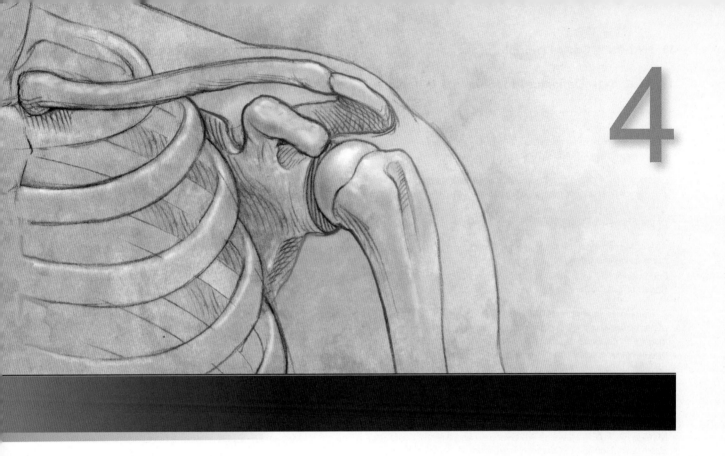

CLASSIFICATION OF SHOULDER INSTABILITY

John E. Kuhn

INTRODUCTION

The classification of disease states serves many important functions with regard to the care of patients. Clear and concise classification systems are important because they can (1) allow health care providers to communicate the condition of a patient accurately, (2) provide prognostic information with regard to the natural history of a disorder, (3) allow physicians to pool similar patient populations to conduct studies on the best methods of treatment, and (4) help payers determine appropriate reimbursement for care.

Shoulder instability as a disease state is no exception; however, our classification systems have not been clear and have led to some controversy. The purpose of this chapter is to review the definitions and classification systems for shoulder instability that have been used in the past, identify where commonly used classification systems are flawed and produce confusion, and finally to recommend a method of classifying instability that has been shown to be reliable.

DEFINING SHOULDER INSTABILITY

Defining shoulder instability is the foundation upon which a classification system can be constructed; however, defining instability is not as clear as one might think.

TABLE 4-1 Definitions for Shoulder Instability

"Instability is defined as excessive symptomatic translation of the humeral head relative to the glenoid articular surface during active motion."
Allen AA. Clinical evaluation of the unstable shoulder. In: Warren RF, Craig EV, Altchek DW, eds. *The Unstable Shoulder*. Philadelphia, PA: Lippincott-Raven; 1999:93–106.

"Instability is a pathologic condition that manifests as pain or discomfort in association with excessive translation of the humeral head on the glenoid fossa during active shoulder motion."
Cole JB, Warner JJP. Anatomy, biomechanics, and pathophysiology of glenohumeral instability. In: Ianotti JP, Williams GR, eds. *Disorders of the Shoulder: Diagnosis and Management*. Philadelphia, PA: Lippincott Williams & Wilkins; 1999:208.

"Glenohumeral instability can be defined as pain associated with the loss of shoulder function as a result of excessive translation of the humeral head on the glenoid fossa."
Friedman RJ. Glenohumeral capsulorrhaphy. In: Matsen FA, Fu FH, Hawkins RJ, eds *The Shoulder: A Balance of Mobility and Stability*. Rosemont, IL: American Academy of Orthopaedic Surgeons; 1993:446.

"Instability is an abnormal limit of motion associated with a functional deficit (dynamic instability) or subluxation/dislocation (static or dynamic instability). A dynamically unstable configuration of load state would be one in which an increment of load will cause pain and inability to continue the function; in other words, "functionally buckling." A statically unstable configuration and load state would be the one in which an incremental increase in load leads to a large displacement with subsequent subluxation or dislocation."
Lew WD, Lewis JL, Craig EV. Stabilization by capsule, ligaments, and labrum: Stability at the extremes of motion. In: Matsen FA, Fu FH, Hawkins RJ, eds. *The Shoulder: A Balance of Mobility and Stability*. Rosemont, IL: American Academy of Orthopaedic Surgeons; 1993:84.

"...the inability to maintain the humeral head centered in the glenoid fossa."
Matsen FA, Fu FH, Hawkins RJ. Overview and directions of future research. In: Matsen FA, Fu FH, Hawkins RJ, eds. *The Shoulder: A Balance of Mobility and Stability*. Rosemont, IL: American Academy of Orthopaedic Surgeons; 1993:3.

"This is a condition of a joint characterized by an abnormal increased amount of mobility secondary to injury of the ligaments, capsule, bone, etc.; when applied to the shoulder, instability typically is used to describe a clinical condition characterized by physical signs and related patients' symptoms of increased or excessive displacement of the glenohumeral joint."
Rodkey WG, Noble JS, Hintermeister RA. Laboratory methods of evaluating the shoulder. In: Matsen FA, Fu FH, Hawkins RJ, eds. *The Shoulder: A Balance of Mobility and Stability*. Rosemont, IL: American Academy of Orthopaedic Surgeons; 1993:570.

"Instability is a clinical diagnosis manifest as excessive translation of the humeral head on the glenoid occurring during active shoulder rotation in association with symptoms."
Warner JJP, Boardman ND III. Anatomy, biomechanics, and pathophysiology of glenohumeral instability. In: Warren RF, Craig EV, Altchek DW, eds. *The Unstable Shoulder*. Philadelphia, PA: Lippincott-Raven; 1999:51–52.

Different authors define instability in different ways—even in the same text! To avoid confusion, the definition must be clear and accepted universally before the disorder can be classified.

In surveying a variety of texts it is clear that different experts define instability differently (1–7) (Table 4-1). These different perspectives of instability are part of the reason there is controversy on how best to classify this condition. For example, does the patient with a painful labral tear have "instability" (8)? Does a thrower with shoulder pain, but no sense of abnormal glenohumeral joint, have "subtle instability" (9)? Clearly, if a patient presents with a shoulder that feels "unstable," he or she is describing a sense of looseness that results from excessive glenohumeral joint translation. Pain as a symptom confuses this diagnosis. We recognize that the diagnostic accuracy for physical examination tests for instability is improved when fear or reproduction of the patient's shifting is used as a positive test when compared to using pain (10,11). As there are many disorders in the shoulder capable of producing pain, pain should not be used as a symptom to define instability; rather, a clear definition of instability would be one where patients have a sensation of their shoulder as "loose" or "going out" or "slipping." While it is possible that a patient may have pain with these events, the criteria to define instability should include these sensations of excessive translation, and not rely on pain as the sole criterion for defining the condition.

HISTORICAL METHODS OF CLASSIFYING SHOULDER INSTABILITY

Historically, a variety of descriptive terms have been used to classify glenohumeral instability leading to a virtual potpourri of terms (Fig. 4-1). Unfortunately, it

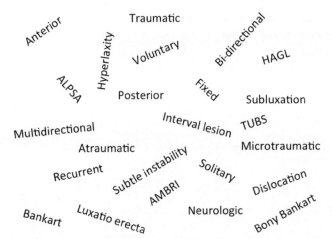

▲ FIGURE 4-1: The potpourri of terms used to describe shoulder instability. Without organization into meaningful concepts, it is nearly impossible to compare the outcomes of treatment.

TABLE 4-2 Patient Characteristics in Neer's Classic Study on Multidirectional Instability

Feature		Number of Patients (N = 40 Total)
Frequency	Solitary episode	0
	More than one episode	40
Etiology	Traumatic	29
	Atraumatic	7
Direction	Anterior	29
	Inferior	40
	Posterior	29
Severity	Subluxation	38
	Dislocation	2
Other	Hyperlaxity	17
	Bankart lesion	5

The heterogeneity in the population is the concern with treatment-based studies.

From: Neer CS 2nd, Foster CR. Inferior capsular shift for involuntary inferior and multidirectional instability of the shoulder: A preliminary report. *J Bone Joint Surg Am.* 1980;62:897–908.

becomes difficult to classify patients and combine them into distinct groups. In some ways this is a result of the approaches used historically to produce manuscripts for publication. In the older literature on instability, the authors used a *treatment-based* approach—pooling patients who have had the same treatment for study (e.g., "Let's review all of my inferior capsular shift patients") (12). The *treatment-based* approach typically will include a heterogeneous population of patients (Table 4-2), some of whom do well and some do not after a particular treatment. This may help in defining the indications for a particular treatment, but it does not help us define which treatment would be best for a given patient. An example of a *treatment-based* approach that has led to confusion in the classification of instability is Neer's work on the inferior capsular shift for "multidirectional instability" (13–15). Another example that has led to confusion is when an instability operation (anterior capsular labral reconstruction) is used for treating throwing athletes with shoulder pain but who may not have instability symptoms (16). To justify the use of an instability operation, Jobe and Pink (16) and Garth et al. (17) defined throwers with pain as having "subtle" or "occult" instability. In a similar approach, Rowe (18) suggested that patients with a "dead arm syndrome" were suffering from a subtle form of instability. Advances in our understanding of the dysfunctional thrower's shoulder allow us to appreciate that there are many sources of shoulder pain, and these throwers may not have instability as a source of their symptoms (19–22).

Instead, a *condition-based* approach to conduct and report research is preferred. In a *condition-based* approach, similar patients who have had different treatments are compared to find the best treatment for that type of patient (e.g., "Let's review all of my

patient with traumatic, solitary dislocation events and compare two treatments"). Meaningful and reliable classification systems for disease states help us define populations of patients that can then be used for these comparative treatment studies.

FLAWS AND CONTROVERSY IN THE CLASSIFICATION OF SHOULDER INSTABILITY

Most classification systems in the literature have not been developed systematically, rather they are proposed by a particular author, usually in the discussion section of a manuscript, or as a chapter or a review article (1,2,23–38). Unfortunately, this represents the lowest level of evidence and is germane only to that author's perception of the world, which may be biased and inaccurate. As can be seen in Table 4-3, these biases led to different authors emphasizing different components of instability. Without standardization and agreement, confusion will exist.

The Concept of Multidirectional Instability

For example, the concept of multidirectional instability, which is extremely popular, is significantly flawed,

TABLE 4-3   Features Used by Authors to Classify Instability

Feature Ranked by Popularity	Authors Using It in Their Classification System (Reference Listed)	Total N = 18
Etiology	1,2,23–32,34–37	16 (89%)
Severity	1,2,23–25,30–34,36,38	14 (78%)
Direction	1,2,23–26,29–32,35–38	12 (67%)
Frequency	1,2,24,29–32,34,35,37,38	11 (61%)
Voluntary Nature	23,25,26,29,32,34,36	7 (39%)
Static vs. Dynamic	1,25,26,38	4 (22%)
Hyperlaxity	26–28,35	4 (22%)
Surgical Pathology	26,28,37	3 (17%)
Imaging Findings	26	1 (6%)
Treatment Rendered	37	1 (6%)
Muscle Patterning	28	1 (6%)
Bilaterality	37	1 (6%)

None of the proposed classification systems were developed systematically, and all represent the opinions and bias of each author. It is interesting to note that there is substantial disagreement on which features should be included when describing patients with the same disorder.

and leads to confusion in the literature. In 1980, Neer and Foster described this disorder (12). The original manuscript is a classic example of a *treatment-based* approach. In this manuscript, Neer described a collection of patients who all had in common a procedure he called the inferior capsular shift. Unfortunately, this collection of patients had a variety of features of instability and by no means represents a homogeneous population (Table 4-2). The one thing they did have in common was a sulcus sign—a physical examination finding. This *treatment-based* approach and the heterogeneous population described in the manuscript have led to confusion in the literature, and different authors have subsequently defined multidirectional instability in a variety of ways. Some suggest that these patients do not have a history of trauma, have generalized ligamentous laxity, and respond well to rehabilitation. Others suggest that patients with traumatic instability, labral tears, and symptoms in more than one direction fit the diagnosis. The controversy exists because the population of patients was mixed and not well classified.

Chahal et al. (13), who surveyed shoulder experts with regard to their diagnosis and treatment for a series of patient scenarios, demonstrated this confusion. These authors found particularly poor agreement in diagnosis and treatment in scenarios that involved "subtle" and "multidirectional" forms of instability. In a different approach, McFarland et al. (14) used four

different recommended approaches to classify instability (1,12,26,39) in assessing a cohort of 168 patients. Interestingly, he found significant differences existed in the proportion of patients who were diagnosed as having "multidirectional instability," prompting an editorial on the problem with classifying instability and the difficulties that arise in conducting research and interpreting the literature (15).

The Concept of Voluntary Instability

While other authors identified an emotional or psychological disorder may be associated with voluntary instability (40,41), Rowe (42), in 1973, studied this concern with formal psychiatric evaluations in his patients with voluntary shoulder instability. His series included 26 patients who underwent psychiatric interviews (18) or had previous psychiatric treatments (8). He divided this population into two groups: Group I (N = 8) had severe emotional and character problems and Group II (N = 18) had no psychological or social disorders other than the normal emotional disturbances of adolescence. He noted that both nonsurgical and surgical treatments were less successful in the patients with severe emotional or character problems.

After this report, a number of surgeons misinterpreted Rowe's findings and would refuse to operate on any patient who could demonstrate their instability, with concerns that they would all fail. This clearly is not the case, as there are two general classes of patients who can demonstrate their instability. Some patients want their shoulder to go out for psychological or secondary gain issues. This type of voluntary instability is *volitional.* Other patients do not enjoy or want their shoulders to sublux, but will demonstrate it to the clinician in hopes that it will help make the diagnosis. This type of instability is not volitional rather it is *demonstrable.*

Without formal psychiatric testing it may be difficult to distinguish between these two patient groups. If a patient is suspected of volitional instability, psychological testing would be recommended before proceeding with surgery. While this method of stratifying patients is critically important to predict outcomes after treatment, the need for psychiatric evaluation makes this feature of instability less practical for inclusion in a general classification system for shoulder instability.

ICD-9 and ICD-10 Classification of Instability

Perhaps the most widely used and most confusing classification systems for glenohumeral joint instability are those suggested by the authors of the International Classification of Diseases, 9th edition (ICD-9). While these codes are used globally to classify patients for epidemiologic and billing reasons, they are notably poor in classifying glenohumeral joint instability. The ICD-9 codes (Table 4-4) include features such as open versus closed dislocations, and developmental and pathologic dislocations, which have little meaning to clinicians. It is therefore not surprising that interobserver agreement is poor when using this classification system (43).

The ICD-10 classification is scheduled to be implemented in October 2014, and will invariably be more complex and specific than ICD-9 (the ICD-10 has over 141,000 codes, which is eight times the 17,000 codes in ICD-9). With regard to shoulder instability, the version currently proposed includes classes for instability that define frequency (recurrent or not), direction (anterior, inferior, and posterior), and severity (dislocation or subluxation) (Table 4-5). It appears that it remains to be seen if this system for classifying instability has high agreement. If the ICD-10 system is reliable, it should allow for large, population-based epidemiologic studies on patients with glenohumeral joint instability.

THE FEDS CLASSIFICATION—A SYSTEM DEVELOPED METHODOLOGICALLY

Recognizing the difficulties that currently exist in classifying glenohumeral joint instability, Kuhn et al. attempted a methodologic approach to develop a system

TABLE 4-4   ICD-9 Codes for Glenohumeral Joint Instability

Code	Description
718.21	Pathologic dislocation shoulder
718.31	Recurrent dislocation shoulder
718.71	Developmental dislocation shoulder
718.81	Joint derangement not elsewhere classified shoulder
718.91	Joint derangement NOS shoulder
719.81	Other specified disorders of joint of shoulder region
726.2	Other affections of shoulder region not elsewhere classified
831.00	Closed dislocation of shoulder, unspecified site
831.01	Closed anterior dislocation of humerus
831.02	Closed posterior dislocation of humerus
831.03	Closed inferior dislocation of humerus
831.10	Open dislocation of humerus NOS
831.11	Open anterior dislocation of humerus
831.12	Open posterior dislocation of humerus
831.13	Open inferior dislocation of humerus
831.19	Open dislocation of humerus not elsewhere classified
840.7	Superior glenoid labrum lesion

for classifying instability (44,45). First, a systematic review of the literature was performed to identify features used by others to classify instability and ascertain their frequency (Table 4-3). The following features of instability were used by more than 50% of the authors who proposed classification systems: Frequency, etiology, direction, and severity (FEDS). All other features were used by fewer than 40% of the authors. The authors also surveyed the members of the American Shoulder and Elbow Surgeons using a 7-point Likert scale to rank the importance of a number of features in guiding the diagnosis of glenohumeral joint instability. Interestingly, the features of the patient's history (etiology) and physical examination (using provocative testing) were deemed extremely important. None of the radiographic techniques, nor findings during examination under anesthesia scored as extremely important. Because FEDS can be obtained by the history and physical examination, the authors used these criteria to develop a classification system. Each feature was then subclassified into clinically meaningful groups as determined by an expert panel (Table 4-6).

TABLE 4-5 Potential ICD-10 Codes for Glenohumeral Instability

Code	Description	Code	Description
M24.2	Disorder of ligament: Instability secondary to old ligament injury. Ligamentous laxity NOS	S43.004	Unspecified dislocation of right shoulder joint
		S43.005	Unspecified dislocation of left shoulder joint
M24.20	Disorder of ligament, unspecified site	S43.006	Unspecified dislocation of unspecified shoulder joint
M24.21	Disorder of ligament, shoulder	S43.01	Anterior subluxation and dislocation of humerus
M24.211	Disorder of ligament, right shoulder	S43.011	Anterior subluxation of right humerus
M24.212	Disorder of ligament, left shoulder	S43.012	Anterior subluxation of left humerus
M24.219	Disorder of ligament, unspecified shoulder	S43.013	Anterior subluxation of unspecified humerus
M24.3	Pathologic dislocation of joint, not elsewhere classified	S43.014	Anterior dislocation of right humerus
		S43.015	Anterior dislocation of left humerus
M24.30	Pathologic dislocation of unspecified joint, not elsewhere classified	S43.016	Anterior dislocation of unspecified humerus
M24.31	Pathologic dislocation of shoulder, not elsewhere classified	S43.02	Posterior subluxation and dislocation of humerus
		S43.021	Posterior subluxation of right humerus
M24.311	Pathologic dislocation of right shoulder, not elsewhere classified	S43.022	Posterior subluxation of left humerus
		S43.023	Posterior subluxation of unspecified humerus
M24.312	Pathologic dislocation of left shoulder, not elsewhere classified	S43.024	Posterior dislocation of right humerus
		S43.025	Posterior dislocation of left humerus
M24.319	Pathologic dislocation of unspecified shoulder, not elsewhere classified	S43.026	Posterior dislocation of unspecified humerus
M24.4	Recurrent dislocation of joint	S43.03	Inferior subluxation and dislocation of humerus
M24.40	Recurrent dislocation, unspecified joint	S43.031	Inferior subluxation of right humerus
M24.41	Recurrent dislocation, shoulder	S43.032	Inferior subluxation of left humerus
M24.411	Recurrent dislocation, right shoulder	S43.033	Inferior subluxation of unspecified humerus
M24.412	Recurrent dislocation, left shoulder	S43.034	Inferior dislocation of right humerus
M24.419	Recurrent dislocation, unspecified shoulder	S43.035	Inferior dislocation of left humerus
M24.81	Other specific joint derangements of shoulder, not elsewhere classified	S43.036	Inferior dislocation of unspecified humerus
M24.811	Other specific joint derangements of right shoulder, not elsewhere classified	S43.08	Other subluxation and dislocation of shoulder joint
		S43.081	Other subluxation of right shoulder joint
M24.812	Other specific joint derangements of left shoulder, not elsewhere classified	S43.082	Other subluxation of left shoulder joint
		S43.083	Other subluxation of unspecified shoulder joint
M24.819	Other specific joint derangements of unspecified shoulder, not elsewhere classified	S43.084	Other dislocation of right shoulder joint
		S43.085	Other dislocation of left shoulder joint
M25.3	Other instability of joint	S43.086	Other dislocation of unspecified shoulder joint
M25.30	Other instability, unspecified joint	S43.30	Subluxation and dislocation of unspecified parts of shoulder girdle
M25.31	Other instability, shoulder		
M25.311	Other instability, right shoulder	S43.301	Subluxation of unspecified parts of right shoulder girdle
M25.312	Other instability, left shoulder	S43.302	Subluxation of unspecified parts of left shoulder girdle
M25.319	Other instability, unspecified shoulder	S43.303	Subluxation of unspecified parts of unspecified shoulder girdle
S43.0	Subluxation and dislocation of shoulder joint		
S43.00	Unspecified subluxation and dislocation of shoulder joint	S43.304	Dislocation of unspecified parts of right shoulder girdle
S43.001	Unspecified subluxation of right shoulder joint	S43.305	Dislocation of unspecified parts of left shoulder girdle
S43.002	Unspecified subluxation of left shoulder joint	S43.306	Dislocation of unspecified parts of unspecified shoulder girdle
S43.003	Unspecified subluxation of unspecified shoulder joint		

These are not due to be adopted until October 2014, and may undergo revision; however, with descriptors for direction, severity, and frequency, the ICD-10 codes will have more clinical meaning than the ICD-9 codes.

TABLE 4-6   **The FEDS Classification of Glenohumeral Joint Instability**

Frequency	Solitary—1 event Frequent—2–5 events/yr Recurrent—>5 events/yr
Etiology	Traumatic—history of injury Atraumatic—no history of injury
Direction	Anterior Inferior Posterior
Severity	Subluxation—reduced without help Dislocation—required help to reduce

Frequency, etiology, and severity can be determined by the history. Direction refers to the primary direction and is determined by physical examination using provocative testing to determine the one most symptomatic direction.

Frequency

Frequency of events is obtained by the history. It represents the number of events that occur over the course of a year due to the seasonal nature of sports. It is divided into three subclasses: Solitary (one event), frequent (2 to 5 events/year), and recurrent (more than 5 events/year).

Etiology

Etiology is also derived from the history. It can be either traumatic if the patient has a history of injury, or atraumatic if there is no history of injury. The formerly described class of microtraumatic instability would fall under the atraumatic subclass.

Direction

Direction is determined by provocative testing under physical examination. Provocative tests for instability that reproduce the patient's symptoms have higher sensitivity and specificity and better agreement than tests that produce pain, measure the amount of translation or examination under anesthesia (46–51). Provocative tests are performed for anterior instability (e.g., apprehension testing), inferior instability (e.g., sulcus sign), and posterior instability (e.g., jerk test). The one direction that the patient describes as most reproducing his or her symptoms would be the *primary direction* of the instability.

Severity

Severity is determined by the history. If a patient never has required assistance to have the shoulder reduced, he or she would fall under the subluxation subclass. If a patient has required assistance in reducing the shoulder, he or she would fall under the dislocation subclass.

The authors then assessed the inter- and intraobserver agreement of the FEDS classification system in a consecutive series of patients with instability as defined by a feeling that the shoulder is "slipping, falling out, dislocating, or loose." They found the FEDS classification system had high levels of agreement (44).

The advantages of the FEDS system for classifying glenohumeral joint instability are the following: (1) it creates mutually exclusive classes of patients with features that are the most popular among shoulder experts giving it content validity, (2) it does not require imaging or surgical pathology to place patients in a class, (3) it has high

TABLE 4-7   **Classes of the FEDS System for Classifying Glenohumeral Joint Instability**

Solitary, traumatic, anterior, subluxation	Solitary, traumatic, anterior, dislocation	Solitary, traumatic, inferior, subluxation	Solitary, traumatic, inferior, dislocation	Solitary, traumatic, posterior, subluxation	Solitary, traumatic, posterior, dislocation
Solitary, atraumatic, anterior, subluxation	*Solitary, atraumatic, anterior, dislocation*	Solitary, atraumatic, inferior, subluxation	Solitary, atraumatic, inferior, dislocation	Solitary, atraumatic, posterior, subluxation	*Solitary, atraumatic, posterior, dislocation*
Occasional, traumatic, anterior, subluxation	Occasional, traumatic, anterior, dislocation	Occasional, traumatic, inferior, subluxation	*Occasional, traumatic, inferior, dislocation*	Occasional, traumatic, posterior, subluxation	*Occasional, traumatic, posterior, dislocation*
Occasional, atraumatic, anterior, subluxation	*Occasional, atraumatic, anterior, dislocation*	Occasional, atraumatic, inferior, subluxation	*Occasional, atraumatic, inferior, dislocation*	Occasional, atraumatic, posterior, subluxation	*Occasional, atraumatic, posterior, dislocation*
Frequent, traumatic, anterior, subluxation	Frequent, traumatic, anterior, dislocation	Frequent, traumatic, inferior, subluxation	*Frequent, traumatic, inferior, dislocation*	Frequent, traumatic, posterior, subluxation	*Frequent, traumatic, posterior, dislocation*
Frequent, atraumatic, anterior, subluxation	*Frequent, atraumatic, anterior, dislocation*	Frequent, atraumatic, inferior, subluxation	*Frequent, atraumatic, inferior, dislocation*	Frequent, atraumatic, posterior, subluxation	*Frequent, atraumatic, posterior, dislocation*

While there are 36 potential classes, nearly half (*noted in italics*) would be extremely uncommon.

inter- and intraobserver agreement, and (4) it parallels the ICD-10 codes fairly well. However, the FEDS system for classifying shoulder instability does have some limitations. First, the system creates a large number of potential classes that a patient could fall into (Table 4-7). Second, features that are important (e.g., volitional instability) would require further subclassification within each class. Despite these limitations, the FEDS system is the only method of classifying instability that has been systematically developed and has been shown to have high reliability.

S U M M A R Y

Shoulder instability historically has been described using a variety of features with little agreement on definitions and classifications. This makes it extremely difficult to interpret the literature, and makes it impossible to conduct systematic reviews and meta-analyses. It is of critical importance that definitions of instability are agreed upon, and that instability can classify patients into similar mutually exclusive groups, so that different treatments can be compared using populations of people with the same types of instability. The requirement to have symptoms of translation can help clarify the definition of instability. Classifying patients with instability using the FEDS system can produce groups of similar patients and allow for comparative trials in *treatment-based* research. Hopefully, the newest edition of the ICD will be found to be reliable so that meaningful large population studies of patients with glenohumeral joint instability can be performed.

References

1. Allen AA. Clinical evaluation of the unstable shoulder. In: Warren RF, Craig EV, Altchek DW, eds. *The Unstable Shoulder.* Philadelphia, PA: Lippincott-Raven; 1999: 93–106.
2. Cole JB, Warner JJP. Anatomy, biomechanics, and pathophysiology of glenohumeral instability. In: Ianotti JP, Williams GR, eds. *Disorders of the Shoulder: Diagnosis and Management.* Philadelphia, PA: Lippincott Williams & Wilkins; 1999:208.
3. Friedman RJ. Glenohumeral capsulorrhaphy. In: Matsen FA, Fu FH, Hawkins RJ, eds. *The Shoulder: A Balance of Mobility and Stability.* Rosemont, IL: American Academy of Orthopaedic Surgeons; 1993:446.
4. Lew WD, Lewis JL, Craig EV. Stabilization by capsule, ligaments, and labrum: Stability at the extremes of motion. In: Matsen FA, Fu FH, Hawkins RJ, eds. *The Shoulder: A Balance of Mobility and Stability.* Rosemont, IL: American Academy of Orthopaedic Surgeons; 1993:84.
5. Matsen FA, Fu FH, Hawkins RJ. Overview and directions of future research. In: Matsen FA, Fu FH, Hawkins RJ, eds. *The Shoulder: A Balance of Mobility and Stability.* Rosemont, IL: American Academy of Orthopaedic Surgeons; 1993:3.
6. Rodkey WG, Noble JS, Hintermeister RA. Laboratory methods of evaluating the shoulder. In: Matsen FA, Fu FH, Hawkins RJ, eds. *The Shoulder: A Balance of Mobility and Stability.* Rosemont, IL: American Academy of Orthopaedic Surgeons; 1993:570.
7. Warner JJP, Boardman ND III. Anatomy, biomechanics, and pathophysiology of glenohumeral instability. In: Warren RF, Craig EV, Altchek DW, eds. *The Unstable Shoulder.* Philadelphia, PA: Lippincott-Raven; 1999:51–52.
8. Bradley JP, Baker CL 3rd, Kline AJ, et al. Arthroscopic capsulolabral reconstruction for posterior instability of the shoulder: A prospective study of 100 shoulders. *Am J Sports Med.* 2006;34:1061–1071.
9. Jobe FW, Kvitne RS, Giangarra CE. Shoulder pain in the overhand or throwing athlete. The relationship of anterior instability and rotator cuff impingement. *Orthop Rev.* 1989;18(9):963–975.
10. Lo IK, Nonweiler B, Woolfrey M, et al. An evaluation of the apprehension, relocation, and surprise tests for anterior shoulder instability. *Am J Sports Med.* 2004;32: 301–307.
11. Speer KP, Hannafin JA, Altchek DW, et al. An evaluation of the shoulder relocation test. *Am J Sports Med.* 1994;22:177–183.
12. Neer CS 2nd, Foster CR. Inferior capsular shift for involuntary inferior and multidirectional instability of the shoulder: A preliminary report. *J Bone Joint Surg Am.* 1980;62:897–908.
13. Chahal J, Kassiri K, Dion A, et al. Diagnostic and treatment differences among experienced shoulder surgeons for instability conditions of the shoulder. *Clin J Sport Med.* 2007;17:5–9.
14. McFarland EG, Kim TK, Park HB, et al. The effect of variation in definition on the diagnosis of multidirectional instability of the shoulder. *J Bone Joint Surg Am.* 2003;85A:2138–2144.
15. Richards RR. The diagnostic definition of multidirectional instability of the shoulder: Searching for direction. *J Bone Joint Surg Am.* 2003;85A:2145–2146.
16. Jobe FW, Pink M. Classification and treatment of shoulder dysfunction in the overhead athlete. *J Orthop Sports Phys Ther.* 1993;18:427–432.
17. Garth WP Jr, Allman FL Jr, Armstrong WS. Occult anterior subluxations of the shoulder in noncontact sports. *Am J Sports Med.* 1987;15:579–585.
18. Rowe CR. Recurrent transient anterior subluxation of the shoulder. The "dead arm" syndrome. *Clin Orthop Relat Res.* 1987;223:11–19.
19. Burkhart SS, Morgan CD, Kibler WB. The disabled throwing shoulder: Spectrum of pathology. Part I: Pathoanatomy and biomechanics. *Arthroscopy.* 2003;19:404–420.

20. Burkhart SS, Morgan CD, Kibler WB. The disabled throwing shoulder: Spectrum of pathology. Part II: Evaluation and treatment of SLAP lesions in throwers. *Arthroscopy.* 2003;19:531–539.

21. Burkhart SS, Morgan CD, Kibler WB. The disabled throwing shoulder: Spectrum of pathology. Part III: The SICK scapula, scapular dyskinesis, the kinetic chain, and rehabilitation. *Arthroscopy.* 2003;19:641–661.

22. Kibler WB, Kuhn JE, Wilk K, et al. The disabled throwing shoulder: Spectrum of pathology-10-year update. *Arthroscopy.* 2013;29(1):141–161.

23. Cofield RH, Irving JF. Evaluation and classification of shoulder instability. With special reference to examination under anesthesia. *Clin Orthop Relat Res.* 1987;223:32–43.

24. Friedman RJ. Glenohumeral capsulorrhaphy. In: Matsen FA, Fu FH, Hawkins RJ, eds. *The Shoulder: A Balance of Mobility and Stability.* Rosemont, IL: American Academy of Orthopaedic Surgeons; 1993:446.

25. Gallinat BJ, Warren RF. Shoulder: Trauma and related instability. In: *Orthopaedic Knowledge Update 3.* Park Ridge, IL: American Academy of Orthopaedic Surgeons; 1990:303.

26. Gerber C, Nyffeler RW. Classification of glenohumeral joint instability. *Clin Orthop Relat Res.* 2002;400:65–76.

27. Joseph TA, Williams JS Jr, Brems JJ. Laser capsulorrhaphy for multidirectional instability of the shoulder. An outcomes study and proposed classification system. *Am J Sports Med.* 2003;31:26–35.

28. Lewis A, Kitamura T, Bayler JIL. The classification of shoulder instability: New light through old windows! *Current Orthopaedics.* 2004;18:97–108.

29. Maruyama K, Sano S, Saito K, et al. Trauma-instability-voluntarism classification for glenohumeral instability. *J Shoulder Elbow Surg.* 1995;4:194–198.

30. Nebelung W. [Classification of recurrent shoulder joint instability]. *Z Orthop Ihre Grenzgeb.* 2001;139:M84–M87.

31. Ozkan M, Ekin A, Bolukbasi S, et al. [Shoulder instability: classification and methods of clinical examination]. *Acta Orthop Traumatol Turc.* 2005;39(suppl 1):14–23.

32. Pollock RG, Flatow EL. Classification and evaluation. In: Bigliani LU, ed. *The Unstable Shoulder.* Rosemont, IL: American Academy of Orthopaedic Surgeons; 1996:25–36.

33. Protzman RR. Anterior instability of the shoulder. *J Bone Joint Surg Am.* 1980;62:909–918.

34. Rockwood CA. Subluxation of the shoulder: The classification, diagnosis, and treatment. *Orthop Trans.* 1979;4:306.

35. Schneeberger AG, Gerber C. [Classification and therapy of the unstable shoulder]. *Ther Umsch.* 1988;55(3):187–191.

36. Silliman JF, Hawkins RJ. Classification and physical diagnosis of instability of the shoulder. *Clin Orthop Relat Res.* 1993;291:7–19.

37. Thomas SC, Matsen FA 3rd. An approach to the repair of avulsion of the glenohumeral ligaments in the management of traumatic anterior glenohumeral instability. *J Bone Joint Surg Am.* 1989;71:506–513.

38. Wirth MA, Rockwood CA. Traumatic glenohumeral instability: Pathology and pathogenesis. In: Matsen FA, Fu FH, Hawkins RJ, eds. *The Shoulder: A Balance of Mobility and Stability.* Rosemont, IL: American Academy of Orthopaedic Surgeons; 1993:279–305.

39. Matsen FA 3rd, Thomas SC, Rockwood CA Jr, et al. Glenohumeral instability. In: Rockwood CA Jr, Matsen FA 3rd, eds. *The Shoulder.* 2nd ed. Philadelphia, PA: WB Saunders; 1998:611–754.

40. Howorth MB. General relaxation of the ligaments. With special reference to the knee and the shoulder. *Clin Orthop Relat Res.* 1963;30:133–143.

41. Keiser RP, Wilson CL. Bilateral recurrent dislocation of the shoulder (atraumatic) in a thirteen-year-old girl. Report of an unusual case. *J Bone Joint Surg.* 1961;43A:553–554.

42. Rowe CR, Pierce DS, Clark JG. Voluntary dislocations of the shoulder. A preliminary report on a clinical, electromyographic, and psychiatric study of twenty-six patients. *J Bone Joint Surg Am.* 1973;55:445–460.

43. Throckmorton TW, Dunn W, Holmes T, et al. Intraobserver and interobserver agreement of ICD-9 codes in classifying shoulder instability. *J Shoulder Elbow Surg.* 2009;18:199–203.

44. Kuhn JE, Helmer TT, Dunn WR, et al. Development and reliability testing of the frequency, etiology, direction, and severity (FEDS) system for classifying glenohumeral instability. *J Shoulder Elbow Surg.* 2011;20:548–556.

45. Kuhn JE. A new classification system for shoulder instability. *Br J Sports Med.* 2010;44:341–346.

46. Lo IK, Nonweiler B, Woolfrey M, et al. An evaluation of the apprehension, relocation, and surprise tests for anterior shoulder instability. *Am J Sports Med.* 2004;32(2):301–307.

47. Speer KP, Hannafin JA, Altchek DW, et al. An evaluation of the shoulder relocation test. *Am J Sports Med.* 1994;22:177–183.

48. Tzannes A, Murrell GA. Clinical examination of the unstable shoulder. *Sports Med.* 2002;32:447–457.

49. Tzannes A, Paxinos A, Callanan M, et al. An assessment of the interexaminer reliability of tests for shoulder instability. *J Shoulder Elbow Surg.* 2004;13:18–23.

50. Ellenbecker TS, Bailie DS, Mattalino AJ, et al. Intrarater and interrater reliability of a manual technique to assess anterior humeral head translation of the glenohumeral joint. *J Shoulder Elbow Surg.* 2002;11:470–475.

51. Levy AS, Lintner S, Kenter K, et al. Intra- and interobserver reproducibility of the shoulder laxity examination. *Am J Sports Med.* 1999;27:460–463.

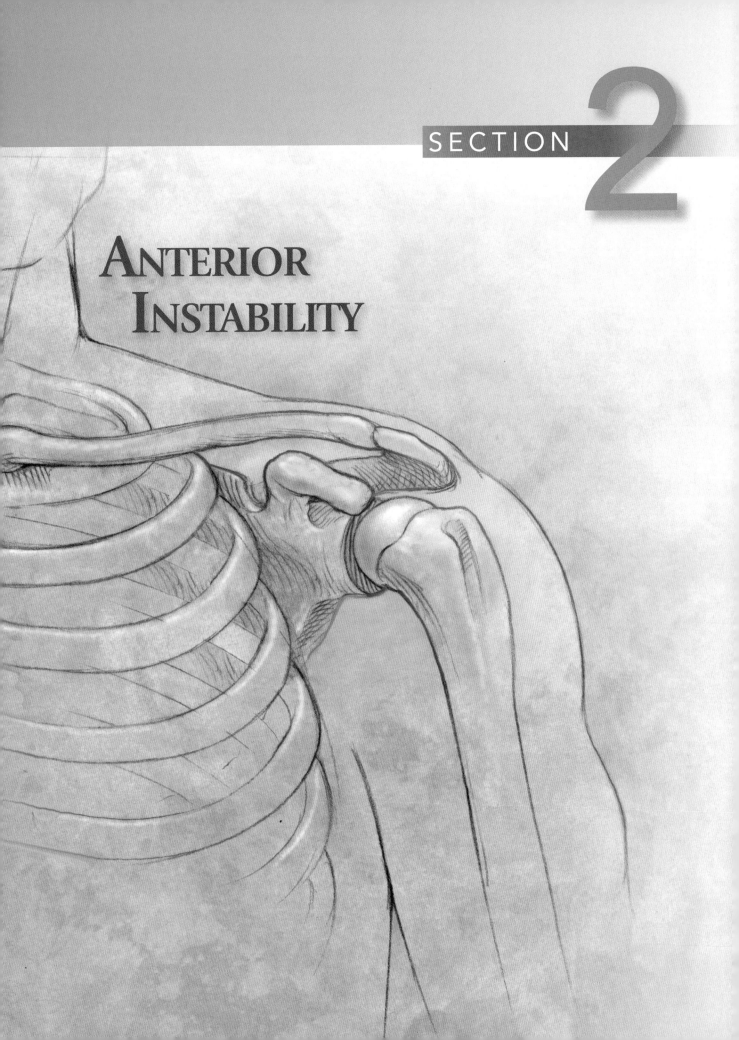

ANTERIOR INSTABILITY

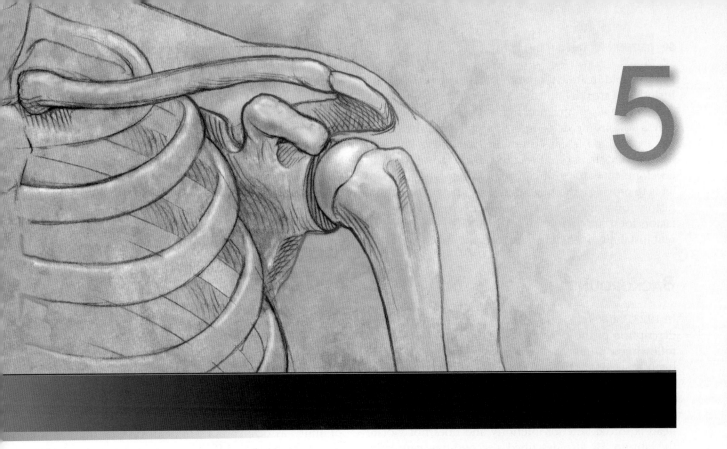

NATURAL HISTORY OF ANTERIOR SHOULDER INSTABILITY

Matthew Mendez-Zfass / Bryson P. Lesniak /
Asheesh Bedi

The shoulder is the most commonly dislocated large joint. The humeral head articulates with a relatively small glenoid providing significant freedom of motion with both rotation and translation, but this comes with the associated risk of potential instability. The potential for recurrent instability following a first-time dislocation is often a significant factor in the development of an appropriate treatment plan. However, because the natural history of these injuries is heterogeneous, a full understanding of the risk factors associated with recurrence is essential to develop the optimal, individualized management plan.

Simonet et al. (1) reported that a primary or recurrent traumatic shoulder dislocation occurs at least 11 to 24 times per 100,000 person-years (1–4). In a population study in Sweden, anterior primary glenohumeral dislocations occurred in 1.7% of the population. Of these dislocations, approximately 96% were anterior dislocations (5).

After appropriate management of the acute dislocation, patient-specific variables and the degree of bony and soft-tissue injuries are assessed to define the risk of recurrent dislocation and instability. Determining the patient-specific risk of recurrence is the primary diagnostic objective. The patient and physician are presented with the challenge of achieving a stable, pain-free shoulder with a full range of motion with the least morbid treatment option. Patient-specific variables include but are not limited to age, occupation, functional demands, and compliance. Injury-specific variables also play a role in the decision-making process. The degree of capsular and labral disruptions, glenoid or humeral fracture, and status of the rotator cuff are all important in development of the treatment plan. The goal of this chapter is to provide a thorough understanding of the natural history following primary shoulder dislocation, the risk factors for recurrent instability, and the sequelae of recurrent instability, including posttraumatic arthropathy.

BACKGROUND

In 1923, Bankart (6) attempted to provide a mechanistic description of the etiology behind recurrent instability following a primary anterior shoulder dislocation. He hypothesized that the dislocation occurred by means of two distinct entities. The first is what he termed an "ordinary dislocation" caused by a fall on an abducted arm. This, he reasoned, did not cause recurrence because the head is forced anterior-inferiorly and does not violate the labrum. He also described a second type caused by a fall directly on the shoulder or elbow (6). This injury pattern, Bankart believed at the time, led to recurrent dislocation and potential damage to the anterior "fibro-cartilaginous glenoid ligament" or labrum. Bankart's mechanistic description is today known to be erroneous; however, his emphasis on an anterior labral lesion as one potential cause of recurrent instability allowed him to describe an operation that led to its treatment.

Rowe (7) expanded on Bankart's work by publishing data on the prognosis of first-time shoulder dislocations. Furthermore, he proposed that the mechanism of injury in dislocations occurs along a spectrum with variable rates of recurrence. Rowe reported a rate of redislocation of 56% in "ordinary" dislocations caused by a twisting injury or fall on an abducted arm. In contrast to Bankart's theory, patients who fell directly on the anterior shoulder actually sustained a lower rate of recurrence of 19% (7).

Contrary to Bankart's initial description, the main risk factors for recurrent instability are not simply limited to mechanism of injury. Multiple studies have confirmed age as the most significant and consistent risk factor for recurrent instability (1,7–13). In addition, male gender has been found to be independently predictive of recurrent instability, while other variables that have been associated with recurrence include functional demand and the postreduction immobilization protocol (14,15).

AGE

Age has long been known to be an important risk factor for recurrence following primary anterior shoulder dislocations (7). Younger age has been borne out in the literature as the most significant and consistent risk factor for recurrent dislocations (1,7,16–19). Many retrospective analyses have concluded that the risk of recurrent instability is inversely proportional to age. McLaughlin and Cavallaro (19) evaluated 101 cases retrospectively and stratified risk by age. Patients younger than 20 years had an 88% (7 of 8) risk of recurrence, patients between 20 and 40 years old had a 58% risk of recurrence (10 of 17), and patients older than 40 years had only an 11% risk of recurrence (2 of 19). The decreasing risk with age was postulated to be secondary to changes in the relative strengths of the anterior and posterior soft tissue restraints that may occur over time (19). They further postulated that the strong relationship with age is incompatible with theories that mechanism of injury or treatment protocol is an important factor in recurrence as suggested by Bankart (6). Following the results of McLaughlin and Cavallaro (19), Rowe (7) evaluated 398 patients with primary anterior shoulder dislocation admitted to a single institution. He stratified their prognosis based on the mechanism of injury, associated bony or neurovascular injuries, the age of the patient, difficulty or ease of reduction, postoperative treatment protocol, patient handedness, and pathologic findings at surgery. His age-related recurrence results mirrored McLaughlin and Cavallaro's with 83% recurrence before 20 years of age, 63% recurrence from 20 to 40 years of age, and only 16% recurrence in patients who had their primary dislocation after 40 years of age (7).

Marans et al. (20) evaluated 21 patients with open physes (4 to 16 years old) with primary anterior dislocations that were stratified to treatment with immobilization or early motion. All of the 21 patients had at least one recurrence and 62% (13 of 21) of patients had undergone anterior stabilization surgery by time of publication.

Hoelen et al. (21) retrospectively evaluated 168 patients following primary anterior shoulder dislocation. They found a rate of recurrence in patients younger than 30 years of 64% (35 of 55). Of those patients who recurred, 83% did so at 2 years and 98% did so at 3 years.

Simonet and Cofield (12) reported on 116 patients with first-time anterior glenohumeral dislocation. Eighty-four percent (27 of 32) of patients younger than 20 years had either a recurrence of dislocation or symptomatic instability, compared to 49% (21 of 43) of patients between 20 and 40 years old. Of those older than 40 years, none had recurrent dislocation and only 10% (4 of 41) had recurrent instability (12).

Gumina and Postacchini (22) evaluated 95 patients aged 60 years and older with first-time anterior dislocations. They found an overall rate of recurrence of 22% (21 of 95), and a 61% incidence (58 of 95) of rotator cuff tears in these patients. Of note, 11% sustained multiple recurrences. In these patients with multiple recurrences, magnetic resonance imaging (MRI) uniformly demonstrated anterior labral injury. This is consistent with the anterior labrum's role as a main soft tissue stabilizer of the shoulder (22).

The previous studies were all retrospective analyses; however, Hovelius et al. (18) published a prospective study of recurrence in patients 40 years of age and younger with 25-year follow-up. In their series, 50% (10 of 20) of patients aged 12 to 16 years underwent surgery due to instability, and this percentage decreased to 14% in patients 30 to 40 years old at the time of their initial dislocation. Overall, 67% (66 of 98) of patients aged 12 to 22 years sustained a recurrence. In the age group 23 to 29 years, 54% (29 of 54) recurred and in the age group 30 to 40 years, only 23% (18 of 77) had a recurrence (18). This finding challenged the notion that young patients uniformly incur recurrent instability and led the authors to not recommend routine surgical stabilization for younger patients who are first-time dislocators.

GENDER

Gender has frequently been analyzed to identify a potential correlation with recurrence of glenohumeral instability. Men are reported to have a higher incidence of shoulder dislocations than females and account for 72% of emergency room visits (4). This increased incidence is thought to stem from a greater rate of recurrent dislocations as well as riskier behavior and does not represent an inherently greater risk of primary dislocation (23,24). Another study was able to demonstrate a 41% recurrence rate in males compared to a 12% recurrence rate in females. However, once matched for age, the relative risk of male gender disappeared (1). A female to male odds ratio of recurrence of 3.2 was identified in a study by te Slaa et al. (13) of 129 primary anterior shoulder dislocations. Robinson et al. (15) used survival analysis to determine the interval risk for recurrence in 252 first-time dislocators aged 15 to 35 years. Using multivariate analysis, only male gender and younger age were found to be independent risk factors for recurrent instability (15). The probability of 2-year recurrence in males who experienced a first-time dislocation at age 15 years was 86% and decreased to 29% for those who had their first-time dislocation at age 35 years. Females had a 2-year probability of recurrence of 54% when they suffered a first-time dislocation at age 15 years and this decreased to 13% when the first-time dislocation occurred at age 35 years (15).

Interestingly, Hovelius et al. (16–18) did not demonstrate a difference between male and female patients with respect to recurrence at 5-, 10-, or 25-year follow-up of the original study population.

ATHLETIC ACTIVITY AND WORK

A significant number of glenohumeral instability events occur during athletic activity. Nordqvist and Petersson (3) studied injuries to the shoulder girdle in an urban population and found that in adults 35% of dislocations were due to sport. In younger patients, this number may be as high as 85% (15). Studies on the role of athletic activity in recurrence following a primary dislocation have been conflicting. Previous retrospective series have demonstrated that patients participating in sports, in particular shoulder-straining sports, have an increased recurrence risk (10,12,25). Simonet and Cofield (12) reported that athletic injury was a significant cause of recurrent instability. In their study, athletes had an 82% (27 of 33) recurrence rate compared to nonathletes with a rate of 30% (8 of 27). In contrast, Hovelius et al. (18) were unable to find a significant difference in the rates of recurrence based upon participation in sports. In their cohort, the highest rates of recurrence were found in those who participated in no sports at all. However, this result did not reach statistical significance. Hoelen et al. (21) found results similar to those of Hovelius et al. regarding athletic activity. In a cohort of 196 patients, there was no statistically significant difference in recurrence with respect to participation in athletics, with the nonathletes trending to have a higher rate of recurrence (21). While Sachs et al. (26) did not find a statistically significant correlation between athletic activity or contact sport activity and redislocation, they did find that patients whose occupation required them to use the arm at or above chest level were more likely to sustain a subsequent instability event. Another retrospective review demonstrated that the presence or type of athletic activity had no influence on redislocation rate. However, approximately one-third of subjects changed their postdislocation sport to one that placed less stress on the shoulder (11). Once a patient sustains an instability event he or she may self-modify activity level and shoulder movements to protect against recurrence.

In high-risk populations such as soldiers and alpine and water sport enthusiasts, recurrent instability may have disastrous and even mortal consequences. Wheeler et al. (27) evaluated the natural history of military cadets at the United States Military Academy following a primary anterior shoulder dislocation. Nine cadets were treated with surgical stabilization following their initial dislocation and 38 were treated nonoperatively. Twenty-two percent (2 of 9) of those treated surgically had evidence of recurrent instability compared to 92% (35 of 38) of those treated nonoperatively. The authors concluded that this provided a rationale for early surgery in these high-risk populations (27).

In a prospective study, te Slaa et al. (28) evaluated 31 patients and found no difference in recurrent instability between those who participated in sports and those who did not. They did; however, find that participation decreased at 5-year follow-up from 71% (22 of 31) to 42% (13 of 31). The same group also looked at patients' return to work following initial dislocation in a separate retrospective study (13). They found that 36 of 105 patients (34%) did not return to the same level of work as before the dislocation. However, of these only 5% (5 of 107) modified their work primarily because of complaints with activity of the affected shoulder (13,28).

ROTATOR CUFF TEAR

A traumatic rotator cuff tear following shoulder dislocation is relatively common and a source of significant disability in older patients (29–34). The incidence of concomitant rotator cuff tears in patients older than 40 years has been estimated to be between 38% and 100%, with an increasing incidence and severity seen with advancing age (32–35).

Berbig et al. (29) used ultrasonography to evaluate the rate of rotator cuff tear following anterior dislocation. Fifteen percent of patients (25 of 167) suffered acute large tears and another 14% (24 of 167) suffered massive tears.

Asymptomatic small tears in the rotator cuff that are more common with advancing age are theorized to contribute to the formation of larger tears following a dislocation. Subsequent dislocation episodes are thought to contribute to increasing rotator cuff tears (36). Porcellini et al. (36) demonstrated in an arthroscopic case series that patients with an increasing number of dislocations had a significantly greater number of tears in the rotator cuff.

An ultrasound study demonstrated that 50% of asymptomatic individuals over the age of 60 years had a partial or full-thickness rotator cuff tear (37). Sher et al. (38) performed MRI of the shoulder on a series of asymptomatic individuals. Overall, 54% of those older than 60 years had a partial or a full-thickness rotator cuff tear. The younger asymptomatic patients had a significantly lower incidence of partial or full-thickness tears than the older cohort (38).

Patients with symptomatic rotator cuff tear following a dislocation are of clinical interest because operative intervention may improve functional outcomes and reduce the risk of recurrent instability episodes. Pevny et al. (39) evaluated 125 consecutive patients 40 years or older who sustained primary anterior shoulder dislocations. Those with dislocation and isolated rotator cuff tears treated nonoperatively had significantly lower Rowe shoulder scores at 5-year follow-up (39).

A study by Neviaser et al. (40) demonstrated that 30% of patients (11 of 37) older than 40 years experienced recurrent instability following a primary

dislocation with an associated subscapularis and anterior capsule tear.

Subscapularis tears have been shown to have significant rates of recurrence in the literature. Another study by Neviaser et al. (34) evaluated 31 patients aged 35 years or greater who had loss of abduction following dislocation. All 31 patients had tears of the rotator cuff. Of these, 8 patients developed recurrent instability, all of whom had documented subscapularis tears (34).

NERVE INJURY

During the evaluation of patients following shoulder dislocation, it is imperative to evaluate not only the reduction and stability of the injured shoulder, but also the neurovascular status of the extremity. While recurrent instability is a significant source of morbidity, nerve injuries are also common, with rates of nerve injury following dislocation ranging from 5.4% to 65% (7,13,31,35).

Nerve injuries to the shoulder have been found to occur more frequently in older individuals, with an incidence as high as 65% (33). Because of the relatively high incidence of associated rotator cuff tears in the older patient, the inability to abduct the arm in a patient following a primary anterior shoulder dislocation may be diagnosed as a rotator cuff tear when it, in fact, represents a nerve injury.

The axillary nerve is most commonly involved, and it is most commonly a solitary lesion (35). It is theorized that in a dislocation the traction force on the brachial plexus is borne primarily by the infraclavicular plexus, which, being nearest to the distal anchorage, has a propensity for injury (41). An electromyography (EMG) study by Toolanen (33) performed on 55 patients with a mean age of 64 years following first-time anterior shoulder dislocation demonstrated that 65% (36 of 55) of patients had EMG findings of one or more nerve lesions. Thirty-five patients had involvement of the axillary nerve, and five of these demonstrated concomitant injury to other nerves in the brachial plexus (33). Of those with axillary denervation, 74% (26 of 35) had either slight or moderate denervation and 26% (9 of 35) had either pronounced or total denervation. In contrast to the high rates of nerve lesions seen with dislocation by Toolanen (33) and Gumina and Postacchini (22) reported a rate of axillary nerve injury of only 9.3% (10 of 109) in patients aged 60 years or older. However, in this study, only the patients with clinical evidence of nerve injury underwent EMG, which may have understated the incidence of nerve injury in the sample population (22). In their study, Neviaser et al. (34) demonstrated that 100% of patients older than 35 years with inability to abduct the arm after primary anterior dislocation suffered a tear of the rotator cuff. In addition,

9.8% of these patients also suffered from nerve injury (34). Fortunately, most of these injuries are thought to recover spontaneously and have been reported to have an 85% to 100% rate of recovery within 6 to 12 months from the time of injury (42,43). A retrospective case series by Travlos et al. (44) of 28 patients who presented to a brachial plexus clinic following anterior shoulder dislocation demonstrated the importance of maintaining joint mobility. In the study, patients with isolated axillary nerve lesions who also had joint stiffness prior to full neurologic recovery tended to have poorer prognoses (44).

GREATER TUBEROSITY FRACTURE

Many studies have demonstrated that an associated greater tuberosity fracture correlates with a reduced risk of recurrent instability following a traumatic first-time anterior dislocation (7,11,13,16,17,19,31). This phenomenon was first described by Hermodsson (45). Landmark studies by Rowe (7) and McLaughlin and Cavallaro (19) identified fractures of the greater tuberosity as protecting against recurrence. In Rowe's original sample of 500 patients, 75 sustained greater tuberosity fractures. Only 7% (3 of 44) of the patients who completed follow-up were found to have recurrent dislocation (7). McLaughlin and Cavallaro (19) demonstrated an even lower rate of recurrence. In the 34 patients with fractures of the greater tuberosity, 0% recurred. This study and Rowe's study (7) were both able to demonstrate an age-related risk of greater tuberosity fracture with higher rates of fracture in older patients.

While the precise etiology of the reduction in recurrence risk is unknown, it is hypothesized that the absorption of force by the fracture may dampen and protect the capsule and labrum from irreversible damage (46). Additional explanations divide the shoulder into anterior joint restraints consisting of the subscapularis and capsuloligamentous and labral complexes and posterior joint constraints, consisting of the greater tuberosity and the posterior rotator cuff. In this view, the damage to the posterior joint constraints both shields the anterior joint constraints from damage *and may* have a greater capacity to heal than anterior soft tissue structures. McLaughlin and MacLellan (31) further extrapolated a correlation of greater tuberosity fracture with age in hypothesizing that greater tuberosity fractures and failure in posterior support structures are more common in older patients secondary to the cumulative effect of wear and tear. This, they proposed, leads to a relative weakness of these structures and their preferential failure in older patients (31).

Kralinger et al. (11) reported on 241 patients and found greater tuberosity fractures in 25% (61 of 241). There was no age-related increase in fractures in these patients and the overall rate of redislocation was 4.9% (3 of 61). In contrast to the view of McLaughlin et al., the hypothesis by Kralinger et al. (11) as to why the greater tuberosity fracture is associated with a risk reduction stems from a loss of external rotation, both at neutral and in 90 degrees of abduction. In comparing the injured extremity to the contralateral side there was an average loss of 3.3 degrees of external rotation at 90 degrees of abduction, and this loss of external rotation in the position of apprehension was thought to correlate with the reduced risk of recurrence. No recurrences were found by te Slaa et al. (13) in 14 patients with greater tuberosity fractures. In this study, patients presenting with a greater tuberosity fracture were found to be older, with a mean age of 53 years compared to a study with a mean age of 40 years.

Hovelius et al. (16,17) reported on 257 patients aged 12 to 40 years with primary anterior dislocations. In this cohort, 12% (32 of 257) sustained a fracture of the greater tuberosity. The incidence of greater tuberosity fractures decreased in the teen years to a nadir in the 20- to 22-year age group. Of the patients aged 12 or 13, 44% (3 of 7) sustained greater tuberosity fractures.

GLENOID FRACTURE AND BONE LOSS

As the humeral head forcibly dislocates over the anterior rim of the glenoid damage can occur to the anterior labrum, anterior bony glenoid, or both. In addition, recurrent dislocations may cause erosive bony changes of the anterior glenoid that can be further destabilizing (47). This bone loss is a known factor in and sequelae of primary and recurrent glenohumeral instability, respectively. The loss of the anterior bone also compromises glenoid concavity that impairs the static restraints of the joint (48). Glenoid fractures have been reported in a study by Taylor and Arciero (49) to occur in 22% of first-time anterior dislocations as judged by plain radiographs.

To quantify the nature of bony defects seen in patients with recurrent instability, Sugaya et al. (50) performed three-dimensional (3D) computed tomography (CT) scans of 100 consecutive patients with recurrent instability. In their series, 10% (10 of 100) demonstrated no glenoid lesion, 50% (50 of 100) had a true osseous fragment or bony Bankart, and 40% (40 of 100) had erosive changes or abnormal morphology when compared to the contralateral side (50).

Bigliani et al. (51) classified anterior glenoid rim lesions into two main groups depending on whether the lesion represented a fracture fragment or rather chronic erosion. A type I lesion has a stable labral attachment to a distinct displaced fracture fragment. A type II lesion has a malunited fracture fragment with detached labrum and a type III lesion has glenoid bone loss. Type IIIa has less than 25% bone loss while type IIIb has greater than 25% glenoid bone loss. The severity and type of glenoid bone loss was reported to have implications for the surgical approach for stabilization surgery (51).

Historically, there have been conflicting reports in the literature with regard to the impact of glenoid rim lesions on the risk of recurrent instability. While Rowe (7) demonstrated an increased rate of instability with glenoid fractures, studies by Hovelius et al. (18) did not report the same correlation. Rowe (7) reported recurrence in 62% of 27 patients with an associated anterior glenoid fracture following dislocation. This is in contrast to the findings published by Hovelius et al. (18), in which, at 25-year follow-up, small glenoid rim fractures at the time of primary dislocation were not found to influence the rates of recurrence.

The discrepancies in the literature may stem from a difficulty in accurately recognizing, quantifying, and diagnosing these lesions with plain radiographs (51). The most sensitive projections in evaluating glenoid bone loss are those that are angled relative to the face of the glenoid such as the West Point view. To identify and characterize glenoid rim lesions more reliably, CT scans have been advocated and found to be sensitive and specific for glenoid rim pathology (52). The use of 3D CT reconstruction combined with digital subtraction of the humeral head allow for image quantification of the glenoid deficiency as a percentage of the normal inferior glenoid surface area. It has been shown that the amount of glenoid bone loss correlates with future anterior instability (53).

In an attempt to quantify the critical value that leads to instability, Itoi et al. (54) performed a biomechanical study on 10 cadavers. Sequential osteotomies were made at 45 degrees to the long axis of the glenoid and the peak forces required to translate the humeral head were measured both before and after capsulolabral repair. An osseous defect greater than 21% of glenoid length led to significantly decreased forces causing anterior translation and subluxation (54). Further, Saito et al. (53) used 3D CT to determine the precise location of the bony defect in 123 patients with recurrent anterior instability. The mean location of the defect was at the 3-o'clock position on the face of the glenoid, indicating that the defect may actually most commonly occur in a directly anterior location (53).

Untreated glenoid rim lesions may also contribute to recurrent instability and failure despite arthroscopic capsulolabral repair. Burkhart and De Beer (55) demonstrated that untreated "significant" bony defects of the glenoid and humeral head led to a rate of recurrence after arthroscopic Bankart repair of 67%. This was significantly higher than the 6.5% recurrence in patients who did not have these "significant" bony defects (55).

Traditionally, loss of roughly 25% of the anterior glenoid had been associated with recurrent instability and treated with a soft tissue repair. Burkhart and De Beer (55) retrospectively evaluated the role of soft tissue Bankart repair in patients with an "inverted pear glenoid" or large glenoid bony defects. In their study, 67% (14 of 21) of patients who suffered from recurrent instability had significant bony defects. Another retrospective study on a series of active duty armed forces personnel did not report such unfavorable results with arthroscopic soft tissue Bankart repair (56). Of 21 patients noted to have a 20% to 30% bony deficiency at the time of arthroscopic stabilization, only 14% (3 of 21) sustained recurrent instability. The authors' contributed their success to their specific technique of anterior capsular plication that has the consequence of improving stability at the expense of a mean 8-degree loss in external rotation.

HILL-SACHS LESION

Flower in 1861 (57) first described the anatomic defect of the posterolateral humeral head following anterior dislocation and originally called it "the grooved defect in the humeral head." In 1963, Hermodsson et al. (45) attributed the defect to anterior dislocation. He also noted that the defect size was proportional to the time the humeral head was dislocated and generally increased with recurrent dislocations. Further, he noted that the lesion is generally larger in anteroinferior than straight anterior dislocations. Hill and Sachs (58) in 1940 described the "grooved defect" as an actual compression fracture of the posterolateral humeral head after forceful contact with the dense anterior glenoid. Historically, difficulties in evaluating the lesion on radiographs may have led to an underreporting of the true incidence of the Hill-Sachs lesion as well as its association with recurrent instability. Also, direct arthroscopic evaluation was not available in the past to evaluate the lesion and much discussion was based on the proper radiographic projection to evaluate the defect. To determine the true incidence, Calandra et al. (59) evaluated first-time dislocators between 15 and 28 years of age and found that 15 of 32 patients (47%) had evidence of Hill-Sachs lesions. Hill and Sachs (58) and Hermodsson et al. (45) both emphasized the importance of the anterior–posterior view with the arm in maximal internal rotation for identifying the lesion.

To better identify the best projections to diagnose and evaluate Hill-Sachs lesions, Danzig et al. (60) created Hill-Sachs lesions in cadaveric humeri and under fluoroscopy identified the best projections to detect these lesions. The projections were then evaluated on human subjects with a known history of anterior dislocation. Of all projections tested, the anteroposterior view with the humerus in 45 degrees of internal rotation, the notch (Stryker) view and the modified Didee view were confirmed to be the optimal methods for detection (60).

Hill-Sachs lesions have been known to correlate with an increased risk of recurrent instability. These lesions have the potential to engage the glenoid rim and cause dislocation if they become large enough and extend into the zone of contact between the humeral head and the glenoid in the position of apprehension (61). In a study by Cetik et al. (62), patients with recurrent instability were grouped by their total number of dislocations and the head involvement and depth of the Hill-Sachs defect were recorded by double-contrast CT arthrography. Patients with one to five dislocations had an average of 11.9% head involvement and an average depth of 4.14 mm. In patients with 6 to 20 previous dislocations, the average head involvement was 25.4% and the average depth 5.13 mm. In patients with greater than 20 previous dislocations, the average involvement was 26% and the average depth was 4.38 mm (62).

Kralinger et al. (11) were also able to correlate the size of the lesion with the likelihood of recurrence. After calculating the Hill-Sachs quotient or volume by multiplying the surface area and depth of the Hill-Sachs lesion on two radiographic projections, the lesion was graded depending on size as grade I, grade II, or grade III. Patients with grade I or grade II lesions suffered a 20% (32 of 160) rate of recurrence while those with grade III lesions suffered a 67% chance of recurrence (4 of 6) (11).

If left untreated, large bony defects in both the glenoid and the humeral head have been associated with a high rate of failed stabilization in arthroscopic soft tissue repair.

IMMOBILIZATION

Nonoperative treatment protocols and immobilization have traditionally been recommended following primary dislocation with the goal of "allowing the injury time to heal," followed by progressive strengthening of the rotator cuff and dynamic stabilizers of the glenohumeral joint. Itoi et al. (63) published a study demonstrating that immobilization in external rotation may provide benefit in reducing the risk of recurrence. They performed MRI studies on cadavers that demonstrated that the Bankart lesion was significantly less separated and displaced from the glenoid neck in a position of external rotation compared to one of internal rotation (63). In a randomized controlled trial, 198 patients were assigned to immobilization in either internal rotation or external rotation for a period of 3 weeks. In the external rotation group, recurrence was 26% (22/85) and in the internal rotation group recurrence was 42% (31/74). The reduction in the rate of recurrence with external rotation reached statistical significance. Immobilization in external rotation also trended to show lower rates of

recurrence when age groups were stratified, although this did not reach statistical significance (14).

Seybold et al. (64) performed an MRI study of first-time anterior dislocators to determine which soft tissue lesions are amendable to coaptation via immobilization in external rotation. A distinction was made between labral lesions with intact scapular periosteum and those without. A Bankart lesion is defined in the article as a separation of the labrum from the glenoid rim with rupture of the attachment of the scapular periosteum from the labrum. In contrast, a Perthes lesion is defined as a separation of the labrum from the glenoid rim with continuity between the labrum and the periosteum. They determined that Perthes lesions with a mild degree of labroligamentous plastic deformation showed the best reduction in the position of external rotation (64).

A recent randomized controlled study by Liavaag et al. (65) of 188 patients randomized to either internal or external rotation immobilization following primary anterior shoulder dislocation failed to establish a benefit to external rotation bracing. Finestone et al. (66) also failed to find a benefit to external rotation.

In Liavaag et al. (65) and Finestone et al. (66), patients were placed in 15 to 20 degrees of external rotation for a period of 3 to 4 weeks. Patients in Itoi et al.'s (14) study were older with an average age of 37 years and of different cultural habits than those in Liavaag et al.'s and Finestone et al.'s populations. This has been proposed as a possible explanation for the discrepancies between the two studies (67).

Paterson et al. (68) performed a systematic review of the literature and a meta-analysis of the position and duration of immobilization. They found no benefit to immobilization in a conventional internal rotation sling for greater than 1 week in patients younger than 30 years. Although immobilization in external rotation did show a trend in reducing recurrence, the data did not reach significance (68).

POSTTRAUMATIC GLENOHUMERAL ARTHROSIS

Dislocation and instability in other joints are known to lead to posttraumatic degeneration, and it has been theorized that traumatic shoulder dislocations may lead to similar changes (69,70). In fact, the risk of recurrence and associated irreversible injury to chondral surfaces and soft tissue of the glenohumeral joint has largely provided the impetus for surgical intervention after first-time dislocation in at-risk individuals based on systematic reviews of the literature (71).

Much of the early inference of glenohumeral dislocation-induced arthrosis was derived from direct observation of the joint injury at the time of open stabilization surgery (72,73). Samilson and Prieto (69) coined the term "dislocation arthropathy" and described a radiographic grading criteria. In their study, they inferred a higher rate of arthrosis than previously believed.

It is known from arthroscopy of first-time shoulder dislocations that a discrete set of pathologic changes may be encountered. These are believed to contribute to the development of osteoarthrosis. Taylor and Arciero (49) reported on a series of 63 patients with first-time dislocation, and identified 34 patients with humeral head osteochondral lesions and an additional 23 with high-grade chondral damage.

Hovelius and Saeboe (74) collected prospective data with an impressive 25-year follow-up on patients after glenohumeral instability episodes. In their cohort of 223 patients repeat radiographs 25 years after the initial dislocation demonstrate that 29% had mild arthropathy, 9% had moderate arthropathy, and 17% had severe changes. Only 44% had "normal" radiographs. Recurrence was correlated with a higher percentage of moderate or severe changes than solitary dislocations (39% vs. 18%). In addition, older age at initial dislocation, alcoholism, and high-energy sporting were all correlated with increased development and severity of arthropathy. This prospective study perhaps provides the greatest insight on the risk and incidence of dislocation arthropathy (74).

In a case-control study by Marx et al. (75), 91 patients who had undergone a shoulder arthroplasty for osteoarthrosis were compared with a group of 282 controls who had undergone total knee arthroplasty. Questionnaires for history of previous shoulder dislocation were sent to both groups and the results demonstrated an overall odds ratio of 19.3, indicating that patients who had undergone a shoulder arthroplasty had a 19.3 times higher history of dislocation than the controls. Excluding the patients with a history of shoulder surgery before total shoulder arthroplasty, a shoulder dislocation increased the risk of developing arthrosis by a factor of 10 (75).

CONCLUSION

The treatment of patients with a primary glenohumeral dislocation presents a difficult problem for the physician. Understanding the factors that influence rates of recurrence provides the shoulder surgeon with useful information that can help guide treatment on an individualized basis. A significant risk of recurrence and the potential for irreversible chondral and soft-tissue injuries to the glenohumeral joint have provided significant impetus for surgical stabilization after first-time instability events in active, young patients.

Interestingly, in the prospective 25-year follow-up by Hovelius et al. (18), the possibility of a shoulder becoming stable after multiple instability events

was evaluated. Sixty-five percent of patients (33 of 51) who had at least three events of instability did not sustain any recurring instability events in the final 10 years of follow-up. The possibility of a return to stability in patients following a history of multiple instability episodes has called into question the necessity of routine surgical stabilization in first-time dislocators who are at the highest risk for recurrence, notably young males.

Decision making on performing early surgical stabilization has traditionally been based on mitigating recurrent dislocation while only secondarily considering functional ability and quality of life. Younger, active patients who dislocate may become limited by subjective instability without ever sustaining a true "recurrence." Therefore, while the natural history for a young male with a primary dislocation may not be doomed to recurrent dislocations, there is evidence that outcome scores are improved with surgical stabilization and repair. Current recommendations for younger, active first-time dislocators include obtaining advanced imaging in patients who are considered high risk for recurrent instability or who have a potential for functional limitation. This includes younger male patients who are active in contact sports and have glenohumeral bone loss suspected on plain radiographs (51). Treatment is then based on anatomic restoration, with repair of the damaged bony and soft tissue structures dictated by the severity of injury and the ability to maximize functional results.

Additional research is needed to evaluate immobilization in external rotation as a mechanism to modify the natural history in high-risk populations. While the original work by Itoi et al. (14,63) is promising, follow-up studies have failed to find a significant benefit.

In older patients, the primary goal remains the maximization of functional results. While this is generally accomplished by a physical therapy protocol to preserve motion and strength, there does appear to be a role for surgical repair of older patients with rotator cuff tears if these tears are symptomatic or contribute to recurrent instability.

References

1. Simonet WT, Melton LJ 3rd, Cofield RH, et al. Incidence of anterior shoulder dislocation in Olmsted County, Minnesota. *Clin Orthop Relat Res.* 1984;186:186–191.
2. Kroner K, Lind T, Jensen J. The epidemiology of shoulder dislocations. *Arch Orthop Trauma Surg.* 1989;108(5):288–290.
3. Nordqvist A, Petersson CJ. Incidence and causes of shoulder girdle injuries in an urban population. *J Shoulder Elbow Surg.* 1995;4(2):107–112.
4. Zacchilli MA, Owens BD. Epidemiology of shoulder dislocations presenting to emergency departments in the United States. *J Bone Joint Surg Am.* 2010;92(3):542–549.

5. Hovelius L. Incidence of shoulder dislocation in Sweden. *Clin Orthop Relat Res.* 1982;166:127–131.

6. Bankart AS. Recurrent or habitual dislocation of the shoulder-joint. *Br Med J.* 1923;2(3285):1132–1133.

7. Rowe CR. Prognosis in dislocations of the shoulder. *J Bone Joint Surg Am.* 1956;38-A(5):957–977.

8. Arciero RA, Taylor DC. Primary anterior dislocation of the shoulder in young patients. A ten-year prospective study. *J Bone Joint Surg Am.* 1998;80(2):299–300.

9. Chalidis B, Sachinis N, Dimitriou C, et al. Has the management of shoulder dislocation changed over time? *Int Orthop.* 2007;31(3):385–389.

10. Henry JH, Genung JA. The natural history of glenohumeral dislocation—revisited. *Am J Sports Med.* 1982;10(3):135–137.

11. Kralinger FS, Golser K, Wischatta R, et al. Predicting recurrence after primary anterior shoulder dislocation. *Am J Sports Med.* 2002;30(1):116–120.

12. Simonet WT, Cofield RH. Prognosis in anterior shoulder dislocation. *Am J Sports Med.* 1984;12(1):19–24.

13. te Slaa RL, Wijffels MP, Brand R, et al. The prognosis following acute primary glenohumeral dislocation. *J Bone Joint Surg Br.* 2004;86(1):58–64.

14. Itoi E, Hatakeyama Y, Sato T, et al. Immobilization in external rotation after shoulder dislocation reduces the risk of recurrence. A randomized controlled trial. *J Bone Joint Surg Am.* 2007;89(10):2124–2131.

15. Robinson CM, Howes J, Murdoch H, et al. Functional outcome and risk of recurrent instability after primary traumatic anterior shoulder dislocation in young patients. *J Bone Joint Surg Am.* 2006;88(11):2326–2336.

16. Hovelius L, Augustini BG, Fredin H, et al. Primary anterior dislocation of the shoulder in young patients. A ten-year prospective study. *J Bone Joint Surg Am.* 1996;78(11):1677–1684.

17. Hovelius L, Eriksson K, Fredin H, et al. Recurrences after initial dislocation of the shoulder. Results of a prospective study of treatment. *J Bone Joint Surg Am.* 1983;65(3):343–349.

18. Hovelius L, Olofsson A, Sandstrom B, et al. Nonoperative treatment of primary anterior shoulder dislocation in patients forty years of age and younger. A prospective twenty-five-year follow-up. *J Bone Joint Surg Am.* 2008; 90(5):945–952.

19. Mclaughlin HL, Cavallaro WU. Primary anterior dislocation of the shoulder. *Am J Surg.* 1950;80(6):615–621.

20. Marans HJ, Angel KR, Schemitsch EH, et al. The fate of traumatic anterior dislocation of the shoulder in children. *J Bone Joint Surg Am.* 1992;74(8):1242–1244.

21. Hoelen MA, Burgers AM, Rozing PM. Prognosis of primary anterior shoulder dislocation in young adults. *Arch Orthop Trauma Surg.* 1990;110(1):51–54.

22. Gumina S, Postacchini F. Anterior dislocation of the shoulder in elderly patients. *J Bone Joint Surg Br.* 1997; 79(4):540–543.

23. Owens BD, Agel J, Mountcastle SB, et al. Incidence of glenohumeral instability in collegiate athletics. *Am J Sports Med.* 2009;37:1750–1754.

24. Owens BD, Dawson L, Burks R, et al. Incidence of shoulder dislocation in the United States military: Demographic considerations from a high-risk population. *J Bone Joint Surg Am.* 2009;91(4):791–796.

25. Arciero RA, Wheeler JH, Ryan JB, et al. Arthroscopic Bankart repair versus nonoperative treatment for acute, initial anterior shoulder dislocations. *Am J Sports Med.* 1994;22(5):589–594.

26. Sachs RA, Lin D, Stone ML, et al. Can the need for future surgery for acute traumatic anterior shoulder dislocation be predicted? *J Bone Joint Surg Am.* 2007;89(8):1665–1674.

27. Wheeler JH, Ryan JB, Arciero RA, et al. Arthroscopic versus nonoperative treatment of acute shoulder dislocations in young athletes. *Arthroscopy.* 1989;5(3): 213–217.

28. te Slaa, RL, Brand R, Marti RK. A prospective arthroscopic study of acute first-time anterior shoulder dislocation in the young: A five-year follow-up study. *J Shoulder Elbow Surg.* 2003;12(6):529–534.

29. Berbig R, Weishaupt D, Prim J, et al. Primary anterior shoulder dislocation and rotator cuff tears. *J Shoulder Elbow Surg.* 1999;8(3):220–225.

30. Hawkins RJ, Bell RH, Hawkins RH, et al. Anterior dislocation of the shoulder in the older patient. *Clin Orthop Relat Res.* 1986;206:192–195.

31. McLaughlin HL, MacLellan DI. Recurrent anterior dislocation of the shoulder. II. A comparative study. *J Trauma.* 1967;7(2):191–201.

32. Simank HG, Dauer G, Schneider S, et al. Incidence of rotator cuff tears in shoulder dislocations and results of therapy in older patients. *Arch Orthop Trauma Surg.* 2006;126(4):235–240.

33. Toolanen G, Hildingsson C, Hedlund T, et al. Early complications after anterior dislocation of the shoulder in patients over 40 years. An ultrasonographic and electromyographic study. *Acta Orthop Scand.* 1993;64(5):549–552.

34. Neviaser RJ, Neviaser TJ, Neviaser JS. Concurrent rupture of the rotator cuff and anterior dislocation of the shoulder in the older patient. *J Bone Joint Surg Am.* 1988;70(9):1308–1311.

35. Robinson CM, Shur N, Sharpe T, et al. Injuries associated with traumatic anterior glenohumeral dislocations. *J Bone Joint Surg Am.* 2012;94(1):18–26.

36. Porcellini, G., Paladini, P., Campi, F., et al. Shoulder instability and related rotator cuff tears: Arthroscopic findings and treatment in patients aged 40 to 60 years. *Arthroscopy.* 2006;22(3):270–276.

37. Milgrom C, Mann G, Finestone A. A prevalence study of recurrent shoulder dislocations in young adults. *J Shoulder Elbow Surg.* 1998;7(6):621–624.

38. Sher JS, Uribe JW, Posada A, et al. Abnormal findings on magnetic resonance images of asymptomatic shoulders. *J Bone Joint Surg Am.* 1995;77(1):10–15.

39. Pevny T, Hunter RE, Freeman JR. Primary traumatic anterior shoulder dislocation in patients 40 years of age and older. *Arthroscopy.* 1998;14(3):289–294.

40. Neviaser RJ, Neviaser TJ, Neviaser JS. Anterior dislocation of the shoulder and rotator cuff rupture. *Clin Orthop Relat Res.* 1993;291:103–106.

41. Leffert RD. Nerve lesions about the shoulder. *Orthop Clin North Am.* 2000;31(2):331–345.

42. Blom S, Dahlback LO. Nerve injuries in dislocations of the shoulder joint and fractures of the neck of the humerus. A clinical and electromyographical study. *Acta Chir Scand.* 1970;136(6):461–466.

58 SECTION 2 Anterior Instability

43. Safran MR. Nerve injury about the shoulder in athletes, part 1: Suprascapular nerve and axillary nerve. *Am J Sports Med.* 2004;32(3):803–819.

44. Travlos J, Goldberg I, Boome RS. Brachial plexus lesions associated with dislocated shoulders. *J Bone Joint Surg Br.* 1990;72(1):68–71.

45. Hermodsson I, Moseley HF, Overgaard B. *Hermodsson's Roentgenological Studies of Traumatic and Recurrent Anterior and Inferior Dislocations of the Shoulder Joint.* Montreal: McGill University Press; 1963.

46. Bedi A, Ryu RK. The treatment of primary anterior shoulder dislocations. *Instr Course Lect.* 2009;58:293–304.

47. Piasecki DP, Verma NN, Romeo AA, et al. Glenoid bone deficiency in recurrent anterior shoulder instability: Diagnosis and management. *J Am Acad Orthop Surg.* 2009;17(8):482–493.

48. Murray IR, Ahmed I, White NJ, et al. Traumatic anterior shoulder instability in the athlete. *Scand J Med Sci Sports.* E-pub 28 June 2012. doi:10.1111/j.1600-0838.2012.01494.x.

49. Taylor DC, Arciero RA. Pathologic changes associated with shoulder dislocations. Arthroscopic and physical examination findings in first-time, traumatic anterior dislocations. *Am J Sports Med.*1997; 25(3):306–311.

50. Sugaya H, Moriishi J, Dohi M, et al. Glenoid rim morphology and recurrent anterior glenohumeral instability. *J Bone Joint Surg Am.* 2003;85:878–884.

51. Bigliani LU, Newton PM, Steinmann SP, et al. Glenoid rim lesions associated with recurrent anterior dislocation of the shoulder. *Am J Sports Med.* 1998;26(1):41–45.

52. Singson RD, Feldman,F, Bigliani LU. CT arthrographic patterns in recurrent glenohumeral instability. *AJR Am J Roentgenol.* 1987;149:749–753.

53. Saito H, Itoi E, Sugaya H, et al. Location of the glenoid defect in shoulders with recurrent anterior dislocation. *Am J Sports Med.* 2005;33(6):889–893.

54. Itoi E, Lee SB, Berglund LJ, et al. The effect of a glenoid defect on anteroinferior stability of the shoulder after Bankart repair: A cadaveric study. *J Bone Joint Surg Am.* 2000;82(1):35–46.

55. Burkhart SS, De Beer JF. Traumatic glenohumeral bone defects and their relationship to failure of arthroscopic Bankart repairs: Significance of the inverted-pear glenoid and the humeral engaging Hill-Sachs lesion. *Arthroscopy.* 2000;16(7):677–694.

56. Mologne TS, Provencher MT, Menzel KA, et al. Arthroscopic stabilization in patients with an inverted pear glenoid: Results in patients with bone loss of the anterior glenoid. *Am J Sports Med.* 2007;35(8):1276–1283.

57. Flower WH. On the pathological changes produced in the shoulder-joint by traumatic dislocations, as derived from an examination of all specimens illustrating this injury in the museums of London. *Trans Pathol Soc London.* 1861;12:179.

58. Hill HA, Sachs MD. The grooved defect of the humeral head: A frequently unrecognized complication of dislocations of the shoulder joint. *Radiology.* 1940;35:690–700.

59. Calandra JJ, Baker CL, Uribe J. The incidence of Hill-Sachs lesions in initial anterior shoulder dislocations. *Arthroscopy.* 1989;5(4):254–257.

60. Danzig LA, Greenway G, Resnick D. The Hill-Sachs lesion. An experimental study. *Am J Sports Med.* 1980; 8(5):328–332.

61. Yamamoto N, Itoi E, Abe H, et al. Contact between the glenoid and the humeral head in abduction, external rotation, and horizontal extension: A new concept of glenoid track. *J Shoulder Elbow Surg.* 2007;16(5):649–656.

62. Cetik O, Uslu M, Ozsar BK. The relationship between Hill-Sachs lesion and recurrent anterior shoulder dislocation. *Acta Orthop Belg.* 2007;73(2):175–178.

63. Itoi E, Sashi R, Minagawa H, et al. Position of immobilization after dislocation of the glenohumeral joint. A study with use of magnetic resonance imaging. *J Bone Joint Surg Am.* 2001;83-A(5):661–667.

64. Seybold D, Schliemann B, Heyer CM, et al. Which labral lesion can be best reduced with external rotation of the shoulder after a first-time traumatic anterior shoulder dislocation? *Arch Orthop Trauma Surg.* 2009;129(3):299–304.

65. Liavaag S, Brox JI, Pripp AH, et al. Immobilization in external rotation after primary shoulder dislocation did not reduce the risk of recurrence: A randomized controlled trial. *J Bone Joint Surg Am.* 2011;93(10):897–904.

66. Finestone A, Milgrom C, Radeva-Petrova DR, et al. Bracing in external rotation for traumatic anterior dislocation of the shoulder. *J Bone Joint Surg Br.* 2009;91(7):918–921.

67. Miller BS. Commentary on an article by Sigurd Liavaag, MD, et al.: "Immobilization in external rotation after primary shoulder dislocation did not reduce the risk of recurrence. A randomized controlled trial". *J Bone Joint Surg Am.* 2011;93(10):e56.

68. Paterson WH, Throckmorton TW, Koester M, et al. Position and duration of immobilization after primary anterior shoulder dislocation: A systematic review and meta-analysis of the literature. *J Bone Joint Surg Am.* 2010;92(18):2924–2933.

69. Samilson RL, Prieto V. Dislocation arthropathy of the shoulder. *J Bone Joint Surg Am.* 1983;65(4):456–460.

70. Brophy RH, Marx RG. Osteoarthritis following shoulder instability. *Clin Sports Med.* 2005;24(1):47–56.

71. Handoll HH, Almaiyah MA, Rangan A. Surgical versus non-surgical treatment for acute anterior shoulder dislocation. *Cochrane Database Syst Rev.* 2004;1:CD 0043245.

72. Hastings DE, Coughlin LP. Recurrent subluxation of the glenohumeral joint. *Am J Sports Med.* 1981;9(6):352–355.

73. Hindmarsh J, Lindberg A. Eden-Hybbinette's operation for recurrent dislocation of the humero-scapular joint. *Acta Orthop Scand.* 1967;38(4):459–478.

74. Hovelius L, Saeboe M. Neer Award 2008: Arthropathy after primary anterior shoulder dislocation–223 shoulders prospectively followed up for twenty-five years. *J Shoulder Elbow Surg.* 2009;18(3):339–347.

75. Marx RG, McCarty EC, Montemurno TD, et al. Development of arthrosis following dislocation of the shoulder: A case-control study. *J Shoulder Elbow Surg.* 2002;11(1):1–5.

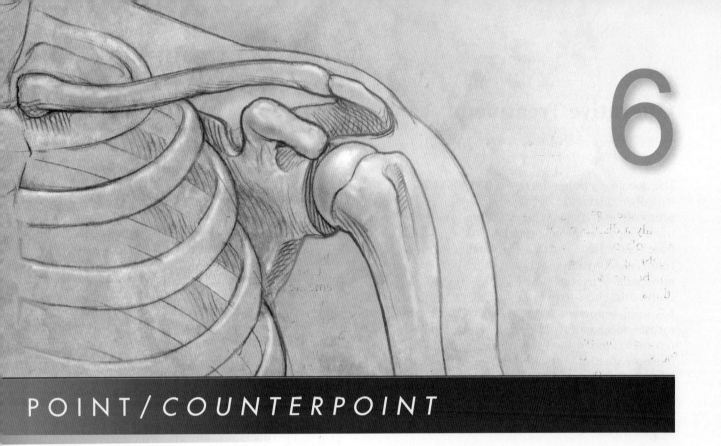

POINT / COUNTERPOINT

FIRST-TIME DISLOCATORS

*T*he ideal treatment of first-time dislocators is controversial. While high recurrence rates have been well documented in younger patients, many surgeons will allow these patients to declare themselves to be recurrent dislocators before proceeding with surgical intervention. In many cases, this approach will save some individuals from ever needing surgery. Unfortunately, each dislocation is not a benign event. Intra-articular pathology, including bone loss, may worsen with each event. And, some studies have shown that patients who have multiple dislocations prior to surgical stabilization are at a higher risk for revision surgery. The following sections will make the case for and against stabilization of the first-time dislocator.

Operative Treatment

Matthew J. White / Jeffrey R. Dugas

The debate regarding the first-time shoulder dislocator is really a discussion of the advancement of treatment protocols over time. Whereas conservative nonoperative therapy was the gold standard of the past, questions have been raised recently as to whether treatment algorithms may be shifting (1). We plan to demonstrate that nonoperative treatment leaves something to be desired both in the short-term as well as long-term future. This has been supported in the most recent literature and focuses on a handful of clinically relevant topics: Rate of recurrence, progression to arthritis, return to sport, and outcome metrics. Any one of these topics in isolation could make a case that surgical management of the first-time dislocator is viable and should be considered. The combination of these topics pushes surgical repair as the possible new gold standard in treatment.

RATE OF RECURRENCE

The concept of the "first-time dislocator" is probably limited in its definition. This could be interpreted as "first and only time dislocator," when in reality it is much more in line with "first of multiple dislocations." Jakobsen et al. (2) in a longitudinal study demonstrated that recurrent instability was present in 54% of patients treated nonoperatively at 2 years compared to 2.7% of patients treated with open surgical management. This has been corroborated in other studies with recurrence rates for nonoperatively at 2 years nearing 50% compared to 7% for those treated surgically (3). Similarly, Chahal et al. (4) found in a systematic review that the risk of recurrent shoulder instability following anatomic Bankart repair was approximately one-fifth the risk of all other treatment options. Furthermore, young age has been shown in multiple studies throughout the years to be a consistent prognostic factor in recurrence (5–8). This is particularly worse in the extremely young patient with open physes as demonstrated by Marans et al. (9) with 100% of first-time dislocators in this demographic sustaining subsequent recurrence. Military cadets make up another at-risk group that has been studied. In this population, recurrence rates after first-time dislocation are between 75% and 90% in nonoperative treatment protocols (10,11). Recurrence of shoulder dislocation can become a vicious cycle in which the labral-ligamentous complex is repeatedly further injured with each incident (12). This progression of injury begs the question, "What is happening to the integrity of the glenohumeral joint?"

PROGRESSION TO ARTHRITIS

One of the main tenets of orthopedic surgery surrounds joint preservation. Surgical techniques with this central theme are found in cartilage restoration surgeries, irrigation and debridement of chondrotoxic infections, and joint fractures and dislocations treated with prompt and anatomic reductions. Despite our best efforts, much of what we do is trying to chase cartilage damage as opposed to preventing it. We can, however, work to prevent it in some areas. Common sense would dictate that frequent instability, whether it be subluxation or frank dislocation, will over time damage the structural integrity of the shoulder joint including the cartilage. Anecdotally, we see this in patients that present late (Fig. 6-1). This is not limited to the cartilage as it has been shown in MRI and CT studies that recurrent dislocators have a significantly higher prevalence of anterior–inferior labral lesions as well as bone loss (13,14). Though not evaluated to the point of arthropathy, recently, it was demonstrated that recurrent instability does increase the presence of concomitant pathology (i.e., SLAP, rotator cuff tears) noted at the time of definitive arthroscopy (15). Such intra-articular damage could predispose to early and more prevalent arthropathy. One study by Hovelius and Saeboe (16) demonstrated recurrent dislocators presented with more arthritic changes than those individuals who had not sustained a recurrence. Another group found that postoperative arthritis in those individuals who were surgically fixed correlated strongly with the number of preoperative dislocations (17). Even nonoperative patients who became "stable"

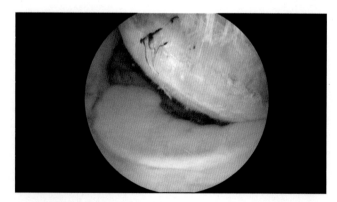

▲ **FIGURE 6-1:** Arthroscopic picture of the glenohumeral joint of a collegiate football player with recurrent instability over several years. Notice the loss of articular cartilage on both the humeral head and the glenoid, along with the anterior glenoid bone loss.

over time demonstrate more arthropathy than their surgical counterparts (16). Based on these studies, we can state that the volume of instability episodes matters.

RETURN TO SPORT

Many of the individuals that sustain shoulder dislocations are involved in athletic competition or desire to participate athletically. The initial question is often, "When can I get back?" The prognosis in active individuals treated conservatively is not favorable. Buss et al. (18) found that athletes had a nonoperative recurrence rate of 1.4 episodes per athlete per season and 66% of these eventually underwent surgical stabilization by 6 months. Robinson et al. (19) noted in a study from the United Kingdom that the risk of discontinuing contact sports within the first 2 years following primary dislocation was significantly higher in those treated with arthroscopic lavage (essentially equivalent nonoperative treatment) versus arthroscopic Bankart repair. Kirkley et al. (20) advocated for immediate stabilization in younger, active patients who participate in athletic activities presenting risk, such as football and rugby. In the athletically active patient population, nature of the sport and timing play a huge role in decision making. Patients that are mid-season can be treated conservatively so as to complete the season with subsequent stabilization in the off-season. This can often be facilitated with bracing that prevents the patient from at-risk positions. Contact sports can increase risk of recurrence as noted above and this risk should be fully explained to patients and their families.

OUTCOMES

As orthopedics and medicine in general moves to a more evidence-based mission, we must consider outcomes as they provide guidance for patient care algorithms. There are a number of different scores available to evaluate shoulder function and they are often used in an inconsistent manner. Nonetheless, there is some increasing outcome score evidence regarding treatment of first-time shoulder dislocators. Chahal et al. (4), in a systematic review, noted that in pooled analysis arthroscopic shoulder stabilization leads to improved disease-specific quality of life (Western Ontario Shoulder Instability questionnaire [WOSI]) over a short period of 2 to 6 years. Similarly, a prospective trial by Kirkley et al. (20), found a small but clinical significant difference in the WOSI outcomes favoring repair. Robinson et al. (19) reported a significant difference in DASH score at 2 years between patients undergoing arthroscopic Bankart repair versus lavage alone. Another study regarding 10-year follow-up noted a 74% unsatisfactory score in the Oxford

Shoulder score for those patients treated nonoperatively (2). Recently, two studies have come out that attempt to create novel and predictive models to help with decisions regarding treatment based upon previous outcome scores and recurrence rates (21,22). In the future, decision analysis and predictive modeling such as these may help fill in some of the gaps that currently exist in outcome score data.

SURGICAL TECHNIQUE (PEARLS AND PITFALLS)

We perform arthroscopic stabilization of the shoulder in first-time dislocators in the lateral position. A standard posterolateral arthroscopic portal is established 1-cm medial and 2-cm distal to the posterolateral corner of the acromion. An anterior portal can be placed in the rotator interval (RI) with either a switching stick or outside-in technique. While many surgeons will utilize multiple anterior portals at the RI level, we prefer one. A thorough diagnostic arthroscopy can be performed at this point taking inventory of the pathology present, including the anterior glenolabral complex. We then transition the scope to the anterior portal to evaluate the anterior aspect of the shoulder from a different perspective. At this time, we can also view our posterolateral portal and ensure that our cannula is set just lateral to the posterior glenoid rim so as to maximize our view of the anterior shoulder. We then move the scope back to the posterolateral portal and begin preparation for repair of the anterior labrum. We typically will use a combination of a shaver and/or elevator to abraid the glenoid neck and rim to encourage a good bleeding bed so as to maximize healing (Fig. 6-2). Sometimes running a shaver or burr on forward will tend to "kick" the instrument onto the glenoid and potentially damage the cartilage surface. Running the instrument of reverse can prevent this and often will obtain a similar bleeding surface.

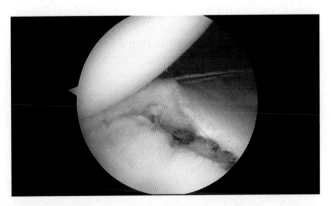

▲ **FIGURE 6-2:** The anterior glenoid rim is abraided back to bleeding bone to create a more biologically advantageous healing response.

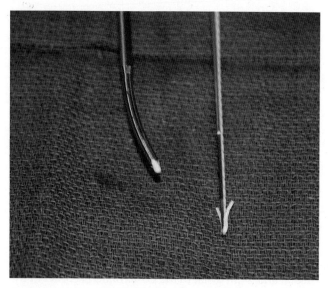

▲ **FIGURE 6-3:** Small anchors (1.5 mm) and curved cannulas allow for accurate placement of multiple suture anchors to create a more mechanically sound repair.

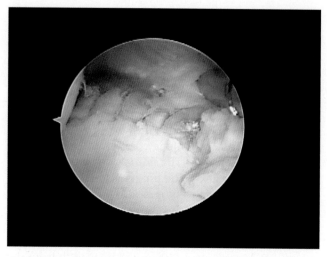

▲ **FIGURE 6-4:** An arthroscopic view of an anterior labral repair with multiple anchors placed at the articular margin.

With the glenolabral complex ready for repair, we then need to lay out a plan of anchors and repair style. Typically, we place an anchor at the inferior apex of the tear. The key is being able to reach this position. If the tear reaches a true inferior position, a subscapularis portal is an excellent way of reaching that position. Curved drill guides and flexible anchors allow for greater ease of insertion (Fig. 6-3). At this position, it is nearly impossible to place a knotless anchor. We utilize a 70-degree suture passer to place a horizontal mattress knot in this position. If the pass is particularly difficult from the anterior portal, one option is to view from the anterior portal and pass from the posterior portal. These passes can be shuttled and tied (standard sliding knot followed by series of half hitches) through our anterior portal. Once that inferior "bumper" has been re-established, we proceed proximally and tend to place an anchor at each hour on the clockface (Fig. 6-4). We are generous in our placement of anchors as we feel that this reinforces our repair and ensures good contact with our previously prepared bleeding bone surface reducing spotweld healing. One study has shown a lower recurrence rate for first-time stabilization in the group that had the most anchors placed (23). It is surgeon's discretion on whether horizontal mattress or simple suture passes are placed while moving proximally. The greatest utility for a horizontal mattress is to roll the labrum and capsule back up. If tissue is redundant or only mildly displaced, then simple sutures are more than adequate. In addition, we feel that as the repair moves proximally, knotless repair is a possibility though we tend to tie knots as we feel that gives us greater control over the position of the labrum in the repair. If it is difficult to manage a fully detached labrum, a traction stitch can be placed in the proximal portion of the labrum and out the anterior portal to "reduce" the labrum before attempting to repair it.

CONCLUSIONS

First-time dislocation of the shoulder can set in motion a series of events that can lead to both immediate and long-term concerns. The previous gold standard of initial conservative treatment puts a significant portion of the injured population at risk for recurrence and progression of shoulder pathology. Initial arthroscopic stabilization allows for return to function and sport with less recurrence and better outcomes. We would submit that the standard treatment for first-time shoulder dislocators has indeed changed.

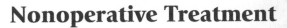

Nonoperative Treatment

Curtis Bush / Stephen C. Hamilton /
Gabriel J. Rulewicz / Richard J. Hawkins

INTRODUCTION

First-time anterior shoulder dislocations (FTASD) occur in approximately 2% of the population with 80% of dislocations occurring in younger patients (24). Data from the National Collegiate Athletic Association Injury Surveillance System determined that 45% of instability events resulted in more than 10 days lost to sport (25). Recurrent instability after an FTASD is common, approaching even 90% in high-risk populations by some reports (26). Controversy exists over the best treatment of young, in-season athletes and overhead laborers following their first-time anterior dislocation. In this chapter we will make the argument that nonoperative treatment is an acceptable, and often preferred, treatment of FTASD.

When deciding between immediate surgical stabilization and nonoperative treatment, the choice may be tailored to the individual patient and circumstances. Proponents of nonoperative treatment cite the following advantages: (1) Avoidance of surgical risks; (2) earlier return to activity and less time away from sport or work; (3) a nonbinding treatment option that gives the patient and surgeon the choice of converting to operative treatment as needed. On the other side of the debate, proponents of immediate surgical treatment cite the following concerns with nonoperative treatment: (1) High recurrent dislocation rates associated with nonoperative treatment in young patients, collision athletes, and overhead laborers; (2) risk that recurrent instability might lead to progressive degeneration of soft tissue stabilizers, glenoid bone loss and perhaps compromise the quality of delayed repairs; (3) risk that recurrent instability may lead to posttraumatic arthritis. This chapter will take a critical look into the literature on the nonoperative treatment of FTASD, and will review the risks and benefits of nonoperative and operative treatments' options. This chapter is not intended to advocate nonoperative management for every patient. The goal is to provide readers with a fair and balanced approach that can be tailored to the individual patient.

NATURAL HISTORY

Follow-up studies on nonoperative treatment of FTASD are numerous (Tables 6-1 and 6-2). The data from these studies show variably high rates of recurrent instability, most notably in young, male patients. Hovelius et al. (35) published a series with perhaps the largest numbers ($n = 229$) and length of follow-up (minimum 25 years). In this population, taking all-comers with an FTASD, 43% did not redislocate, 7% had only one recurrence, and 14.4% became stable over time (which means they experienced one or more repeat dislocations in the first 10 years following initial dislocation but none in the subsequent 15 years). Twenty-seven percent underwent surgical stabilization for recurrent instability and 7.9% continued to be unstable. The operative rate was higher in younger age groups (38% in patients 12 to 25 years old compared to 18% in patients 26 to 40 years old). Patients with recurrent instability had worse DASH outcome scores. The authors concluded that if one operates on all FTASD then over half of those patients would be undergoing unnecessary surgery.

TABLE 6-1   Recurrence Rates in Young Patients

	Age	Recurrence (%)
Rowe (27)	<20	94
McLaughlin (28)	<20	95
Henry and Genung (7)	17–23	90
Simonet et al. (29)	Athletes <30	82
Marans et al. (9)	Open physes	100
Postacchini et al. (30)	Adolescents	92

TABLE 6-2   Recurrence Rates in Contact Athletes

	Age	Recurrence (%)
Larrain et al. (31)	17–27	94
Wheeler et al. (11)	17–22	92
Arciero et al. (32)	17–23	86
Hovelius (33)	<20	90
Henry and Genung (7)	17–23	90
Simonet and Cofield (34)	<30	82

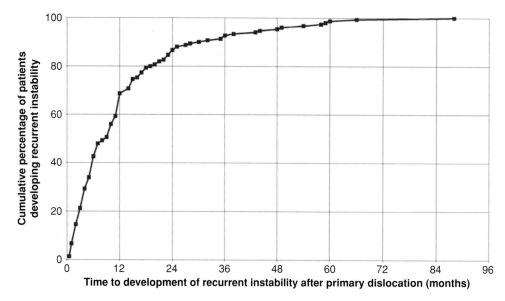

◀ FIGURE 6-5: Graph depicting the timing of the onset of instability in patients who had recurrent instability after a primary dislocation. (Reprinted from Robinson CM, Howes J, Murdoch H, et al. Functional outcome and risk of recurrent instability after primary traumatic anterior shoulder dislocation in young patients. *J Bone Joint Surg Am.* 2006;88:2326–2336.)

Robinson et al. (36) published a prospective study involving 25 patients between ages 15 and 35 which excluded patients with multi-directional instability. Recurrence, as defined by a subluxation or dislocation episode, was found to be 56% at 2 years and 67% at 5 years. The rate was higher among younger patients, 87% between ages 15 and 20. Most recurrent episodes occurred within the first 2 years (see Fig. 6-5), and most shoulders seemed to stabilize within a period of 2 years.

Sachs et al. (37) published a series with 131 patients with FTASD with 4 years of follow-up. Recurrence rates were lower in this study compared to those by Robinson et al. (36) and Hovelius et al. (35). The total rate of recurrent instability was 33%, but when broken down by age, the rate was 56% between ages 12 and 19, and 38% between ages 20 and 29. Of the patients who experienced a recurrence, 51% had only a single episode and almost all were involved in contact sports or an occupation requiring overhead activity. Among the younger patients (aged 12 to 19) in the study by Sachs et al. (37), 49% underwent surgical stabilization. The authors concluded that initial surgical stabilization is not warranted following acute dislocation. In a prospective, randomized trial published by Bottoni et al. (11) involving a very active, military population, 75% of patients treated nonoperatively had recurrent instability, and 67% of recurrent instability required subsequent open Bankart repair. However, of all the patients treated nonoperatively in this study only 50% came to surgery. Data from this study and Hovelius' study advocate that immediate surgical stabilization for FTASD may not be the best choice for many patients. In fact, if one were to operate on all FTASD, then many patients would face undue surgical risks since many shoulders stabilize over time without surgery.

PREDICTING RECURRENT INSTABILITY

In the aforementioned study by Sachs et al., patients younger than 25 years had significantly higher recurrence rates. Other factors that trended toward significance in this study were an occupation involving use of the arm above shoulder level, participation in collision sports, and greater pain associated with the initial dislocation. Among the studies on the topic, younger age seems to be the most important risk factor in predicting recurrent instability (6,8,35,38). Divergent results are reported on gender (8,35), though male gender trends as a risk factor as well.

MANAGEMENT OPTIONS

The relative indications for nonoperative treatment are listed in Table 6-3. Nonoperative management involves a brief period of immobilization immediately followed by rehabilitation. In regard to the length of immobilization, there is variability in practice patterns where immobilization may range from 3 days to 3 weeks. Hovelius et al. (35) divided their treatment groups into one that was immobilized for 3 to 4 weeks and another that wore a sling as needed for approximately 1 week. Paterson et al. (39) used this data with 2, 5, 10, and 25-year follow-up to determine the recurrence rates and found no difference between the groups. In another study, Kiviluoto et al. (40) found no difference in recurrence rates when comparing patients younger than 30 years treated with either 1 week of immobilization or 3 weeks. Paterson et al. (39) published a meta-analysis showing that recurrence rates were similar between two groups of patients less than 30 years old immobilized for either 1 week or 3 weeks.

TABLE 6-3   Indications for Nonsurgical Management of FTASD

Injury Characteristics	Player- and Sport-specific Characteristics
Initial shoulder dislocation	Athlete desires return to sport in season
Absence of bony injury that precludes joint stability	Nonoverhead or nonthrowing athlete
Absence of fracture or soft tissue injury, for example, rotator cuff tear, that requires surgery	Athlete plays a noncontact sport
	Athlete can complete sport-specific drills without instability

Adapted from Owens BD, et al. Management of mid-season traumatic anterior shoulder instability in athletes. *J Am Acad Orthop Surg.* 2012; 20:518–526.

TABLE 6-4   Relative Indications for Early Surgical Treatment

Associated injury
>50% Rotator cuff tear
Glenoid osseous defects >25%
Humeral head osseous defects contributing to persistent instability
Proximal humerus fracture requiring surgery
Irreducible dislocation
Interposed tissue or nonconcentric reduction
Failed trial of rehabilitation
Inability to tolerate shoulder restrictions
Inability to perform sport-specific drills without instability
Greater than two dislocations during the season
Overhead or throwing athletes

Adapted from Owens BD, Dickens JF, Kilcoyne KG, et al. Management of mid-season traumatic anterior shoulder instability in athletes. *J Am Acad Orthop Surg.* 2012;20:518–526.

In addition to the length of immobilization, questions arise regarding the best position of immobilization for FTASD. Itoi et al. (41) showed that immobilization in external rotation may better approximate the anterior soft tissue stabilizers than internal rotation, that is, conventional sling. Studies by Miller et al. (42) and Itoi et al. (43) suggest that immobilization in external rotation likely places these structures in a more anatomic position for healing. Liavaag et al. (44) reported improved healing of Bankart lesions and reduced separation with immobilization in external rotation. Itoi et al. (45) evaluated recurrence rates in 40 patients immobilized in either external rotation or internal rotation for a period of 3 weeks and found higher recurrence rates in those immobilized in internal rotation. In contrast to those findings, Finestone et al. (46) found no difference in recurrence rates between patients immobilized for 4 weeks in external rotation or internal rotation. In the aforementioned meta-analysis by Paterson et al. (39), there was no significant difference between immobilization in external rotation versus internal rotation; however, there was a trend toward less recurrence with external rotation. One drawback to immobilizing in external rotation is the issue of patient compliance, as this position may be more difficult from a practical standpoint (44).

Rehabilitation following immobilization is intended to achieve full pain-free range of motion and strength. Reaching these parameters facilitates return to sport or work in as little as 1 to 3 weeks, although return may be delayed up to 6 weeks in contact athletes. Bracing, in conjunction with rehabilitation, may decrease recurrence and is particularly beneficial in contact athletes who tolerate the restricted range of motion. In the opinion of the senior author (RJH), patients who continue to experience apprehension following a rehabilitation program have a poor prognosis and have a higher likelihood of requiring surgical stabilization.

There is controversy over the appropriate surgical indications for the young, contact athlete with FTASD. Less controversial indications for surgical treatment of instability are listed in Table 6-4. Surgical management might involve either open or arthroscopic techniques depending on circumstances and surgeon preference. Surgical management of FTASD significantly reduces recurrence rates but entails longer recovery periods and more time away from sport or work. The dilemma in managing FTASD comes when measuring the risk of recurrent instability associated with nonoperative treatment against the risk of exposing a significant number of patients to undue surgery by routinely operating on *all* FTASD.

RESULTS OF OPERATIVE AND NONOPERATIVE TREATMENT

There are various reports in the literature comparing operative and nonoperative treatments of FTASD. In a systematic review involving three level I studies and one quasi-level II study (a total of 228 patients), Chahal et al. (4) showed that the risk of recurrent instability following arthroscopic Bankart repair is one-fifth that of controls, which included rehabilitation or arthroscopic lavage. A summary of this review is depicted in Table 6-5.

Of these studies, only those by Kirkley et al. (20) and Robinson et al. (36) showed improved outcome scores (WOSI score) with anatomic Bankart repair at the 2- to 6-year mark. In a Cochrane review, Handoll and AlMaiyah (47) showed 68% to 80% reduction in relative risk for recurrent instability after surgery compared with nonoperative treatment and significantly higher outcome scores in the surgical group. Approximately half of patients treated nonoperatively subsequently underwent surgery.

TABLE 6-5 Characteristics of Included Studies

Study	Study Design	Treatment Groups	Technique and Fixation Method	Sample Size[a] (% Male)	Mean Age[a] (yr)	Rate of F/U[a,b] (%)	Length of F/U[a,b] (mo)	Outcome Measures
Bottoni et al. (11)	Level II quasi-randomized	(1) Bankart repair (2) Rehabilitation	Arthroscopic repair Bioabsorbable tacks	24 (100)	22.4	87.5	36 (range, 16–56)	Recurrent instability SANE score L'Insalata score Satisfaction
Kirkley et al. (20)	Level I randomized	(1) Bankart repair (2) Rehabilitation	Arthroscopic repair Transglenoid suture fixation (Caspari)	40 (87.5)	22.4	77.5	79 (range, 51–102)	Recurrent instability WOSI score DASH score ASES score
Jakobsen et al. (2)	Level I randomized	(1) Bankart repair (2) Lavage	Open repair Suture anchors	76 (81.6)	21.5	98.7	120	Recurrent instability Oxford score
Robinson et al. (19)	Level I randomized	(1) Bankart repair (2) Lavage	Arthroscopic suture anchors	88 (93.2)	24.8	95.4	24	Recurrent instability WOSI score DASH score SF-36 score Satisfaction

[a]No significant difference between treatment groups at baseline.

[b]Follow-up for primary outcome (recurrent instability).

ASES, American Shoulder and Elbow Surgeons; F/U, follow-up; SANE, Single Assessment Numeric Evaluation; SF-36, Short Form 36

Reprinted from Chahal J, Marks PH, MacDonald PB, et al. Anatomic bankart repair compared with nonoperative treatment and/or arthroscopic lavage for first-time trauma shoulder dislocation. *Arthroscopy.* 2012;28(4):565–575.

Brophy and Marx (3) authored a systematic review of studies comparing nonoperative and operative treatments. The authors' inclusion of certain studies was based upon the use of suture anchor fixation in the surgical technique. As a result, this review may represent contemporary surgical techniques better than some earlier publications. The mean patient age was 24 years. At 2 years, the nonoperative group had 46% recurrence rate and the operative group 7%. The conclusion of this review was that early surgical intervention leads to significantly lower recurrence rates for younger, active patients, though it results in "some patients having unnecessary surgery." According to a Cochrane review and the data reported by Bottoni et al. (11) if one were to operate on all first-time dislocators then approximately 50% of patients would receive surgery that never would have required surgery. Half the patients in the nonoperative treatment groups never required surgical intervention for recurrent instability.

CURRENT TRENDS IN TREATMENT

There appears to be a growing trend in the treatment of FTASD toward operative treatment. Malhotra et al. (48)

surveyed the British Elbow and Shoulder Society regarding their current treatment preferences. In 2002, 35% of participants preferred operative treatment, and in 2009 that percentage rose to 68%. This trend is probably related to high recurrence rates reported with nonoperative treatment, but may also be attributable to increasing surgeon comfort with arthroscopy and improved arthroscopic techniques.

IN-SEASON DISLOCATION/ RETURN TO PLAY

The goal of treatment for the collision athlete in season is to preserve function, minimize time away from competition, return to play safely, and minimize the risk of further injury. The collision athlete is at high risk for recurrent instability, but the question remains whether that athlete is better managed with immediate surgery, as suggested by Kirkley et al. (20), or with an initial trial of nonoperative treatment that may allow earlier return to play. Nonoperative treatment typically consists of a short period of immobilization (3 to 10 days) followed by rehabilitation to restore ROM and strength. Return to sport may range from 1 to 6 weeks with a brace to limit abduction and external rotation. Surgical management is thought to be the definitive treatment in terms of preventing recurrence. When chosen as the initial treatment, surgery removes the athlete from competition for the remainder of the current season and an additional 6 to 9 months for rehabilitation.

Buss et al. (18) reviewed the outcomes of contact athletes treated nonoperatively to determine success in returning to play and finishing the season. In this study 30 athletes with a dislocation (19 of 30) or subluxation (11 of 30) were treated with a brace and physical therapy. Twenty-seven of 30 patients were able to return to part or all of the same season and 26 completed the season. The average time away from competition was 10.2 days. Ten patients (37%) had one sport-related recurrence between 0 and 8 years from the index event, and only one patient had two recurrences. Of the 26 patients who completed the season, 12 eventually underwent delayed surgical stabilization in the offseason, and 14 did not. It may be worthwhile to consider, in light of this study, the utility that may be gained from the opportunity to return to activity more quickly and in doing so perhaps complete the ongoing season. The patient may value the opportunity to return to play in season more than the disutility associated with a second dislocation. These considerations are specific to each patient and should be an integral part of the decision-making process for both the surgeon and the patient.

RECURRENT INSTABILITY

The senior author (RJH) commonly encounters the following questions when treating athletes who sustain an FTASD: Can I return to play? Will a repeat dislocation increase the damage to my shoulder? And will the outcome of surgical treatment differ after multiple dislocations? Buss et al. showed that an athlete may safely return to play in the same season. Less evident are the answers for the latter two questions, which both relate to recurrent instability. In this portion of the chapter we will take a critical look at some important publications addressing the risks associated with recurrent instability.

The primary risk associated with nonoperative treatment is recurrent instability. After a second or third redislocation, surgery becomes a suitable option for most patients and is advocated by the senior author (RJH). An important question regarding nonoperative treatment of FTASD is whether further risk is incurred in the event of a second or third dislocation. The debate surrounding the management of FTASD largely revolves around this question, but unfortunately the current body of literature is somewhat unclear as to the answer. For those who believe that a second or third dislocation causes further and/or irreparable damage to

the joint (i.e., articular cartilage, stabilizing soft tissue structures), then it might seem reasonable to pursue immediate operative repair. For those who believe that a second or third dislocation does not necessarily put the joint at further risk then it is reasonable to pursue nonoperative treatment, leaving open the possibility of avoiding surgery altogether. Detailed below is a review of the literature discussing the pathology associated with recurrent instability. Based upon this information there does not seem to be overwhelming evidence that a second or third dislocation would add significant risk to the shoulder joint or at least enough to justify routine surgery for all FTASD. This is especially true given that approximately half of FTASD would never come to surgery.

RISKS TO STABILIZING STRUCTURES?

Several studies (12,17,49,50) have suggested that instability episodes may lead to progressive deterioration of joint stabilizing structures, specifically the glenoid labrum and inferior glenohumeral ligaments. The implication of these studies is that progressive deterioration of joint stabilizing structures from recurrent instability might contribute to inferior surgical results compared to early or immediate surgical treatment. As point in fact, Grumet et al. (23) found no difference in recurrence or complications between the treatment for FTASD and recurrent instability. In contrast, Jakobsen et al. (2) found that recurrent episodes may have a deleterious affect on outcomes. Only 63% of delayed repairs following recurrent episodes among their patients led to good or excellent results. Some might also argue that if recurrent instability should cause additional damage to labral, capsular, or bony structures then delayed surgical treatment becomes more technically challenging. While there is relatively weak evidence to the fact that persistent shoulder instability may put joint structures at risk, there is no good evidence that a *second* or *third* instability episode adds substantive risk to those structures or compromises surgical outcome. For this reason the senior (RJH) author advocates nonoperative treatment as an initial course and surgical treatment only when the instability proves itself recurrent, that is, following a second episode.

RISK OF OSTEOARTHRITIS?

Posttraumatic osteoarthritis (OA) is thought to be a sequela of recurrent instability of the knee, hip, ankle, etc. It is less clear whether a similar causal relationship exists between shoulder instability and shoulder OA. The literature provides conflicting results on the subject, and there is considerable doubt as to which is a greater cause of OA, recurrent instability or the surgery to treatment it.

Cameron et al. (51) reported on 422 patients with a diagnosis of shoulder instability and no history of previous shoulder surgery that underwent an arthroscopic procedure. The authors found a low prevalence of OA related to shoulder instability, and no difference in the prevalence of OA between patients with chronic or acute instability. Patients with evidence of chondral damage in this study, according to the Outerbridge classification, were older and had a greater time period from the first episode to surgery (referred to as anamnesis). Rachbauer et al. (52) found that the degree of OA does not relate to anamnesis or the number of dislocations before surgery.

Samilson and Prieto (53) introduced a shoulder OA classification based on the AP radiograph and subsequently used in many studies. Mild arthrosis was defined as inferior humeral and/or glenoid exostosis less than 3 mm, moderate arthrosis as exostosis measuring 3 to 7 mm and slight glenohumeral joint irregularity, and severe arthrosis as exostosis greater than 7 mm with glenohumeral joint narrowing and sclerosis. In this study, 24% of recurrent disclocators and 71% of solitary dislocators developed moderate or severe OA, and the authors found no relationship between the number of instability episodes and severity of arthrosis. The severity of arthrosis was correlated only with age at the time of dislocation. Of the patients who did not undergo surgery, 16/29 developed moderate or severe OA; however, 6 of the 16 had chronic locked posterior dislocations with delayed diagnosis and treatment. When you exclude the subset of posterior dislocations from the nonoperative group, 34% developed moderate or severe OA, compared to 29% (13/45) in the operative group. This study reported a higher prevalence of moderate and severe OA than other studies in the literature, which is most likely due to the inclusion of locked posterior dislocations in the FTASD group.

Perhaps the highest quality study on the subject is by Hovelius et al. (35) who reported 25 years of follow-up on 223 patients with shoulder instability. Radiographically 44% of patients were normal, 29% had mild arthrosis, 9% moderate, and 17% severe arthrosis. The authors found that the rate of arthrosis following a single dislocation is 18%, the rate following two or more dislocations was 40%, and the rate following surgical stabilization was 21%. The authors could not demonstrate a statistical relationship between the degree of arthropathy at 25 years and the treatment of the initial dislocation or presence of an impression fracture of the humeral head or glenoid rim fracture (resulting from the initial dislocation). It should be noted that many of the surgical procedures used in this study were open techniques that have mostly been abandoned because of the potential to overconstrain the joint and increase shear forces.

In the Hovelius et al. (35) study, the shoulders that became stable over time, (one or more repeat dislocations in the first 10 years following initial dislocation but none in the subsequent 15 years), had similar rates of arthrosis as patients with recurrent instability but higher rates than patients with an isolated dislocation. Patients with an isolated dislocation had similar rates of arthrosis as patients that were surgically stabilized. Patients who had a solitary dislocation and patients who became stable over time had similar DASH scores. High-energy athletic injuries (37% rate of moderate/severe arthropathy), and older age at the time of initial dislocation were correlated with arthropathy. The clinical significance of arthropathy seen on radiography in this study was minimal as there was no difference in subjective function or DASH scores between groups. No patient in this study necessitated surgery due to arthropathy, although two patients reported decreased activity and two patients changed occupations due to their arthropathy. The authors concluded that patients 23 to 33 years old with primary dislocation caused by high-energy trauma are at risk of developing arthropathy, regardless of the initial treatment, and especially if dislocation recurs.

Ogawa et al. (54) performed preoperative radiographs and CT scans on 282 patients with a history of shoulder instability scheduled to undergo shoulder surgery (presumably for instability) on average 3.7 years following onset. Using CT scan the authors were able to detect a significantly higher rate of arthrosis compared to radiographs (31.2% vs. 11.3%). Similar to the findings of some of the aforementioned studies, this study found that older age at the time of the initial dislocation was related to higher incidence of OA. The authors found that mild OA was more likely in patients with a glenoid bone defect greater than 20% of the glenoid compared to lesser bone defects. They did not, however, correlate larger glenoid defects with the number of dislocations/subluxations. It is unclear whether a second or third recurrence might cause progressively larger glenoid bone defects. The authors also found that the total number of dislocations and/or subluxations and frequency of dislocation and/or subluxations in osteoarthritic joints (classified by radiograph and CT scan) *were* significantly larger and higher, respectively, than those of nonosteoarthritic joints. This marks one of the few findings in the reported literature that correlates recurrent shoulder instability and arthrosis. Notably, all the shoulders determined to have developed arthrosis in this study were classified as mild or moderate and clinically asymptomatic. According to a case-control study by Marx et al. (55), the odds ratio for developing OA with a history of instability compared to no instability is 10. However, when excluding solitary dislocations from the group, thereby considering only recurrent dislocators, the odds ratio falls to 7.

Buscayret et al. (17) also evaluated patients undergoing surgery for recurrent instability for the presence of OA. The type of surgical intervention in this study included arthroscopic Bankart, Latarjet, and open capsulolabral repair/shift. They found that 8.5% of 570 patients had developed arthrosis prior to surgical intervention. The severity of OA was grade 3 or less (according to the Samilson and Prieto (53) classification) for most patients. Factors associated with the development of OA were: Age at the time of the initial dislocation, bony lesions of the anterior glenoid rim and humeral head, and tearing of the rotator cuff. The number of dislocation episodes was *not* associated with higher risk of developing OA. Among the patients without preoperative signs of OA, 20% developed radiographic evidence of OA postoperatively. These findings may raise the question whether the surgical intervention has more to do with developing OA than does the number of preoperative instability episodes, though no definitive conclusions can be made based on the data available. In the senior author's experience, hundreds of TSA have been performed for patients who have had previous surgery or instability. The number of TSA performed on patients with a history of instability who never had surgery is very small. The more common scenario involves patients who developed OA due to an open stabilization procedure in which the joint was overconstrained and shear forces were increased.

In a study by Hindmarsh and Lindberg (56) on FTASD treated with surgery (using notably older, mostly abandoned surgical techniques), 72% of patients developed postoperative OA. The authors are quoted as saying, "Even if the causes of arthrosis are many and difficult to evaluate, one can scarcely avoid the impression that the operation (Eden–Hybbinette) as such plays a part in its appearance." Franceschi et al. (57) evaluated the outcomes of arthroscopic Bankart repairs, which better represent current techniques compared to the series by Buscayret et al. (17) and Hindmarsh and Lindberg (56) (which together included several different open techniques). Of the patients in this study, 22% developed or progressed in OA stage. The authors found several risk factors associated with OA including age, increased time period from the initial event, increased number of dislocations, increased number of anchors, and presence of a degenerative labrum. It should be noted that most subjects in both series developed low-grade (grades 1 to 3) arthrosis, the clinical significance of which is likely minimal. In a case series on arthroscopic repairs with 13-year follow-up, Kavaja et al. (58) found that 60% of 72 patients developed arthrosis, though 80% of those cases were considered mild. Mean WOSI and WOOS scores were good and 75% of patients were satisfied with the results. Those who were dissatisfied cited loss of motion as the reason.

In a series published by Neer et al. (59) that included 273 shoulders with end-stage OA undergoing total shoulder arthroplasty, only 26 had a history of shoulder dislocation. Of those 26, 22 had a prior surgery

to treat instability. Matsoukis et al. (60) reported on 55 shoulders that had a history of previous anterior dislocation out of a total of 1,542 primary total shoulder replacements over 7 years. Of the 55, 27 had previously undergone stabilization surgery and 28 had not prior to arthroplasty. The authors did not find any difference between shoulders previously treated with stabilization surgery and those treated nonoperatively.

In summary, there is inconclusive data to support a strong relationship between recurrent shoulder instability and OA. Some degree of chondral damage may result from instability, but it seems the damage is related mostly to the initial dislocation and not heavily affected by subsequent recurrence. Chondral pathology seems likely to worsen with time but not necessarily with each recurrence, and it is unclear how quickly and in which patients it progresses. The notion that surgical stabilization will minimize or prevent the occurrence of posttraumatic OA is not well supported in the literature. Based upon the foregoing studies, surgical intervention (using open or arthroscopic techniques) seems to have little preventive effect and perhaps a deleterious effect on the development of OA. The argument that FTASD should be managed with immediate Bankart repair for the purpose of preventing OA (by preventing recurrence) is not well supported.

DECISION MAKING

The introduction of predictive disease modeling may be part of the future in tailoring treatment to individual patients. Disease modeling is a useful decision-making tool that helps clinicians provide better information to patients during treatment discussions and improve patients' ability to formulate treatment preferences. One example is the model constructed by Mather et al. (22). It is a Markov decision model of the natural history of an FTASD. "The model was constructed to provide, for a defined population, the likelihood of a variety of outcomes of potential importance to decision makers, such as number of patients experiencing recurrent instability, stabilization procedures, revision stabilizations, and stability at 10 years, as well as disease-specific quality of life." The model factors in variables such as age, gender, time lost from work or sport from surgery (defined as disutility of an intervention), and outcome of a treatment intervention are described in Tables 6-6 and 6-7.

Bishop et al. (21) published another type of decision-making model based upon expected value decision analysis. The expected value is derived from the utility of each outcome multiplied by the probability of that outcome. Utility values were derived from patient surveys and outcome probabilities derived from the literature. This model may allow surgeons and patients to arrive at the preferred treatment choice based upon the

TABLE 6-6 Base Case Model Parameters

Population	Base Case	Source
Age	23.4 (15–35)	15
Sex	87% men	15
Utility (WOSI)		
Stable shoulder	84	5
Recurrent instability	69	5
Revision stabilization	75	5
Disutility (WOSI)		
Stabilization of recurrent instability	25	Expert opinion
Revision stabilization	40	Expert opinion
Probabilities		
Recurrence after primary dislocation	**Age and gender dependent (Appendix)**	
Risk of failure from primary stabilization	8%	17
Age (odds ratio, age >22)	0.46	17
Gender (odds ratio, male)	3.65	17
Time from initial dislocation (odds ratio, >6 mos)	2.62	17
Rate of surgery for instability	23%	5
Failure of revision surgery	11%	18, 23
Length of model	10 yrs	15

Reprinted from Mather, RC, Orlando, LA, Henderson, RA, et al. A predictive model of shoulder instability after a first-time anterior shoulder dislocation. *J Shoulder Elbow Surg.* 2011;20:259–266.

TABLE 6-7 Results of Microsimulation of the Base Model Representing a Cohort of the Annual Incidence of First-time Anterior Shoulder Dislocation

	Raw Numbers	Probability
WOSI	70 (60–73)	N/A
Recurrent dislocations		
Year one	19,504	39%
Total	31,452	63%
Primary stabilization	6,301	12.6%
Revision stabilization	0.43	0.1%
Stable shoulder at 10 yrs	23,900	48%

Reprinted from Mather, RC, Orlando, LA, Henderson, RA, et al. A predictive model of shoulder instability after a first-time anterior shoulder dislocation. *J Shoulder Elbow Surg.* 2011;20:259–266.

patients' individual utility for nonoperative treatment, recurrent dislocation, and successful surgical treatment. This model suggests that a patient would be best served with nonoperative treatment if his or her chance of recurrent instability were less than 32% (see Fig. 6-6).

AUTHOR'S PREFERRED TREATMENT

The senior author's (RJH) preference is to treat most FTASD nonoperatively with aggressive rehabilitation avoiding the provocative position of external rotation and abduction. This approach allows the athlete

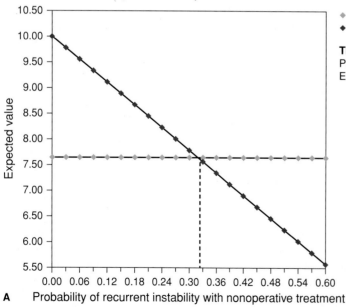

Sensitivity analysis on probability of recurrent instability with nonoperative treatment

◆ Arthroscopic stabilization
◆ Nonoperative treatment

Threshold values:
Probability of recurrent instability with nonoperative treatment = 0.32
Expected value = 7.63

▲ **FIGURE 6-6: A:** Sensitivity analysis on probability of recurrent instability with nonoperative treatment. *Green line,* utility from surgical stabilization; *blue line,* utility from nonoperative treatment over varying probabilities of redislocation. Based upon this patient's utility from either treatment option, the patient would be best suited for nonoperative treatment if his or her probability of recurrence is less than 32%. If his or her probability of recurrence is greater than 32%, then the patient would derive greater utility from arthroscopic stabilization.

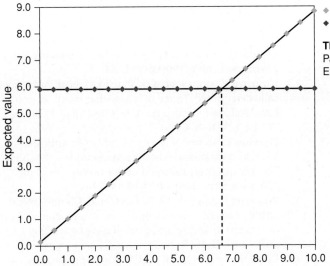

B   Payoff of having surgery and no complications or recurrence

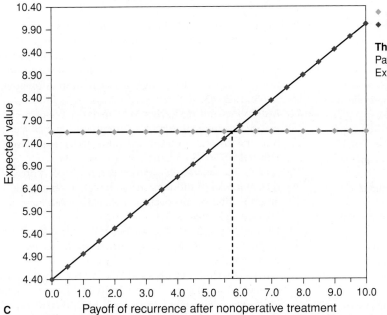

C   Payoff of recurrence after nonoperative treatment

▲ FIGURE 6-6: (*Continued*) **B:** Sensitivity analysis on payoff of having surgery and no complications or recurrence. This model illustrates that if a patient derives >5.6 utility from recurrence, then nonoperative treatment is the preferred choice. **C:** Sensitivity analysis on payoff of recurrence after nonoperative treatment. Based upon this model, if the patient were to derive >6.6 utility from a successful surgery then arthroscopic stabilization is the preferred choice, whereas if the utility from successful surgery is <6.6 then nonoperative treatment is preferred. (Reprinted from Bishop JA, Crall TS, Kocher MS. Operative versus nonoperative treatment after primary traumatic anterior glenohumeral dislocation: Expected-value decision analysis. *J Shoulder Elbow Surg.* 2011;20(7):1087–1094.)

to return to sport when ready (weeks) and offers the opportunity to return with a brace during the same season. The majority of athletes who suffer a mid-season FTASD are able to return and participate in the same season with nonoperative treatment. Surgery is considered when the instability becomes recurrent and a disability, usually following a second or third episode. The literature does not definitively show that a second or third dislocation causes additional damage to the shoulder joint or that surgery following a second or third dislocation leads to worse outcomes compared to surgery following an initial dislocation. Immediate surgery following the first dislocation is considered in selected athletes determined by circumstance and timing in the season.

References

1. Boone JL, Arciero RA. First-time anterior shoulder dislocations: Has the standard changed? *Br J Sports Med.* 2010;44:355–360.
2. Jakobsen BW, Johannsen HV, Suder P, et al. Primary repair versus conservative treatment of first-time traumatic anterior dislocation of the shoulder: A randomized study with 10-year follow-up. *Arthroscopy.* 2007;23(2):118–123.
3. Brophy RH, Marx RG. The treatment of traumatic anterior instability of the shoulder: Nonoperative and surgical treatment. *Arthroscopy.* 2009;25(3):298–304.
4. Chahal J, Marks PH, MacDonald PB, et al. Anatomic bankart repair compared with nonoperative treatment and/or arthroscopic lavage for first-time traumatic shoulder dislocation. *Arthroscopy.* 2012;28(4):565–575.
5. te Slaa RL, Brand R, Marti RK. A prospective arthroscopic study of acute first-time anterior shoulder dislocation in the young: A five year follow-up study. *J Shoulder Elbow Surg.* 2003;12:529–534.
6. Rowe CR. Prognosis in dislocations of the shoulder. *J Bone Joint Surg Am.* 1956;38:957–977.
7. Henry JH, Genung JA. Natural history of glenohumeral dislocation. *Am J Sports Med.* 1982;10:135–137.
8. Hovelius L, Augustini BG, Fredin H, et al. Primary anterior dislocation of the shoulder in young patients. A ten-year prospective study. *J Bone Joint Surg Am.* 1996;78:1677–1684.
9. Marans HJ, Angel KR, Schemitsch EH, et al. The fate of traumatic anterior dislocation of the shoulder in children. *J Bone Joint Surg Am.* 1992;74:1242–1244.
10. Wheeler JH, Ryan JB, Arciero RA, et al. Arthroscopic versus non-operative treatment of acute shoulder dislocations in young athletes. *Arthroscopy.* 1989;5(3):213–217.
11. Bottoni CR, Wilckens JH, DeBerardino TM, et al. A prospective, randomized evaluation of arthroscopic stabilization versus nonoperative treatment in patients with acute, traumatic, first-time shoulder dislocation. *Am J Sports Med.* 2002;30(4):576–580.
12. Habermeyer P, Gleyze P, Rickert M. Evolution of lesions of the labrum-ligament complex in posttraumatic anterior shoulder instability: A prospective study. *J Shoulder Elbow Surg.* 1999;8:66–74.

13. Kim DS, Yoon YS, Yi CH. Prevalence comparison of accompanying lesions between primary and recurrent anterior dislocation in the shoulder. *Am J Sports Med.* 2010;38:2071–2076.
14. Griffith JF, Antonio GE, Yung PS, et al. Prevalence, pattern, and spectrum of glenoid bone loss in anterior shoulder dislocation: CT analysis of 218 patients. *AJR Am J Roentgenol.* 2008;190:1247–1254.
15. Gutierrez V, Monckeberg JE, Pinedo M, et al. Arthroscopically determined degree of injury after shoulder dislocation relates to recurrence rate. *Clin Orthop Relat Res.* 2012;470:961–964.
16. Hovelius L, Saeboe M. Neer Award 2008: Arthropathy after primary anterior shoulder dislocation–223 shoulders prospectively followed up for twenty-five years. *J Shoulder Elbow Surg.* 2009;18:339–347.
17. Buscayret F, Edwards TB, Szabo I, et al. Glenohumeral arthrosis in anterior instability before and after surgical treatment: Incidence and contributing factors. *Am J Sports Med.* 2004;32:1165–1172.
18. Buss DD, Lynch GP, Meyer CP, et al. Nonoperative management for in-season athletes with anterior shoulder instability. *Am J Sports Med.* 2004;32(6):1430–1433.
19. Robinson CM, Jenkins PJ, White TO, et al. Primary arthroscopic stabilization for a first-time anterior dislocation of the shoulder. *J Bone Joint Surg Am.* 2008;90:708–721.
20. Kirkley A, Werstine R, Ratjek A, et al. Prospective randomized clinical trial comparing the effectiveness of immediate arthroscopic stabilization versus immobilization and rehabilitation in first traumatic anterior dislocations of the shoulder: Long-term evaluation. *Arthroscopy.* 2005;21:55–63.
21. Bishop JA, Crall TS, Kocher MS. Operative versus nonoperative treatment after primary traumatic anterior glenohumeral dislocation: Expected-value decision analysis. *J Shoulder Elbow Surg.* 2011;20(7):1087–1094.
22. Mather RC, Orlando LA, Henderson RA, et al. A predictive model of shoulder instability after a first-time anterior shoulder dislocation. *J Shoulder Elbow Surg.* 2011;20:259–266.
23. Grumet RC, Bach BR, Provencher MT. Arthroscopic stabilization for first-time versus recurrent shoulder instability. *Arthroscopy.* 2010;26(2):239–248.
24. Owens BD, Duffey ML, Nelson BJ, et al. The incidence and characteristics of shoulder instability at the United States Military Academy. *Am J Sports Med.* 2007;35:1168–1173.
25. Owens BD, Agel J, Mountcastle SB, et al. Incidence of glenohumeral instability in collegiate athletics. *Am J Sports Med.* 2009;37(9):1750–1754.
26. Burns TC, Owens BD. Management of shoulder instability in in-season athletes. *Phys Sportsmed.* 2010;38(3):55–60.
27. Rowe CR. Acute and recurrent anterior dislocation of the shoulder. *Orthop Clin North Am.* 1980;11(2):253–270.
28. McLaughlin HL. *Trauma.* Philadelphia, PA: W B. Saunders Company; 1959.
29. Simonet WT, Melton LJ, Cofield RH, et al. Incidence of anterior shoulder dislocation in Olmsted County, Minnesota. *Clin Orthopaedics and Rel Research.* 1984;186:186–191.

30. Postacchini F, Gumina S, Cinotti G. Anterior shoulder dislocation in adolescents. *J Shoulder Elbow Surg.* 2000;9(6):470–474.

31. Larrain MV, Botto GJ, Montenegro HJ, et al. Arthroscopic repair of acute traumatic anterior shoulder dislocation in young athletes. *Arthroscopy.* 2001;17(4):373–377.

32. Arciero RA, Wheeler JH, Ryan JB,et al. Arthroscopic bankart repair versus nonoperative treatment for acute, initial anterior shoulder dislocations. *Am J Sports Med.* 1994;22(5):589–594.

33. Hovelius, L. Shoulder dislocation in swedish ice hockey players. *Am J Sports Med.* 1978;6(6):373–377.

34. Simonet WT, Cofield RH. Prognosis in anterior shoulder dislocation. *Am J Sports Med.* 1984;12(1):19–24.

35. Hovelius L, Olofsson A, Sandström B, et al. Nonoperative treatment of primary anterior shoulder dislocation in patients forty years of age and younger. *J Bone Joint Surg Am.* 2008;90(5):945–952.

36. Robinson CM, Howes J, Murdoch H, et al. Functional outcome and risk of recurrent instability after primary traumatic anterior shoulder dislocation in young patients. *J Bone Joint Surg Am.* 2006;88:2326–2336.

37. Sachs RA, Lin D, Stone ML, et al. Can the need for future surgery for acute traumatic anterior shoulder dislocation be predicted? *J Bone Joint Surg Am.* 2007;89:1665–1674.

38. Kalinger FS, Golser K, Wischatta R, et al. Predicting recurrence after primary anterior shoulder dislocation. *Am J Sports Med.* 2002;30:116–120.

39. Paterson WH, Throckmorton TW, Koester M, et al. Position and duration of immobilization after primary anterior shoulder dislocation: A systematic review and meta-analysis of the literature. *J Bone Joint Surg Am.* 2010;92(18):2924–2933.

40. Kiviluoto O, Pasila M, Jaroma H, et al. Immobilization after primary dislocation of the shoulder. *Acta Orthop Scand.* 1980;51:915–919.

41. Itoi E, Hatakeyama Y, Urayama M, et al. Position of immobilization after dislocation of the shoulder : A cadaveric study. *J Bone Joint Surg.* 1999;81(3):385–390.

42. Miller BS, Sonnabend DH, Hatrick C, et al. Should acute anterior dislocations of the shoulder be immobilized in external rotation? A cadaveric study. *J Shoulder Elbow Surg.* 2004;13:589–592.

43. Itoi E, Sashi R, Minagawa H, et al. Position of immobilization after dislocation of the glenohumeral joint. A study with use of magnetic resonance imaging. *J Bone Joint Surg Am.* 2001;83:661–667.

44. Liavaag S, Stiris MG, Lindland ES, et al. Do Bankart lesions heal better in shoulders immobilized in external rotation? A randomized single-blind study of 55 patients examined with MRI. *Acta Orthop.* 2009;80(5):579–584.

45. Itoi E, Hatakeyama Y, Sato T, et al. Immobilization in external rotation after shoulder dislocation reduces the risk of recurrence. A randomized controlled trial. *J Bone Joint Surg Am.* 2007;89:2124–2131.

46. Finestone A, Milgrom C, Radeva-Petrova DR, et al. Bracing in external rotation for traumatic anterior dislocation of the shoulder. *J Bone Joint Surg Br.* 2009;91:918–921.

47. Handoll HH, Al-Maiyah MA, Rangan A. Surgical versus non-surgical treatment for acute anterior shoulder dislocation. *The Cochrane Database of Systematic Reviews.* 2004; Issue 1. Art. No.:CD004325. doi: 10.1002/14651858. CD004325.pub2.

48. Malhotra A, Freudmann MS, Hay SM. Management of traumatic anterior shoulder dislocation in the 17 to 25-year age group: A dramatic evolution of practice. *J Shoulder Elbow Surg.* 2012;21:545–553.

49. Urayama M, Itoi E, Sashi R, et al. Capsular elongation in shoulders with recurrent anterior dislocation: Quantitative assessment with MRI arthrography. *Am J Sports Med.* 2003;31:64–67.

50. Levine WN, Arroyo JS, Pollock RG, et al. Open revision stabilization surgery for recurrent anterior glenohumeral instability. *Am J Sports Med.* 2000;28(2):156–160.

51. Cameron ML, Kocher MS, Briggs KK, et al. The Prevalence of glenohumeral osteoarthrosis in unstable shoulders. *J Shoulder Elbow Surg.* 2003;31(1):53–55.

52. Rachbauer F, Ogon M, Wimmer C, et al. Glenohumeral osteoarthritis after the Eden-Hybbinette procedure. *Clin Orthop.* 2000;373:135–140.

53. Samilson RL, Prieto V. Dislocation arthropathy of the shoulder. *J Bone Joint Surg Am.* 1983;65(4):456–460.

54. Ogawa K, Yoshida A, Ikegami H. Osteoarthritis in shoulders with traumatic anterior instability: Preoperative survey using radiography and computed tomography. *J Shoulder Elbow Surg.* 2006;15(1):23–29.

55. Marx RG, McCarty EC, Montemurno TD, et al. Development of arthrosis following dislocation of the shoulder: A case-control study. *J Shoulder Elbow Surg.* 2002;11:1–5.

56. Hindmarsh J, Lindberg A. Eden-Hybbinette's operation for recurrent dislocation of the humero-scapular joint. *Acta Orthop Scand.* 1967;38(4):459–478.

57. Franceschi F, Papalia R, Del Buono A, et al. Glenohumeral osteoarthritis after arthroscopic Bankart repair for anterior instability. *Am J Sports Med.* 2011;39(8):1653–1659.

58. Kavaja L, Pajarinen J, Sinisaari I, et al. Arthrosis of glenohumeral joint after arthroscopic Bankart repair: A long-term follow-up of 13 years. *J Shoulder Elbow Surg.* 2012;21(3):350–355.

59. Neer CS 2nd, Watson KC, Stanton FJ. Recent experience in total shoulder replacement. *J Bone Joint Surg Am.* 1982;64:319–337.

60. Matsoukis J, Tabib W, Guiffault P, et al. Shoulder arthroplasty in patients with a prior anterior shoulder dislocation: Results of a multicenter study. *J Bone Joint Surg Am.* 2003;85-A:1417–1424.

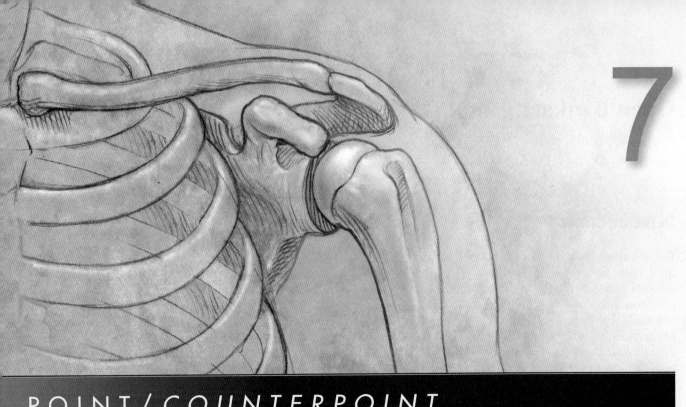

TECHNIQUE FOR ANTERIOR STABILIZATION

Open Bankart repair has long been considered the gold standard treatment for anterior instability. Over the last decade, arthroscopic stabilization results have approached those obtained with open repairs. Several studies have shown higher rates of recurrence in those with significant bone loss. Based on these results, many surgeons routinely use bone block techniques as their primary means of treating anterior instability. Then there are surgeons who, based on the rotator cuff literature highlighting the benefits of double-row repairs, have shifted toward arthroscopic or open double-row repairs as a means of better recreating the capsulolabral anatomy while strengthening the repair. The following chapters will highlight the benefits of each technique sharing technical pearls and elucidating the ideal indications for each repair construct described.

Open Bankart

Moira M. McCarthy / Samuel A. Taylor /
Anne M. Kelly / Edward V. Craig

INTRODUCTION

The shoulder is the most commonly dislocated major joint with an annual incidence of 11.2 per 100,000 patients (1). Anterior shoulder instability is the most common direction of instability (95%) and is the most common reason for instability intervention (2,3). The recurrence risk of anterior dislocation is particularly high in young and active athletes. Up to 87% of athletes will develop recurrent instability compared to 30% of nonathletes (4–8). The disability spectrum of anterior instability ranges from pain and apprehension with overhead activities to subluxation and to recurrent dislocation (9,10). Options for surgical treatment of anterior shoulder instability include a variety of arthroscopic techniques as well as open repair, often dependent on related pathology.

Open Bankart repair has been regarded as the gold standard for treatment of anterior shoulder instability (6,11–14). A Bankart lesion consists of avulsion of the anterior shoulder capsule, inferior glenohumeral ligament (IGHL), and glenoid labrum from the anterior glenoid rim. It is most commonly associated with a shoulder dislocation (15). Bankart lesions are found in 65% to 90% of shoulders at the time of surgery to correct anterior instability (16–19). A redundant anterior capsule (20), deficient subscapularis muscle (20), and a large opening in the rotator interval (10) may also contribute to anterior instability. Indications for operative management of anterior instability include an initial shoulder dislocation in a high-demand patient, recurrent dislocations or symptomatic subluxations, or refractory pain and instability after completion of a physical therapy protocol. Pagnani and Dome (21) followed 58 American football players at an average 37-month follow-up after open Bankart repair, and 3.4% experienced a recurrent subluxation, 94.8% of patients were rated as good or excellent, and 89.6% of patients were able to return to sport for at least 1 year. With the advancement of arthroscopic techniques and tools, however, many Bankart lesions previously treated with the open technique can be addressed arthroscopically with the risk of increased recurrence rate. Open Bankart repair remains the gold standard treatment for anterior shoulder instability in the setting of deficient anterior capsule, a glenoid rim fracture or defect greater than 25% (22–24), failed arthroscopic Bankart repair (25), association with humeral avulsion of glenohumeral ligament (HAGL) lesions, and failed prior surgery in which the Bankart lesion was not addressed (26).

SURGICAL TECHNIQUE

Examination of the shoulder under anesthesia is essential to determine the degree and direction of laxity of the shoulder prior to operative intervention. The deltopectoral approach is routinely employed for open Bankart repair (Fig. 7-1A). The anterior axillary fold is identified and an approximately 5-cm skin incision is made in-line with that fold. After the deep fascia is exposed, the deltopectoral groove is identified. The cephalic vein is a guide to the deltopectoral groove and should be mobilized and retracted laterally with the deltoid muscle. The pectoralis major muscle is retracted medially. The lateral border of the conjoint tendon is identified and retracted medially along with the pectoralis major, taking care to protect the musculocutaneous nerve.

The subscapularis tendon can be divided in either a vertical incision (20), an L-shaped incision (27), or a transverse incision (28). It is important to leave a 1- to 2-cm cuff of tendon off the lesser tuberosity for later repair. The subscapularis tendon should be incised carefully to avoid damage to the underlying capsule (Fig. 7-1B). The subscapularis is then elevated off the anterior capsule, taking care to properly ligate the vessels at the inferior border of the subscapularis. Inspection of the rotator cuff and the rotator interval is then performed. If the rotator interval is torn or enlarged such that the interval extends lateral to the humeral head it can be repaired in a side-to-side fashion. The capsule is then divided either vertically 5 mm lateral to the glenoid rim, in a T-shaped fashion, or transversely in the midportion of the capsule (Fig. 7-1C). Making the transverse limb of the T-shaped incision first allows evaluation of the distance from the glenoid rim to ensure that 5 mm of capsule is left attached to the rim (29). The edges of the capsule are tagged for retraction and later repair.

The Bankart repair offers the most reliable results in patients with anterior instability and a Bankart lesion. This technique repairs the avulsed capsule and labrum back to the glenoid rim (17,20,30,31). The anterior glenoid rim is debrided with a Cobb elevator down to the bleeding bone. Three curved bone tunnels or, alternatively, suture anchors are placed at the 2-o'clock,

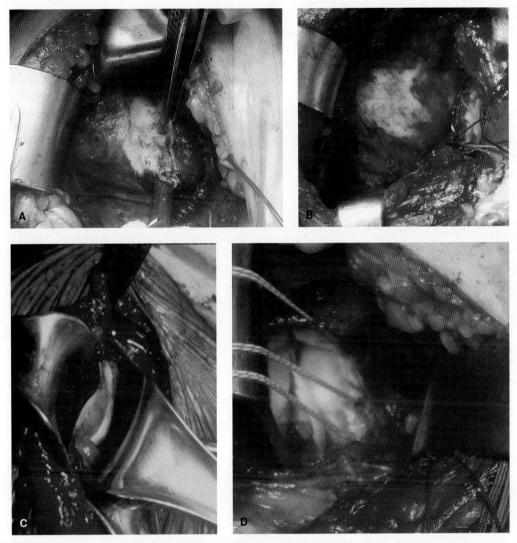

▲ **FIGURE 7-1:** Open Bankart repair. **A:** Deltopectoral approach with subscapularis tagged with ethibond. Clamp is used to define the interval between subscapularis and capsule. **B:** Subscapularis is released while the capsule beneath is left intact. **C:** Bankart lesion. **D:** Suture anchor placement on glenoid.

4-o'clock, and 6-o'clock positions for the right shoulder or 10-o'clock, 8-o'clock, and 6-o'clock positions for the left shoulder (9). Nonabsorbable sutures are then passed through the bone tunnels and through the avulsed labral and capsular tissue. Using the tagging sutures placed on the capsular edges, the capsule is retrieved and pulled medially. The sutures from either the suture anchors or the bone tunnels are then used to repair the capsule and labrum to the glenoid. Each suture is tightened and tied successively from inferior to superior (Fig. 7-1D). Warner et al. (32) prefer a modification of the Bankart in which the inferior capsule is shifted superiorly while the arm is held in a position of abduction and external rotation. To prevent loss of rotation with this technique the capsular incision is made with the arm in maximal external rotation. If there is excessive capsular laxity the capsule can be imbricated

or overlapped in a "pants-over-vest" technique. The subscapularis is anatomically repaired using absorbable suture.

There are several methods of attachment of the Bankart lesion to the glenoid rim. The curved drill holes provide a strong repair, but are technically demanding (33). The pull-out strength of drill holes is 98 N compared to 90 N for suture anchors (34,35). Suture anchors are advantageous in their ease of use except potentially at the 6-o'clock position where placement may be difficult. Suture anchors may have a potential to pull out and become loose bodies within the joint and they may also provide less contact surface area between the capsule and the glenoid rim than the drill hole technique (33). In an effort to increase contact surface area, some surgeons use a mattress technique with suture anchors.

Postoperative rehabilitation is critical for successful outcomes. Pendulum motion begins on postoperative day one. A sling is not necessary but the elbow must be kept forward of the coronal plane for 6 weeks. Passive elevation to 90 degrees and external rotation to 0 degree are allowed immediately. Gradual increase in full elevation, full internal rotation, and external rotation are regained over the first 6 weeks with the goal to achieve 50% external rotation of the contralateral extremity by 6 weeks and 100% external rotation by 12 weeks. Contact sports are allowed between 4 and 6 months and overhead throwing permitted at 6 to 9 months (33).

DISCUSSION

Open stabilization remains the gold standard procedure for treatment of anterior instability especially for severe instabilities, revision procedures (25,26), and athletes who participate in contact sports (11,36,37). Rowe et al. (20) were one of the first to report on the outcomes of the open Bankart procedure in 1978. At an average 6-year follow-up of 145 shoulders treated with open Bankart repairs, there were five recurrences (3.5% patients). The authors advocated that early return of motion and function can be expected with anatomic dissection, identification and repair of the lesion responsible for instability, and early postoperative immobilization (20). With these guidelines, Rowe reported 98% of patients had good or excellent results and resumption of athletic activity was possible. Pelet et al. (38) concluded that open Bankart repair provides reliable, long-term glenohumeral stability in a study of 29-year follow-up of 30 patients. All returned to their preinjury level of activity. Three patients (10%) had recurrent dislocation and one underwent reoperation (38). Hovelius et al. (39) retrospectively reviewed 26 open Bankart procedures at a mean 17.5-year follow-up and found that one patient had a revision surgery for recurrent instability and one patient had a positive apprehension test. Seventeen patients were "very satisfied" and seven patients were "satisfied." They concluded that open Bankart repair remains the "gold standard" (39).

While the open technique may remain the gold standard overall, advances in arthroscopic technique have provided acceptable outcomes for primary repair of anterior shoulder instability (40,41). In the revision setting, however, open treatment is generally favored. Cho et al. (25) reported the results of open Bankart revision surgery following failed arthroscopic repair and found that 88.5% of patients reported good or excellent results, three patients (11.5%) had redislocation all associated with an engaging Hill-Sachs lesion and hyperlaxity. In revision settings the open Bankart technique is appropriate and can provide satisfactory outcomes with a low recurrence rate, but with the risk of decreased postoperative range of motion.

In addition, the open technique is of particular importance to contact athletes. Rhee et al. (37) reported on a cohort study in contact athletes treated with open Bankart repair (32 shoulders) and arthroscopic repair (16 shoulders). At an average 72-month follow-up, the arthroscopic group had a higher failure rate (25%) compared to the open repair group (12.5%), and thus Rhee recommended open repair for anterior shoulder instability in contact athletes. In an earlier study, Cho reported an unacceptably high recurrent instability rate after arthroscopic stabilization for anterior instability. They enrolled 29 athletes; 14 contact athletes and 15 noncontact athletes. 65.5% returned to near preinjury sports activity level. Five athletes (17.2%) experienced postoperative instability with one subluxation and four redislocations. Four cases (28.6%) of postoperative instability occurred in the contact group whereas one was in the noncontact group (6.7%). There is a high recurrence rate of shoulder dislocations among athletes (17.2%) and the rate is higher among contact athletes (28.6%) as compared to noncontact athletes (6.7%) (36). The recurrence rate of 28.6% for contact athletes is in stark comparison to Pagnani and Dome's (21) data of 3.4% recurrence in football players who had open stabilization. This data combined with Rhee et al.'s (37) data suggest that open Bankart repair is particularly important for young contact athletes.

Several studies have been performed comparing outcomes following open and arthroscopic intervention for anterior instability. Bottoni et al. (42) reported a randomized controlled trial evaluating patients with recurrent anterior shoulder instability who received either arthroscopic (32 patients) or open (29 patients) stabilization. Of the 61 patients evaluated at 32 months postoperatively, there were three clinical failures (two open and one arthroscopic stabilization). No difference was found between open and arthroscopic groups. Both groups were equivalent subjectively. However, the mean loss of motion was greater in the open procedures. Bottoni et al. (42) recommended that arthroscopic stabilization for anterior instability was comparable to the outcomes achieved with the open technique dependent on the patient type and the activity level. In addition, Fabbriciani et al. (43), in a prospective, randomized controlled trial, compared 30 patients with an arthroscopic Bankart repair to 30 patients with an open Bankart procedure. At 2-year follow-up there were no treatment failures in either group. Rowe and Constant scores were similar between the groups. More recently, Archetti et al. (44) reported a randomized controlled trial of arthroscopic versus open techniques in the setting of traumatic anterior instability. There were no significant differences in UCLA or Rose scores nor were there differences in complications or range of motion suggesting that the open and arthroscopic techniques are equivalent.

Several meta-analyses and systematic reviews have been performed looking at the outcomes between open and arthroscopic Bankart repairs. Freedman et al. (45), in a meta-analysis of six studies comparing open Bankart with arthroscopic repair, found there was a higher rate of recurrence of instability with arthroscopic Bankart repair with transglenoid sutures or bioabsorbable tacks (20.3%) as compared to the open Bankart technique (10.3%). More patients undergoing open repair had a good or excellent (88%) Rowe score as compared to arthroscopic repairs (71%) (45). Hobby et al. (46) reported in a systematic review and meta-analysis that there was a significantly higher failure rate after arthroscopic Bankart stabilization using staples or transglenoid sutures as compared to open Bankart repair or arthroscopic repair using suture anchors or bioabsorbable tacks. They reported the rates of failure to be comparable at 2-year follow-up between open repair and arthroscopic repair using suture anchors. Finally, Lenters et al. (47) performed a meta-analysis of 18 studies and reported that open Bankart repair was more effective than arthroscopic procedures in preventing recurrent anterior instability and in enabling patients to return to work and sports. However, they also reported that the arthroscopic repairs resulted in better function in the form of Rowe scores (47).

CONCLUSION

The open Bankart remains the "gold standard" of treatment for anterior instability. The advancement of arthroscopic techniques makes arthroscopic management of anterior instability with a Bankart lesion possible in many cases with comparable outcomes to open repair. However, in revision cases, cases with glenoid bone loss greater than 25%, associated lesions such as the HAGL lesion, and in contact athletes, the open technique remains the treatment of choice and can reliably provide subjective and objective outcomes.

The Arthroscopic Bankart Procedure

Edward S. Chang / Bradford Tucker /
Christopher C. Dodson

INTRODUCTION AND EARLY ARTHROSCOPIC BANKART TECHNIQUE

Historically, the open Bankart repair has been regarded as the gold standard in the treatment of traumatic anterior instability (48). Rowe et al. (20) reported on 161 patients with 162 shoulders that underwent open stabilization. Of the 145 followed, there were five recurrences (3.5%) with 98% of patients rating their results as excellent or good. Rockwood (49) reviewed literature around the world and found a 3% recurrence rate in 2,300 patients who underwent open stabilization, regardless of the technique.

Over the past few decades, the advent of arthroscopy has provided surgeons with a superior view of the glenohumeral joint while minimizing trauma to the surrounding structures. Even with a planned open stabilization, a diagnostic arthroscopy is often implemented during the same surgical setting (50).

As arthroscopy became more widely implemented, surgeons began to develop techniques to treat shoulder instability without an open approach. As with any surgical advancement, the goal of arthroscopic stabilization was to improve on open results, while minimizing complications. This procedure was believed to be advantageous due to decreasing surgical morbidity and improved postoperative range of motion (5).

With improving technology coevolving with arthroscopic techniques incorporating open treatment principles, the arthroscopic Bankart procedure has become a mainstay in treating traumatic anterior instability.

Staple Capsulorrhaphy

The use of open staple capsulorrhaphy was implemented in the early mid 20th century. Although early, short-term results were favorable, O'Driscoll and Evans (51) reported a 22% dislocation rate, which increased in frequency with the duration of follow-up. Hardware loosening and migration was significant (12%), and pain and arthrosis were more frequent with these complications.

Arthroscopic staple capsulorrhaphy was met with a similar fate (52,53). The high failure rate along with potentially devastating complications led the surgeons to all but abandon the procedure.

Transglenoid Suture

As with staple capsulorrhaphy, transglenoid suture fixation of the capsulolabral lesion was first described as an open technique by Viek and Bell (54) in 1959. Morgan and Bodenstab (55) later popularized an arthroscopic procedure. The main advantage of the technique was the ability to stabilize the capsule–labral junction extra-articularly, leaving no hardware in the glenohumeral joint. The authors reported excellent early results with no recurrences.

Other results (56,57) have been less favorable and it was believed that tying sutures over the posterior infraspinatus fascia did not allow for consistent tensioning of the anterior structures, as well as placing the suprascapular nerve at risk.

O'Neill (58) had superior results, employing a modified technique of bluntly exposing the posterior scapula, ensuring advancement of the knot to the bone, without entrapment of the soft tissue. Of the 41 patients prospectively studied, 40 went on to return to their sports, with two patients experiencing recurrent instability (5%). However, due to the variable recurrence rate as well as the risk of nerve injury, this technique has fallen out of favor.

Bioabsorbable Tacks

The development of bioabsorbable tacks was triggered by the desire to repair Bankart lesions arthroscopically while avoiding the complications associated with metal implants and the transglenoid technique (59). Bioabsorbable tacks were employed with some success (recurrence rate 10% to 21%) (60), specifically in patients with isolated Bankart lesions without capsular laxity or redundancy. The authors also noted that patients requiring a capsulorrhaphy or capsular shift had a high likelihood of failing this procedure.

Suture Anchors

The introduction of arthroscopic fixation of capsular and labral tissues to the glenoid via suture anchors is the culmination of arthroscopic instrumentation and technique advancement. This procedure, first described by Wolf (35), combines the technique of open stabilization with arthroscopic technology. It also avoids the limitations and complications experienced by previous arthroscopic methods without compromising fixation. In a biomechanics study using a canine model, McEleney et al. (61) showed suture anchor repair to be superior compared to other techniques.

The clinical results of suture anchor repair have been favorable as well. Gartman et al. (62) reported on

53 patients treated with a minimum of 2-year follow-up. Ninety-two percent had good-to-excellent outcomes, with four patients experiencing recurrent instability. It was also noted that capsular tension by suture technique was supplemented by thermal capsulorrhaphy in 48 patients. The authors attributed their low recurrence rate to repair of any additional labral lesions along with rotator interval closure.

Kim et al. (41) prospectively evaluated 167 patients with traumatic, recurrent anterior instability treated with suture anchors. 159 patients (95%), with a mean follow-up of 44 months, had good-to-excellent outcomes with a recurrence rate of 4%.

Arthroscopic stabilization in the high-demand patient, including contact athletes, was also reported to be successful. Bacilla et al. (63) followed 40 patients with a mean follow-up of 30 months. Thirty-seven of the 40 returned to normal activities, including 29 of 32 patients involved in athletics, by 6 months. The recurrence rate was 7%.

Mazzocca et al. (7) reviewed 18 patients involved in contact or collision sports who underwent arthroscopic suture anchor repair. All returned to organized sports with two patients (11%) experiencing recurrent instability (both collision athletes). The overall recurrence rate for collision athletes was 15% (2 of 13 patients), leading the authors to conclude that participating in collision or contact sports was not a contraindication to arthroscopic anterior stabilization.

The biomechanical and clinical literature suggests that arthroscopic Bankart repair with suture anchors is a reliable operation in the setting of anterior traumatic instability. Furthermore, recent studies show that it can be a successful procedure in contact and collision athletes. Currently, most orthopedic surgeons employ suture anchors when performing arthroscopic Bankart repairs. Whether or not the outcomes are superior to open anterior stabilization remains an area of debate.

The Case for Arthroscopic Stabilization

Arthroscopic Bankart repair has become increasingly popular in the treatment of anterior instability. Historically, open shoulder stabilization has been associated with a lower recurrence rate. However, long-term studies show that many patients had significant decreases in range of motion, most notably external rotation (17). This is likely due to the violation of the subscapularis during the exposure.

The advantages of an arthroscopic procedure are improved cosmesis and decreased surgical morbidity, leading to better overall range of motion (5). With improved surgical techniques, likely from a combination of instrument development and greater surgeon experience and comfort, arthroscopic stabilization has become ever increasingly popular.

Early arthroscopic techniques (e.g., transglenoid sutures, bioabsorbable tacks) did not fare well compared to open techniques. Gaunche et al. (64) compared open and arthroscopic stabilization in 27 patients with anterior instability. Transglenoid suture technique was mostly employed. With a mean follow-up of 26 months, there was a higher recurrence rate in the arthroscopic group (5 of 15) versus the open group (1 of 12).

Freedman et al. (45) performed a meta-analysis comparing the results of arthroscopic stabilization (172 patients) with transglenoid sutures or bioabsorbable tacks versus open stabilization (156 patients). The arthroscopic group had a significantly higher recurrence rate (12.6% vs. 3.4%).

With the introduction of the arthroscopic suture anchor, recent studies have suggested that arthroscopic repair with suture anchors may be a viable alternative to open stabilization. Kim et al. (65) compared arthroscopic suture anchor repair (58 patients) to open Bankart repair (30 patients) over a mean follow-up of 39 months. Both groups showed good-to-excellent results in greater than 85% of patients. The arthroscopic group had slightly higher Rowe and UCLA scores. Two patients (6.7%) in the open group and two patients in the arthroscopic group (3.4%) demonstrated a recurrent dislocation. Overall residual instability was similar (10% in the open group vs. 10.2% in the arthroscopic group).

A prospective, randomized clinical trial conducted by Bottoni et al. (42) compared open stabilization versus arthroscopic stabilization with suture anchors by a single surgeon. Both groups had statistically significant improvement and subjective satisfaction. The open group experienced two failures, compared to one failure in the arthroscopic group. The mean surgical time was 59 minutes in the arthroscopic group versus 149 minutes in the open group. There was a greater loss of motion versus the contralateral side in the open group. The authors concluded that clinical outcomes of arthroscopic stabilization are comparable to open stabilization.

The most recent meta-analysis of the literature was conducted by Pulavarti et al. (66). The authors included three randomized controlled trials comparing open versus arthroscopic repair of anterior traumatic instability. All the three trials had a minimum of 2-year follow-up. Pooled results revealed no significant difference between the two groups regarding recurrent instability in subsequent instability-related surgery. There was also no significant difference regarding the functional outcome.

The lack of randomized controlled trials comparing arthroscopic to open repair for recurrent anterior shoulder instability makes it difficult to come to a definitive conclusion. However, more recent evidence shows arthroscopic stabilization has a slightly inferior recurrence rate with decreased surgical morbidity and better overall range of motion as compared to open stabilization. It is in our opinion, that with careful patient selection and awareness of technical considerations, the clinical results of an arthroscopic Bankart repair can approach those of the open repair.

INDICATIONS FOR ARTHROSCOPIC STABILIZATION

At our institution, we routinely perform arthroscopic anterior stabilization in patients with primary recurrent anterior instability as well as patients with failed stabilization without significant glenoid bone loss or other risk factors known to have poor arthroscopic results (i.e., large Hill-Sachs lesions, HAGL lesions, capsular deficiency). Patients who participate in contact sports are not a contraindication to arthroscopic stabilization. However, these patients are counseled that they are at a higher risk for recurrence should they return to their previous level of activity.

Treatment of the Young, Active First-time Dislocator

There is also an increasing trend to stabilize first-time dislocators in the young athlete, especially those involved in high-risk activities. Recent literature has supported acute operative intervention in this group.

Bottoni et al. (67) randomized 21 young, active patients in the military sustaining a first-time anterior dislocation. These patients either received arthroscopic stabilization with a bioabsorbable tack or nonoperative treatment with immobilization followed by supervised rehabilitation. At 3-year follow-up, the redislocation rate was 11% in the operative group and 75% in the nonoperative. Furthermore, a majority of the recurrent dislocators in the nonoperative group required open anterior stabilization.

The in-season athlete can be managed with immobilization followed by early range of motion and therapy directed at strengthening the dynamic glenohumeral stabilizers (68). It is important to counsel the athletes returning to play about the risk of further damage to the shoulder should recurrent dislocations occur.

Return to play with bracing is then appropriate as long as the athlete does not experience any recurrent instability events and is able to safely perform sport-specific activities. If the athlete redislocates or is unable to participate in drills, surgical stabilization is generally recommended.

AUTHORS' PREFERRED METHOD OF TREATMENT

Based on results published using suture anchors for arthroscopic stabilization and our experience with them, we generally treat traumatic anterior instability via this approach. As mentioned earlier, the goal of surgery is to reattach the labrum, capsule, and ligaments to their anatomic position. The diagnosis is made in the office following an extensive history and physical and review of the radiographs. Advanced preoperative imaging such as an MRI or MRI arthrogram is routinely obtained to verify the diagnosis and aid in surgical planning.

Setup and Patient Positioning

An interscalene block on the operative side is generally administered prior to surgery. Once identified, the patient is brought back into the operating theatre and induction of general anesthesia occurs. The patient is then placed in the beach chair position. The kidney rests should be tightly positioned on both sides of the patient. Before sitting the patient up, a pillow is placed under the knees of the patient and the foot of the bed is lowered approximately 45 degrees. In certain individuals at risk for orthostatic hypotension, the patient should be brought up half way first and blood pressure should then be recorded. Once the vital signs are deemed appropriate by anesthesia, the patient is then brought up the rest of the way.

Examination Under Anesthesia and Prep and Drape

Antibiotics are administered and a time-out is performed. An examination under anesthesia is performed. Range of motion and stability in multiple directions (anterior, posterior, and inferior) are tested and recorded. The ability to perform an accurate and thorough examination under anesthesia is paramount in the treatment of patients with shoulder instability. The patient is then prepped and draped sterilely.

Anatomic landmarks are then marked out including the scapular spine, acromion, clavicle, acromioclavicular joint, and the coracoid process. The arm is then placed in a McConnell arm holder (McConnell Orthopedic Manufacturing Company, Greenville, Tex).

Diagnostic Arthroscopy

A posterior portal is established 2 cm inferior and 2 cm medial to the posterolateral acromion. We prefer a slightly more medial portal for anterior instability cases to aid in visualization of the Bankart lesion. The arthroscope is placed atraumatically into the glenohumeral joint and an anterolateral rotator interval viewing portal is created under direct visualization.

A diagnostic arthroscopy is performed prior to any intervention (Fig. 7-2). Once the Bankart lesion and associated pathology are identified, it is important to rule out other conditions including rotator cuff tears, labral tears at the posterior and anterior–superior

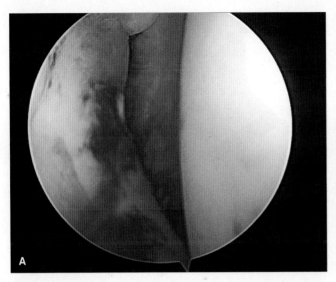
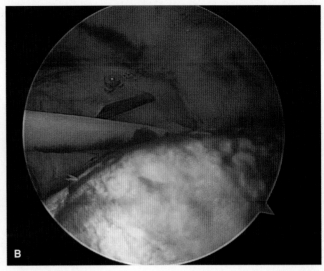

▲ **FIGURE 7-2:** Arthroscopic view demonstrating a Bankart lesion. **A:** Standard posterior viewing portal. **B:** A superolateral rotator interval viewing portal is then established under direct visualization.

glenoid, and large bony loss in the glenoid or in the humerus (Hill-Sachs lesion). Glenoid bone loss greater than 20% or a large engaging Hill-Sachs lesion during external rotation warrants consideration to convert to an open procedure. A drive-through sign is also performed to confirm glenohumeral instability.

Arthroscopic Bankart Repair

Once the diagnosis is established and there is no associated bony loss requiring an open repair or reconstruction, an anterior–inferior portal is established. The placement of this portal is critical and a spinal needle is first used to confirm access to both the anterior–inferior

glenoid and the glenoid face. A second anterior superolateral portal is then established and using a switching stick the scope is placed through this portal. This portal is critical because it allows for an "anterior view" of the glenoid and the labrum (Fig. 7-3A). The detached labrum is mobilized from the glenoid using a tissue elevator via the standard anterior portal. The pictures need to be changed to reflect the changes in text. We typically mobilize the capsulolabral complex until the underbelly of the subscapularis muscle is visualized. This results in labrum "floating" next to the glenoid indicating adequate mobilization. A rasp and a motorized shaver are then used to create a bleeding surface to enhance tissue healing (Fig. 7-3B).

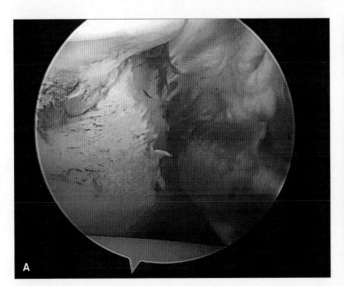
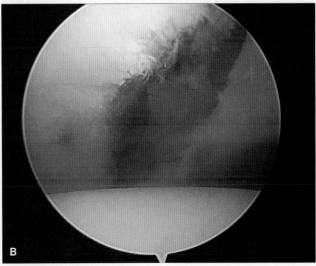

▲ **FIGURE 7-3:** Arthroscopic view from superolateral rotator interval viewing portal. **A:** An arthroscopic elevator is used to mobilize the capsule–labral complex from the glenoid. **B:** Mobilized labral complex and glenoid following the introduction of an arthroscopic shaver and rasp to create a healing surface on the glenoid.

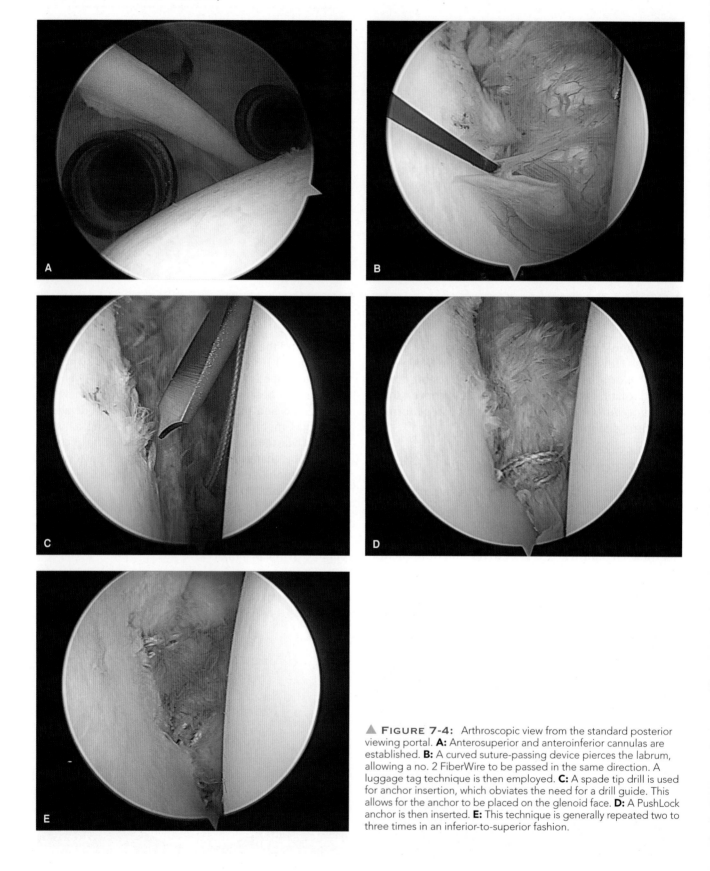

▲ FIGURE 7-4: Arthroscopic view from the standard posterior viewing portal. **A:** Anterosuperior and anteroinferior cannulas are established. **B:** A curved suture-passing device pierces the labrum, allowing a no. 2 FiberWire to be passed in the same direction. A luggage tag technique is then employed. **C:** A spade tip drill is used for anchor insertion, which obviates the need for a drill guide. This allows for the anchor to be placed on the glenoid face. **D:** A PushLock anchor is then inserted. **E:** This technique is generally repeated two to three times in an inferior-to-superior fashion.

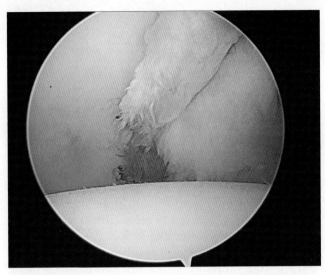

▲ FIGURE 7-5: Arthroscopic view from superolateral rotator interval viewing portal demonstrating completed Bankart repair.

A curved suture-passing device is introduced via the anterior portal and pierces the capsule and the labrum below the desired anchor position, ensuring a capsular shift will occur during the repair. A no. 2 Fiber-Wire (Arthrex Inc., Naples, FL) is then passed through, with both strands retrieved and stored through the anteroinferior cannula (Fig. 7-4B,C) in a luggage tag fashion.

A 2.9-mm Biocomposite PushLock anchor (Arthrex Inc., Naples, FL) is then introduced to the glenoid face superior to the previously captured tissue. During insertion, tensioning of the capsule and the labrum can be adjusted by pulling on the ends of the no. 2 suture (Fig. 7-4D,E). Generally, this is repeated two to three times, with each anchor placed more superior on the glenoid rim (Fig. 7-5).

Following the Bankart repair, anterior stability is then reassessed as well as the need for further capsular plication or closure specifically in the rotator interval. A drive-through sign is also repeated as another measure to ensure stability.

Postoperative Rehabilitation

Following surgery, patients are placed in an abduction sling for 4 weeks, coming out of the sling only for elbow range of motion and basic scapular retraction exercises. After 4 weeks, the sling is discontinued and formal physical therapy is initiated. Generally speaking, therapy continues for 3 to 4 months at which point patients transition to a home exercise program. Return to full athletics begins at 5 months and contact sports are prohibited until 6 to 7 months post op.

SUMMARY

The advances in arthroscopic techniques have allowed for the surgeons to perform many procedures arthroscopically while preserving the principles that made open techniques highly successful. The literature has started to demonstrate that arthroscopic anterior stabilization is comparable to open stabilization and future prospective studies will most likely support this.

We believe that arthroscopic anterior stabilization is a highly effective procedure to eliminate anterior shoulder instability. It should not be considered in patients with significant bone loss, capsular deficiency, or HAGL lesions and in certain cases of previously failed stabilizations.

Double-Row Capsulolabral Repair

Matthew M. Thompson / Joshua S. Dines /
David W. Altchek

Shoulder stabilization techniques have progressed from open procedures such as those described by Bankart, Helfet, and Latarjet more than 60 years ago to arthroscopic techniques using suture anchors (33,69). Unfortunately, recent studies describing even the most modern arthroscopic techniques and implants are still reporting recurrent instability rates >10% (70–72). Burkhart and De Beer (23) have elucidated the fact that instability in the setting of significant glenoid bone loss or inverted pear-shaped glenoids treated arthroscopically are at higher risk of recurrence (73). In these situations, a bone graft type operation is very appropriate. Improved outcomes have been reported in these situations with the Latarjet procedure (74,75), but the procedure is not without complications including nerve injury, arthritis, and hardware issues (76). In an effort to improve surgical outcomes in anterior shoulder instability, double-row capsulolabral repair techniques, similar in concept to double-row rotator cuff repair, are being investigated.

To determine the best repair technique for capsulolabral injuries associated with anterior shoulder instability, it is important to understand both the injury pattern and the anatomy of the capsulolabral attachment to the anterior–inferior glenoid. This chapter focuses on (1) the anatomy of the capsule and labrum by reviewing recent anatomical and biomechanical studies; (2) the indications for which double-row labral repair may be considered; and (3) reviewing open and arthroscopic double-row repair techniques.

ANATOMY AND BIOMECHANICS

The anatomy of the capsular attachment to the glenoid and the labrum has been delineated in several studies, and variations in attachment have been described. Capsular attachment primarily to the labrum was found in 80% of adult specimens (77) and 77% of embryos (78), which has been termed a type 1 origin. A type 2 origin was found in the other 20% and 23% of shoulders, in which the capsule is attached solely to the glenoid neck. Another study looking at the attachment of the entire capsulolabral complex found it to be attached to cartilage and bone in 88% of shoulders and only to bone in 12% of shoulders (79), though separate capsular and labral attachments were not distinguished. This type 2 capsular origin could have implications in performing a Bankart repair if the labrum is repaired but inadequate attention is given to the capsular repair, since in about 20% of shoulders the capsule appears to attach primarily to the bone and not the labrum.

Also described is the medial-to-lateral width of the attachment of the capsulolabral complex to the bone. The attachment was noted to range from a width of 4.3 to 11.5 mm between the 2-o'clock and 6-o'clock positions, with the widest attachment between the 3-o' clock and 4-o'clock positions (77,79,80). This relatively broad width of attachment suggests that a double-row labral repair would recreate the native capsulolabral footprint better than a single-row repair. In fact, this was shown in a study in which recreation of the capsulolabral footprint was measured after performing single- and double-row repairs (80). For the single-row repair, four anchors were placed along the glenoid rim from 2:30 to 5:30 clock positions, with simple knots placed around 1 cm of capsulolabral tissue. For the double-row technique, four medial anchors were placed on the anterior glenoid neck, and then the sutures were passed laterally into four knotless anchors on the glenoid rim, compressing the capsule onto the anterior glenoid as well as fixing the capsulolabral tissue to the rim. The surface area covered by the double-row repair was 103% larger, or twice the size of the single-row repair. The single-row repair recreated only 42% of the native capsulolabral attachment, while the double-row repair recreated 86% of the attachment.

A similar study was done comparing mean contact pressure in double-row and single-row repairs (81) using a similar anchor configuration and repair technique as reported by Ahmad et al. (80). The mean contact pressure in the double-row repair was 38% greater than that in the single-row repair, and the double-row repair also covered a larger surface area (78% vs. 39%) of the native capsulolabral attachment.

Another cadaver study (82,27) assessed load to failure of double-row versus single-row capsulolabral repairs, and found a significantly greater load to failure in the double-row repair (374 N) versus the single-row repair (225 N). In this study, the single-row repair was done with three anchors placed along the anteroinferior glenoid rim with simple knots placed around 1 cm of capsulolabral tissue. The double-row repair was done with three anchors placed along the anteroinferior glenoid rim, tying a simple knot around the labrum for the middle anchor and then feeding the two suture limbs from each of the end anchors around capsulolabral tissue and into knotless anchors placed 1 cm medially on

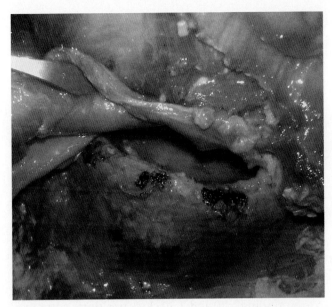

▲ **FIGURE 7-6:** Positions marked for three glenoid rim anchors and two medial knotless anchors.

the anterior glenoid in a suture bridge configuration (Figs. 7-6 and 7-7). This "W" configuration is similar to the Cassiopeia technique described by Lafosse et al. (83), except that knotless anchors were used medially to bridge the suture over the capsulolabral complex on the anterior glenoid in a mattress fashion.

Several biomechanical studies have shown that the creation of a Bankart lesion, by releasing the capsulolabral attachment off the anterior–inferior glenoid, increases humeral translation but does not result in an anterior shoulder dislocation (84–87). Further capsular injury superiorly and posteriorly is required in order for complete dislocation of the shoulder to occur. This is an important concept to consider—more than just a labral tear must occur to result in shoulder dislocation. This has implications when performing an anterior stabilization

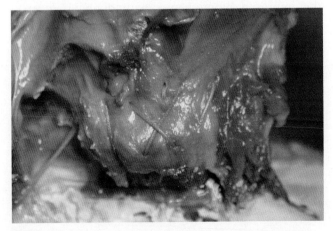

▲ **FIGURE 7-7:** Double-row capsulolabral repair showing a mattress configuration with suture limbs from the superior and inferior glenoid rim anchors secured medially with knotless anchors.

procedure, in that capsular injury needs to be adequately assessed and then addressed in the repair, rather than directing too much attention on fixing the labral tear without regard to the capsule. In regards to this concept, a double-row capsulolabral repair may provide for an overall improved healing environment, with evidence of stronger pull-out strength of the initial repair, better recreation of the native footprint (80), and increased mean contact pressure in the repaired area (81).

SURGICAL INDICATIONS

When determining which surgical technique to use, it is important to assess for glenoid fracture/deficiency, engaging Hill-Sachs defect, HAGL lesion, anterior labral periosteal sleeve avulsion (ALPSA) lesion, glenolabral articular disruption (GLAD) lesion, rotator cuff tear (particularly in older patients) and patient factors such as age, ligamentous laxity, recurrent dislocations, prior stabilization surgery and playing contact sports. These factors may require changing the surgical plan, and some have been associated with a higher recurrence rate, particularly with arthroscopic procedures (23,73,88). It is in some of these circumstances that a double-row repair may be beneficial. In the ALPSA lesion where extensive capsulolabral release and mobilization is required, a double-row repair may offer better healing potential by opposing a larger amount of capsulolabral tissue to its insertion than a single-row repair would. Double-row arthroscopic repair of bony Bankart lesions has also been described (89–92), with the benefits of two-point fixation of the bony fragment, and avoiding splitting of the fragment which may occur with the use of screws or a penetrator to pass a suture through the fragment. When performing open anterior stabilization for any of these situations, a double-row repair has potential benefits in that a greater amount of the capsulolabral footprint is restored and the pull-out strength of the repair appears to be greater (80,82,93).

SURGICAL TECHNIQUES

Capsulolabral repair techniques have evolved with improved understanding of anatomy and the development of more versatile fixation methods. Similar to recent research on double-row rotator cuff repair, several techniques have been described for both open and arthroscopic double-row labral repairs (83,89–95). Lafosse et al. (83) first described a technique for arthroscopic double-row labral repair with two anchors placed medially on the anterior glenoid and three anchors on the glenoid rim in a "W" configuration, terming it the Cassiopeia technique. The technique was developed out of concern for healing of the capsulolabral complex more medially along the glenoid neck, which is not conventionally addressed with a single-row technique with fixation only at the glenoid rim. One of the more technically difficult aspects of the procedure is that a more medial and inferior trans-subscapularis portal was used to place the medial anchors. Simple knots were tied with each suture. With short-term follow-up no complications were noted in 12 patients. The concept behind the technique is that the capsule fixed to the anterior labrum with medial anchors provides a greater surface area for healing than just fixing the labrum at the glenoid rim. This technique does not use knotless anchors and sutures are not passed from the medial to lateral row to achieve compression of the tissue between the anchors. In relation to rotator cuff repair, this technique is similar to a standard double-row repair in contrast to a transosseous-equivalent technique, with a potential drawback being that optimal compression of the tissue between the medial and lateral anchors may not be achieved.

Ahmad et al. (80) describes an arthroscopic double-row labral repair technique which is similar to a transosseous-equivalent rotator cuff repair, using knotless anchors on the glenoid rim to secure sutures from the medial anchors. Specific technical aspects of the procedure include thorough mobilization of the capsulolabral complex off the anterior glenoid, placement of two to three 2.4-mm anchors 10 mm medial to the glenoid rim either percutaneously or through a low anterior portal just above the subscapularis tendon, use of a suture lasso to shuttle the sutures around the medial aspect of the capsulolabral tissue, and fixation of both suture limbs with a corresponding 2.9-mm knotless anchor on the glenoid rim. Viewing through the anterosuperior portal for placement of the medial anchors is helpful, and suture management is a crucial aspect of the procedure. At an average of 6 months follow-up, there had been no complications in six patients who underwent this procedure. Other similar arthroscopic double-row capsulolabral repair techniques have been described, which can be used with or without the presence of a small-to-moderate-sized bony Bankart lesion.

For open double-row capsulolabral repair, Altchek has described the use of two medial row and two lateral row anchors with a suture bridge configuration (93). In this technique, after incising and tagging the subscapularis, the capsule is incised laterally along its humeral attachment, exposing the joint. The capsulolabral complex is elevated from the anteroinferior glenoid rim and neck, and a pitchfork retractor is placed deep to the capsule exposing the glenoid neck. Two 3-mm suture anchors are placed at the 5:30 and 4:30 clock positions 10 mm medial to the glenoid rim. The pitchfork retractor is then placed outside the capsule and deep to the subscapularis, and the sutures are passed around the medial edge of the capsulolabral complex. The sutures are not tied. They are then secured with two 2.9-mm PushLock knotless anchors on the glenoid rim at the corresponding 4:30 and 5:30 clock positions, compressing the capsulolabral complex over its native insertion. Capsular shift can then be performed as indicated when repairing the capsule laterally to the humerus.

Just as double-row repair has shown biomechanical advantages in the rotator cuff, studies are showing the same benefits in capsulolabral repair. The benefits shown so far in the limited studies that are available are greater coverage of the native footprint (89), higher mean contact pressure over this area (81), and higher pull-out strength. It is uncertain yet whether these benefits will translate to improved clinical results. The double-row technique may be well suited for more complex situations, such as when an ALPSA lesion or bony Bankart is present, or in higher risk patients such as contact athletes or those with multiple prior dislocations or failed stabilization surgery. With improved surgical techniques and suture anchors, double-row capsulolabral repair is becoming a more viable option for the surgeons. Further research, especially clinical outcome studies, will be needed to assess its utility in specific situations, though the improved biomechanics with double-row repair should spur the surgeons to consider repair options beyond the standard single-row technique.

Bone Block/Latarjet Procedure

Thomas Obermeyer / Brad Parsons

INTRODUCTION

Glenoid bone loss after anterior glenohumeral dislocation can occur due to acute fracture or a more chronic process of bony resorption and compression after recurrent anterior instability. Anterior glenoid fracture after traumatic glenohumeral dislocation results in disruption of the osseous concavity of the glenoid as well as the IGHL complex , termed the bony Bankart lesion (22). These "separation fractures," readily apparent on imaging, contrast with "compression fractures" or a more chronic abrasive process, where anterior glenoid deficiency exists without an identifiable fracture fragment (96). The latter situation of glenoid bone loss without a repairable bony fragment has been identified as a risk factor in failure of arthroscopic and open soft tissue stabilization procedures (23,88,97,98), and is frequently underappreciated on routine imaging. Glenoid bone loss can be effectively managed by glenoid reconstruction by transferring the osteotomized coracoid process to the area of glenoid deficiency, first described by Latarjet in 1954 (96).

As experience with Latarjet's procedure grew in the years following the initial description, modifications have been proposed. In 1958, Helfet (99) described the Bristow technique, in which the tip of the coracoid is sutured to the capsuloperiosteal attachments of the anterior glenoid, which was later modified to include screw fixation. The Bristow technique utilized one screw and the tip of the coracoid was placed end-on onto the glenoid neck, while the Latarjet procedure utilized a larger length of coracoid, two screws, and the inferior surface of the coracoid was oriented toward the glenoid neck. Early success with the Latarjet procedure was hypothesized to occur via three primary mechanisms (100): The effect of the tensioned conjoint tendon when the shoulder is abducted and externally rotated, creating a "sling" of glenohumeral support on the inferior capsule; the structural support of the bone block; and the capsular tension generated by suturing capsule to the conjoint tendon. The original technique involved cutting the subscapularis tendon, but this has been modified to a subscapularis split, so the tendon and muscle fibers remain in continuity.

PREOPERATIVE EVALUATION

As detailed in prior chapters, a complete history including age at initial dislocation, mechanism for dislocation, and maneuvers/force required for dislocation and reduction is important to obtain. Specifically, a history of recurrent instability, especially when associated with progressively less force required to induce instability, such as dislocation during activities of daily living or while sleeping, should raise suspicion for anterior glenoid erosion. Examination should assess the ease of instability (how much abduction, external rotation results in apprehension) and provocative tests such as anterior load and shift or the apprehension/relocation signs are helpful. The finding of a Gagey sign indicates IGHL attenuation or rupture, either at the capsular attachment at the glenoid or via an unstable bony Bankart lesion (101). Axillary nerve function should always be assessed (including lateral arm sensation and ability to fire all three deltoid heads). Signs for multidirectional hyperlaxity should also be evaluated (elbow and metacarpophalangeal hyperextension), including assessment for a sulcus sign, as these may further indicate the potential failure of a soft tissue stabilization procedure.

Routine radiographs should include orthogonal views of the scapula with the shoulder in neutral and in external rotations, which may help to identify a Hill-Sachs lesion (102), as well as axillary and outlet views. Bernageau et al. (103) described a profile view of the glenoid, which has been demonstrated to be of benefit in identifying anterior glenoid bone fracture fragments and understanding the degree of compression/rounding of the anterior glenoid rim (104). It may be helpful to compare radiographs (particularly glenoid profile views) with the contralateral unaffected shoulder. CT scanning with three-dimensional reconstructions (with humeral head subtraction) allows for excellent characterization of osseous anatomy (104) (Fig. 7-8), although MRI (often with arthrogram) may assist in identifying the severity of the capsulolabral injury as well as in identifying concomitant pathology (e.g., SLAP or rotator cuff tears). Although these studies are helpful, none has prospectively evaluated a critical threshold of bone loss requiring augmentation, although several authors have developed criteria and scoring systems to assist in determining the significance of the bone loss and its contribution to instability (102).

INDICATIONS

Previous studies have cited that glenoid bone loss of less than 20% may be amenable to arthroscopic soft tissue repair alone (22,23). One biomechanical study showed

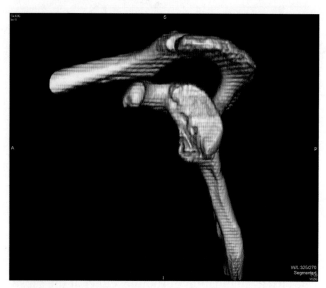

▲ **FIGURE 7-8:** Three-dimensional reconstruction of the scapula (with humeral head subtraction) demonstrating the extent of anterior bone loss.

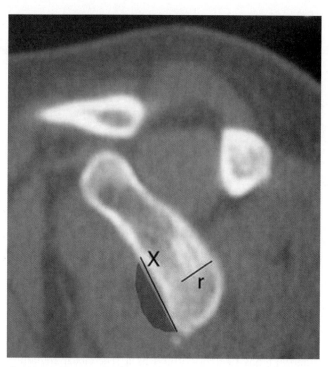

▲ **FIGURE 7-9:** Gerber's CT-based method of assessing bone loss. Here the width of the defect (x) is greater than half the maximum width of the glenoid (r), and therefore, bony augmentation is indicated using these criteria.

that when the width of the glenoid osseous defect is less than 21% of the glenoid length, significantly less force is required to anteriorly translate the glenohumeral joint (105). Another biomechanical study similarly showed that the translational force was significantly decreased after soft tissue capsulolabral repair when 19% or more of the glenoid length was removed (106). Other authors suggest that the arthroscopic appearance of the glenoid as an "inverted pear" represents 25% to 27% loss of width of the inferior glenoid and use this as an indication for a bone grafting procedure (107). No studies have prospectively evaluated the "critical" limit of glenoid bone loss necessitating osseous reconstruction, although recent studies have confirmed that the presence of 20% glenoid bone loss is a risk factor for recurrence following soft tissue repair (97).

Chuang et al. (108) demonstrated that preoperative three-dimensional CT scanning could accurately predict the need for an open bone grafting procedure when compared with the gold standard of arthroscopic evaluation of bone loss. These authors used 25% as the threshold of requiring glenoid bone grafting. The CT scan evaluating for bone loss should ideally be analyzed using objective area measurements of bone loss on the sagittal CT scan *en face* through the glenoid, as some authors have noted that bone loss can easily be underestimated if not measured, especially if axial CT views are used for estimating bone loss (108). When analyzing the sagittal CT scans and objective area measurements are not available, the method used by Gerber and Nyffeler (98) of comparing the radius of the inferior glenoid to the length of the defect may be helpful (Fig. 7-9). These authors have suggested that if the length of the defect (X) is greater than half the maximum width of the glenoid (W/2), consideration should be given to bony augmen-

tation. It should also be noted that many patients with glenoid lesions have corresponding Hill-Sachs lesions that may further increase the effect of glenoid deficiency on success of repair (109). It is important to identify the cumulative effect of both glenoid and humeral head bony deficits on the instability of the shoulder when determining the best treatment plan. For example, some have advocated the utilization of glenoid bone augmentation (such as the Latarjet procedure) to treat the unstable shoulder with moderate glenoid bone loss (<20%) but associated moderate to large Hill-Sachs defects, with the premise that by widening the glenoid with the coracoid transfer, the Hill-Sachs is no longer able to engage the rim of the glenoid and induce instability (23).

When used in conjunction with careful scrutiny of CT scans, scoring systems may be useful to identify patients at high risk of instability after soft tissue capsulolabral repair. Balg and Boileau (102) developed the instability severity index score (ISIS) based on retrospective analysis of risk factors for recurrent instability after soft tissue Bankart repair. Their scoring system uses factors of initial dislocation at age <20, involvement in overhead throwing or collision sports, hyperlaxity, and anteroposterior radiographic identification of Hill-Sachs or glenoid lesions as factors important in recurrent instability. Boileau et al. (110) have furthered the indications for Latarjet to include those patients who have undergone failed prior capsulolabral repair, with good results in this subset of previously operated patients (111).

CONTRAINDICATIONS

While the presence of glenoid osseous defects is very common in shoulders with recurrent unilateral glenohumeral instability, defects large enough to require coracoid transfer is only among a small subpopulation of these patients. Sugaya et al. (104) showed that among 100 recurrently unstable shoulders, 50% had the presence of a glenoid osseous lesion, but only one patient had a lesion greater than 20% of the glenoid surface area. Patients with smaller glenoid lesions (less than 20% of the surface area of the glenoid) may be amenable for arthroscopic or open soft tissue stabilization. Patients who are first-time dislocators or have glenoid fractures amenable to reduction and fixation generally do not warrant coracoid transfer or bony augmentation. Other contraindications include axillary neuropathy with incompetent deltoid function, uncontrolled seizures or movement disorders (112), infection, and advanced pre-existent osteoarthritis.

SURGICAL TECHNIQUE

Various alterations of technique have been described for the Latarjet procedure in the literature, including the surgical approach (skin incision, subscapularis management, and recently, open vs. arthroscopic techniques) as well as the orientation of the transferred coracoid process. We utilize the classic "French" technique as advocated by Young et al. (113) which utilizes a limited deltopectoral approach, a subscapularis split, and a classic orientation of the coracoid, placing the inferior decorticated surface against the neck of the glenoid, such that the lateral coracoid surface articulates with the glenohumeral joint. We describe this technique below.

The patient is placed in the beach chair position with the arm supported. We often utilize intraoperative neuromonitoring (continuous EMG and SSEP) throughout the procedure to protect the brachial plexus, especially the musculocutaneous and axillary nerves. A bump is placed along the thoracic spine along the medial scapula to prevent scapular protraction and make the coracoid as prominent as possible. A limited deltopectoral approach is used with the incision extending from the tip of the coracoid process inferiorly to the axillary crease (Fig. 7-10). The cephalic vein is taken laterally. Dissection is carried through the clavipectoral fascia and the coracoid is exposed with the arm in abduction and external rotation to relax deltoid tension. A Hohmann retractor is then placed over the top of the coracoid process. The lateral coracoid is freed by incising the coracoacromial ligament approximately 1 cm from its coracoid attachment (Fig. 7-11). The coracohumeral ligament, lying deep to the coracoacromial ligament, is incised.

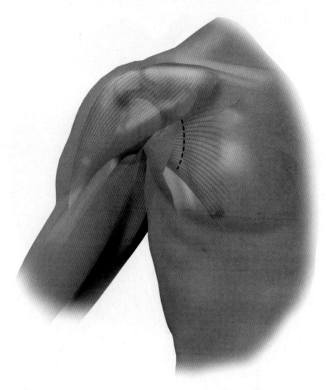

▲ **FIGURE 7-10:** The skin incision extends from the coracoid tip to the axillary crease.

The arm is then abducted and internally rotated to expose the medial coracoid. The pectoralis minor is released from its coracoid attachment with electrocautery, with care taken not to devascularize the tendon. The soft tissue on the inferior undersurface of the coracoid is removed with a periosteal elevator. Using a

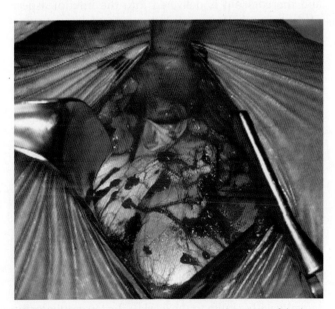

▲ **FIGURE 7-11:** Retractor placement with incision of the coracoacromial ligament using electrocautery.

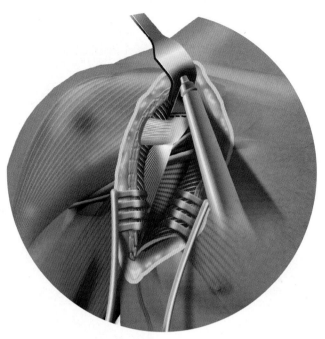

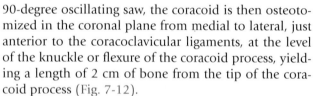

▲ **FIGURE 7-12:** The coracoid is osteotomized at the "knee" with a right-angle oscillating saw.

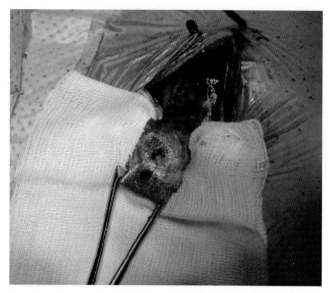

▲ **FIGURE 7-13:** The coracoid is elevated into the wound and prepared with a burr or oscillating saw and 3.2-mm drill holes are placed approximately 1 cm apart.

90-degree oscillating saw, the coracoid is then osteotomized in the coronal plane from medial to lateral, just anterior to the coracoclavicular ligaments, at the level of the knuckle or flexure of the coracoid process, yielding a length of 2 cm of bone from the tip of the coracoid process (Fig. 7-12).

To complete the coracoid harvest, the arm is abducted and externally rotated and the coracoid is freed from attachments to the coracohumeral ligament. The arm is then returned to a neutral position and the coracoid is delivered into the inferior aspect of the wound. The coracoid is prepared by removing soft tissue attachments at the graft site using a knife, and an oscillating saw or burr is used to decorticate the undersurface of the coracoid to optimize bony healing. An osteotome is placed to protect the skin and two drill holes are made 1 cm apart, with the holes in the central axis of the coracoid approximately 1 cm apart (Fig. 7-13). The coracoid is then pushed underneath the pectoralis major to expose the underlying subscapularis muscle.

The superior and inferior margins of the subscapularis muscle are identified to determine the location of the muscle split, which may be localized by a raphe often found between the midsubstance of the muscle and the lower one-third of the muscle (Fig. 7-14). A mayo scissors is used to create the split just medial to the muscle/tendon junction, and the split is extended medially approximately 3 cm, and then extended laterally with a knife to the level of the lesser tuberosity. The superior subscapularis is bluntly elevated from the

subscapularis fossa and retracted. The inferior subscapularis is retracted with a blunt cobra (or similar) retractor to fully expose the underlying capsule. The capsule is incised at the level of the joint longitudinally from the 2-o'clock position to just inferior to the glenoid. An intra-articular retractor is placed inferior to the glenoid

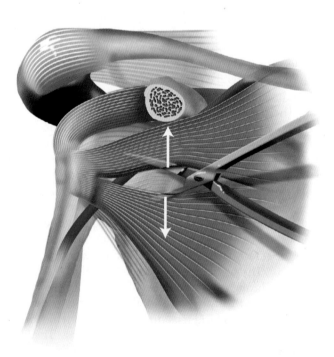

▲ **FIGURE 7-14:** The subscapularis is split longitudinally at the junction of the upper two-thirds and inferior one-third. The split is extended laterally to the level of the lesser tuberosity.

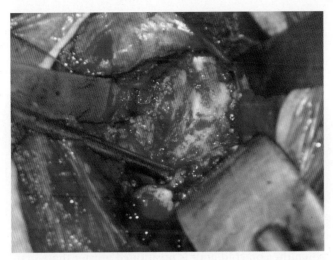

▲ **FIGURE 7-15:** Glenoid exposure.

such as a Fukuda. A Hohmann is placed in a supero-medial orientation on the glenoid which is now fully exposed (Fig. 7-15).

The anteroinferior labrum and periosteum are excised from approximately 2-o'clock to 5-o'clock positions in a right shoulder from the articular surface medially for 2 cm, which is facilitated by the common presence of a Bankart lesion at this location. The antero-inferior surface of the glenoid is prepared with a burr to create a bed for transfer of the coracoid graft. The coracoid is now retrieved from its location under the pectoralis major and provisionally placed into position to determine the location of the glenoid drill holes, with care taken to place the coracoid sufficiently medially so that no graft will overhang in the joint. The orientation of the coracoid is confirmed, which can be with either the lateral or inferior surfaces acting as the glenoid face. A recent study has suggested that placing the coracoid flush to the glenoid face with the inferior coracoid surface as the glenoid face completely restores the surface area of a 30% anterior glenoid defect to the intact state (114).

The coracoid is returned to its retracted position under the pectoralis tendon and the inferior glenoid drill hole is made at the 5-o'clock position, penetrating the posterior scapular cortex. The depth of the drill hole is measured and added to the depth of the coracoid (for a screw length typically around 35 to 40 mm). The coracoid is retrieved and placed into position, and an appropriately sized partially threaded screw is placed into the inferior drill hole and tightened. Care should be taken to ensure the graft lies parallel to the anterior border of the glenoid with no lateral overhang. Rotation of the coracoid is confirmed prior to final screw tightening, and the remaining superior drill hole is made through the superior hole already drilled in the coracoid. Rotation of the graft should be avoided while drilling. The hole is measured and the correct-sized 4.5-mm partially threaded screw is placed into position and tightened

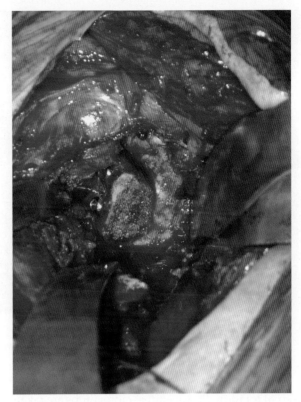

▲ **FIGURE 7-16:** Placement and fixation of coracoid bone graft.

(Fig. 7-16). Care should be taken not to overtighten the screws to avoid coracoid fracture. The capsule is repaired to the stump of the coracoacromial ligament (Fig. 7-17) with the arm in maximum external rotation to avoid overtensioning the capsule and postoperative loss of

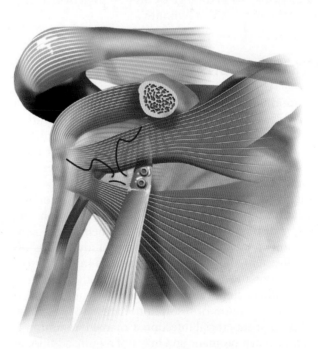

▲ **FIGURE 7-17:** The stump of the coracoacromial ligament is sutured to the capsule. The split in the subscapularis is not repaired.

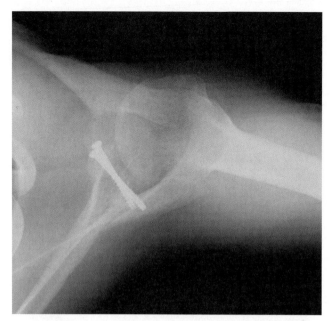

▲ **FIGURE 7-18:** Postoperative radiographs demonstrating the final construct.

external rotation. Postoperative radiographs are taken to confirm graft placement (Fig. 7-18).

POSTOPERATIVE CARE

Patients are placed into a sling for 6 weeks, with only gentle active-assisted range of motion exercises. Return to sport is permitted at 3 months.

COMPLICATIONS

Complications are not infrequent following the Latarjet procedure. One recent series reported a complication rate of 25% (85), with neurologic injury occurring in 10% of patients with roughly equal numbers of musculocutaneous, radial, and axillary nerve injuries. It should be noted that a high percentage (73%) of the patients in this study had undergone failed prior stabilization procedures, and thus the complication rate may be disproportionately high. Most neurologic complications resolve. A recent anatomic study reports on the consistent and significant alterations in the musculocutaneous and axillary nerves following the procedure (115). Other complications include recurrent instability, coracoid nonunion or resorption, hardware loosening, and deep or superficial infection. Coracoid nonunion is not always symptomatic and may not require additional intervention. Coracoid lysis has been documented to occur and may be prevented by preserving vascular

attachments to the coracoid during medial dissection (116). Glenohumeral osteoarthritis is a possible long-term sequela, particularly with a graft that is overhanging (85,114).

OUTCOMES

Allain, in a series of 58 shoulders followed for a mean of 14 years, reported a complication rate of only 7% with no recurrent instability and good or excellent outcomes in 88% (85). Recent studies have demonstrated mixed results with regard to returning to high-impact sporting activities (117,118). Recurrent instability is uncommon in most series (85,119,120), with an increased incidence when the coracoid graft is positioned greater than 1 cm medial to the glenoid (120). Osteoarthritis has been reported in ~15% of patients at long-term follow-up (121). Patients who have undergone failed primary stabilization procedures have predictably good-to-excellent subjective outcome scores, with diminished subjective outcomes in patients with higher levels of postoperative pain (111).

CONCLUSIONS

The Latarjet procedure is effective at restoring glenohumeral stability in patients with glenoid bone deficiency by restoring the glenoid bone cavity and by tensioning the soft tissues without sacrificing motion. With an appropriately planned and executed coracoid transfer, excellent outcomes can be achieved in the appropriately selected patient with limited surgical morbidity.

References

1. Simonet WT, Melton LJ 3rd, Cofield RH, et al. Incidence of anterior shoulder dislocation in Olmsted County, Minnesota. *Clin Orthop Relat Res.* 1984;(186):186–191.
2. Burkhead WZ Jr, Rockwood CA Jr. Treatment of instability of the shoulder with an exercise program. *J Bone Joint Surg Am.* 1992;74(6):890–896.
3. Goss TP. Anterior glenohumeral instability. *Orthopedics.* 1988;11(1):87–95.
4. Arciero RA, Wheeler JH, Ryan JB, et al. Arthroscopic Bankart repair versus nonoperative treatment for acute, initial anterior shoulder dislocations. *Am J Sports Med.* 1994;22(5):589–594.
5. Cole BJ, L'Insalata J, Irrgang J, et al. Comparison of arthroscopic and open anterior shoulder stabilization. A two to six-year follow-up study. *J Bone Joint Surg Am.* 2000;82-A(8):1108–1114.
6. Karlsson J, Magnusson L, Ejerhed L, et al. Comparison of open and arthroscopic stabilization for recurrent shoulder dislocation in patients with a Bankart lesion. *Am J Sports Med.* 2001;29(5):538–542.

7. Mazzocca AD, Brown FM Jr, Carreira DS, et al. Arthroscopic anterior shoulder stabilization of collision and contact athletes. *Am J Sports Med.* 2005;33(1):52–60.
8. Simonet WT, Cofield RH. Prognosis in anterior shoulder dislocation. *Am J Sports Med.* 1984;12(1):19–24.
9. Liu SH, Henry MH. Anterior shoulder instability. Current review. *Clin Orthop Relat Res.* 1996;(323):327–337.
10. Rowe CR, Zarins B. Recurrent transient subluxation of the shoulder. *J Bone Joint Surg Am.* 1981;63(6):863–872.
11. Geiger DF, Hurley JA, Tovey JA, et al. Results of arthroscopic versus open Bankart suture repair. *Clin Orthop Relat Res.* 1997;(337):111–117.
12. Guanche CA, Quick DC, Sodergren KM, et al. Arthroscopic versus open reconstruction of the shoulder in patients with isolated Bankart lesions. *Am J Sports Med.* 1996;24(2):144–148.
13. Levine WN, Richmond JC, Donaldson WR. Use of the suture anchor in open Bankart reconstruction. A follow-up report. *Am J Sports Med.* 1994;22(5):723–726.
14. Pollock RG, Owens JM, Flatow EL, et al. Operative results of the inferior capsular shift procedure for multidirectional instability of the shoulder. *J Bone Joint Surg Am.* 2000;82-A(7):919–928.
15. Bankart AS, Cantab MC. Recurrent or habitual dislocation of the shoulder-joint. 1923. *Clin Orthop Relat Res.* 1993;(291):3–6.
16. Detrisac DA, Johnson LL. Arthroscopic shoulder capsulorrhaphy using metal staples. *Orthop Clin North Am.* 1993;24(1):71–88.
17. Gill TJ, Micheli LJ, Gebhard F, et al. Bankart repair for anterior instability of the shoulder. Long-term outcome. *J Bone Joint Surg Am.* 1997;79(6):850–857.
18. Rowe CR. Acute and recurrent anterior dislocations of the shoulder. *Orthop Clin North Am.* 1980;11(2):253–270.
19. Rowe CR, Zarins B, Ciullo JV. Recurrent anterior dislocation of the shoulder after surgical repair. Apparent causes of failure and treatment. *J Bone Joint Surg Am.* 1984;66(2):159–168.
20. Rowe CR, Patel D, Southmayd WW. The Bankart procedure: A long-term end-result study. *J Bone Joint Surg Am.* 1978;60(1):1–16.
21. Pagnani MJ, Dome DC. Surgical treatment of traumatic anterior shoulder instability in American football players. *J Bone Joint Surg Am.* 2002;84-A(5):711–715.
22. Bigliani LU, Newton PM, Steinmann SP, et al. Glenoid rim lesions associated with recurrent anterior dislocation of the shoulder. *Am J Sports Med.* 1998;26(1):41–45.
23. Burkhart SS, De Beer JF. Traumatic glenohumeral bone defects and their relationship to failure of arthroscopic Bankart repairs: Significance of the inverted-pear glenoid and the humeral engaging Hill-Sachs lesion. *Arthroscopy.* 2000;16(7):677–694.
24. Pagnani MJ. Open capsular repair without bone block for recurrent anterior shoulder instability in patients with and without bony defects of the glenoid and/or humeral head. *Am J Sports Med.* 2008;36(9):1805–1812.
25. Cho NS, Yi JW, Lee BG, et al. Revision open Bankart surgery after arthroscopic repair for traumatic anterior shoulder instability. *Am J Sports Med.* 2009;37(11):2158–2164.
26. McAuliffe TB, Pangayatselvan T, Bayley I. Failed surgery for recurrent anterior dislocation of the shoulder. Causes and management. *J Bone Joint Surg Br.* 1988;70(5):798–801.
27. Matsen FA, Thomas SC, Rockwood CA, et al. Glenohumeral instability. In: Rockwood CA, Matsen FA, eds. *The Shoulder.* New York, NY: Churchill Livingstone; 1998:717.
28. Zarins B, Rowe C. Modifications of the Bankart procedure. In: Post M, Morrey BF, Hawkins RJ, eds. *Surgery of the Shoulder.* St. Louis, MO: Mosby-Year Book; 1990:170–177.
29. Vezeridis PS, Zarins B. Open Bankart procedure for recurrent anterior shoulder dislocation. In: Neviaser RJ, Lee DH, eds. *Shoulder and Elbow Surgery.* Philadelphia, PA: Elsevier Saunders; 2011:297.
30. Zarins B, Daly PJ. Bankart repair of anterior shoulder dislocation and subluxation. In: Craig EV, ed. *Master Techniques in Orthopaedic Surgery: The Shoulder.* New York, NY: Raven Press; 1995:71–87.
31. Zarins B. Anterior shoulder stabilization using the bankart procedure. *Sports Med Arthrosc.* 1993;1(4):259–265.
32. Warner JJ, Johnson D, Miller M, et al. Technique for selecting capsular tightness in repair of anterior-inferior shoulder instability. *J Shoulder Elbow Surg.* 1995;4(5):352–364.
33. Gill TJ, Zarins B. Open repairs for the treatment of anterior shoulder instability. *Am J Sports Med.* 2003;31(1):142–153.
34. Wirth MA, Blatter G, Rockwood CA Jr. The capsular imbrication procedure for recurrent anterior instability of the shoulder. *J Bone Joint Surg Am.* 1996;78(2):246–259.
35. Wolf EM. Arthroscopic capsulolabral repair using suture anchors. *Orthop Clin North Am.* 1993;24(1):59–69.
36. Cho NS, Hwang JC, Rhee YG. Arthroscopic stabilization in anterior shoulder instability: Collision athletes versus noncollision athletes. *Arthroscopy.* 2006;22(9):947–953.
37. Rhee YG, Ha JH, Cho NS. Anterior shoulder stabilization in collision athletes: Arthroscopic versus open Bankart repair. *Am J Sports Med.* 2006;34(6):979–985.
38. Pelet S, Jolles BM, Farron A. Bankart repair for recurrent anterior glenohumeral instability: Results at twenty-nine years' follow-up. *J Shoulder Elbow Surg.* 2006;15(2):203–207.
39. Hovelius LK, Sandstrom BC, Rosmark DL, et al. Long-term results with the Bankart and Bristow-Latarjet procedures: Recurrent shoulder instability and arthropathy. *J Shoulder Elbow Surg.* 2001;10(5):445–452.
40. Ee GW, Mohamed S, Tan AH. Long term results of arthroscopic Bankart repair for traumatic anterior shoulder instability. *J Orthop Surg Res.* 2011;6:28.
41. Kim SH, Ha KI, Cho YB, et al. Arthroscopic anterior stabilization of the shoulder: Two to six-year follow-up. *J Bone Joint Surg Am.* 2003;85-A(8):1511–1518.

42. Bottoni CR, Smith EL, Berkowitz MJ, et al. Arthroscopic versus open shoulder stabilization for recurrent anterior instability: A prospective randomized clinical trial. *Am J Sports Med.* 2006;34(11):1730–1737.

43. Fabbriciani C, Milano G, Demontis A, et al. Arthroscopic versus open treatment of Bankart lesion of the shoulder: A prospective randomized study. *Arthroscopy.* 2004;20(5):456–462.

44. Archetti Netto N, Tamaoki MJ, Lenza M, et al. Treatment of Bankart lesions in traumatic anterior instability of the shoulder: A randomized controlled trial comparing arthroscopy and open techniques. *Arthroscopy.* 2012; 28(7):900–908.

45. Freedman KB, Smith AP, Romeo AA, et al. Open Bankart repair versus arthroscopic repair with transglenoid sutures or bioabsorbable tacks for recurrent anterior instability of the shoulder: A meta-analysis. *Am J Sports Med.* 2004;32(6):1520–1527.

46. Hobby J, Griffin D, Dunbar M, et al. Is arthroscopic surgery for stabilisation of chronic shoulder instability as effective as open surgery? A systematic review and meta-analysis of 62 studies including 3044 arthroscopic operations. *J Bone Joint Surg Br.* 2007;89(9):1188–1196.

47. Lenters TR, Franta AK, Wolf FM, et al. Arthroscopic compared with open repairs for recurrent anterior shoulder instability. A systematic review and meta-analysis of the literature. *J Bone Joint Surg Am.* 2007;89(2):244–254.

48. Bankart, A: The pathology and treatment of recurrent dislocation of the shoulder joint. *Br J Surg.* 1938;26:23–29.

49. Rockwood CA Jr. Subluxations and dislocations about the shoulder. In: Rockwood CA Jr, Green DP, eds. *Fracture in Adults, 2nd ed.* Philadelphia, PA: JB Lippincott; Vol 1, 1984:722–985.

50. Gamradt SC, Williams RJ, Warren RF. Arthroscopic treatment of shoulder instability. In: Rockwood CA, ed. *The Shoulder, 4th ed.* Philadelphia, PA: Saunder-Elsevier. Vol 2, 940–960.

51. O'Driscoll SW, Evans DC. Long-term results of staple capsulorrhaphy for anterior instability of the shoulder. *J Bone Joint Surg Am.* 1993;75:249–258.

52. Cook M, Richardson AB. Arthroscopic staple capsulorrhaphy for treatment of anterior shoulder instability [abstract]. *Orthop Trans.* 1991;15:1.

53. Lane JG, Sachs RA, Riehl B. Arthroscopic staple capsulorrhaphy: A long term follow up. *Arthroscopy.* 1993; 9(2):190–194.

54. Viek P, Bell BT. The Bankart Shoulder Reconstruction; the use of pullout wires and other practical details. *J Bone Joint Surg Am.* 1959;41(2):236–242.

55. Morgan CD, Bodenstab AB. Arthroscopic Bankart suture repair: Technique and early results. *Arthroscopy.* 1983;3:111–122.

56. Grana WA, Buckley PD, Yates CK. Arthroscopic Bankart suture repair. *Am J Sports Med.* 1993;21:348–353.

57. Green MR, Christensen KP. Arthroscopic Bankart procedure: Two- to five-year follow-up with clinical correlation to severity of glenoid labral lesion. *Am J Sports Med.* 1995;23:276–281.

58. O'Neill DB. Arthroscopic Bankart Repair of Anterior Detachments of the Glenoid Labrum: A prospective study. *J Bone Joint Surg Am.* 1999;81(10):1357–1365.

59. Fealy S, Drakos MC, Allen AA, et al. Arthroscopic Bankart repair: Experience with an absorbable, transfixing implant. *Clin Orthop Relat Res.* 2001; 390:31–41.

60. Speer KP, Warren RF, Pagani M, et al. An arthroscopic technique for anterior stabilization of the shoulder with a bioabsorbable tack. *J Bone Joint Surg Am.* 1996; 78(12):1801–1807.

61. McEleney ET, Donovan MJ, Shea KP, et al. Initial failure strength of open and arthroscopic Bankart repairs. *Arthroscopy.* 1995;11:426–431.

62. Gartman GM, Roddey TS, Hammerman SM. Arthroscopic treatment of anterior-inferior glenohumeral instability. Two to five-year follow up. *J Bone Joint Surg Am.* 2000;82(7):991–1003.

63. Bacilla P, Field LD, Savoie FH3rd. Arthrosopic Bankart repair in a high demand patient population. *Arthroscopy.* 1997;13(1): 51–60.

64. Gaunche CA, Quick DC, Sodergren KM, et al. Arthroscopic versus open reconstruction of the shoulder in patients with isolated Bankart lesions. *Am J Sports Med.* 1996;24:144–148.

65. Kim SH, Ha KI, Kim SH. Bankart repair in traumatic anterior instability: Open versus arthroscopic technique. *Arthroscopy.* 2002;18(7):755–763.

66. Pulavarti RS, Symes TH, Rangan A. Surgical Intervention for anterior shoulder instability in adults. *Cochrane Database Syst Rev.* 2009;7(4):CD005077.

67. Bottoni CR, Wilcklens JH, DeBerardino TM, et al. A prospective, randomized evaluation of arthroscopic stabilization versus nonoperative treatment in patients with acute, traumatic, first-time shoulder dislocations. *Am J Sports Med.* 2002;30:576–580.

68. Owens BD, Dickens JF, Kilcoyne KG, et al. Management of mid-season traumatic anterior shoulder instability in athletes. *J Am Acad Orthop Surg.* 2012;20:518–526.

69. Diduch DR, Scanelli J, Tompkins M, et al. Tissue anchor use in arthroscopic glenohumeral surgery. *J Am Acad Orthop Surg.* 2012;20:459–471.

70. Mohtadi NGH, Chan DS, Hollinshead R, et al. An expertise-based randomised clinical trial comparing arthroscopic versus open stabilization for recurrent anterior shoulder instability: Two-year post-operative disease-specific quality of life outcomes. *J Bone Joint Surg Br.* 2012;94:166–166.

71. Voos JE, Livermore RW, Feeley BT, et al. Prospective evaluation of arthroscopic Bankart repairs for anterior instability. *Am J Sports Med.* 2010;38:302–307.

72. Van der Linde JA, van Kampen DA, Terwee CB, et al. Long-term results after arthroscopic shoulder stabilization using suture anchors: An 8- to 10-year follow-up. *Am J Sports Med.* 2011;39:2396–2403.

73. Piasecki DP, Verma NN, Romeo AA, et al. Glenoid bone deficiency in recurrent anterior shoulder instability: Diagnosis and management. *J Am Acad Orthop Surg.* 2009;17:482–493.

74. Walch G, Boileau P. Latarjet-Bristow procedure for recurrent anterior instability. *Tech Shoulder Elbow Surg.* 2000;1:256–261.

75. Allain J, Goutallier D, Glorion C. Long-term results of the Latarjet procedure for the treatment of anterior

instability of the shoulder. *J Bone Joint Surg Am.* 1998; 80:841–852.

76. Shah AA, Butler RB, Romanowski J, et al. Short-term complications of the Latarjet procedure. *J Bone Joint Surg.* 2012;94:495–501.

77. Eberly VC, McMahon PJ, Lee TQ. Variation in the glenoid origin of the anteroinferior glenohumeral capsulolabrum. *Clin Orthop Relat Res.* 2002;400:26–31.

78. Uhthoff HK, Piscopo M. Anterior capsular redundancy of the shoulder: Congenital or traumatic? An embryological study. *J Bone Joint Surg Br.* 1985;67:363–366.

79. Itoigawa Y, Itoi E, Sakoma Y, et al. Attachment of the anteroinferior glenohumeral ligament-labrum complex to the glenoid: An anatomic study. *Arthroscopy.* 2012;28:1628–1633.

80. Ahmad CS, Galano GJ, Vorys GC, et al. Evaluation of glenoid capsulolabral complex insertional anatomy and restoration with single-and double-row capsulolabral repairs. *J Shoulder Elbow Surg.* 2009;18:948–954.

81. Kim DS, Yoon YS, Chung HJ. Single-row versus doublerow capsulolabral repair: A comparative evaluation of contact pressure and surface area in the capsulolabral complex-glenoid bone interface. *Am J Sports Med.* 2011;39:1500–1506.

82. Thompson MM, Dines JS, McGarry MH, et al. Biomechanical evaluation of capsulolabral repairs: Double-row compared with single-row fixation. Publication Pending

83. Lafosse L, Baier GP, Jost B. Footprint fixation for arthroscopic reconstruction in anterior shoulder instability: The Cassiopeia double-row technique. *Arthroscopy.* 2006;22:231.e1–231.e6.

84. Speer KP, Deng X, Borrero S, et al. Biomechanical evaluation of a simulated Bankart lesion. *J Bone Joint Surg Am.* 1994;76:1819.

85. Black KP, Schneider DJ, James RY, et al. Biomechanics of the Bankart repair: The relationship between glenohumeral translation and labral fixation site. *Am J Sports Med.* 1999;27:339–344.

86. Pouliart N, Marmor S, Gagey O. Simulated capsulolabral lesion in cadavers: Dislocation does not result from a Bankart lesion only. *Arthroscopy.* 2006;22: 748–754.

87. Bigliani LU, Pollock RG, Soslowsky LJ, et al. Tensile properties of the inferior glenohumeral ligament. *J Orthop Res.* 1992;10:187–197.

88. Boileau P, Villalba M, Hery JY, et al. Risk factors for recurrence of shoulder instability after arthroscopic Bankart repair. *J Bone Joint Surg.* 2006;88:1755–1763.

89. Millett PJ, Braun S. The "bony Bankart bridge" procedure: A new arthroscopic technique for reduction and internal fixation of a bony Bankart lesion. *Arthroscopy.* 2009;25:102–105.

90. Jiang KN, Byram IR, Hsu SH, et al. Double-row labral repair: Knotless suture-bridge technique. *TSES.* 2012;13: 107–110.

91. Kim KC, Rhee KJ, Shin HD. Arthroscopic three-point double-row repair for acute bony Bankart lesions. *Knee Surg Sports Traumatol Arthrosc.* 2009;17:102–106.

92. Zhang J, Jiang C. A new "double-pulley" dual-row technique for arthroscopic fixation of bony Bankart lesion. *Knee Surg Sports Traumatol, Arthrosc.* 2011;19:1558–1562.

93. Mauro CS, Hammoud S, Dawson CK, et al. Double-row capsulolabral repair. *Shoulder Instability: Springer Milan.* 2011:69–88.

94. Lee CS, Abboud JA, Hsu JE. Parallel bridge fixation for Bankart lesions: An arthroscopic technique for anatomic fixation and true restoration of the labroligamentous bumper. *Curr Orthop Pract.* 2011;22:208.

95. Iwaso H, Uchiyama E, Sakakibara SI, et al. Modified double-row technique for arthroscopic Bankart repair: Surgical technique and preliminary results. *Acta Orthop Belg.* 2011;77:252–257.

96. Latarjet, M. A propos du traitement des luxations recidivantes de l'epaule. *Lyon Chir.* 1954;49:994–1003.

97. Milano G, et al. Analysis of risk factors for glenoid bone defect in anterior shoulder instability. *Am J Sports Med.* 2011;39(9):1870–1876.

98. Gerber C and Nyffeler RW. Classification of glenohumeral joint instability. *Clin Orthop Relat Res.* 2002;(400):65–76.

99. Helfet AJ. Coracoid transplantation for recurring dislocation of the shoulder. *J Bone Joint Surg Br.* 1958; 40-B(2):198–202.

100. Patte, Luxations recidivantes de l'epaule. Encycl Med Chir. *Paris-Technique chirurgicale.* 1980;44265:4.4–02.

101. Gagey OJ, Gagey N. The hyperabduction test. *J Bone Joint Surg Br.* 2001;83(1):69–74.

102. Balg F, Boileau P. The instability severity index score. A simple pre-operative score to select patients for arthroscopic or open shoulder stabilisation. *J Bone Joint Surg Br.* 2007;89(11):1470–1477.

103. Bernageau J, Patte D, Debeyre J, et al. [Value of the glenoid profil in recurrent luxations of the shoulder]. *Rev Chir Orthop Reparatrice Appar Mot.* 1976;62(2 suppl): 142–147.

104. Sugaya H, Moriishi J, Dohi M, et al. Glenoid rim morphology in recurrent anterior glenohumeral instability. *J Bone Joint Surg Am.* 2003;85-A(5):878–884.

105. Itoi E, et al. The effect of a glenoid defect on anteroinferior stability of the shoulder after Bankart repair: A cadaveric study. *J Bone Joint Surg Am.* 2000;82(1): 35–46.

106. Yamamoto N, et al. Stabilizing mechanism in bonegrafting of a large glenoid defect. *J Bone Joint Surg Am.* 2010;92(11):2059–2066.

107. Lo IK, Parten PM, Burkhart SS. The inverted pear glenoid: An indicator of significant glenoid bone loss. *Arthroscopy.* 2004;20(2):169–174.

108. Chuang TY, Adams CR, Burkhart SS. Use of preoperative three-dimensional computed tomography to quantify glenoid bone loss in shoulder instability. *Arthroscopy.* 2008;24(4):376–382.

109. Calandra JJ, Baker CL, Uribe J. The incidence of Hill-Sachs lesions in initial anterior shoulder dislocations. *Arthroscopy.* 1989;5(4):254–257.

110. Boileau P, Mercier N, Roussanne Y, et al. Arthroscopic Bankart-Bristow-Latarjet procedure: The development and early results of a safe and reproducible technique. *Arthroscopy.* 2010;26(11):1434–1450.

111. Schmid SL, Farshad M, Catanzaro S, et al. The Latarjet procedure for the treatment of recurrence of anterior instability of the shoulder after operative repair: A

retrospective case series of forty-nine consecutive patients. *J Bone Joint Surg Am.* 2012;94(11):e75.

112. Raiss P, Lin A, Mizuno N, et al. Results of the Latarjet procedure for recurrent anterior dislocation of the shoulder in patients with epilepsy. *J Bone Joint Surg Br.* 2012;94(9):1260–1264.

113. Young AA, Maia R, Berhouet J, et al. Open Latarjet procedure for management of bone loss in anterior instability of the glenohumeral joint. *J Shoulder Elbow Surg.* 2011;20(2 Suppl):S61–S69.

114. Ghodadra N, Gupta A, Romeo AA, et al. Normalization of glenohumeral articular contact pressures after Latarjet or iliac crest bone-grafting. *J Bone Joint Surg Am.* 2010;92(6):1478–1489.

115. Freehill MT, et al. The Latarjet coracoid process transfer procedure: Alterations in the neurovascular structures. *J Shoulder Elbow Surg.* 2013;22(5):695–700.

116. Hamel A, Hamel O, Ploteau S, et al. The arterial supply of the coracoid process. *Surg Radiol Anat.* 2012;34(7):599–607.

117. Boileau P, Fourati E, Bicknell R. Neer modification of open bankart procedure: What are the rates of recur-rent instability, functional outcome, and arthritis? *Clin Orthop Relat Res.* 2012;470(9):2554–2560.

118. Neyton L, Young A, Dawidziak B, et al. Surgical treatment of anterior instability in rugby union players: Clinical and radiographic results of the Latarjet-Patte procedure with minimum 5-year follow-up. *J Shoulder Elbow Surg.* 2012;21(12):1721–1727.

119. Burkhart SS, De Beer JF, Barth JR, et al. Results of modified Latarjet reconstruction in patients with anteroinferior instability and significant bone loss. *Arthroscopy.* 2007;23(10):1033–1041.

120. Hovelius L, Sandström B, Olofsson A, et al. The effect of capsular repair, bone block healing, and position on the results of the Bristow-Latarjet procedure (study III): Long-term follow-up in 319 shoulders. *J Shoulder Elbow Surg.* 2012;21(5):647–660.

121. Hovelius L, Sandstrom B, Saebo M. One hundred eighteen Bristow-Latarjet repairs for recurrent anterior dislocation of the shoulder prospectively followed for fifteen years: Study II-the evolution of dislocation arthropathy. *J Shoulder Elbow Surg.* 2006;15(3):279–289.

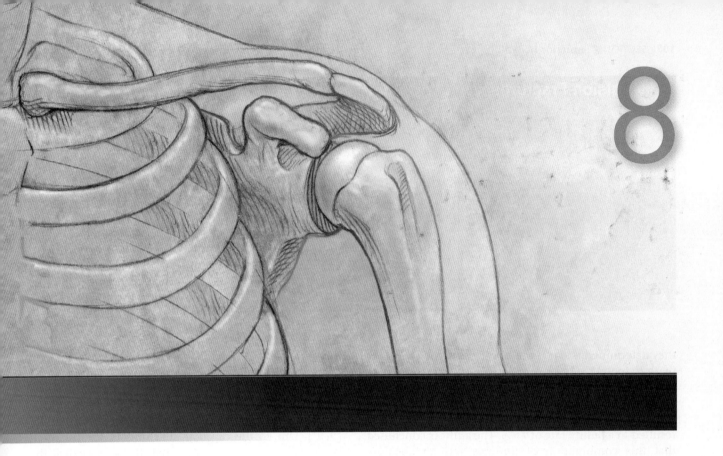

Bone Loss in the Unstable Shoulder: The Glenoid

Pascal Boileau / Walter B. McClelland, Jr /
Charles-Edouard Thélu

Introduction

The etiology of recurrent anterior glenohumeral instability can be divided into three categories: Those cases due to deficient soft tissue stability, those resultant from deficient bony stability, and those with a combined deficiency. As surgical techniques to treat shoulder instability have evolved, the role of each stabilizing structure has been further evaluated, with increased attempts to contour surgical treatment appropriately for each patient.

Historically, recurrent shoulder instability has been addressed by open surgery, with predictable results from open Bankart repairs, bone block procedures, and coracoid transfer (1). The rise of arthroscopy gave promise for quicker recovery, less postoperative scar tissue, and improved postoperative range of motion. However, early attempts to treat recurrent shoulder instability arthroscopically were met with disappointing results and high rates of recurrence (2–5). As more and more effort has been directed at improving these techniques, increased focus has been directed to analyzing causes of failure.

Multiple studies have identified glenoid bone deficiency as a cause of recurrent glenohumeral instability and a contributor to surgical failure after isolated Bankart repair (1,6–8). Boileau et al. (1) evaluated the risk factors for recurrent instability following isolated arthroscopic Bankart repair/capsular shift for recurrent, traumatic, anterior glenohumeral instability. In a consecutive series of 91 patients,

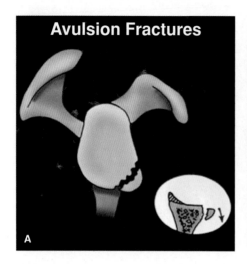

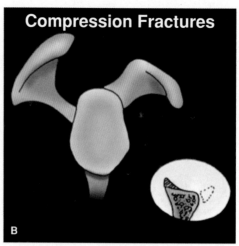

◀ FIGURE 8-1: Two types of glenoid fracture associated with recurrent anterior instability must be differentiated: Avulsion or separation fractures **(A)** with avulsion of a bone fragment, often secondary to true recurrent dislocations, and compression fractures **(B)** without any bone fragment, often secondary to recurrent subluxations.

they determined that glenoid bone loss involving >25% of the glenoid surface (erosion or compression fracture) posed a significant risk for recurrent instability ($p = 0.01$). The combination of significant glenoid bone loss with a stretched inferior glenohumeral ligament resulted in a failure rate of 75%. The authors concluded that this combination of findings was an absolute contraindication to arthroscopic Bankart repair alone. Interestingly, the presence of a glenoid avulsion fracture was not associated with increased risk of recurrent instability.

Kim et al. (6) found a similar impact of anterior glenoid wear on instability recurrence. In a cohort of 174 arthroscopic anterior stabilization procedures, the authors determined that glenoid bone loss of >30% of the glenoid circumference was significantly related to risk of recurrence ($p < 0.001$). The authors recommended open Bankart repair with glenoid augmentation in this population.

It is essential for shoulder surgeons to (1) identify glenoid pathology during the preoperative workup, and (2) adjust their treatment plans accordingly. Known glenoid deficiency must be corrected at the time of surgical intervention, or surgical outcomes will be disappointing.

MECHANISMS OF INSTABILITY

The shoulder is the most mobile but also the most unstable joint in the body. This is a consequence of the differential in both size and congruency between the small flat surface of the glenoid and the large spherical surface of the humeral head. The labrum compensates for the difference between the radius of curvature of the humeral head and the glenoid.

Glenoid deficiency can develop in an acute or chronic manner. Acutely, this is resultant from antero-

inferior glenoid rim fractures following a forceful dislocation episode, often referred to as a "bony Bankart." This represents a disruption of both bony and soft tissue restraints on the shoulder, and has long been understood as a risk factor for recurrent shoulder instability (9,10). Due to the capsular attachments, the fragment is typically displaced in a medial direction against the glenoid neck. The reported incidence of this lesion in acute shoulder instability varies widely between studies (8% to 73%), likely due to differing imaging protocols and modalities used (11,12).

Chronic glenoid erosion develops with increasing instability episodes, as the softer subchondral bone of the glenoid becomes progressively impacted or eroded. We draw a distinction between *separation or avulsion fractures* and *compression fractures,* which corresponds to true glenoid erosion (Fig. 8-1). The former are often secondary to recurrent dislocations while the latter are secondary to recurrent subluxations. As the anterior to posterior width of the glenoid shrinks, the distance traveled by the humeral head before reaching a position of dislocation is shortened. This is compounded by the capsular deficiency that often accompanies patients with multiple subluxations (Fig. 8-2).

PREOPERATIVE EVALUATION: CLINICAL

Complete discussion of the clinical examination for the unstable shoulder will be highlighted in another chapter. However, several elements of the history and examination may clue the practitioner in to the type of glenoid injury one can expect to see on preoperative imaging.

We draw a distinction between patients who dislocate and those who subluxate. Dislocators tend to have appropriate soft tissue restraints with a robust anterior capsule and glenohumeral ligaments. An instability

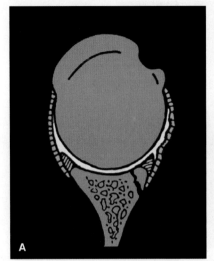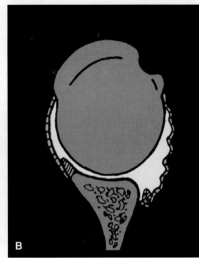

▶ **FIGURE 8-2:** When the capsule is strong and of good quality, an instability episode results in a fracture separation without substantial capsular stretching: The weak link in the chain is the bone and not the ligament **(A)**. In contrast, if the capsule is weak, it will elongate and the glenoid rim will be compressed and eroded by the recurrent subluxations or dislocations leading to a compression fracture **(B)**. In this situation, two weak links in the chain are the loose capsule and the glenoid bone loss; the risk for recurrent instability is higher.

episode in this population is more likely to result in an acute glenoid rim fracture or deep Hill–Sachs defect, due to the restraining force compressing the humeral head against the glenoid during anterior translation. Subluxators tend to have lax anterior capsules and may be found to be hyperlax on clinical examination (≥90 degrees of external rotation with the arm in an adducted position). These patients, the so-called subluxators, have a higher risk for recurrent instability and have a larger number of instability episodes, as compared to dislocators. This results in a progressive wear of the anteroinferior glenoid rim, resulting in progressive bony insufficiency. If a Hill–Sachs defect is present in this population, it tends to be wider and shallower.

The number of dislocations/subluxations has been shown to correlate with the degree of glenoid bone loss (13). A thorough history should determine the number of instability episodes, but it is important to realize that many instability episodes are not perceived as such by patients. If a patient reports pain, apprehension, or mechanical symptoms during certain positions or activities, this may actually represent a small episode of subluxation.

PREOPERATIVE EVALUATION: IMAGING STUDIES

The presence of glenoid bone loss can have a direct impact on the strategy, technique, or procedure used to surgically stabilize the shoulder. With this in mind, it is essential to have a full understanding of the defect before entering the operating room. Standard shoulder radiographs in most clinics consist of an AP view (in neutral or neutral/internal rotation/external rotation), an axillary view, and an outlet or scapular Y view. Because this combination of radiographs is considered inadequate to fully evaluate the status of the anteroinferior glenoid,

several special radiographic views have been described to assess the presence and degree of glenoid bone loss in the setting of instability.

The Bernageau glenoid profile view is an effective way to evaluate the anteroinferior angle of the glenoid rim (14). The arm is positioned overhead with the hand resting on the top of the head. The cassette is placed in the axilla, with the x-ray beam directed 20 to 30 degrees inferiorly and in line with the plane of the scapula. Critics would argue that this position may be symptomatic for patients with glenohumeral instability, but we have not found this to be a limitation in the use of this view. Sugaya has proposed a modified position with the patient lying on the table. The primary advantage of the Bernageau view is that it clearly shows the anterior glenoid rim (Fig. 8-3).

Edwards et al. (15) described three types of pathology identifiable on the Bernageau glenoid profile view—glenoid rim fractures, the "cliff" sign, and the "blunted angle" sign. The "cliff" sign, felt to be resultant from resorption of an avulsion fracture fragment, was defined as a loss of the anterior triangle of the glenoid without appreciable displaced bone. The "blunted angle" sign was defined as a rounded appearance to the anterior triangle, and was felt to represent an impaction fracture from multiple instability episodes. These findings were compared to the patient's unaffected contralateral shoulder when possible. The overall incidence of osseous abnormalities seen on the Bernageau view was 79%. In addition, they noted a high percentage of inferior glenoid rim fractures identified on the AP internal rotation view, with this view being more effective at identifying far inferior fractures than the Bernageau view. When the findings from the AP and Bernageau views were combined, 87% of shoulders demonstrated an osseous glenoid abnormality. It is important to perform bilateral Bernageau views to compare affected and unaffected sides (Fig. 8-4).

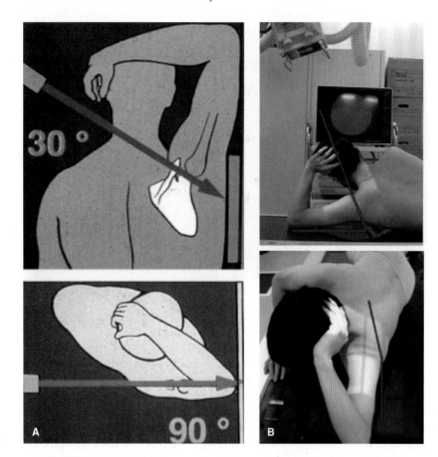

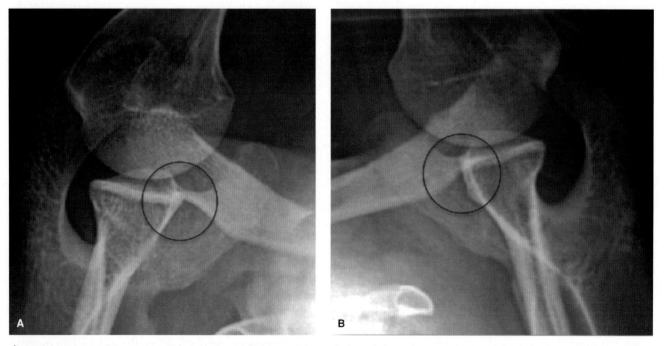

◀ **FIGURE 8-3:** Position of the patient and the beam for the classical Bernageau view with the patient standing **(A)** and the modified laying position proposed by Sugaya **(B)**.

▲ **FIGURE 8-4:** Comparative Bernageau (or profile) views: A normal glenoid demonstrates a sharp anterior angle with a triangle **(A)**; when a glenoid erosion is present, the anterior triangle disappears **(B)**.

The apical oblique, or Garth view (16), can be taken with the patient standing or supine. The cassette is positioned posterior to the shoulder in the plane of the scapula. The x-ray beam is directed 45-degree lateral and 45-degree caudal, providing a coronal profile view of the glenohumeral joint. This view can be helpful in both evaluation of the acutely dislocated shoulder and postreduction evaluation of the glenohumeral bony structures.

The West Point view is an additional modification of the axillary view (17). The patient is placed in the prone position with the shoulder abducted 90 degrees. The x-ray beam is directed into the axilla, angled downward and medially 25 degrees each. This provides a tangential view of the glenoid rim, allowing evaluation of both posterior and anterior aspects. Rokous et al. identified glenoid abnormalities in 53 of 63 patients with a history of instability in their initial description of the technique. In their description of the apical oblique view, Garth et al. (16) acknowledged that the West Point view was more sensitive in identifying small marginal fractures of the glenoid rim and ossification along the anterior glenoid rim (i.e., chronic Bankart lesion), indicating that the effectiveness of these special views may be variable.

With all of the radiographic techniques, evaluating the "sharpness" of the anteroinferior glenoid rim can be key in detecting subtle bony defects. A normal glenoid should demonstrate a sharp angle both anteriorly and posteriorly. If the margin appears rounded or blunted, further investigation may be warranted for possible glenoid insufficiency.

CT scan has been suggested as a way to improve the sensitivity of glenohumeral imaging in cases of dislocation or subluxation. Seltzer and Weissman (18) highlighted the sensitivity of two-dimensional (2D) CT in identifying lesions in patients with instability. They acknowledged the inability to fully evaluate the capsulolabral structures in the absence of intra-articular contrast. Bigliani et al. (19) highlighted the use of CT arthrograms as an adjunct to their instability workup. They utilized CT arthrograms to better define a lesion incompletely viewed on plain x-rays, or in the setting of negative x-rays but a high-clinical suspicion for glenoid rim pathology. They noted accurate and clear assessment of the lesion in all cases in which the CT arthrogram was performed.

More recently, CT scan with three-dimensional (3D) reconstruction has gained in popularity for the evaluation of the unstable shoulder (Fig. 8-5). Stevens et al. (20) compared pathologic findings after imaging 11 patients (12 shoulders) with plain XR (AP and axial views) and CT scan (axial images, oblique coronal and oblique sagittal reformats, and 3D reconstructions). Specific to the glenoid, they identified glenoid rim fractures in 50% of patients and periosteal new bone formation along the glenoid neck in 42% based on CT imaging. None of these abnormalities were identified using plain x-ray, indicating the superior sensitivity of CT in detecting lesions of the glenoid. It should be noted, however, that no special x-ray views were included in their assessment. The authors argued that the complex techniques needed to obtain these special views eliminated the opportunity for uniformity between centers. They concluded that the 3D reconstructions offered excellent information for preoperative planning, and

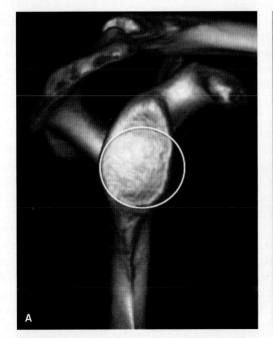
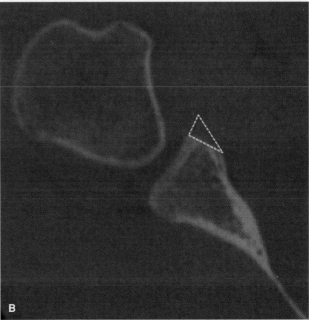

▲ **FIGURE 8-5:** Compression fracture (i.e., anterior glenoid bone loss), as seen on 3D CT scan with en face view **(A)**, and on axial view **(B)**; same patient as Figure 8-4.

that the oblique coronal and sagittal reformatted images offered no additional information.

Despite the positive experience with CT scan in this clinical situation, downsides to this technology do exist, including additional expense and radiation exposure. We find CT to be an integral portion of our preoperative planning, particularly the "en face sagittal oblique view" of the glenoid and the 3D reconstruction images with the humeral head eliminated. These views also provide an excellent way to evaluate bone placement and union in coracoid transfer or bone grafting procedures, if post-operative evaluation is needed.

SURGICAL PLANNING

While the results of isolated arthroscopic Bankart repair alone have been disappointing in patients with significant glenoid rim defects, the definition of "significant" varies greatly between authors. Burkhart and De Beer (7,21) recommend bone grafting in the presence of an inverted pear glenoid. In cadavers, a lesion involving ≥25% the diameter of the inferior glenoid was necessary to produce this conformation (22). This number is in agreement with that put forth by Bigliani et al. (19), who suggested a loss of 25% of the glenoid width as an appropriate cutoff. Itoi et al. (23) referenced a glenoid width-to-length ratio of less than 79%. Sugaya et al. (24), referencing the work of Itoi, considered ≥20% to be the cutoff for bone grafting, although they recommended fixing displaced bony Bankart fragments if present, even if the defect was smaller.

In an effort to provide some objective data to assist in the decision-making process, Boileau et al. (25) developed the Instability Severity Index Score (ISIS). They reviewed 131 consecutive patients who underwent arthroscopic Bankart repair for recurrent anterior shoulder instability to determine risk factors for recurrence. Six factors were identified, including loss of glenoid contour seen on the AP x-ray, which were used to construct the ten-point scale (Table 8-1). The scoring system was then reapplied to the study population to stratify risk. The authors determined that an ISIS >6 points resulted in a 70% risk for recurrent instability. They concluded that these patients were inappropriate candidates for arthroscopic Bankart alone. Depending on the type of bony lesions found, they recommended a coracoid transfer in case of glenoid erosion or an associated Hill–Sachs remplissage in case of isolated deep impaction fracture of the humerus.

INTRAOPERATIVE ASSESSMENT

While imaging modalities can provide a good idea of the status of the glenoid rim preoperatively, it is

TABLE 8-1 **Instability Severity Index Score** (Based on preoperative questionnaire, clinical examination and radiographs)

Prognostic Factors		Points
Age at surgery	≤20 yrs	2
	>20 yrs	0
Degree of sport practice	Competition	2
	Recreational or no sports	0
Type of sports	Contact or forced ABD-ER	1
	Other	0
Shoulder hyperlaxity	Shoulder hyperlaxity	1
	Normal laxity	0
Hill–Sachs on AP x-ray	In external rotation	2
	Not visible in ER	0
Glenoid loss of contour on AP x-ray	Loss of contour	2
	No lesion	0

necessary to confirm these findings with a thorough intraoperative assessment. If there is a delay between imaging study and surgery, or if the patient has experienced additional instability episodes in the interim, the appearance of the glenoid may have evolved from that seen on imaging studies. However, these lesions are not always easy to identify. Bigliani et al. (19) identified glenoid rim defects in only 11% of 200 patients undergoing open stabilization surgery for recurrent, traumatic glenohumeral instability, a number well below the known incidence of these lesions. We believe identification of these defects is easier with newer arthroscopic techniques.

Bony Bankart fragments are often visible with the detached anterior labrum. In the subacute or chronic setting, these fragments may be malunited against the glenoid neck. If the goal is to mobilize and restore the native position of these fragments, care must be taken to carefully define the plane between displaced fragment and native glenoid, so as not to truncate the size of the fragment or disrupt its capsulolabral attachments. If the goal is to neglect or replace the bony Bankart with an isolated soft tissue repair or arthroscopic coracoid transfer, one must be careful to gently release the capsulolabral tissues from the bony margin to maintain as much integrity as possible for later labral repair/capsular shift.

The description of the glenoid in the recurrently unstable shoulder as an inverted pear is attributed to Burkhart and De Beer (7). As progressive bone loss at the anteroinferior glenoid occurs, the appearance of the glenoid changes, with increased width superiorly versus inferiorly. This is termed the "inverted pear." This conformation is indicative of significant bone loss and can provide an intraoperative assessment as to the degree of glenoid insufficiency.

While first described as a subjective description of the glenoid shape when viewed from the anterosuperior portal (7), the degree of bone loss needed to result in an inverted pear glenoid was later quantified (26). The authors used a graduated probe intraoperatively inserted through the posterior portal to measure from the central bare spot to determine the width of bone missing from the anterior glenoid. They also replicated inverted pear glenoids in cadavers and measured the amount of bone resected. Their conclusions were that 25% to 27% loss of the inferior glenoid AP diameter was needed before an inverted pear glenoid was created.

The authors have demonstrated the clinical relevance of this finding (7). In a retrospective review of 194 patients undergoing Bankart repair for recurrent anterior instability, the recurrence rate was 4% in those patients without an inverted pear glenoid and 61% in those patients with such a deformity. However, the inverted pear glenoid in patients with recurrent anterior instability is not a universally accepted finding. In their CT study of unstable shoulders, Griffith et al. (13) found the majority of bone loss to be anterior as opposed to anteroinferior, and did not observe the inverted pear morphology.

As an alternative to measuring from the glenoid bare spot, Kim et al. (6,27) have proposed dividing the glenoid face into four quadrants, with a vertical line between 12-o'clock and 6-o'clock, and a horizontal line at the midglenoid notch. The margin of the glenoid in each quadrant, therefore, represents 25% of the circumference of the glenoid. They felt this was a more reproducible technique than attempting to determine the area of the defect, but they acknowledged the potential subjectivity of this technique.

Boileau et al. (1) agreed with the quadrant technique of Kim, but chose to divide the glenoid face into six sections in hopes of increasing the reproducibility of the glenoid defect estimate. The authors agreed with Kim, however, that 25% of the circumference of the glenoid should be considered a significant lesion.

SURGICAL INTERVENTION

While the Bankart procedure (28) is capable of restoring the anterior glenoid bumper, it has been shown to be inadequate in cases of glenoid bone loss. The Bristow–Latarjet procedure (29,30) successfully addresses glenoid deficiency, but has been implicated in the development of shoulder arthritis due to its nonanatomic nature. The association of the Bristow–Latarjet with the Bankart repair (2B3 procedure) (31) benefits of both, and avoids the downsides.

Bony Bankart—Acute Repair

When fixed acutely, bony Bankart lesions can be repaired in identical fashion to their soft tissue counterpart. Care should be taken to either penetrate the bony fragment during the capsulolabral repair, or loop a suture around the bony fragment for firm fixation (Fig. 8-6). Holding the bony fragment in a reduced position with a grasper during the process of suture tying can assist reduction and avoid undue strain and friction on the suture material.

Bony Bankart—Subacute or Chronic Repair

Neglected bony Bankart lesions will often heal to the glenoid neck in a medialized position, the so-called

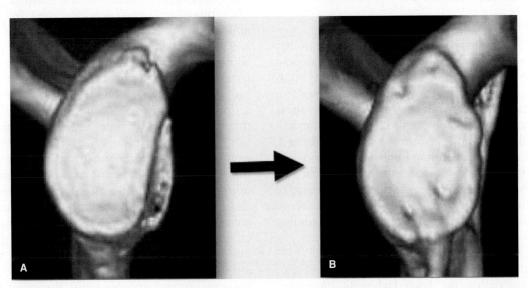

▲ **FIGURE 8-6:** 3D CT scan images demonstrate a typical avulsion fracture of the anterior glenoid rim after anterior dislocations **(A)**, and the glenoid reconstruction obtained after refixation of the glenoid bone fragment with sutures and anchors, as promoted by Sugaya **(B)**.

ALPSA lesion. The decision to salvage the native bone depends on the size of the displaced bony fragment, as well as the size of the calculated bone loss. With time, the size of the bony Bankart fragment can shrink, whether due to fragment resorption, ongoing compression/erosion from recurrent instability episodes, or both. In their retrospective review on arthroscopic management of chronic bony Bankart lesions, Sugaya et al. (32) documented an average glenoid bone loss of 24.8%, while the bony fragment represented only 9.2%.

If the degree of glenoid bone loss is negligible, the fragment can be ignored and a standard Bankart/capsular shift procedure will suffice. If there is significant glenoid bone loss and the displaced fragment is of adequate size, it can be mobilized to its native position in combination with the soft tissue reconstruction. Sugaya et al. (32) have shown success in separating the bony Bankart fragment from the glenoid neck before proceeding to a repair identical to that of an acute glenoid fracture. In their series of forty-two shoulders, they documented good to excellent results in 93% and a return to sport (contact and overhead) in 95%. Recurrent instability developed in two patients (5%), both occurring during sporting activities.

If glenoid bone loss is deemed to be significant, but the bony fragment does not appear of sufficient size to repair the defect, a separate bone graft or coracoid transfer procedure is necessary.

Glenoid Erosion

In order to reconstruct the glenoid bone loss, the surgeon has the choice between transfer of the coracoid process (Bristow–Latarjet procedure), iliac crest bone graft (Eden–Hybinette procedure), or allograft. The procedures can be done open or under arthroscopy.

The Eden–Hybinette Procedure

The Eden–Hybinette procedure involves transfer of iliac crest autograft to the anteroinferior aspect of the glenoid (33,34). This allows transfer of a large amount of bone, but we feel there are several downsides as compared to a coracoid transfer. First, while the coracoid retains some of its vascularity from the origin of the conjoint tendon, the iliac crest bone is completely devascularized. Second, obtaining iliac crest requires a second incision, with the additional risks of infection, iatrogenic fracture, and neurovascular injury. Finally, iliac crest bone graft stabilizes the shoulder by increasing the bony surface of the glenoid alone. It has no impact on the surrounding soft tissues.

In a series of young athletes, Gebhard et al. (35) demonstrated good to excellent results in only 61% of patients undergoing the Eden–Hybinette procedure. Redislocation rate was 7%, whereas the rate of arthrosis was 25% over a short study period (minimum follow-up

18 months). Complete resorption of the graft material was seen in 30% of cases. Scheibel et al. (36) and Taverna et al. (37) described an all-arthroscopic reconstruction technique of the anteroinferior glenoid that includes an autologous iliac crest bone grafting using screws and a capsulolabral repair using suture anchors. This technique recreates the bony and soft tissue anatomy of the anteroinferior glenoid while preserving the integrity of insertion of the subscapularis tendon. More recently, Provencher et al. (38) have proposed using tibial pilon allograft to reconstruct the anterior glenoid.

The Bristow–Latarjet Procedure

Michael Latarjet, a surgeon in Lyon (France), described a procedure in the 1950s that reconstructs glenoid bony defects by transferring the coracoid process through the subscapularis and fixing it with a screw (30) (Fig. 8-7). Not only does this statically restore the bony volume of the glenoid, but it also dynamically reinforces the weak anterior capsule through a sling effect. The conjoint tendon depresses the inferior portion of the subscapularis, therefore, the more the patient puts their arm in the "at-risk" position (abduction–external rotation), the more the head is pushed posteriorly on the glenoid (Fig. 8-8). In the Latarjet procedure, the bone block is positioned in the "lying" position and fixed with two screws (Fig. 8-9). In the Bristow modification, the bone block is positioned in the "standing" position and fixed with a single screw. Although the two-screw fixation is initially stronger, osteolysis of the proximal bone block has been observed in some cases, putting into question the need for the lying position and the use of two screws (Figs. 8-10 and 8-11).

Bankart–Bristow–Latarjet Procedure

The combined Bankart–Bristow–Latarjet procedure (2B3 procedure) has been described by the senior author (PB) as a way to address the combined bony and soft tissue defects present in this patient population without sacrificing the benefits of an all-arthroscopic technique. Dubbed the 2B3 procedure, this surgery improves the stability of the shoulder through three separate mechanisms: (1) The Bankart repair recreates the anterior glenoid bumper and retentions the lax anterior capsule tissue (bumper effect), (2) the transferred coracoid bone block augments the deficient glenoid rim, increasing the amount of humeral head translation required before dislocation can occur (bony effect), and (3) the transferred conjoint tendon reinforces the anterior soft tissues and creates a sling during positions of abduction/external rotation by lowering the inferior one-third of the subscapularis (belt effect). In order to avoid the complications reported with screws (bending, pull-out, humeral impingement), the senior author has developed a technique of fixation using a double button (Figs. 8-12 and 8-13).

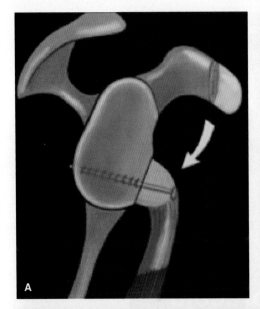

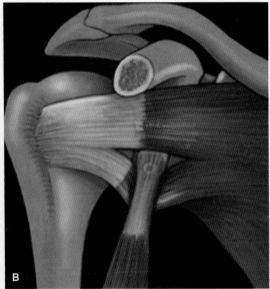

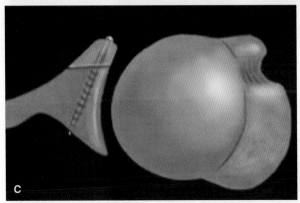

▲ **FIGURE 8-7:** The Bristow–Latarjet procedure transfers the tip of the coracoid to the anterior glenoid neck **(A)** after passing through the subscapularis (upper 2/3 and lower 1/3 junction) **(B)**; the bone block must be below the equator and flush to the glenoid articular surface **(C)**.

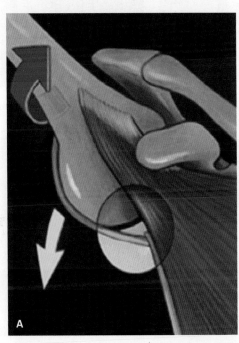

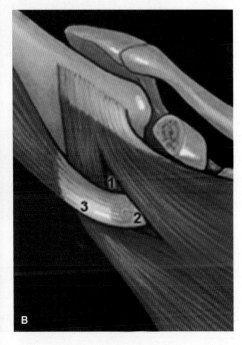

▶ **FIGURE 8-8:   A:** In the throwing (abduction and external rotation) position, the subscapularis slides over the equator, leaving only the weak anteroinferior labrum and capsule to stabilize the humeral head: The 5-o'clock point is truly the vulnerable point of the glenoid rim. **B:** By performing two procedures (Bankart and Bristow–Latarjet), a "triple blocking" of the shoulder is obtained (the so-called 2B3 procedure): (1) bumper (or Bankart) effect, (2) bony (or bone block) effect, and (3) belt (or sling) effect.

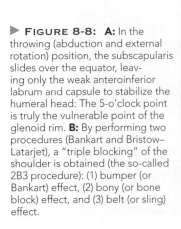

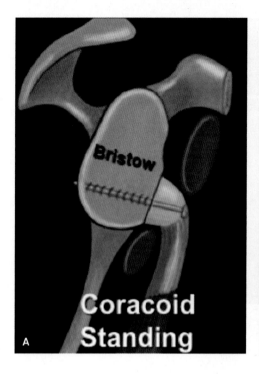
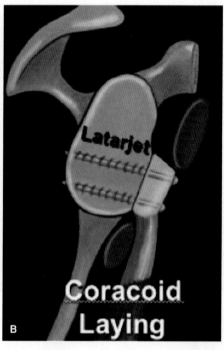

◀ **FIGURE 8-9:** The bone block must be passed through the subscapularis muscle and can be placed either in the standing position **(A)** or in the laying position **(B)**.

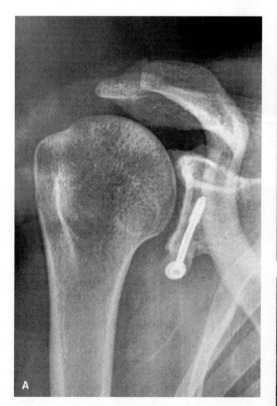
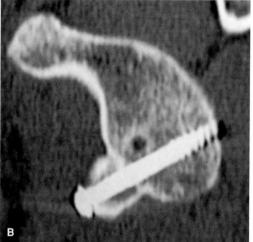
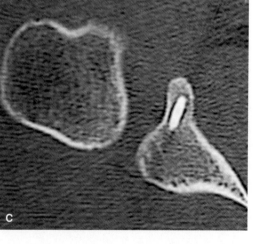

▲ **FIGURE 8-10:** Bristow procedure with fixation of the bone block in the standing position with one screw. Postoperative AP radiograph **(A)**, CT scan coronal (en face) view **(B)**, and axial view **(C)**. Notice the restoration of the glenoid concavity provided by the bone block in the standing position.

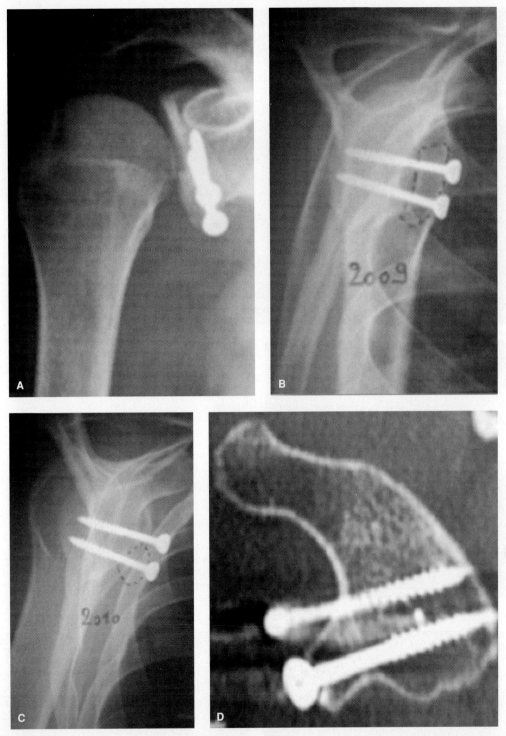

▲ **FIGURE 8-11:** Latarjet procedure with the coracoid process in the lying position fixed with two partially threaded screws as seen on postoperative AP view **(A)** and lateral view **(B)**. The x-ray **(C)** and CT scan **(D)** performed 1 year after surgery demonstrate partial proximal resorption of the bone block, probably because of decreased constraint proximally (Wolff's law).

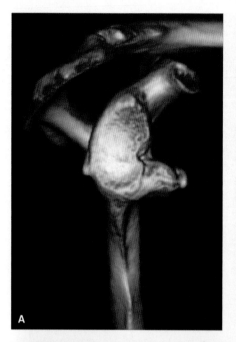

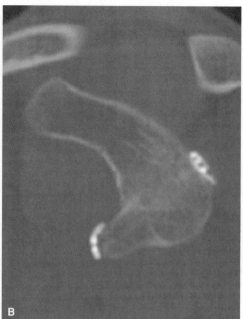

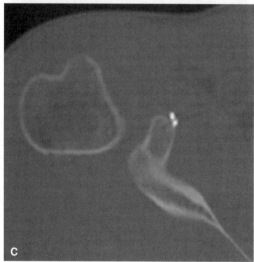

▲ **FIGURE 8-12:** Arthroscopic Bristow procedure using a double button to fix the bone block to the anterior glenoid neck. Anterior glenoid reconstruction, as seen on 3D CT scan **(A)**, en face view **(B)**, and axial view **(C)**; same patient as Figures 8-4 and 8-5.

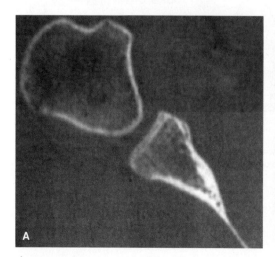

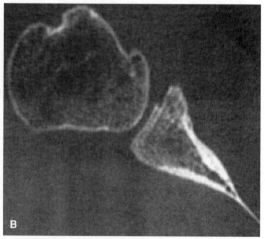

▲ **FIGURE 8-13:** Low-axial views on CT scan demonstrate anterior glenoid deficiency before surgery **(A)**, and glenoid reconstruction after arthroscopic Bristow–Latarjet procedure **(B)**; same patient as Figures 8-4, 8-5, and 8-12.

CONCLUSIONS

Fracture or erosion of the anteroinferior glenoid rim has long been a known etiology of recurrent glenohumeral instability. It has been demonstrated that about 50% of the shoulders with recurrent anterior glenohumeral instability have an osseous Bankart lesion while 40% demonstrate erosion or compression of the glenoid rim; only 10% of symptomatic shoulders have no glenoid bone lesions. A variety of specialized x-ray views have been developed to augment the clinical examination in this patient population. We believe 3D CT to offer the most complete assessment of the status of the glenoid, and use it routinely prior to surgical intervention. The degree of glenoid bone loss needed to contribute to recurrent instability is debatable, but 20% to 25% appears to be a minimum threshold to consider a bone grafting procedure. Surgical intervention should be based on patient variables and surgeon's experience, but we feel appropriate care should address both soft tissue and bony components of the patient's pathology to optimize surgical outcomes. When there is a bone fragment equivalent to the glenoid bone loss and no capsular deficiency, a bony Bankart repair is often sufficient. However, when the bony fragment is partially resorbed or absent, a bone graft is needed. The advantage of the Bristow–Latarjet procedure over an iliac crest (or allograft) bone graft is that the coracoid transfer provides a local, living, vascularized bone graft with the additional benefit of the "seat-belt effect" given by the conjoint tendon. Because patients with glenoid erosion also often have deficient anterior capsules, the Bristow–Latarjet is an optimal procedure, addressing both components of shoulder instability: The glenoid deficiency and the soft tissue deficiency. Today, this procedure can be performed under arthroscopy, in combination with a labrum repair, and is our prefered procedure in cases of recurrent anterior instability with glenoid bone deficiency.

References

1. Boileau P, Villalba M, Héry JY, et al. Risk factors for recurrence of shoulder instability after arthroscopic Bankart repair. *J Bone Joint Surg.* 2006;88A(8):1755–1763.
2. Geiger DF, Hurley JA, Tovey JA, et al. Results of arthroscopic versus open Bankart suture repair. *Clin Orthop.* 1997;337:111–117.
3. Guanche CA, Quick DC, Sodergren KM, et al. Arthroscopic versus open reconstruction of the shoulder in patients with isolated Bankart lesions. *Am J Sports Med.* 1996;24:144–148.
4. Steinbeck J, Jerosch J. Arthroscopic transglenoid stabilization versus open anchor suturing in traumatic anterior instability of the shoulder. *Am J Sports Med.* 1998;26:373–378.
5. Hobby J, Griffin D, Dunbar M, et al. Is arthroscopic surgery for stabilisation of chronic shoulder instability as effective as open surgery? A systematic review and meta-analysis of 62 studies including 3044 arthroscopic operations. *J Bone Joint Surg Br.* 2007;89(9):1188–1196.
6. Kim SH, Ha KI, Cho YB, et al. Arthroscopic anterior stabilization of the shoulder: Two to six-year follow-up. *J Bone Joint Surg.* 2003;85A(8):1511–1518.
7. Burkhart SS, DeBeer JF. Traumatic glenohumeral bone defects and their relationship to failure of arthroscopic Bankart repairs: significance of the glenoid's "inverted pear" and the humeral "engaging Hill-Sachs lesion." *Arthroscopy.* 2000;16:677–694.
8. Rowe CR. Prognosis in dislocations of the shoulder. *J Bone Joint Surg.* 1956;38A:957–977.
9. Kummel BM. Fractures of the glenoid causing chronic dislocation of the shoulder. *Clin Orthop.* 1970;69:189–191.
10. Aston JW Jr, Gregory CF. Dislocation of the shoulder with significant fracture of the glenoid. *J Bone Joint Surg.* 1973;55A(7):1531–1533.
11. Hovelius L, Eriksson K, Fredin H, et al. Recurrences after initial dislocation of the shoulder. Results of a prospective study of treatment. *J Bone Joint Surg.* 1983;65A:343–349.
12. Rowe CR, Patel D, Southmayd WW. The Bankart procedure: A long-term end-result study. *J Bone Joint Surg.* 1978;60A:1–16.
13. Griffith JF, Antonio GE, Tong CWC, et al. Anterior shoulder dislocation: Quantification of glenoid bone loss with CT. *AJR.* 2003;180:1423–1430.
14. Bernageau J, Patte D, Bebeyre J, et al. Intérêt du profil glénoïdien dans les luxations récidivantes de l'épaule. *Rev Chir Orthop Reparatrice Appar Mot.* 1976;62(suppl 2):142–147.
15. Edwards TB, Boulahia A, Walch G. Radiographic analysis of bone defects in chronic anterior shoulder instability. *Arthroscopy.* 2003;19(7):732–739.
16. Garth WP, Slappey CE, Ochs CW. Roentgenographic demonstration of instability of the shoulder: The apical oblique projection. A technical note. *J Bone Joint Surg.* 1984;66A(9):1450–1453.
17. Rokous JR, Feagin JA, Abbott HG. Modified axillary roentgenogram. A useful adjunct in the diagnosis of recurrent instability of the shoulder. *Clin Orthop.* 1972;82:84–86.
18. Seltzer SE, Weissman BN. CT findings in normal and dislocating shoulders. *J Can Assoc Radiol.* 1985;36(1):41–46.
19. Bigliani LU, Newton PM, Steinmann SP, et al. Glenoid rim lesions associated with recurrent anterior dislocation of the shoulder. *Am J Sports Med.* 1998;26:41–45.
20. Stevens KJ, Preston BJ, Wallace WA, et al. CT imaging and three-dimensional reconstructions of shoulders with anterior glenohumeral instability. *Clin Anat.* 1999;12:326–336.
21. Burkhart SS, De Beer JF, Tehrany AM, et al. Quantifying glenoid bone loss arthroscopically in shoulder instability. *Arthroscopy.* 2002;18(5):488–491.
22. Tehrany AM, Burkhart SS. The bare spot: A method of evaluating bone loss in glenohumeral instability. Presented at the 20th Annual Meeting of the Arthroscopy Association of North America, Seattle, WA, April 20, 2011.
23. Itoi E, Lee SB, Berglund LJ, et al. The effect of a glenoid defect on anteroinferior stability of the shoulder after

Bankart repair: A cadaveric study. *J Bone Joint Surg.* 2000;82A:35–46.

24. Sugaya H, Moriishi J, Dohi M, et al. Glenoid rim morphology in recurrent anterior glenohumeral instability. *J Bone Joint Surg.* 2003;85A(5):878–884.

25. Balg F, Boileau P. The instability severity index score: A simple pre-operative score to select patients for arthroscopic or open shoulder stabilization. *J Bone Joint Surg.* 2007;89B(11):1470–1477.

26. Lo IKY, Parten PM, Burkhart SS. The inverted pear glenoid: An indicator of significant glenoid bone loss. *Arthroscopy.* 2004;20(2):169–174.

27. Kim SH, Ha KI, Kim YM. Arthroscopic revision Bankart repair: A prospective outcome study. *Arthroscopy.* 2002; 18(5):469–482.

28. Bankart ASB. Recurrent or habitual dislocation of the shoulder joint. *Br Med J.* 1923;2:1132–1133.

29. Helfet AJ. Coracoid transplantation for recurrent dislocation of the shoulder. *J Bone Joint Surg Br.* 1958;40B:198–202.

30. Latarjet M. Traitement de la luxation récidivante de l'épaule. *Lyon Chir.* 1954;49(8):986–993.

31. Boileau P, Mercier N, Roussanne Y, et al. Arthroscopic Bankart-Bristow-Latarjet procedure: The development and early results of a safe and reproducible technique. *Arthroscopy.* 2010;26(11):1434–1450.

32. Sugaya H, Moriishi J, Kanisawa I, et al. Arthroscopic osseous Bankart repair for chronic recurrent traumatic anterior glenohumeral instability. *J Bone Joint Surg.* 2005;87A(8):1752–1760.

33. Eden R. Zur Operation der habituellen Schulterluxation unter Mitteilung eines neuen Verfahrens bei Abriss am inneren Pfannenrand. *Dtsch Z Chir.* 1918;144: 268–280.

34. Hybinette S. De la transplantation d'un fragment osseux pour remédier aux luxations récidivantes de l'épaule; consultations et résultats opératoires. *Acta Chir Scand.* 1932;71:411–445.

35. Gebhard F, Draeger M, Steinmann R, et al. Functional outcome of Eden-Hybinette-Lange operation in post-traumatic recurrent should dislocation. *Unfallchirurg.* 1997;100(10):770–775 (in German).

36. Scheibel M, Kraus N, Diederichs G, et al. Arthroscopic reconstruction of chronic anteroinferior glenoid defect using an autologous tricortical iliac crest bone grafting technique. *Arch Orthop Trauma Surg.* 2008;128(11): 1295–1300.

37. Taverna E, Golano P, Pascale V, et al. An arthroscopic bone graft procedure for treating anterior-inferior glenohumeral instability. *Knee Surg Sports Traumatol Arthrosc.* 2008;16(9):872–875.

38. Provencher MT, Ghodadra N, LeClere L, et al. Anatomic osteochondral glenoid reconstruction for recurrent glenohumeral instability with glenoid deficiency using a distal tibia allograft. *Arthroscopy.* 2009;25(4):446–452.

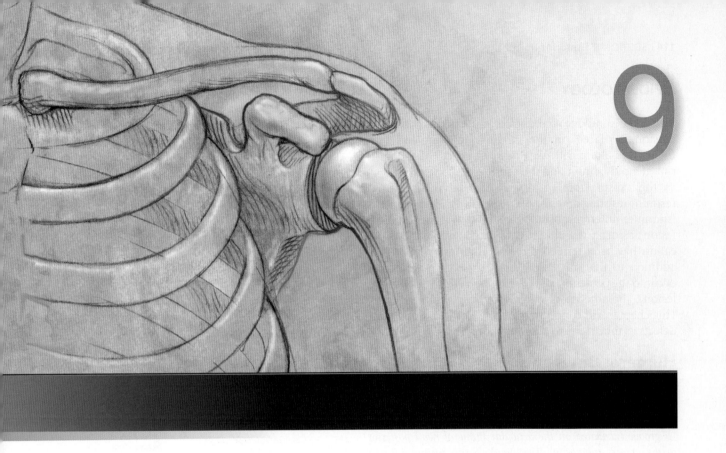

Bone Loss in the Unstable Shoulder: The Humeral Head

Michael J. Griesser / Waqas M. Hussain / Brett W. McCoy /
Aaron J. Bois / Anthony Miniaci

Introduction

The glenohumeral joint is one of the most frequently dislocated joints in the human body secondary to its inherent lack of osseous stability (1). Shoulder stability is critical for precise positioning and function of the upper extremity and is dependent on the interplay between static and dynamic stabilizers (2). Glenohumeral bone loss plays a critical role in recurrent instability by altering joint contact area, congruency, and function of the static restraints (3). Re-establishment of normal articular geometry is important to create a stable platform when critical bone loss exists, particularly in cases of failed soft tissue stabilization procedures.

The purpose of this chapter is to review the available evidence regarding the epidemiology, pathophysiology, evaluation, and management of humeral head bone loss as it pertains to anterior shoulder instability. This chapter will also review the biomechanical and clinical data that address "critical" thresholds for stability and the treatment algorithms for humeral head bone loss derived from these findings. This remains a challenging clinical scenario and limitation in the current literature and areas for future investigation will be discussed as they pertain to the evaluation and management of bone loss. Glenoid bone loss in the setting of anterior and posterior instability will be discussed in the appropriate chapter(s).

EPIDEMIOLOGY

When the shoulder is abducted and externally rotated, tension is placed on the inferior glenohumeral ligament. This along with the "bumper effect" of the anterior glenoid labrum and the capsule (collectively known as the capsulolabral complex) are the main passive restraint resisting anterior dislocation (4). The characteristic anteroinferior capsulolabral injury (Perthes–Bankart lesion) associated with an acute anterior shoulder dislocation has been termed the "essential lesion" (5,6). In addition to this soft tissue injury, osseous injuries can occur to the posterior–superior humeral head (Hill-Sachs lesion), the anterior or anteroinferior glenoid, or both. This chapter will concentrate on the humeral head bony defects as they relate to anterior shoulder instability.

Humeral Bone Loss

In 1861, Flower (7) described the anatomical lesions commonly found in the setting of recurrent anterior glenohumeral instability; included in this description was that of *"a groove excavated on the articular humeral head posterior to the greater tuberosity."* This lead to the humeral head defect being labeled the *"typical defect."* In 1940, Hill and Sachs (8) utilized radiographic analysis of the humeral head to thoroughly evaluate and describe *"compression fractures."* This pathology, which is commonly referred to as a *"Hill-Sachs lesion"* was evident in 74% of patients with recurrent anterior glenohumeral instability. Subsequent studies demonstrate similar rates of humeral head defects (as defined radiologically) ranging from 67% to 81% of patients following an initial dislocation (9–11), and from 70% to 87% of patients following recurrent instability (9,11,12). Advanced imaging and arthroscopy may provide a more sensitive method for assessing intra-articular pathology, including glenohumeral bone loss. Not surprisingly, several authors have noticed slightly higher incidence of Hill-Sachs defects with arthroscopy compared to radiological studies following both first-time dislocations (47% to 100%) (13–17) and recurrent glenohumeral instability (84% to 93%) (16,17).

PATHOPHYSIOLOGY AND PATHOANATOMY OF GLENOHUMERAL BONE LOSS

The mechanisms involved in anterior shoulder instability correlate with the pathoanatomy created at the time of injury. An understanding of the pathoanatomy facilitates judicious surgical planning as neglect of "critical" bone loss, either unipolar or bipolar, has been correlated with higher recurrence rates following isolated repairs of the capsulolabral complex.

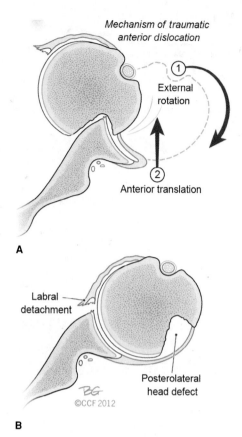

▲ **FIGURE 9-1:** Mechanism of traumatic anterior shoulder dislocation. **A:** Combined forces in external rotation and anterior translation overcome internal restraints resulting in anterior dislocation. **B:** This results in compression of the posterolateral aspect of the humeral head onto the anterior glenoid rim. (Adapted from: Matsen FA 3rd, Chebli C, Lippitt S. Principles for the evaluation and management of shoulder instability. *J Bone Joint Surg Am.* 2006;88:648–659.)

Humeral Bone Loss

Mechanism of Injury

The most common mechanism for an initial, traumatic anterior dislocation is an indirect force with the arm in the abducted and externally rotated position. The dislocation occurs when the restraint provided by the static and dynamic stabilizers has been exceeded. In 1940, Hill and Sachs (8) postulated that the compression fracture of the humeral head was a result of "impingement of the weakest portion of the humeral head (the posterolateral aspect of the articular surface) against the anterior rim of the glenoid fossa" (Fig. 9-1). This mechanism of injury has since been confirmed in both clinical and biomechanical studies.

Morphology of Humeral Head Defects (Location, Orientation, and Size)

Richards et al. (18) provided a thorough description of the depth and location of arthroscopically confirmed

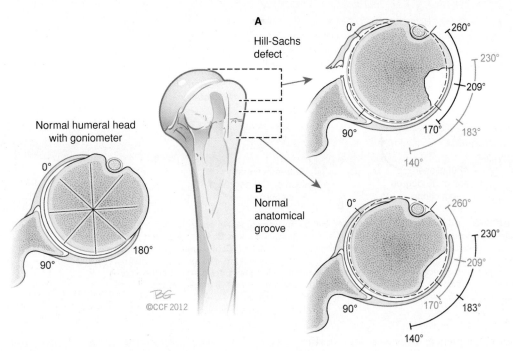

▲ **FIGURE 9-2:** **A:** Typical location of Hill-Sachs lesion. **B:** Anatomic groove. (Adapted from: Richards RD, Sartoris DJ, Pathria MN, et al. Hill-Sachs lesion and normal humeral groove: MR imaging features allowing their differentiation. *Radiology*. 1994;190:665–668.)

Hill-Sachs lesions in 28 patients with anterior shoulder instability based on transaxial MRI with a 360-degree frame of reference. Using this imaging technique, the Hill-Sachs defect was located axially within the range of 170 to 260 degrees, with an average midpoint of 209 degrees (Fig. 9-2). Proximally, Hill-Sachs defects were found within the top 5 mm of the humeral head and extended up to 18 mm distally from the top of the humeral head (average 12 mm). Depth varied in relation to overall lesion size, ranging from 2 to 6 mm (average 4 mm). In contrast, the normal anatomical groove was located slightly more posterior (articular arc location, 140 to 230 degrees) and extended more distally on humeral shaft, with the upper limit extending between 20 and 32 mm from the top of the humeral head (Fig. 9-2). The average depth of the anatomical groove was 3 mm.

In a more recent study, Saito et al. (19) utilized axial CT to map the location and size of Hill-Sachs lesions in reference to the location of the bare area of the proximal humerus. Using the top of the humeral head as a reference point, Hill-Sachs lesions were observed between 0 and 24 mm, whereas the bare areas were found at 19 to 21 mm and extended to the 37- to 39-mm slice level. Interestingly, the bare area was deeper on average than the Hill-Sachs lesions in this cohort of 34 patients with recurrent anterior instability (average depth of the sulcus 6 ± 4.9 mm and average depth of the Hill-Sachs lesion 5 ± 4 mm). This study supports the theory by Richards et al. (18) that Hill-Sachs defects can be easily differentiated from normal anatomical bare areas found

along the posterolateral aspect of the proximal humerus using the superior-to-inferior extent of the humeral head depression found on routine axial imaging.

Burkhart and De Beer (20) provided the first detailed description of the pathoanatomy of significant glenohumeral bone defects which correlated with surgical failure of arthroscopic Bankart repairs. In this study, the orientation of a Hill-Sachs defect was used as the main criterion to decide whether a humeral head defect was considered "significant or critical." The orientation of a Hill-Sachs lesion is determined by the position of the humeral head when it comes into contact with the anterior glenoid. A critical defect, referred to as an "engaging" Hill-Sachs lesion, is a defect with the long axis parallel to the anterior glenoid with the shoulder in a "functional" position of 90-degree abduction and 0- to 130-degree external rotation (Fig. 9-3A).

In contrast, insignificant or "nonengaging" lesions have their long axis diagonal to the anterior glenoid when the shoulder is in a functional position, and the "engagement point" only occurs when the shoulder is in a nonfunctional position of less than 70-degree abduction (Fig. 9-3B,C).

From a biomechanical standpoint, the concept of engaging and nonengaging lesions has been recently challenged by the concept of the glenoid track (21), which is discussed later in this chapter.

The magnitude of bone loss in a Hill-Sachs or reverse Hill-Sachs lesion is dependent on multiple factors including dislocation frequency, chronicity, and force. Several authors have correlated the incidence of Hill-Sachs defects

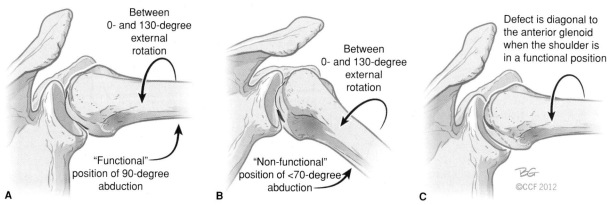

▲ **FIGURE 9-3:** Engaging and nonengaging Hill-Sachs lesions. **A:** An engaging lesion is parallel to the anterior glenoid rim when the shoulder is in a functional position. **B:** The "engagement point" of a nonengaging lesion occurs with the arm in a nonfunctional position. **C:** In a functional position, a nonengaging lesion is diagonal and nonparallel to the anterior glenoid rim. (Adapted from: Burkhart SS, De Beer JF. Traumatic glenohumeral bone defects and their relationship to failure of arthroscopic Bankart repairs: Significance of the inverted-pear glenoid and the humeral engaging Hill-Sachs lesion. *Arthroscopy.* 2000;16:677–694.)

with dislocation frequency; however, few studies have attempted to correlate dislocation frequency with defect size (11,13,16,22). Cetik et al. (22) used CT arthrography to assess the relationship between the number of shoulder dislocations and the magnitude of humeral head bone loss in a series of 30 patients who underwent open surgery for recurrent anterior shoulder dislocation. Patients were divided into three groups based on dislocation frequency; the mean percentage of articular surface involvement was 11.9% in the first group (1 to 5 dislocations), 25.4% in the second group (6 to 20 dislocations), and 26% in the third group (over 20 dislocations). The average depth of the Hill-Sachs lesions was 4.14 mm in the first group, 5.13 mm in the second group, and 4.38 mm in the third group. Griffith et al. (23) also noted that Hill-Sachs lesions were more severe in patients with recurrent instability. Based on these results, an obvious association exists between dislocation frequency and the extent and depth of Hill-Sachs lesions.

Humeral head defect size is also affected by dislocations of longer duration, as seen with neglected and locked shoulder dislocations (24–28).

Large bipolar erosions can be found at sites of osseous contact between the malpositioned humeral head on the anterior glenoid rim in patients with chronic dislocations (Fig. 9-4). The patients will make adjustments to facilitate glenohumeral motion coupled with abnormal contact forces produced by periscapular muscles. In a study using both cadaveric specimens and patients with chronically locked shoulder dislocations, Kirtland et al. (25) evaluated the size of Hill-Sachs defects and found that on average, defects were 26 mm wide, 43 mm long, and 18 mm deep. The large cavitary lesions formed by chronic dislocations often require some form of biological or artificial reconstruction to restore the normal articular arc of the humeral head.

The size of the humeral head defect often correlates with the magnitude of the force producing the instability. Miniaci and Gish (29) reported on a series of patients with Hill-Sachs defects involving 25% or more of the humeral articular surface following multiple traumatic dislocations from contact sports or seizures. Many of these patients had a history of failed soft tissue repairs and ultimately underwent osteoarticular allograft reconstruction. Robinson et al. (30) reported on a series of 26 patients with complex posterior fracture-dislocations of the shoulder and the etiologies were seizures or falls from a height. In all patients, a large reverse Hill-Sachs lesion was found along the anterior aspect of the humeral head. Traumatic dislocation is the most common mechanism responsible for producing large Hill-Sachs defects.

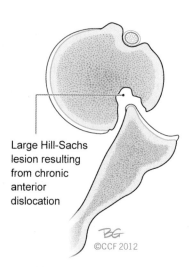

Large Hill-Sachs lesion resulting from chronic anterior dislocation

▲ **FIGURE 9-4:** Chronic anterior shoulder dislocation with associated large Hill-Sachs lesion. (Adapted from: Mehta V. Humeral head plasty for a chronic locked anterior shoulder dislocation. *Orthopedics.* 2009;32:52.)

Microinstability, as seen in the overhead athlete and in patients with anterior subluxation, may generate enough contact pressures between the humeral head and the glenoid rim to create a smaller Hill-Sachs defect (31,32). Miniaci et al. (33) reported on the clinical and MRI results of 14 professional baseball pitchers who had no history of previous shoulder injury, symptoms, or surgery; 29% of the throwing shoulders had evidence of Hill-Sachs lesions. More recently, Owens et al. (34) reported on a cohort of 27 military cadets with a diagnosis of anterior shoulder subluxation only and found MRI evidence of Hill-Sachs lesions in 93% of these patients. Patients may also present without any apparent history of instability, but with deep anterior shoulder pain, hyperlaxity, and soft tissue and/or bone loss consistent with instability; a condition referred to as the unstable painful shoulder (UPS) (35). These findings demonstrate that the pathoanatomy of a Hill-Sachs lesion is complex and multifactorial and they may develop in the absence of a traumatic shoulder dislocation. These small Hill-Sachs defects are generally not thought to be a major risk factor for recurrent anterior instability in patients who undergo soft tissue stabilization procedure (13).

SIGNIFICANCE OF BONE LOSS: BIOMECHANICAL DATA

Humeral Bone Loss

Bone Loss as a Risk for Recurrent Instability— Biomechanical Rationale

In their original series, Burkhart and De Beer (20) described a patient who underwent second look arthroscopy where a normal appearing capsulolabral complex was found, but on dynamic examination the glenoid rim "dropped" into the large Hill-Sachs lesion at 30-degree external rotation. This mode of failure was defined as a humeral articular arc length deficit (36). A similar concept was described in 1948 by Palmer and Widen (37).

Biomechanical Studies of Humeral Bone Loss

There is a limited number of in vitro studies that have assessed the effects of humeral bone loss on glenohumeral stability. Sekiya et al. (38) analyzed the anterior translation and stability ratio (displacing force divided by compressive load) in a cadaveric study by varying the amount of shoulder abduction and external rotation following creation of sequentially larger posterolateral humeral head defects. Defects that were 25% of the humeral head diameter or larger revealed significantly less anterior translation before dislocation and decreased stability ratios compared to the intact specimens. The stability ratio normalized following osteoar-

ticular allograft repair. Kaar et al. (39) noted that defects involving ~60% of the humeral head radius, or larger (5/8 and 7/8 defects respectively, centered at 209 degrees on the axial plane), lead to decreased glenohumeral stability when tested in external rotation and abduction and suggested reconstruction of such defects in addition to a standard capsulolabral repair.

SIGNIFICANCE OF HUMERAL BONE LOSS: CLINICAL DATA

Humeral

In 1978, Rowe et al. (24) analyzed the long-term results of Bankart repairs for recurrent instability and found an overall recurrence rate of 3.4% (5/145); the recurrence rates were 4.7% and 6% for patients with "moderately severe" and "severe" Hill-Sachs lesions, respectively. In two of the five cases deemed as failures there were associated glenoid rim lesions (i.e., presence of bipolar lesions). Hovelius et al. (40) reported a similar trend between Hill-Sachs lesions and recurrent instability. Of the 107 patients found with a Hill-Sachs lesion, 39 (36%) had recurrent instability; however, this finding was not statistically significant. Shortly thereafter, Rowe et al. (41) reviewed the intraoperative findings of 32 patients who underwent revision surgery for recurrent anterior instability. In this series, a Hill-Sachs lesion was found in 76% of the 29 shoulders at the time of revision surgery. A "mild" Hill-Sachs lesion (3 mm depth) was found in 2 patients (7%), "moderately severe" lesion (5 mm depth) in 17 patients (59%), and "severe" lesion (10 mm depth) in 4 patients (14%). However, the authors state that 22 patients (76%) had glenoid rim defects at the time of their index procedure. In addition, these 29 patients underwent one of six different index instability procedures, further confounding the results of this study.

In a more recent study, Burkhart et al. (42) reported 21 recurrent dislocations and subluxations in their series of 194 patients who underwent a primary soft tissue repair; of these, 14 had significant bone defects including 3 engaging Hill-Sachs lesions and 11 inverted-pear Bankart lesions, for a combined recurrence rate of 67%. Significant bone defects in this study were defined intraoperatively on dynamic arthroscopy and no quantitative radiographic measurements were determined. In 2011, Gerson et al. (43) performed a case-control analysis of 91 patients with recurrent instability to evaluate the risk of Hill-Sachs lesions on the failure of soft tissue stabilization procedures. Using preoperative sagittal and axial MRI, the presence, size, and location of Hill-Sachs lesions were analyzed. Of 91 patients included in analysis, 77 (84.6%) had identifiable Hill-Sachs lesions and 14 (15%) had evidence of glenoid bone loss. Thirty-two patients (35.2%) suffered from failure of soft tissue stabilization. The results of this study showed that larger Hill-Sachs lesions were found in patients who failed surgical intervention when compared to patients that did not fail; however, in this retrospective study, the presence of a glenoid lesion did not correlate with recurrent instability.

EVALUATION OF BONE LOSS

History and Physical Examination

A detailed history should be obtained from all patients who present with recurrent shoulder instability, including hand dominance, occupation, and recreational activities (most notably, involvement in contact sports). Several warning signs and symptoms have been described in patients with shoulder instability and critical bone loss that help differentiate them from more benign episodes of instability. Patients with significant bone deficiency typically sustain high-energy injuries at their index dislocation followed by multiple lower energy episodes, including activities of daily living. Patients with significant humeral head defects may present with a catching or popping sensation when the shoulder is at low levels of abduction (below 70 degrees) and typically avoid overhead activities; however, symptoms arising at midrange may also occur when critical glenoid bone loss is present. Prior unsuccessful soft tissue repairs are often seen in the setting of critical bone deficiency. Although less commonly associated with anterior instability, patients may also present with a history of seizure disorder or a locked, neglected dislocation.

The history should be accompanied by a thorough physical examination including both shoulders and affected upper extremity beginning with inspection to evaluate for scars, deformity, or atrophy. Evaluate active and passive motions, and perform rotator cuff and deltoid strength tests, and neurovascular examination. Ask the patient to demonstrate the position of the shoulder during the initial and subsequent instability episodes, commonly referred to as the "no touch" examination. Incorporate special tests to identify bone loss with the patient sitting or supine. Begin with the "shoulder apprehension test": The arm being examined is placed in abduction, extension, and external rotation; start with the patient's elbow at their side and slowly increase passive abduction and external rotation to the 90–90-degree position. In cases of glenohumeral bone loss (unipolar or bipolar deficiency), patients typically exhibit apprehension in 30 to 70 degrees of abduction and in less than 90 degrees of external rotation; the so-called "bony apprehension test" (29) (Fig. 9-5).

Perform a "load-and-shift test" to assess the status of the glenoid concavity (clinical analogue of the stability ratio). With the patient seated and involved forearm resting on their thigh, the humeral head is pressed into the glenoid fossa while anterior translation is attempted. Easy translation of the humeral head over the glenoid lip may be accompanied by a grinding sensation and/or apprehension and suggests that the lip of the glenoid cavity is deficient (2). During both the shoulder apprehension and load-and-shift tests, patient symptoms typically resolve when the humeral head is centered back onto the glenoid fossa. Although not a direct indicator of bone loss, when shoulder hyperlaxity (external rotation >90 degrees or asymmetric hyperabduction >20 degrees) (44) is found with significant glenoid bone loss, the risk of recurrent instability following a primary

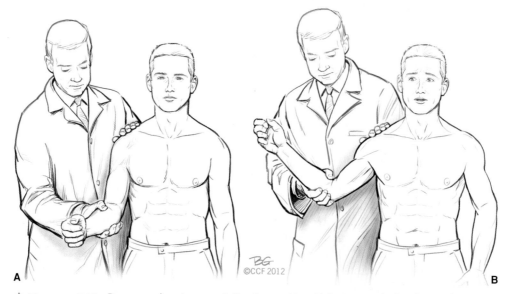

▲ **FIGURE 9-5:** Bony apprehension test. **A:** Starting position. **B:** Patients with glenohumeral bone loss may demonstrate apprehension in a nonfunctional position (<70-degree abduction and <90-degree external rotation). (Adapted from: Bushnell BD, Creighton A, Herring MM. Bony instability of the shoulder: Current concepts. *Arthroscopy.* 2008;24:1061–1073.)

repair is increased and should therefore be incorporated into the clinical examination (45) (see Fig. 9-3).

Noninvasive Imaging and Arthroscopic Evaluation

Preoperative assessment of bone loss in shoulder instability is crucial for surgical decision making as unrecognized bone loss, if significant, often requires additional reconstructive procedures to restore normal glenohumeral mechanics. In addition to the routine radiographic views of the shoulder, specialized radiographic views and advanced imaging techniques have been developed in an attempt to detect and quantify bone defects of the humeral head and the glenoid rim. Although multiple radiographic methods have been described for detecting glenohumeral bone loss, there is no universally accepted method to quantify such defects. A complete overview of the radiographic evaluation of the shoulder will be discussed in the appropriate chapter. Each physician should incorporate some combination of these studies in their evaluation.

Humeral Bone Loss

Hill and Sachs (8) were the first to point out the importance of shoulder rotation for detecting humeral head impression fractures on plain radiographs; suggesting that only in "marked internal rotation" will the posterolateral aspect of the head become viewed in profile for proper evaluation of defect length and depth. They recommended tangential views for assessment of defect width. In 1959, Hall et al. (46) described a special view for identifying Hill-Sachs lesions, which is commonly referred to as the Stryker notch view (47). Both the AP view in internal rotation and the Stryker notch view have good sensitivity for detecting humeral head lesions on plain radiographs (48,49).

Ito et al. (31,50) described a method for measuring defect width and depth on plain radiographs using a variation of the Stryker notch view. Kodali et al. (51) evaluated the accuracy of 2D CT scan measurements of Hill-Sachs lesions and found that observers were more accurate in depth rather than width measurements and that sagittal and axial plane measurements were more accurate for evaluating defects than coronal plane measurements. Humeral head defects have also been quantified on the basis of the percentage of articular involvement using either an axillary radiograph or axial CT imaging (52) (Fig. 9-6). Treatment recommendations based on this calculation were dependent on clinical evidence of defect engagement on the anterior glenoid rim with the shoulder in abduction and external rotation.

Cho et al. (53) used 3D CT from 104 patients (107 shoulders) to preoperatively predict engagement of a Hill-Sachs lesion in patients who were undergoing surgery for recurrent anterior instability. In cases of engaging

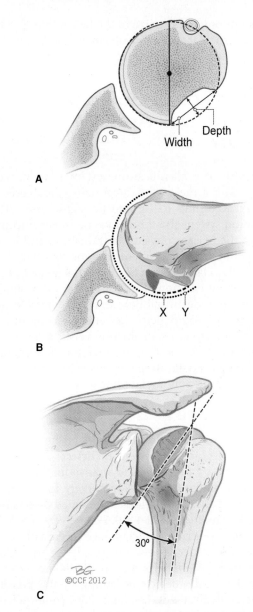

▲ **FIGURE 9-6:** Methods used to quantify Hill-Sachs lesions. **A:** Such defects may be quantified using depth or width measurements, **(B)** percentage of humeral head involvement [(X/Y) × 100], and/or **(C)** by measuring the Hill-Sachs angle. (Adapted from: Cho SH, Cho NS, Rhee YG. Preoperative analysis of the Hill-Sachs lesion in anterior shoulder instability: How to predict engagement of the lesion. *Am J Sports Med.* 2011 and Chen AL, Hunt SA, Hawkins RJ, et al. Management of bone loss associated with recurrent anterior glenohumeral instability. *Am J Sports Med.* 2005;33:912–925.)

lesions, the mean width was 52% (range, 27% to 66%) and depth was 14% (range, 8% to 20%) of the humeral head diameter on axial images. The Hill-Sachs angle was 25.6 degrees (±7.4 degrees) in engaging lesions. Significant differences were found between engaging and nonengaging lesions only for axial plane measurements of width, depth, and Hill-Sachs angle measurements; measurements of defect location were insignificant.

Evaluating the clinical significance of a humeral head defect is a complex and multifactorial process that depends not only on the size of the lesion, but also the amount of articular surface involvement and location of the defect relative to the glenoid track.

CLASSIFICATION OF BONE LOSS ASSOCIATED WITH ANTERIOR INSTABILITY

The purpose of a classification system is to provide clinicians with a means for categorizing the degree of pathology according to prognostic significance. This classification system should include pertinent information from the history, physical examination, and imaging modalities. The assessment of bone loss may be a portion of this classification but is not adequate to help guide treatment decisions without further information. Specific to shoulder instability and bone loss, ideally a classification would help the surgeon determine a threshold for a larger reconstruction versus a soft tissue procedure. Based on the available literature, few scientifically validated classification systems exist for shoulder instability with glenohumeral bone loss.

Humeral Bone Loss

Rowe and Zarins (54) classified humeral head lesions into three categories according to defect size (length and depth) based on the intraoperative findings of 29 patients who underwent revision surgery for recurrent anterior instability. Mild lesions represented defects that were 2 × 0.3 cm; moderate, 4 × 0.5 cm; severe, 4 × 1 cm or larger. In this series, moderate and severe Hill-Sachs lesions were regarded as a major risk factor for failure of the primary instability procedure. Bigliani et al. (55) classified Hill-Sachs defects according to the percentage of head involvement: Less than 20% (mild defect), between 20% and 45% (moderate defect), and greater than 45% (severe defect). The size of the lesion is based on one axial image slice using CT or MRI. Burkhart et al. (42) found a high failure rate of isolated soft tissue stabilization in patients with recurrent anterior instability with *engaging Hill-Sachs lesions,* and when found recommended additional surgical procedures to address the humeral head defect. Since this landmark paper, most authors classify Hill-Sachs defects using this system; such defects can be classified using either dynamic arthroscopy (gold standard) or preoperative CT imaging (53).

The aforementioned classification systems demonstrate the complex nature of this entity; with criteria including direct intraoperative inspection, physical examination, and advanced imaging. It is important to note that these classification systems have not been validated regarding their prognostic value and therefore, surgical planning in the setting of bone loss will require additional consideration.

SURGICAL INDICATIONS AND TECHNIQUES

Currently there are no prospective randomized trials to assist surgeons in the decision-making process for managing glenohumeral bone loss associated with anterior instability (56). Multiple treatment algorithms have been proposed (3,52,57) that the use of biomechanical data and Level IV and Level V clinical evidence as their foundation. Not surprisingly, surgical management of critical bone loss remains a topic of debate and controversy in the orthopedic community. Despite the lack of high-level studies, there are some general trends that have emerged.

Traditionally, bone loss procedures have been considered only after failure of a primary soft tissue stabilization procedure; however, increased recognition of the negative impact of bone deficiency on the success of a soft tissue repair has lead to a paradigm shift with some authors advocating bone augmentation procedures primarily, with or without a soft tissue repair. Any pathology involving the static and dynamic stabilizers of the shoulder should be identified and when indicated, addressed simultaneously to restore shoulder mechanics. Bone augmentation procedures have been traditionally performed as open surgery; however, arthroscopic examination before open reconstruction allows the surgeon to identify and arthroscopically address associated pathology, if necessary (17,58,59).

Humeral Bone Loss

In 1948, Palmer and Widen (37) reported on their results of the Hybbinette-Eden anterior bone block procedure which was originally intended to prevent dislocation of the humeral head into a "false joint cavity" caused by anterior capsular injury and detached labrum. They stated that "compression fracture of the humeral head was the essential lesion" and "recurrent dislocation occurs when the anterior rim of the glenoid slides into the hollow in the humeral head" (Fig. 9-7). This represents one of the earliest procedures to prevent engagement of a large Hill-Sachs lesion and recurrent instability symptoms.

More recently, surgical reconstruction of a humeral head defect has been recommended in patients who have evidence of defect engagement following soft tissue stabilization (36). Others advocate surgical treatment based solely on defect size or location, including in relation to the glenoid track (53,60). Consideration can also involve multiple clinical parameters to decide if a bone augmentation procedure will be performed (61).

Multiple treatment options address critical humeral head defects to prevent lesion engagement. These procedures can be categorized as those that involve (1) rotation of the defect, (2) filling the defect,

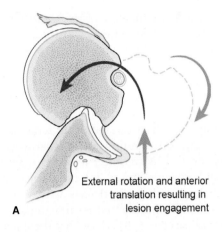

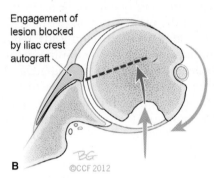

External rotation and anterior translation resulting in lesion engagement

A

Engagement of lesion blocked by iliac crest autograft

B

BG
©CCF 2012

▲ **FIGURE 9-7:** Hybbinette-Eden anterior bone block procedure. **A:** Engagement of the large Hill-Sachs lesion onto the anterior glenoid rim. **B:** Placement of an iliac crest autograft along the anterior glenoid neck limits anterior translation of the humeral head and engagement of the Hill-Sachs lesion. (From: Miniaci A. *Disorders of the Shoulder: Sports Injuries.* Philadelphia, PA: Lippincott Williams & Wilkins; 2013, with permission.)

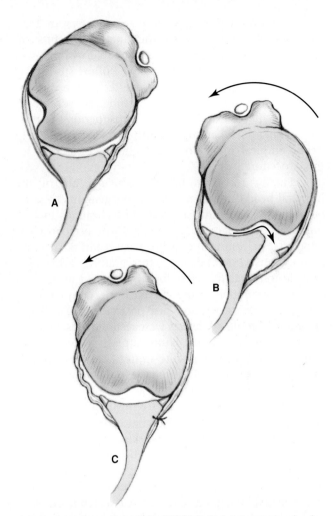

A

B

C

▲ **FIGURE 9-8:** Role of the Hill-Sachs lesion in anterior shoulder instability. **A:** With the arm in internal rotation, the Hill-Sachs lesion is not in contact with the glenoid. **B:** With external rotation, the humeral head translates anteriorly because of the incompetent anterior capsular mechanism. This allows the humeral head to dislocate through the Hill-Sachs lesion. **C:** An adequate Bankart repair keeps the Hill-Sachs lesion contained on the glenoid, unless it is greater than 30% of the humeral articular surface. (Adapted from: Warner JJP, Schulte KR, Imhoff AB. Current concepts in shoulder instability. In: Stauffer RN, Erlich MG, Kostuik JP, Fu FF, eds. *Advances in Operative Orthopaedics.* Vol 3. Philadelphia, PA: Mosby-Year Book: 1995:217–247.)

(3) restoration of the articular arc of the humeral head, and (4) reconstruction of the anterior glenoid. Reconstruction of the glenoid has been recommended in cases without bone loss, to lengthen the glenoid articular arc to prevent engagement (61,62). Two options exist to rotate the lesion away from the anterior glenoid rim; the surgeon can either restrict external rotation by performing an open anterior capsulorrhaphy (63) (Fig. 9-8), or internally rotate the articular surface with a proximal humeral osteotomy (64,65). A capsulorrhaphy procedure is more successful for smaller Hill-Sachs lesions. With larger defects, the amount of overtightening required to limit external rotation and prevent engagement can predispose the patient to late arthrosis (66). Proximal humeral osteotomies are mentioned for historical reasons and have very limited indications due to the potential morbidity associated with this procedure.

Hill-Sachs lesions can also be treated by filling the defect. The term "remplissage" typically refers to procedures that transfer tendon into the defect and thus converts an intra-articular defect into an extra-articular defect. In 1972, Connolly (67) reviewed 90 cases of recurrent anterior instability, of which 10 had "severe"

Hill-Sachs lesions that were surgically treated by an open transfer of the infraspinatus tendon. The stabilization effect was thought to occur as a result of restricted humeral head translation on the glenoid (the so-called "checkrein" effect), rather than restricting external rotation. Only one patient failed this procedure and required further treatment. More recently, Purchase et al. (68) described an arthroscopic "capsulotenodesis" technique utilizing the posterior capsule and infraspinatus tendon with only two failures in 24 patients (7% recurrence rate). Tendon transfer procedures are versatile as they can be performed for acute and chronic instabilities for varying sized lesions. This procedure has been criticized for its nonanatomic nature and concern for recalcitrant loss of motion requiring revision surgery (69). In 2011, Nourissat et al. (70) reported the functional results following a remplissage procedure compared with Bankart repairs alone in a large prospective cohort study. The authors noted that the remplissage technique did not alter the range of motion of the shoulder; however, one-third of patients experienced posterosuperior shoulder pain with forceful motion. Further research will help define surgical indications and clinical outcomes for this procedure.

Finally, reconstituting the articular arc of the humeral head can prevent lesion engagement. This can be accomplished using a variety of techniques including defect disimpaction (humeralplasty), osteoarticular allografts, or resurfacing arthroplasty (partial or complete). Transhumeral disimpaction grafting of humeral head lesions was first described by Kazel et al. (71) in a cadaveric model. Using curved bone tamps passed through a cortical window just posterior to the bicipital groove, simulated defects were restored close to 97% of their original volume. Humeralplasty may be most beneficial following an acute injury (72) and there is minimal information outlining the indications and outcomes for this procedure (28,73).

Osteoarticular allograft reconstruction of Hill-Sachs defects is a viable option that is typically reserved for young patients with large defects with good bone density and the absence of degenerative joint disease (72). Two broad categories exist for allograft reconstruction of humeral lesions; osteochondral plug transfer and size-matched bulk grafts. Only a few case reports exist in the literature (two patients total) describing the technique of osteochondral plug transfer into the base of a humeral defect, both reporting good results after 12 months of follow-up (74,75). In 1997, Gerber (76) was the first to report the use of bulk allografts to reconstruct large Hill-Sachs defects in four patients with chronic anterior dislocations (reference). Yagishita and Thomas (77) later documented successful allograft reconstruction for a large humeral head defect in the setting of a chronic anterior dislocation using a structural allograft taken from the femoral head. Miniaci and Gish (29) described a mathematical method to more precisely size-matched osteoarticular allografts taken from the humeral head in a series of 18 patients who had failed previous instability repairs. All patients had humeral head defects greater than 25% of the articular arc, as measured intraoperatively. At 2-year follow-up, there were no episodes of recurrent instability and 89% of patients returned to work. Osteoarticular allografts have reported complications such as infection, graft resorption, nonunion, or hardware failure. In the experience reported by Miniaci and Gish (29), 2 of 18 patients required screw removal; there were no other complications reported.

Recent interest has emerged in the use of partial resurfacing arthroplasty to address moderate-to-large engaging Hill-Sachs defects. This technique utilizes a round cap-like cobalt-chrome articular component that fills the Hill-Sachs lesion on the posterosuperior humeral head. These techniques avoid some of the potential complications associated with osteoarticular allografts including nonunion and graft resorption; however, possible mismatch between the implant and defect geometry still exists, requiring removal of unaffected bone and surrounding articular cartilage.

Raiss et al. (78) recently reported a series of 10 patients with chronic locked anterior shoulder dislocations with large Hill-Sachs defects who were successfully treated with uncemented resurfacing arthroplasty. However, Scalise et al. (79) advise that there needs to be sufficient quantity and quality of bone in the epiphyseal portion of the humerus to allow stable fixation of the implant. Similarly, Copeland (80) reported that humeral resurfacing requires a minimum of 60% of normal humeral head bone stock and advised conventional stemmed arthroplasty for those with osteopenia. Elderly patients with large (40% or greater) defects and osteoporotic bone or degenerative changes should be considered for a stemmed prostheses (26).

Author's Preferred Surgical Technique

There is no consensus about the degree of humeral or glenoid bone loss that warrants reconstruction. In our practice, we consider bone augmentation procedures when bone loss exceeds approximately 25% of the posterosuperior humeral head (i.e., measured as either the diameter of the humeral head or the articular arc) or anterior glenoid margin (i.e., AP diameter of inferior glenoid). In cases of bipolar bone loss, there is a lower threshold for reconstruction of the humerus or glenoid. In addition to the magnitude of bone loss, clinical patient parameters such as seizure disorder, age, and activity level are paramount to decision making.

Humeral Bone Loss Procedures

The senior author uses either a size-matched humeral head allograft or a partial resurfacing arthroplasty to address critical humeral head defects associated with shoulder instability. Challenges related to allografts including graft availability and potential complications including hardware failure and graft resorption far outweigh those related to resurfacing arthroplasty, and therefore, resurfacing arthroplasty has recently been the procedure of choice for such problems. In the senior author's clinical experience of over 7 years using resurfacing arthroplasty to manage large Hill-Sachs defects in young patients, no long-term complications have been seen with the use of an artificial implant. This may be partly attributed to implant placement in a relatively nonarticular portion of the humeral head.

The surgical approach and superficial exposure is the same for all bone augmentation procedures. The patient is positioned in a modified beach chair position, inclined 45 degrees. An extended deltopectoral approach is used, and following incision of the clavipectoral fascia, the conjoint tendon is retracted medially to expose the subscapularis tendon. With the borders of the subscapularis tendon appropriately defined and the axillary nerve protected (not routinely exposed), the entire tendon is elevated approximately 1 cm from the lesser tuberosity using electrocautery. The anterior humeral circumflex vessels are typically cauterized along the inferior, muscular portion of the subscapularis tendon. At the level of these vessels, the interval between the muscle and the capsule is identified using a narrow elevator, taking care to protect the axillary nerve. This plane of dissection is continued superiorly and medially to a level 1 cm medial to the glenoid rim. The subscapularis tendon is retracted medially with traction sutures and the use of an anterior Bankart-type or Hohmann retractor to facilitate exposure.

The arm is then placed in the plane of the scapula at 45 degrees of abduction and 45 degrees of external rotation to facilitate assessment of capsular redundancy. If the capsule can be easily pulled away from the humeral head in this arm position, a capsular shift procedure may be required to address capsular redundancy. The capsule is incised 5 to 10 mm medial to its insertion on the humeral neck, extending from the rotator interval to the inferior capsular pouch in line with the subscapularis incision. The humeral head is then retracted with a ring retractor and the capsule is retracted medially to inspect the glenoid rim and capsulolabral complex. Hill-Sachs lesions are visualized with the arm in extension and external rotation. If a Bankart lesion is noted, the lesion is elevated from the medial glenoid neck in the usual fashion and repaired at the end of the bone loss procedure using suture anchors.

Following the above-described anterior exposure, the humeral head retractor is removed and the humerus placed into maximal external rotation to expose the Hill-Sachs lesion. A flat narrow retractor (e.g., Darach) is placed around the humeral neck on the deep surface of the posterosuperior rotator cuff to fully expose the defect on the posterolateral head, which now faces toward the glenoid. For cases where an osteoarticular allograft is to be used, a microsagittal saw is used to smooth and reshape the defect into a chevron-type configuration (Fig. 9-9A). The base (X), height (Y), length (Z), and approximate circumference (C) are then measured to the nearest millimeter (Fig. 9-9B). A segment of humeral head allograft that is 2 to 3 mm larger in all dimensions is placed into the Hill-Sachs defect and carefully trimmed and reshaped in all planes until a perfect size-matched graft is achieved. The graft is provisionally secured with two or three 0.045-inch Kirschner wires,

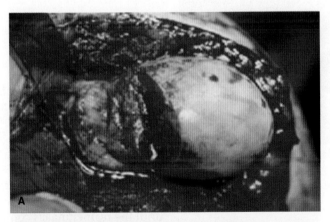

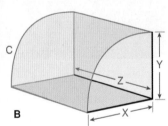

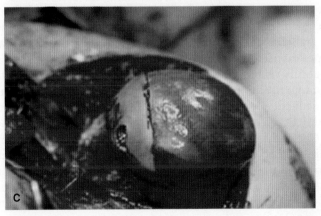

▶ **FIGURE 9-9:** Humeral head allograft reconstruction. **A:** Excised lesion. **B:** Shaping the allograft. **C:** Reconstructed humeral head. (From: Miniaci A. *Disorders of the Shoulder: Sports Injuries*. Philadelphia, PA: Lippincott Williams & Wilkins; 2013, with permission.)

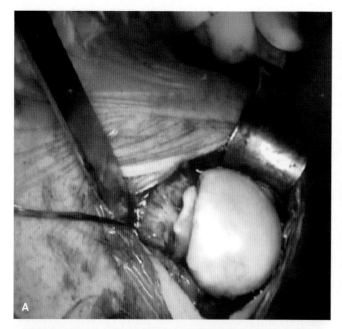

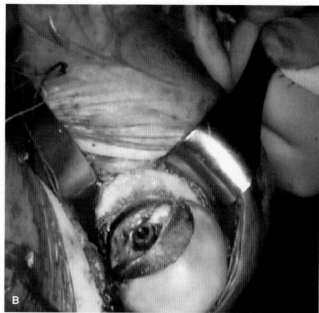

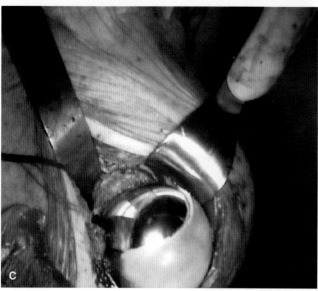

▲ **FIGURE 9-10:** Partial resurfacing of the posterolateral humeral head. **A:** Hill-Sachs defect. **B:** Following insertion of taper post. **C:** Final implant. (From: Miniaci A. *Disorders of the Shoulder: Sports Injuries.* Philadelphia, PA: Lippincott Williams & Wilkins; 2013, with permission.)

and later replaced with 3.5-mm cortical or 4-mm cancellous screws that are lagged and countersunk below the articular surface (Fig. 9-9C).

The surgical approach and exposure of humeral head lesion for partial resurfacing arthroplasty (Hemi-CAP prosthesis; Arthrosurface, Franklin, MA) is similar to that described previously. Once exposed, a drill guide that fully circumscribes the lesion is centered over the defect and a guide pin advanced into the humeral head. A cannulated drill and tap are sequentially placed over the guide pin followed by insertion of a permanent taper post to the appropriate level. Check the height of the taper post to ensure it is flush or slightly below the existing articular cartilage surface to avoid the final component from being placed proud. A sizing probe is inserted into the taper post to obtain the appropriate size of the articular component. A surface reamer is placed over the guide pin and advanced into the cancellous bone until the reamer makes contact with the top of the taper post (Fig. 9-10A,B). After appropriate trialing, the final articular component is placed in the proper orientation and seated into the taper post with an impactor (Fig. 9-10C).

At the time of closure for the above techniques, the joint is irrigated and brought through a range of motion to ensure the reconstructed head provides a smooth congruent articulating surface. A capsulolabral repair is performed if indicated. The capsulotomy is closed with absorbable suture, followed by repair of the subscapularis tendon, which is anatomically reapproximated and secured to its bony footprint using suture anchors along the medial row and nonabsorbable sutures placed laterally. In cases where the humeral head defect was reconstructed with allograft, we routinely obtain a CT scan at 6 months to assess for consolidation and incorporation of the graft.

Postoperative Care

The patient returns for follow-up at 7 to 10 days, at which time the immobilizer can be removed to start rehabilitation. We begin with standard pendulum exercises and isometric shoulder abduction. Full passive range of motion is permitted as tolerated. Activities of daily living are allowed at 6 weeks. Incorporation of internal rotation exercises is dependent on the method of subscapularis dissection. In cases of subscapular detachment, we protect against active and resisted internal rotation and limit external rotation to 30 degrees for 6 weeks. Participation in noncontact or overhead sports is allowed at 4 months; contact sports are permitted at 6 months.

CONCLUSION

Stability of the shoulder results from a delicate balance of static and dynamic factors; the support provided by the bony architecture contributes only a portion of the overall stability. Currently there is a lack of high-level evidence to help guide surgeons with clinical decision making regarding glenohumeral bone loss. This is a multifactorial problem based on the complexity of diagnosis and quantification of the defects as well as the presence of multiple clinical factors that play a role in glenohumeral stability. Further well-conducted studies will help provide clarity to this complex problem.

References

1. Zacchilli MA, Owens BD. Epidemiology of shoulder dislocations presenting to emergency departments in the United States. *J Bone Joint Surg Am.* 2010;92:542–549.
2. Matsen FA 3rd, Chebli C, Lippitt S. Principles for the evaluation and management of shoulder instability. *J Bone Joint Surg Am.* 2006;88:648–659.
3. Bollier MJ, Arciero R. Management of glenoid and humeral bone loss. *Sports Med Arthrosc Rev.* 2010;18:140–148.
4. Turkel SJ, Panio MW, Marshall JL, et al. Stabilizing mechanisms preventing anterior dislocation of the glenohumeral joint. *J Bone Joint Surg Am.* 1981;63:1208–1217.
5. Perthes G. Uber operationen bei habitueller schulterluxation. *Deutsche Zeitschr Chir.* 1906;85:199–227.
6. Bankart ASB. The pathology and treatment of recurrent instability of the shoulder-joint. *Br J Surg.* 1938;26:23–29.
7. Flower WH. On the pathological changes produced in the shoulder-joint by traumatic dislocation: As derived from an examination of all the specimens illustrating this injury in the museums of London. *Trans Pathol Soc London.* 1861;12:179–201.
8. Hill HA, Sachs MD. The grooved defect of the humeral head: A frequently unrecognized complication of dislocations of the shoulder joint. *Radiology.* 1940;35:690–700.
9. Widjaja AB, Tran A, Bailey M, et al. Correlation between Bankart and Hill-Sachs lesions in anterior shoulder dislocation. *ANZ J Surg.* 2006;76:436–438.
10. Antonio GE, Griffith JF, Yu AB, et al. First-time shoulder dislocation: High prevalence of labral injury and age-related differences revealed by MR arthrography. *J Magn Reson Imaging.* 2007;26:983–991.
11. Griffith JF, Antonio GE, Yung PSH, et al. Prevalence, pattern, and spectrum of glenoid bone loss in anterior shoulder dislocation: CT analysis of 218 patients. *AJR Am J Roentgenol.* 2008;190:1247–1254.
12. Edwards TB, Boulahia A, Walch G. Radiographic analysis of bone defects in chronic anterior shoulder instability. *Arthroscopy.* 2003;19:732–739.
13. Calandra JJ, Baker CL, Uribe J. The incidence of Hill-Sachs lesions in initial anterior shoulder dislocations. *Arthroscopy.* 1989;5:254–257.
14. Norlin R. Intraarticular pathology in acute, first-time anterior shoulder dislocation: An arthroscopic study. *Arthroscopy.* 1993;9:546–549.
15. Taylor D, Arciero R. Pathologic changes associated with shoulder dislocations: Arthroscopic and physical examination findings in first-time, traumatic anterior dislocations. *Am J Sports Med.* 1997;25:306–311.
16. Spatschil A, Landsiedl F, Anderl W, et al. Posttraumatic anterior-inferior instability of the shoulder: Arthroscopic findings and clinical correlations. *Arch Orthop Trauma Surg.* 2006;126:217–222.
17. Yiannakopoulos CK, Mataragas E, Antonogiannakis E. A comparison of the spectrum of intra-articular lesions in acute and chronic anterior shoulder instability. *Arthroscopy.* 2007;23:985–990.
18. Richards RD, Sartoris DJ, Pathria MN, et al. Hill-Sachs lesion and normal humeral groove: MR imaging features allowing their differentiation. *Radiology.* 1994;190:665–668.
19. Saito H, Itoi E, Minagawa H, et al. Location of the Hill-Sachs lesion in shoulders with recurrent anterior dislocation. *Arch Orthop Trauma Surg.* 2009;129:1327–1334.
20. Burkhart SS, De Beer JF. Traumatic glenohumeral bone defects and their relationship to failure of arthroscopic Bankart repairs: Significance of the inverted-pear glenoid and the humeral engaging Hill-Sachs lesion. *Arthroscopy.* 2000;16:677–694.
21. Itoi E, Lee SB, Amrami KK, et al. Quantitative assessment of classic anterioinferior bony Bankart lesions by radiography and computed tomography. *Am J Sports Med.* 2003;31:112–118.
22. Cetik O, Uslu M, Ozsar BK. The relationship between Hill-Sachs lesion and recurrent anterior shoulder dislocation. *Acta Orthop Belg.* 2007;73:175–178.
23. Griffith JF, Antonio GE, Tong CWC, et al. Anterior shoulder dislocation: Quantification of glenoid bone loss with CT. *AJR Am J Roentgenol.* 2003;180:1423–1430.
24. Rowe CR, Patel D, Southmayd WW. The Bankart procedure: A long-term end-result study. *J Bone Joint Surg Am.* 1978;60:1–16.
25. Kirtland S, Resnick D, Sartoris DJ, et al. Chronic unreduced dislocations of the glenohumeral joint:

Imaging strategy and pathologic correlation. *J Trauma.* 1988;28:1622–1631.

26. Flatow E, Miller S, Neer CI. Chronic anterior dislocation of the shoulder. *J Shoulder Elbow Surg.* 1993;2:2–10.

27. Loebenberg MI, Cuomo F. The treatment of chronic anterior and posterior dislocations of the glenohumeral joint and associated articular surface defects. *Orthop Clin North Am.* 2000;31:23–34.

28. Mehta V. Humeral head plasty for a chronic locked anterior shoulder dislocation. *Orthopedics.* 2009;32:52.

29. Miniaci A, Gish M. Management of anterior glenohumeral instability associated with large Hill-Sachs defects. *Tech Shoulder Elbow Surg.* 2004;5:170–175.

30. Robinson CM, Akhtar A, Mitchell M, et al. Complex posterior fracture-dislocation of the shoulder: Epidemiology, injury patterns, and results of operative treatment. *J Bone Joint Surg Am.* 2007;89:1454–1466.

31. Ito H, Takayama A, Shirai Y. Radiographic evaluation of the Hill-Sachs lesion in patients with recurrent anterior shoulder instability. *J Shoulder Elbow Surg.* 2000;9:495–497.

32. Werner AW, Lichtenberg S, Schmitz H, et al. Arthroscopic findings in atraumatic instability. *Arthroscopy.* 2004;20: 268–272.

33. Miniaci A, Mascia AT, Salonen DC, et al. Magnetic resonance imaging of the shoulder in asymptomatic professional baseball pitchers. *Am J Sports Med.* 2002;30:66–73.

34. Owens BD, Nelson BJ, Duffey ML, et al. Pathoanatomy of first-time, traumatic, anterior glenohumeral subluxation events. *J Bone Joint Surg Am.* 2010;92:1605–1611.

35. Boileau P, Zumstein M, Balg F, et al. The unstable painful shoulder (UPS) as a cause of pain from unrecognized anteroinferior instability in the young athlete. *J Shoulder Elbow Surg.* 2011;20:98–106.

36. Burkhart SS, Danaceau SM. Articular arc-length mismatch as a cause of failed Bankart repair. *Arthroscopy.* 2000;16: 740–744.

37. Palmer I, Widen A. The bone block method for recurrent dislocation of the shoulder joint. *J Bone Joint Surg Br.* 1948;30:53–58.

38. Sekiya JK, Wickwire AC, Stehle JH, et al. Hill-Sachs defects and repair using osteoarticular allograft transplantation. *Am J Sports Med.* 2009;37:2459–2466.

39. Kaar SG, Fening SD, Jones MH, et al. Effect of humeral head defect size on glenohumeral instability: A cadaveric study of simulated Hill-Sachs defects. *Am J Sports Med.* 2010;38:594–599.

40. Hovelius L, Eriksson K, Fredin H, et al. Recurrences after initial dislocation of the shoulder. Results of a prospective study of treatment. *J Bone Joint Surg Am.* 1983;65:343–349.

41. Rowe CR, Zarins B, Ciullo JV. Recurrent anterior dislocation of the shoulder after surgical repair. Apparent causes of failure and treatment. *J Bone Joint Surg Am.* 1984;66(2):159–68.

42. Burkhart SS, De Beer JF, Tehrany AM, et al. Quantifying glenoid bone loss arthroscopically in shoulder instability. *Arthroscopy.* 2002;18:488–491.

43. Gerson JN, Kodali P, Fening SD, et al. The effect of humeral head defect size on instability of the shoulder. Canadian Orthopaedic Association Annual Meeting. St. John's, 2011.

44. Gagey OJ, Gagey N. The hyperabduction test. *J Bone Joint Surg Br.* 2001;83:69–74.

45. Boileau P, Villalba M, Hery JY, et al. Risk factors for recurrence of shoulder instability after arthroscopic Bankart repair. *J Bone Joint Surg Am.* 2006;88:1755–1763.

46. Hall RH, Isaac F, Booth CR. Dislocation of the shoulder with special reference to accompanying small fractures. *J Bone Joint Surg Am.* 1959;41:489–494.

47. Rockwood CA Jr, Green DP, eds. *Fractures.* 2nd ed. Philadelphia, PA: JB Lippincott; 1984.

48. Pavlov H, Warren RF, Weiss CB, et al. The roentgenographic evaluation of anterior shoulder instability. *Clin Orthop Relat Res.* 1985;194:153–158.

49. Walch G, Boileau P. Latarjet-Bristow procedure for recurrent anterior instability. *Tech Shoulder Elbow Surg.* 2000;1:256–261.

50. Ito H, Shirai Y, Takayama A, et al. A new radiographic projection for the posterolateral notch in cases of recurrent dislocation of the shoulder. *Nihon Ika Daigaku Zasshi.* 1996;63:499–501.

51. Kodali P, Jones MH, Polster J, et al. Accuracy of measurement of Hill-Sachs lesions with computed tomography. *J Shoulder Elbow Surg.* 2011;20:1328–1334.

52. Chen AL, Hunt SA, Hawkins RJ, et al. Management of bone loss associated with recurrent anterior glenohumeral instability. *Am J Sports Med.* 2005;33: 912–925.

53. Cho SH, Cho NS, Rhee YG. Preoperative analysis of the Hill-Sachs lesion in anterior shoulder instability: How to predict engagement of the lesion. *Am J Sports Med.* 2011;39:2389–2395.

54. Rowe CR, Zarins B. Chronic unreduced dislocations of the shoulder. *J Bone Joint Surg Am.* 1982;64:494–505.

55. Bigliani LU, Newton PM, Steinmann SP, et al. Glenoid rim lesions associated with recurrent anterior dislocation of the shoulder. *Am J Sports Med.* 1998;26:41–45.

56. Beran MC, Donaldson CT, Bishop JY. Treatment of chronic glenoid defects in the setting of recurrent anterior shoulder instability: A systematic review. *J Shoulder Elbow Surg.* 2010;19:769–780.

57. Provencher MT, Bhatia S, Ghodadra NS, et al. Recurrent shoulder instability: Current concepts for evaluation and management of glenoid bone loss. *J Bone Joint Surg Am.* 2010;92(suppl 2):133–151.

58. Yin B, Vella J, Levine WN. Arthroscopic alphabet soup: Recognition of normal, normal variants, and pathology. *Orthop Clin North Am.* 2010;41:297–308.

59. Arrigoni P, Huberty D, Brady PC, et al. The value of arthroscopy before an open modified Latarjet reconstruction. *Arthroscopy.* 2008;24:514–519.

60. Yamamoto N, Itoi E, Hidekazu A, et al. Contact between the glenoid and the humeral head in abduction, external rotation, and horizontal extension: A new concept of glenoid track. *J Shoulder Elbow Surg.* 2007;16:649–656.

61. Balg F, Boileau P. The instability severity index score: A simple pre-operative score to select patients for arthroscopic or open shoulder stabilisation. *J Bone Joint Surg Br.* 2007;89:1470–1477.

62. Millett PJ, Clavert P, Warner JJP. Open operative treatment for anterior shoulder instability: When and why? *J Bone Joint Surg Am.* 2005;87:419–432.

63. Neer CS 2nd, Foster CR. Inferior capsular shift for involuntary inferior and multidirectional instability of the shoulder. A preliminary report. *J Bone Joint Surg Am.* 1980;62:897–908.

64. Saha AK, Das AK. Anterior recurrent dislocation of the shoulder: Treatment by rotation osteotomy of the upper shaft of the humerus. *Indian J Orthop.* 1967;1:132–137.

65. Weber BG, Simpson LA, Hardegger F. Rotational humeral osteotomy for recurrent anterior dislocation of the shoulder associated with a large Hill-Sachs lesion. *J Bone Joint Surg Am.* 1984;66:1443–1446.

66. Bigliani L, Weinstein D, Glasgow M, et al. Glenohumeral arthroplasty for arthritis after instability surgery. *J Shoulder Elbow Surg.* 1995;4:87–94.

67. Connolly JF. Humeral head defects associated with shoulder dislocations—their diagnostic and surgical significance. *AAOS Instr Course Lect.* 1972;21:42–54.

68. Purchase RJ, Wolf EM, Hobgood ER, et al. Hill-Sachs "remplissage": An arthroscopic solution for the engaging Hill-Sachs lesion. *Arthroscopy.* 2008;24:723.

69. Deutsh AA, Kroll DG. Decreased range of motion following arthroscopic remplissage. *Orthopedics.* 2008;31:492.

70. Nourissat G, Kilinc AS, Werther JR, et al. A prospective, comparative, radiological, and clinical study of the influence of the "remplissage" procedure on shoulder range of motion after stabilization by arthroscopic Bankart repair. *Am J Sports Med.* 2011;39:2147–2152.

71. Kazel MD, Sekiya IK, Greene JA, et al. Percutaneous correction (humeroplasty) of posterolateral humeral head defects (Hill-Sachs) associated with anterior shoulder instability: A cadaveric study. *Arthroscopy.* 2005;21:1473–1478.

72. Armitage MS, Faber KJ, Drosdowech DS, et al. Humeral head bone defects: Remplissage, allograft, and arthroplasty. *Orthop Clin North Am.* 2010;41:417–425.

73. Re P, Gallo RA, Richmond JC. Transhumeral head plasty for large Hill-Sachs lesions. *Arthroscopy.* 2006;22:798.e1-4.

74. Chapovsky BS, Kelly JD. Osteochondral allograft transplantation for treatment of glenohumeral instability. *Arthroscopy.* 2005;21:1007.

75. Kropf EJ, Sekiya JK. Osteoarticular allograft transplantation for large humeral head defects in glenohumeral instability. *Arthroscopy.* 2007;23:322.e1–322.e5.

76. Gerber C. Chronic, locked anterior and posterior dislocations. In: Warner JJ, Iannotti JP, Gerber C. *Complex and Revision Problems in Shoulder Surgery.* 1st ed. Philadelphia, PA: Lippincott-Raven Publishers; 1997:99–116.

77. Yagishita K, Thomas BJ. Use of allograft for large Hill-Sachs lesion associated with anterior glenohumeral dislocation. A case report. *Injury.* 2002;33:791–794.

78. Raiss P, Aldinger PR, Kasten P, et al. Humeral head resurfacing for fixed anterior glenohumeral dislocation. *Int Orthop.* 2009;33:451–456.

79. Scalise JJ, Miniaci A, Iannotti JP. Resurfacing arthroplasty of the humerus: Indications, surgical technique, and clinical results. *Tech Shoulder Elbow Surg.* 2007;8:152–160.

80. Copeland S. The continuing development of shoulder replacement: "Reaching the surface". *J Bone Joint Surg Am.* 2006;88:900–905.

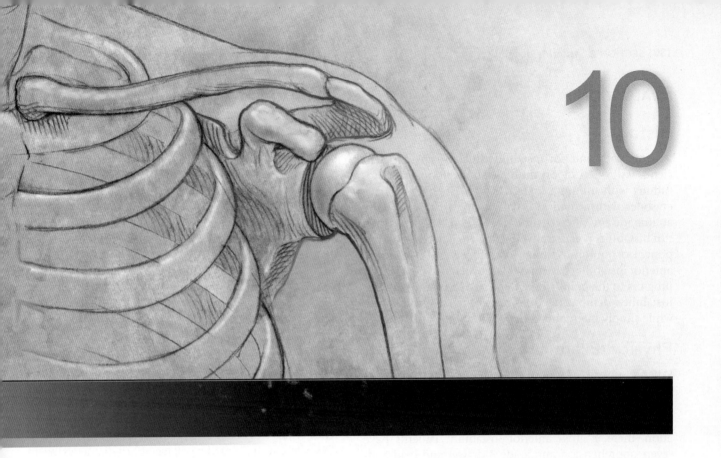

ANTERIOR INSTABILITY WITH CAPSULAR DEFICIENCY

Kenneth A. Kearns / Mark D. Lazarus

INTRODUCTION

The anterior capsule spans from the rotator interval superiorly to the inferior glenohumeral ligament (IGHL) inferiorly and provides an important stabilizing mechanism for the normal shoulder. For most cases of recurrent anterior instability surgery, it is this thick healthy anterior capsule that permits a robust repair. Quality tissue is one of the main reasons why patients who require surgery for recurrent traumatic anterior instability have excellent results and are able to return to near normal function in greater than 90% of primary repairs (1). However, with repeated failed attempts at either arthroscopic or open surgical repair, the glenohumeral capsule may become a thin attenuated remnant incapable of being repaired. Capsular deficiency can also result after electrothermal capsulorrhaphy due to thermal injury and tissue necrosis (2) or hereditary collagen disorders, most commonly Ehlers-Danlos syndrome (EDS) (3). While a deficient anterior capsule is one of the more uncommon causes of recurrent anterior instability, it has long been understood as a major factor in recurrent instability and remains a challenging problem for the surgeons to correct. It requires a thorough preoperative evaluation, specific plan of attack, and alternatives to the standard capsulo-ligamentous repair.

EVALUATION

History

Patients with anterior instability due to capsular deficiency will often report multiple subluxations or dislocations with minimal force. They also frequently have episodes with activities of daily living that are usually atraumatic and often occur in their sleep. Although inferior instability is classically described as a necessary component of multidirectional instability (MDI), recurrent anterior instability patients with capsular deficiencies can progress to the point where they have secondary inferior instability, demonstrated by instability symptoms even while simply maintaining the weight of the arm at rest.

Physical Examination

When a surgeon examines a patient with an intact anterior capsule, the findings that indicate a diagnosis of instability can often be subtle. That is rarely true for the patient with capsular deficiency. During clinical evaluation, there is gross anterior instability. Patients have severe apprehension and grade 3 drawer and load-and-shift tests. It is not uncommon for examination to result in dislocation, particularly if there is associated osseous loss on either the humeral or the glenoid sides. There may be increased passive external rotation that can be in conjunction with a subscapularis deficiency, particularly in patients that have had prior attempts at open repair. For those patients with associated inferior instability, they will have dramatic sulcus signs that may be present even to the force of gravity alone. In addition to these findings, patients with EDS have increased general ligamentous laxity of other joints. There is hyperabduction of the thumb with volar flexion of the wrist and hyperextension of the finger metacarpal joints, elbows, and knees.

Imaging

Standard plain films should include an AP view of the shoulder, a true AP view of the glenoid, a scapulolateral "Y" view, and axillary view to look for any associated bony pathology and/or signs of prior anchor or hardware placement. Clearly, the presence of hardware can significantly influence surgical decision making. Plain MRI may be useful to evaluate the integrity of the rotator cuff, specifically the subscapularis in cases of prior attempted open repair. MR arthrography (MRA) is the main diagnostic tool to assess the integrity of the anterior capsule. Patients with deficiencies of the capsulolabral structures frequently present with patulous joint capsules; hypotrophic anterior labrum; and either stretched or very thin superior, middle, and/or inferior glenohumeral ligaments. MRA may also demonstrate gross capsular rents.

TREATMENT

As stated earlier, patients with anterior capsular deficiency have gross instability. As such, nonsurgical treatment options are limited, consisting of patient counseling on how to live with and limit instability episodes. A key component in the operative treatment of shoulder instability, especially revision surgery, is identification of the quantity and quality of the anterior capsuloligamentous structures (4). In most cases there is sufficient tissue for a standard repair; however, in patients with deficient anterior capsules secondary to multiple failed instability procedures or thermal necrosis, there are insufficient tissue remnants and attempts at repair are futile. Those with EDS who have failed conservative management or operative fixations also often have insufficient anterior capsules that are not amenable to standard repair. Neer and Foster (5) deduced not only an increase in capsular volume in these patients, but also an abnormal capsular compliance. Rodeo et al. found that there was a decreased cysteine content of the capsule, possibly indicating a higher prevalence of less stiff collagen type III. In addition, the skin of these patients had smaller collagen fibril diameters, again suggesting an underlying collagen defect (6). Patients with recurrence of instability after attempted operative fixation often have abnormal healing. Skin incisions heal wider than usual; and on revision open surgery, the amount of deltopectoral and humeral interface scarring appears minimal, often dividable by finger dissection. More importantly, the capsuloligamentous structures are almost always attenuated and deficient. In all these difficult situations, surgeons need a clear approach and a multitude of options in their armamentarium to reconstruct the anterior capsule and stabilize the glenohumeral joint.

Several surgical techniques, both anatomic and nonanatomic have been described to address the reconstruction of the deficient anterior capsule and ligaments. Most authors consider these options a salvage procedure for end-stage shoulder instability and/or treatment of those with instability as a result of collagen disorders (7). Studies report successful restoration of glenohumeral stability without recurrent dislocation in 65% to 96% of patients (7). While controversies remain between the optimal graft selection, allograft versus autograft, method for graft placement and fixation, and postoperative rehabilitation, all revision surgeries for shoulder instability should begin in the same manner.

Regardless of the specific anterior capsule reconstruction technique employed, all open surgical approaches start by defining the humeroscapular motion interface, the plane between the underlying rotator cuff and the overlying deltoid, acromion, and conjoined tendon (8). Initially, the surgeon may be fooled by the intact and often thickened clavipectoral fascia. However, this fascia will not move as one with the humerus during humeral rotation, being clearly differentiated from the subscapularis. All scar and adhesions within this interface are excised and the axillary and musculocutaneous nerves are located. At this juncture, the amount and quality of the subscapularis and anterior capsule can be assessed. A joker or Freer elevator can be passed through the rotator interval and deep to the combined anterior capsule and subscapularis to gauge the combined thickness of these structures.

The simplest solution to a deficient anterior capsule is a coracoid transfer operation, most frequently a Latarjet procedure. This is especially helpful when there is associated anterior glenoid rim loss. Biomechanical studies have demonstrated that approximately 50% of the effectiveness of a Latarjet reconstruction results from the sling effect of the conjoined tendon anteroinferior to the joint (9). This sling effect may be helpful for patients that have anteroinferior capsular deficiencies.

Occasionally, when incising the clavipectoral fascia, it instantly becomes clear that the anterior capsule and subscapularis are completely deficient. In these situations, reconstruction of the capsule is necessary. Capsular reconstruction begins by identifying the interval between the deficient and normal capsules. Typically, the posteroinferior capsule is normally present. By performing a limited posteroinferior

capsular shift, this normal posteroinferior capsule can be mobilized to reconstruct the anteroinferior quadrant. Capsular mobilization should be performed by releasing the posteroinferior capsule from the neck of the humerus instead of the glenoid to obtain the greatest length of tissue. The transferred capsule is sutured to a trough adjacent to the humeral articular surface via bone tunnels (10).

Next, reconstruction of the anterior capsuloligamentous structures is performed. In the past various combinations of tendinous autograft and allograft (e.g., plantaris, gracilis, and achilles) have been used. Gallie and Le Mesurier reported the first attempts at anterior capsular reconstruction and recommended using fascia lata in a nonanatomic fashion. In their series of 175 patients, there were only 7 failures (11). While only a small case study, Warner et al. (4) reported three successful reconstructions using hamstring autograft. Iannotti et al. analyzed seven patients with recurrent anterior instability secondary to capsule deficiency treated with 2-cm strips of the iliotibial band folded on one another to reconstruct the capsule. The most superior strip recreated the rotator interval, while the middle and inferior limbs recreated the middle glenohumeral ligament (MGHL) and anterior inferior glenohumeral ligament (AIGHL), respectively (Fig. 10-1). Bony glenoid defects

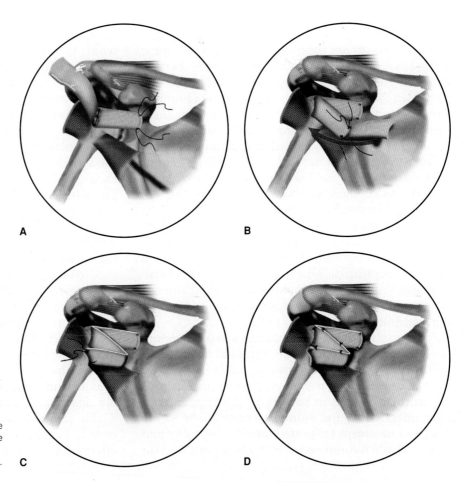

▶ **FIGURE 10-1:** ITB graft reconstruction. **A:** "I" graft rotator interval deficiency. **B:** "V" graft, rotator interval, and middle glenohumeral ligament deficiency. **C:** "Z" graft, rotator interval, middle glenohumeral ligament, and anterior portion of the inferior glenohumeral ligament. **D:** Closure of the horizontal limbs of the graft to each other and to the remaining capsular tissue.

A B C D

were excluded. There were no reports of recurrent instability or range of motion loss at 45-month average follow-up (12). Braun and Millett described the use of a tibialis anterior allograft to reconstruct a deficient labrum and capsule. Using suture anchors, the graft is first used to reconstruct the labrum, then the two free limbs reconstruct the MGHL and anterior band of IGHL through bone tunnels in the superior and inferior humeral heads that run from medial to lateral and exit lateral to the bicipital groove and finally, free ends are tied each other lateral to the bicipital groove (13). At an average follow-up of 3.8 years, 45% remained stable (7).

Lazarus and Harryman (10) described the use of semitendinosus autograft to reconstruct the superior glenohumeral ligament (SGHL) and MGHL. Using a 4-mm pinecone burr, holes are created in the glenoid and the humeral head, these holes corresponding to the origin and insertion sites of the SGHL and MGHL. A single strip of autograft tendon is passed from lateral to medial to recreate the SGHL and then from medial to lateral to reconstruct the MGHL. With the humeral head reduced and the arm in neutral rotation, the graft is tightened. Patients must be aware that this reconstruction with result in permanent motion restrictions, sacrificing normal range of motion for glenohumeral stability. Postoperatively, a sling is placed for 3 weeks, with abduction and external rotation isometrics being the only exercise program. After 3 weeks, the sling is removed three to five times each day for gentle supine active-assisted forward elevation and external rotation exercises. Particularly with external rotation, patients are shown the neutral rotation point and are cautioned against attempting to stretch beyond this range. At 6 weeks postoperative, the sling is discontinued and a gentle rotator cuff and scapular strengthening program is begun. No lifting greater than 4.5 kg (10 lb) is permitted for 6 months. In addition, patients with heavy-labor occupations or those involved in contact sports are encouraged to discontinue these activities permanently. If necessary, the graft can also be simultaneously used to reconstruct a deficient labrum and capsule. Lazarus and Harryman reported this reconstruction technique in 17 patients with capsular insufficiency and recurrent, disabling instability after multiple attempts at anterior stabilization. The procedure was successful in eliminating instability in 70% of cases (10).

As a substitute or an adjunct to allograft tendon, the intra-articular portion of the long head of the biceps (LHB) can be used to reconstruct a deficient rotator interval capsule. This technique, "biceps suspension," is particularly useful in patients with a large inferior component to their instability. First proposed by Nicola (14) as a treatment for posteroinferior instability and most recently recommended by Namdari and Keenan

(15) for the treatment of inferior instability associated with neuromuscular disorders, reverse tenodesis of the LHB can restore anteroinferior stability as well. It is usually done in conjunction with allograft capsular reconstruction. Similar to the technique described above for SGHL reconstruction with allograft, the LHB is left attached at its origin. The LHB is transected just superior to the pectoralis major tendon and a tenodesis is performed between the distal portion of the transected tendon and the pectoralis. The remaining LHB tendon is then converted to a ligament by suturing through bone tunnels in the proximal groove. It is secured with the glenohumeral joint concentrically located and at 0 degree of external rotation, trading range for stability.

For some patients, particularly those with EDS or who have had prior coracoid transfer procedures, an arthroscopic approach to capsular reconstruction might be preferred as

1. avoiding a revision anterior approach through the disrupted tissue planes that result from coracoid transfer will lessen the patient's risk of a neurologic injury.
2. revision anterior approach in EDS and revision patients can jeopardize the already compromised anterior soft tissues.

The procedure begins with a thorough diagnostic examination to assure that there is inferior capsule with which to work and an LHB still present. The inferior capsule can be shifted in an anterosuperior direction to reconstruct the anterosuperior band of the IGHL. The anterosuperior band of the IGHL and the MGHL can also be reconstructed with semitendinosus allograft, similar to the technique described above for open reconstruction. It is helpful to fix the central portion of the allograft to the midglenoid initially and then bring each end individually laterally to the humeral head. The SGHL is reconstructed using the biceps suspension technique described above. Instead of a distal tenodesis, the LHB is simply left attached at its origin and secured into the superior aspect of the biceps groove using suture anchor fixation.

While glenohumeral arthrodesis is a permanent solution to this difficult problem, most patients are unwilling to accept the associated sacrifices of shoulder motion. Furthermore, Richards et al. (16) described the unexpected complication of continued sensations of instability despite radiographic evidence of a solid fusion. Therefore, with a thorough knowledge of the scapular and humeral attachments of the superior, middle, and anterior inferior glenohumeral ligaments, one is able to reconstruct a deficient anterior capsule and provide patients with a moderately successful option, offering fewer restrictions than a fusion.

References

1. Lazarus MD, Walsh M. Complications of instability surgery. In: Iannotti JP, Williams GR, eds. *Disorders of the Shoulder: Diagnosis and Management.* Philadelphia, PA: Lippincott Williams & Wilkins; 2007:487–537.
2. Wong KL, Williams GR. Complications of thermal capsulorrhaphy of the shoulder. *J Bone Joint Surg Am.* 2001;83(suppl 2):151–155.
3. Krishnan SG, Hawkins RJ, Horan MP, et al. A soft tissue attempt to stabilize the multiply operated glenohumeral joint with multidirectional instability. *Clin Orthop Relat Res.* 2004;429:256–261.
4. Warner, JJ, Venegas AA, Lehtinen JT, et al. Management of capsular deficiency of the shoulder. A report of three cases. *J Bone Joint Surg Am.* 2002;84-A(9): 1668–1671.
5. Neer CS 2nd, Foster CR. Inferior capsular shift for involuntary inferior and multidirectional instability of the shoulder. A preliminary report. *J Bone Joint Surg Am.* 1980;62:897–908.
6. Rodeo SA, Suzuki K, Yamauchi M, et al. Analysis of collagen and elastic fibers in shoulder capsule in patients with shoulder instability. *Am J Sports Med.* 1998;26:634–643.
7. Dewing CB, Horan MP, Millett PJ. Two-year outcomes of open shoulder anterior capsular reconstruction for instability from severe capsular deficiency. *Arthroscopy.* 2012;28(1):43–51.
8. Matsen F. Glenohumeral instability. In: C.M.E, ed. *Surgery of the Musculoskeletal System.* New York, NY: Churchill Livingstone; 1990:1439–1469.
9. Giles JW, Boons HW, Elkinson I, et al. Does the dynamic sling effect of the Latarjet procedure improve shoulder stability? A biomechanical evaluation. *J Shoulder Elbow Surg.* 2013;22(6):821–827.
10. Lazarus MD, Harryman DT II. Open repair for anterior instability. In: Warner JJP, Iannotti JP, Gerber C, eds. *Complex and Revision Problems in Shoulder Surgery.* 2nd ed. Philadelphia, PA: Lippincott-Raven; 1997:47–64.
11. Gallie WE, Le Mesurier AB. Recurring dislocation of the shoulder. *J Bone Joint Surg Br.* 1948;30B:9–18.
12. Iannotti JP, Antoniou J, Williams GR, et al. Iliotibial band reconstruction for treatment of glenohumeral instability associated with irreparable capsular deficiency. *J Shoulder Elbow Surg.* 2002;11(6):618–623.
13. Braun S, Millett PJ. Open anterior capsular reconstruction of the shoulder for chronic instability using a Tibialis anterior allograft. *TSES.* 2008;9(2):102–107.
14. Nicola T. Recurrent dislocation of the shoulder. *J Bone Joint Surg Am.* 1934;16:663–670.
15. Namdari S, Keenan MA. Outcomes of the biceps suspension procedure for painful inferior glenohumeral subluxation in hemiplegic patients. *J Bone Joint Surg Am.* 2010;92(15):2589–2597.
16. Richards RR, Beaton D, Hudson AR. Shoulder arthrodesis with plate fixation: Functional outcome analysis. *J Shoulder Elbow Surg.* 1993;2:225–239.

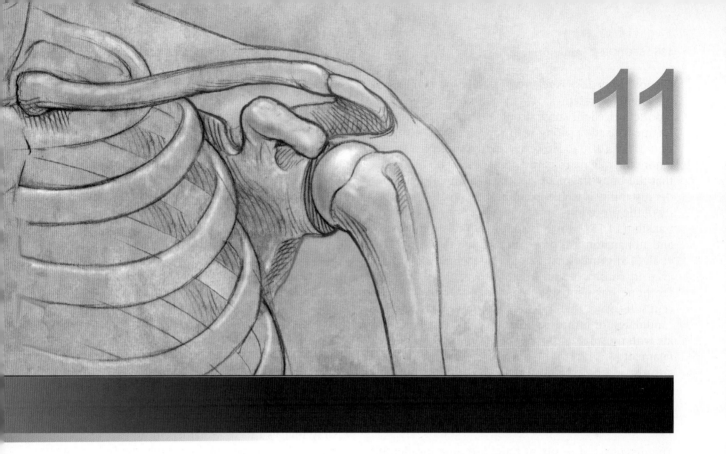

11

ANTERIOR GLENOID RIM FRACTURES

Hiroyuki Sugaya

INTRODUCTION

Glenoid anterior rim fractures, accompanied by acute glenohumeral dislocation and subluxation with tremendous amount of external force (1), usually result in persistent instability of the glenohumeral joint (2). According to a three-dimensionally reconstructed computed tomography (3DCT) study, the prevalence of anterior glenoid bony lesion has been reported as high as 90% in shoulders with chronic recurrent traumatic anterior instability and an associated bony fragment is present in about a half of shoulders with anterior glenoid bony lesion (3). Further, bone loss in shoulders associated with a bony fragment is relatively significant compared to that in shoulders with attritional glenoid without bony fragment (3,4).

In shoulders with bony Bankart lesion, a bone fragment is firmly connected to the labrum because the majority of the anterior glenoid rim fractures are avulsion-type glenoid rim fractures (4–6). In acute cases, it is widely accepted that such glenoid fractures with a large fragment (7), and/or displacement of more than 10 mm (8), and associated instability (2), immediate surgical fragment reduction and fixation using screws (7) or suture anchors (6,9,10), are indicated either open or arthroscopically. On the other hand, in chronic shoulders with recurrent instability, surgeons need to respect entire glenohumeral ligament pathology such as capsular lesions or elongation of the capsule, in addition to the bone loss (11).

Glenoid bone loss is relatively significant when a bony fragment is present (3,4). In addition, some authors reported excellent surgical outcomes after arthroscopic fragment fixation along with capsulolabral reconstruction (4,10,12,13). However, many surgeons tend to ignore the fragment, partly because they do not believe that the bony fragment associated with chronic shoulder instability is viable in addition to possible complexity of the procedure, and prefer to perform the coracoid transfer (14,15), which is simple but relatively invasive and nonanatomical procedure. In the meantime, Fujii et al. (16) proved that these bony fragments are viable even in chronic lesion because their blood supply to the bone fragment was maintained through the adjacent soft tissue. Therefore, these shoulders are favorable candidates for arthroscopic bony Bankart repair associate with capsular tensioning of the entire glenohumeral ligament (4,5,17,18). In this article, technical pearls for arthroscopic bony Bankart repair is described in detail.

HISTORY AND CLINICAL EXAMINATION

The diagnosis of recurrent traumatic anterior glenohumeral instability is usually made easily on the basis of the history of distinct dislocation or subluxation and the positive apprehension sign. The anterior apprehension test is done with the patient in the supine position. In this test, the shoulder is moved passively into maximum external rotation with the arm at side, 30, 60, 90, 120, 150 degrees of abduction, and maximum flexion

(17,18). At the same time, the posterior apprehension test is done with the arm at maximum internal rotation in 90 degrees of abduction. The feeling of apprehension is reported in each arm position. However, the most important and reliable physical examination can usually be done with the patient under anesthesia, comparing stability testing to the contralateral shoulder.

IMAGING

X-ray images are sometimes helpful in detecting the Hill-Sachs lesion and the anterior glenoid rim lesion, especially during the first patient visit. Bernageau (19) described an effective method for detecting an anterior glenoid rim lesion with the patients in the standing position. However, this technique requires fluoroscopic control in order to obtain optimal diagnosable images and; therefore, radiation exposure is an unignorable issue (20). We have developed a modified Bernageau method with the patient lying on their axilla in their most relaxed position (17,18). In this method, clear x-ray images can be obtained more easily with a high probability of ascertaining bony pathology without using fluoroscopic imaging (17,18).

Plain MRI provides only limited information for shoulder instability. However, MR arthrography is helpful when detecting a soft tissue lesion such as a Bankart lesion, capsular pathology, and/or a HAGL (humeral avulsion of the glenohumeral ligament) lesion (Fig. 11-1). Nonetheless, the final diagnosis of soft tissue pathology

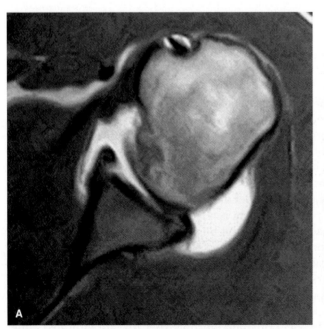
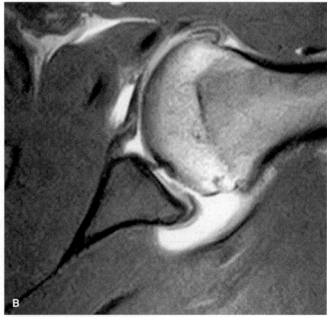

▲ **FIGURE 11-1:** MR arthrography in the shoulder with a bony Bankart lesion. **A:** Axial view. **B:** ABER (abduction and external rotation) view. Although only Bankart lesion is detectable in the axial view, slack IGHL and the humeral head translation in addition to the Bankart lesion are detectable in the ABER view.

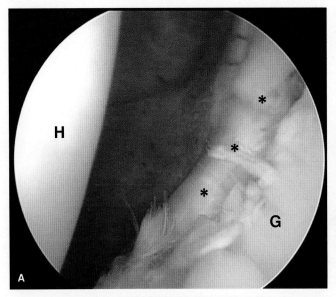 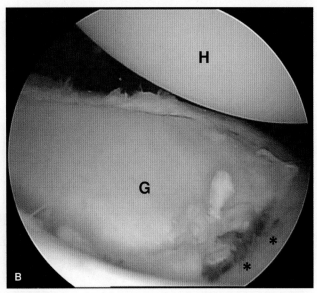

▲ **FIGURE 11-2:** Arthroscopic view of the same shoulder as Figure 11-1. **A:** A view from the posterior portal. **B:** A view from the anterior portal. H, humeral head; G, glenoid. Asterisks indicate bony fragment embedded in the surrounding soft tissue.

can be made most accurately through diagnostic arthroscopy (Fig. 11-2).

3DCT is the most important imaging study in order to assess glenoid morphology accurately (3). In a shoulder with bony Bankart lesion, detecting accurate configuration of the bony fragment during surgery is not easy because the bone fragment is covered by the surrounding soft tissue. Through preoperative 3DCT, surgeons can assess the size and shape of the bony fragment in shoulders with a bony Bankart lesion (Fig. 11-3) (3,4,12).

SURGERY

Regardless of the severity of glenoid bone loss, arthroscopic bony Bankart repair is indicated if an apparent bone fragment is present with 3DCT (4,5). Since the majority of shoulders with a large glenoid bone loss retains bony fragment at the anteroinferior glenoid neck (17,18), this procedure is applicable to most shoulders with significant glenoid bone loss. Normally, in shoulders with bony Bankart lesion, the fragment is medially displaced and partly united to the glenoid neck, and also the fragment is firmly connected to the adjacent labrum or soft tissue (Figs. 11-2–11-4A). Therefore, the bony fragment associated with a bony Bankart lesion can be easily separated from the glenoid neck using standard straight or curved rasps. Although the gap between the fragment and the original glenoid is well demarcated in most shoulders, if otherwise, careful palpation or preoperative 3DCT greatly help surgeons to delineate the gap (Fig. 11-3) (17,18).

Patient Positioning and EUA

All patients are seated in the beach-chair position under general anesthesia and/or interscalene block and joint laxity is assessed by examination of both shoulders prior to surgical intervention. General anesthesia is preferable because surgeons can assess constitutional laxity on the contralateral side during EUA.

Portals and Diagnostic Arthroscopy

A 4-mm arthroscope is introduced through a standard posterior portal and a diagnostic arthroscopy is performed. Then an anterior portal is created just superior to the subscapularis tendon and just lateral to the conjoined tendon using an outside-in technique, in order to facilitate instrument insertion without cannulas (21). Then, arthroscope is switched to the anterior portal and diagnostic arthroscopy is performed in order to evaluate capsular integrity and confirm a bony Bankart lesion (Fig. 11-2). In addition, an anterosuperior portal is established at the anterosuperior margin of the rotator interval utilizing an outside-in technique. This becomes the second working portal. In shoulders with superior labral detachment, a lateral acromial portal, established just lateral to the midpoint of the acromion through the muscle–tendon junction of the infraspinatus, is used instead of the anterosuperior portal.

SURGICAL PROCEDURES

Mobilization of the Complex

After diagnostic arthroscopy from the anterior portal, arthroscope is again switched to the posterior portal.

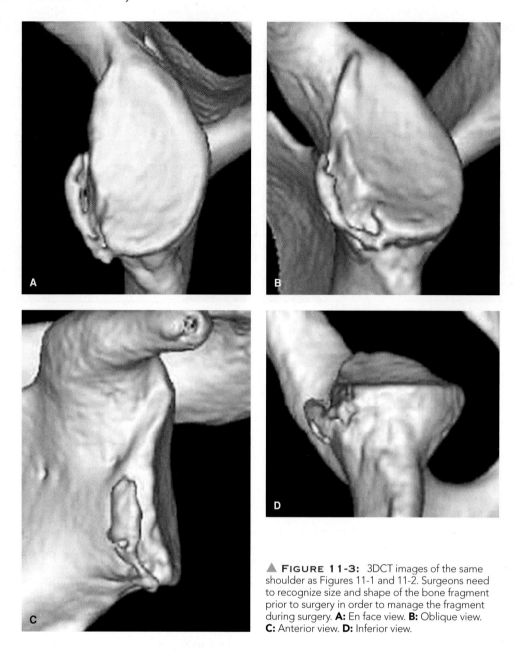

▲ **FIGURE 11-3:** 3DCT images of the same shoulder as Figures 11-1 and 11-2. Surgeons need to recognize size and shape of the bone fragment prior to surgery in order to manage the fragment during surgery. **A:** En face view. **B:** Oblique view. **C:** Anterior view. **D:** Inferior view.

Then, separation and mobilization of the labroligamentous complex together with the bony fragment from the glenoid neck is performed using an elevator, straight and curved rasps, scissors, shavers, and a radiofrequency probe. All of these instrument tools are inserted through a cannulaless anterior portal. This step is a vital part of this procedure.

First, a straight rasp is inserted from the anterior portal and is placed in the small gap between the fragment and the glenoid neck. Then, the gap is expanded by tapping the handle of the rasp (Fig. 11-5A). After separating the fragment from the glenoid neck, the mobilization of the labroligamentous complex is performed up to the 7:30 position in the right shoulder until the complex and the fragment become completely free in

exactly the same way as one would mobilize a Bankart lesion without a bone fragment using the instruments previously described. Further, articular cartilage on the edge of the glenoid is also removed to promote tissue healing after repair (Figs. 11-4B and 11-5B). Normally, the separation of the fragment from the neck can be readily accomplished using only elevators and rasps. If the separation of the fragment is difficult and the fragment is united firmly, a small size chisel can be introduced from the anterior portal to separate it from the glenoid neck.

Pearls

Surgeons should clearly define the gap between the fragment and the glenoid neck, otherwise the fragment or

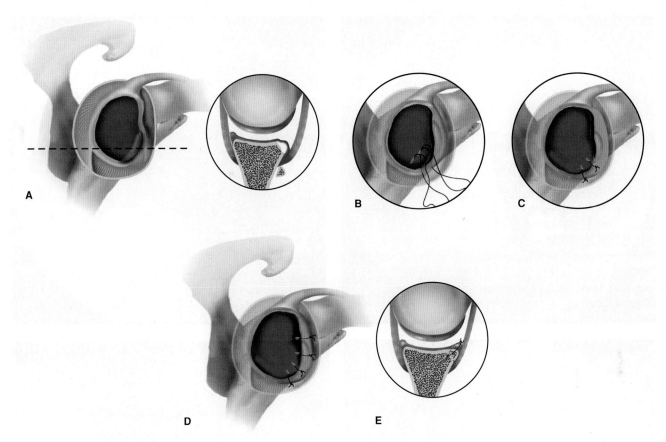

▲ **FIGURE 11-4:** Schematic drawings of entire surgical procedures. In shoulders with bony Bankart lesion, the fragment is normally medially displaced and partly united to the glenoid neck, and also the fragment is firmly connected to the adjacent labrum or soft tissue. The dotted line indicates the plane of the axial section **(A)**. After separation of the fragment and labrum from the glenoid neck, the mobilization of the labroligamentous complex is performed up to the 7:30 position in the right shoulder until the complex and the fragment become completely free. In addition, articular cartilage on the edge of the glenoid is also removed **(B)**. Then, two suture anchors are inserted to the face of the inferior glenoid and the inferior labrum was first reduced. Thanks to this procedure, the bony fragment was automatically brought upward and, therefore, handling of the fragment becomes easier **(C)**. Next, bony fragment is stabilized by pulling the adjacent labrum with a grasper inserted through the anterosuperior portal. Then, a bone penetrating instrument is inserted though the anterior portal and sutures are placed to the fragment. Knot tying provides not just fragment reduction but proper tensioning to the entire inferior glenohumeral ligament **(D,E)**. The gray area on the glenoid indicates the area where articular cartilage is removed. The dark area on the labrum side indicates a bony fragment inside the soft tissue.

native glenoid may be broken during mobilization. In order to avoid this, surgeons need to recognize the size, shape, and location of the bony fragment using preoperative 3DCT prior to surgery (Fig. 11-3). In addition, surgeons need to delineate the gap by exposing the glenoid bone edge using a radiofrequency instrument before inserting a rasp.

Repair of Inferior Labrum Adjacent to the Osseous Fragment

The following procedure is very important in order to obtain optimal fragment reduction and provide proper tension to the inferior glenohumeral ligament (IGHL). The following procedure is performed using the posterior

portal as a viewing portal, and the anterior and anterosuperior portal as working portals.

The first suture anchor loaded with no. 2 high strength suture is inserted on the surface of the glenoid at the 6-o'clock position using a drill guide introduced through the cannulaless anterior portal. Because this portal has no cannula, the angle of approach of the guide can be adjusted easily allowing optimization of the angle to the glenoid (21). After the first anchor insertion, a looped no. 2-0 nylon suture is placed into the labrum at the 6:30 position using a low profile 7-mm Caspari Punch (Conmed Linvatec, Largo, FL, USA) or a Suture Hook (Conmed Linvatec, Largo, FL, USA). A suture relay is then performed intra-articularly (21). The second anchor is inserted into the face of the glenoid at the 4:40 position,

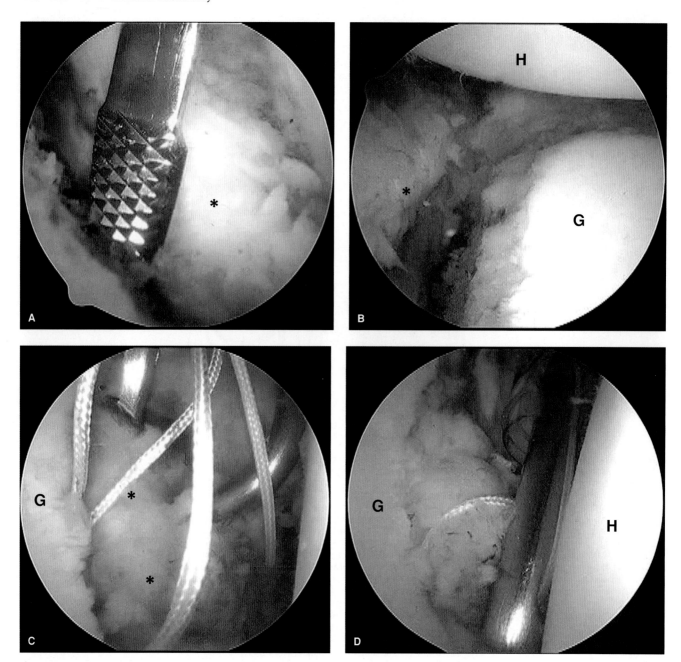

▲ **FIGURE 11-5:** Surgical procedures. A bony fragment and adjacent labrum is separated from the glenoid neck using a rasp **(A)**. Arthroscopic view after complete separation and mobilization of the complex, viewing from the anterior portal. Articular cartilage at the margin of the inferior glenoid face was removed **(B)**. A grasper inserted through the anterosuperior portal stabilizes the bony fragment by pulling the adjacent labrum and a bone penetrating instrument inserted though the anterior portal is trying to penetrate the fragment through the surrounding soft tissue **(C)**. Knot tying after suture placement to the fragment **(D)**. The asterisk indicates the bony fragment embedded in the surrounding soft tissue. H, humeral head; G, glenoid.

followed by the suture placement in the labrum adjacent to the inferior side of the bony fragment using the same technique (Fig. 11-4C). After completion of the suture placement of the inferior two anchors, knot tying is performed using a self-locking sliding knot through a cannula inserted through the anterior portal. To accomplish secure knot tying, the complex, together with the fragment, is held upward and laterally on the glenoid surface by a grasper introduced through the anterosuperior portal to reduce tensile force on the suture.

Osseous Fragment and Superior Labrum Repair

The next step is the suturing of the osseous fragment itself, either by passing the suture through the fragment

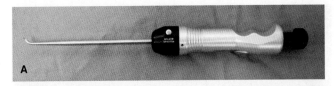

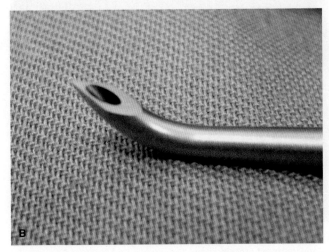

▲ **FIGURE 11-6:** Bone Stitcher (Smith & Nephew, Andover, MA).

or by penetrating it using bone penetrating tools such as a Bone Stitcher (Smith & Nephew, Andover, MA, USA), which is an originally developed bone penetrator with a stiff shaft and large handle (Fig. 11-6), or by passing suture around the fragment using a Suture Hook or Suture Leader (Depuy Mitek, Raynham, MA, USA) and/or Bone Stitcher (5,17,18). It is very important to characterize the fragment shape and size preoperatively by 3DCT evaluation to decide whether passing through or passing around the fragment is most appropriate (Fig. 11-3) (5,17,18). This procedure is facilitated when the bony fragment is reduced and stabilized by grasping cranial portion of the labrum adjacent to the fragment with a grasper introduced from the anterosuperior portal (Fig. 11-5C). Although the number of suture anchors utilized is dependent on the size and shape of the osseous fragment, normally one or two suture anchors are used for stabilizing the bony fragment (5,17,18). Knot tying is performed after placing the sutures through the fragment (Figs. 11-4D and 11-5D). The final step is to suture the labrum adjacent to the cranial side of the fragment to augment the stability of the entire complex. Normally four suture anchors with simple sutures are used to reconstruct the entire labroligamentous complex (Figs. 11-4E and 11-5).

Pearls

Surgeons should use penetrating instrument properly when penetrating the bony fragment, otherwise you cannot penetrate the fragment nicely or may break the instruments. In order to avoid this, surgeons need

to reduce and stabilize a bony fragment by grasping the cranial portion of the labrum adjacent to the fragment with a grasper introduced from the anterosuperior portal. Then, aim the blade of the Bone Stitcher perpendicular to the fragment. After catching the bony fragment by the tip of the penetrating instrument, push the fragment to the neck of the glenoid, and then penetrate it by rotating the blade of the Bone Stitcher applying a force perpendicular to the glenoid neck. During above procedure, the arthroscope need to stay in the portal and both the anterior and anterosuperior portals are used as working portals.

Management of the Associated Pathology

In shoulders with a capsular tear, a capsular repair utilizing two to three side-to-side stitches is performed prior to the bony Bankart repair. Furthermore, in shoulders with a superior labral detachment, arthroscopic reattachment is performed, after the bony Bankart repair is completed, utilizing a lateral acromial portal instead of the anterosuperior portal (Fig. 11-7).

Augmentation

The rotator interval closure and/or Hill-Sachs Remplissage (22) is performed as an augmentation in patients with relatively high-risk shoulders such as contact athletes, young and lax individuals, and those with a large Hill-Sachs lesion. In those patients, the rotator interval is closed by suturing the superior margin of the subscapularis tendon to the superior glenohumeral ligament with the arm held at the side and in maximum external rotation using no. 2 high strength sutures (17,18,23).

POSTOPERATIVE TREATMENT

The shoulders are immobilized for 3 weeks using a sling (Ultra Sling II, Donjoy, Carlsbad, CA). After immobilization, passive and assisted-active exercises are initiated for forward flexion and external rotation avoiding pain. After 6 weeks, patients begin strengthening exercises of the rotator cuff and scapular stabilizers. Three months after the operation, they are permitted to practice non-contact sports. Full return to throwing or contact sports is allowed after 6 months according to each individual's functional recovery. Excessive mechanical stress to the reconstructed site within 3 months after surgery may cause anchor/suture failure. In order to avoid this, instruct patients not to be too active until 3 months after surgery.

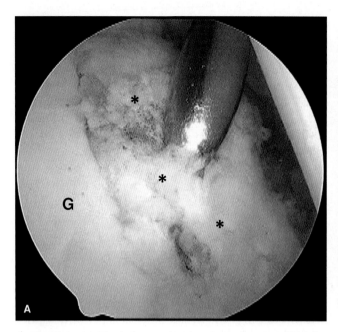
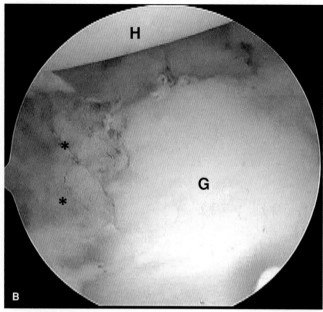

▲ FIGURE 11-7: Arthroscopic appearance after completing bony Bankart repair, viewing from the posterior portal **(A)** and the anterior portal **(B)**. The asterisk indicates the bony fragment embedded in the surrounding soft tissue. H, humeral head; G, glenoid.

SUMMARY

Prevalence of a bony Bankart lesion is as high as 50% in recurrent anterior glenohumeral instability and most of the shoulders with large glenoid defect retain a bony fragment at the anteroinferior glenoid neck. In addition, since a bony Bankart lesion is acute or chronic avulsion-type glenoid rim fracture, normally the fragment and labrum junction is intact even in chronic cases. Therefore, although sometimes techni-cally demanding, arthroscopic bony Bankart repair is technically feasible regardless of fragment or glenoid defect size by incorporating the fragment into labrum and soft tissue repair. If surgeons can understand every single pearls of this procedure described in this article, I believe arthroscopic bony Bankart repair, which is less invasive and anatomical procedure, becomes easy and outcome promising surgery for every surgeons.

References

1. Aston JW, Gregory CF. Dislocation of the shoulder with significant fracture of the glenoid. *J Bone Joint Surg Am.* 1973;55:1531–1533.
2. Ideberg R. Fractures of the scapula involving the glenoid fossa. In: Bateman JE, Welsh RP, eds. *Surgery of the Shoulder.* Toronto, ON: BC Decker; 1984:63–66.
3. Sugaya H, Moriishi J, Dohi M, et al. Glenoid rim morphology in recurrent anterior glenohumeral instability. *J Bone Joint Surg Am.* 2003;85:878–884.
4. Sugaya H, Moriishi J, Kanisawa I, et al. Arthroscopic osseous Bankart repair for chronic recurrent traumatic anterior glenohumeral instability. *J Bone Joint Surg Am.* 2005;87A:1752–1760.
5. Sugaya H, Moriishi J, Kanisawa I, et al. Arthroscopic osseous Bankart repair for chronic traumatic anterior glenohumeral instability. Surgical technique. *J Bone Joint Surg Am.* 2006;88A(suppl 1 part 2):159–169.
6. Sugaya H, Kon Y, Tsuchiya A. Arthroscopic repair of glenoid fractures using suture anchors: Technical note with cases series. *Arthroscopy.* 2005;21:635.e1–635.e5.
7. Rockwood CA, Matsen FA. The scapula. In: Butters, KP, ed. *The Shoulder.* Philadelphia, PA: WB Saunders; 1990:345–353.
8. De Palma AF. Fractures and fracture–dislocations of the shoulder girdle. In: Jacob RP, Kristainsen T, Mayo K, et al., eds. *Surgery of the Shoulder.* 3rd ed. Philadelphia, PA: JB Lippincott; 1983:366–367.
9. Cameron SE. Arthroscopic reduction and internal fixation of an anterior glenoid fracture. *Arthroscopy.* 1998;14:743–746.
10. Porcellini G, Campi F, Paladini P. Arthroscopic approach to acute bony Bankart lesion. *Arthroscopy.* 2002;18:764–769.
11. Shapiro TA, Gupta A, McGarry MH, et al. Biomechanical effects of arthroscopic capsulorrhaphy in line with the fibers of the anterior band of the inferior glenohumeral ligament. *Am J Sports Med.* 2012;40:672–680.

12. Park JY, Lee SJ, Lhee SH, et al. Follow-up computed tomography arthrographic evaluation of bony Bankart lesions after arthroscopic repair. *Arthroscopy.* 2012;28(4):465–473.

13. Mologne TS, Provencher MT, Menzel KA, et al. Arthroscopic stabilization in patients with an inverted pear glenoid: Results in patients with bone loss of the anterior glenoid. *Am J Sports Med.* 2007;35:1276–1283.

14. Latarjet M. Techniques chirugicales dans le trairement de la luxation anteriointerne recidivante de l'epaule. *Lyon Chir.* 1965;61:313–318.

15. Lafosse L, Lejeune E, Bouchard A, et al. The arthroscopic Latarjet procedure for the treatment of anterior shoulder instability. *Arthroscopy.* 2007;23:1242.e1–1242.e5.

16. Fujii Y, Yoneda M, Wakitani S, et al. Histologic analysis of bony Bankart lesions in recurrent anterior instability of the shoulder. *J Shoulder Elbow Surg.* 2006;15:218–223.

17. Sugaya H. Chapter 14. Instability with bone loss. In: Angelo RL, Esch JC, Ryu RK, eds. *AANA Advanced Arthroscopy: The Shoulder.* Philadelphia, PA: Elsevier; 2010:136–146.

18. Sugaya H. Section 2 Anterior instability: Chapter 15 Arthroscopic treatment of glenoid bone loss-surgical technique. In: Provencher M, Romeo A, eds. *Shoulder Instability: A Comprehensive Approach.* Philadelphia, PA: Elsevier; 2011:186–196.

19. Bernageau J. Imaging of the shoulder in orthopedic pathology. *Rev Prat.* 1990;40:983–992. French.

20. Edwards TB, Boulahia A, Walch G. Radiographic analysis of bone defects in chronic anterior shoulder instability. *Arthroscopy.* 2003;19:732–739.

21. Sugaya H, Kon Y, Tsuchiya A. Arthroscopic Bankart repair in the beach-chair position: A cannulaless method using intra-articular suture relay technique. *Arthroscopy.* 2004;20(suppl 2):116–120.

22. Boileau P, O'Shea K, Vargas P, et al. Anatomical and functional results after arthroscopic Hill-Sachs remplissage. *J Bone Joint Surg Am.* 2012;94(7):618–626.

23. Takahashi N, Sugaya H, Matsuki K, et al. Arthroscopic rotator interval closure for recurrent anterior-inferior glenohumeral instability. *Kansetsukyo (Arthroscopy).* 2005;30:57–60. Japanese.

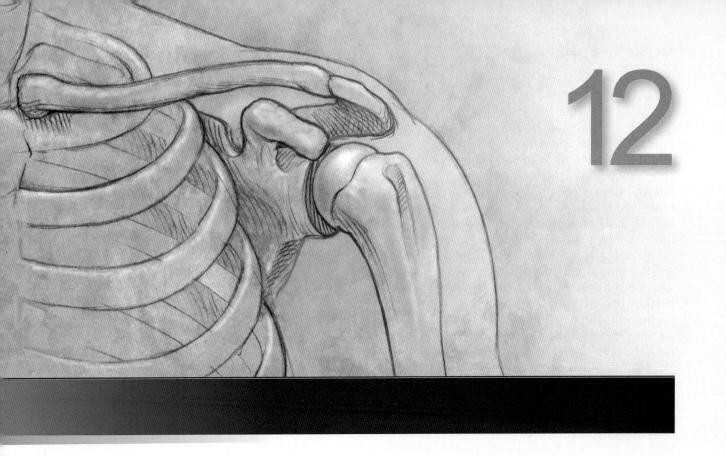

12

Diagnosis and Treatment of Humeral Avulsion of the Glenohumeral Ligament (HAGL) Lesions

Richard K.N. Ryu / John M. Tokish

Introduction

Anterior shoulder instability continues to be among the most common cause of disability in any young population. Failure of the inferior glenohumeral ligament (IGHL) attachment has long been considered the "essential" lesion in this condition (1), and biomechanical studies have revealed this failure as an avulsion occurring most commonly on the glenoid side of the joint (2). Numerous clinical studies have confirmed the intra-articular pathology associated with anterior shoulder dislocations and have identified the Bankart lesion as nearly ubiquitous in its association with shoulder instability (3–5). That said, humeral avulsion of the glenohumeral ligament (HAGL), although uncommon, can be an alternative pathologic entity contributing to shoulder instability. Failure to recognize and address this pathology can lead to persistence of instability even after operative intervention (6–8).

ANATOMY

Stability of the shoulder joint relies upon a complex interplay of static and dynamic stabilizers. An example of this is found in the concavity-compression phenomenon which relies upon an intact labrum to deepen the humeral head–glenoid interface while the rotator cuff musculature provides the dynamic compression component. Loss of integrity of either static or dynamic function increases the risk of instability (9).

The IGHL, the major static stabilizer, relies on an anterior and a posterior band with an axillary pouch suspended by the two main condensations within the IGHL, with attachments spanning the 2- to 4-o'clock position anteriorly, and the 7- to 9-o'clock position posteriorly. The attachment of the IGHL on the humeral neck has been described by Pouliart and Gagey (10) as "V" shaped, originating inferior to both the lesser and greater tuberosities (11). The function of the IGHL has been position dependent, and at 90 degrees of abduction combined with external rotation, the IGHL stabilizes anterior–inferior excursion of the glenohumeral joint (12,13). Similar stability is provided by the posterior band of the IGHL when the shoulder is flexed and internally rotated.

PATHOANATOMY

Several studies have investigated the failure characteristics of the IGHL under load. Stefko et al. (14) studied these characteristics in a cadaveric model with the arm positioned in the abducted, externally rotated position. The authors found that the IGHL strain increased over 7% at failure, and that this failure occurred on the glenoid side in 92% of cases, consistent with clinical observations of the predominance of a Bankart lesion. Another study, however, found that the failure mode was less consistent. Bigliani et al. (2) demonstrated a mixed mode of failure in their experimentally created model, with failure at the glenoid attachment in 40%, midcapsular failure in 35%, and humeral avulsion in 25%. It should be noted that the strain rate in this study was quite low, and other authors have suggested that the rate of loading may play a role in the site of failure of the IGHL. Ticker et al. (11) demonstrated that mechanical failure on the humeral side (an experimentally created HAGL) decreased to 8% when strain rates were increased toward physiologic speeds, lending a pathophysiologic justification to the HAGL mechanism, and offering an explanation as to why it is infrequently seen in the clinical setting.

Clinical investigations have cited a HAGL incidence rate ranging from 1.5% to 9% (7,15,16) (Figs. 12-1 and 12-2). Although these lesions are encountered more often in anterior instability cases, posterior humeral

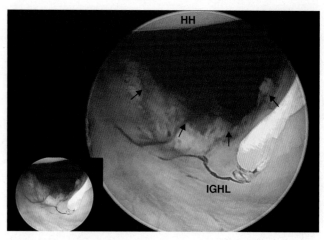

▲ **FIGURE 12-1:** Viewing from anterior-superior portal of a left shoulder, classic appearance of HAGL lesion (*arrows*) with detachment from the humeral side (HH, humeral head; IGHL, inferior glenohumeral ligament).

avulsions of the glenohumeral ligament have been reported as well (15,17,18). Incidence of anterior versus posterior HAGL lesions is felt to be approximately 93% to 7% (15) (Fig. 12-3).

It is also important to note that the HAGL lesion does not have to occur in isolation. Warner and Beim (19) and Field et al. (20) independently reported on the "floating" HAGL in which a Bankart lesion is found in combination with a HAGL lesion. This phenomenon can best be explained on the basis of the evidence of Speer et al. (21). Although creation of a Bankart lesion leads to instability, capsular deformation must accompany the Bankart lesion in order for functional instability to occur. The simultaneous HAGL lesion in conjunction with a Bankart lesion may simply represent a variation of capsular failure. An alternative explanation

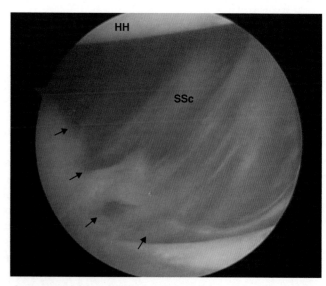

▲ **FIGURE 12-2:** Viewing from posterior portal of a left shoulder, a massive HAGL lesion involving much of the anterior inferior glenohumeral ligament is visualized (*arrows* depict leading edge of the HAGL lesion) (SSc, subscapularis; HH, humeral head).

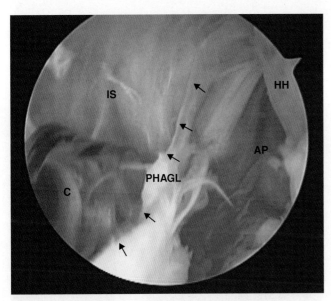

▲ **FIGURE 12-3:** Viewing from the anterior-superior portal of a left shoulder, a posterior HAGL lesion is noted with the avulsed edge (*arrows*) clearly separated from the humeral head (HH) attachment site (AP, axillary pouch; C, cannula; IS, infraspinatus; PHAGL, posterior humeral avulsion of the glenohumeral ligament).

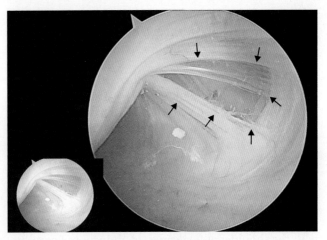

▲ **FIGURE 12-4:** Viewing from an posterior–inferior portal of a right shoulder, an axillary pouch HAGL lesion (*arrows*) is identified (HH, humeral head; IGHL, inferior glenohumeral ligament).

of the "floating" HAGL lesion may represent a metachronous phenomenon is which one lesion occurs after the first predisposes to continuing instability episodes or may simply represent a failure pattern related to the trauma experienced.

Furthermore, although commonly thought to occur in isolation, several studies have reported on a significant rate of associated injuries. Bokor et al. (7) described a 17% incidence of associated pathology while Neviaser et al. (22) reported on 37 cases of anterior dislocation with a high incidence of a subscapularis tear in combination with a humeral avulsion of the IGHL. This pattern of associated pathology is echoed with posterior HAGL lesions as well, with Castagna et al. (18) noting 66% of their posterior HAGL lesions occurring in conjunction with other significant shoulder pathology.

CLASSIFICATION

Six HAGL lesion types were originally included in the West Point classification (15): (1) anterior HAGL, (2) anterior bony HAGL (BHAGL), (3) posterior or reverse HAGL (RHAGL), (4) posterior bony HAGL, (5) anterior "floating" HAGL lesions with detachment at both the glenoid and humeral attachments, and (6) posterior "floating" HAGL lesions with detachment at both the glenoid and humeral attachments. A seventh type of HAGL lesion has recently been described to involve the axillary pouch (APHAGL) (Fig. 12-4), and was postulated to result from repetitive microtrauma and failure of the inferior capsule in female volleyball players (23).

MECHANISM OF INJURY

Most instability episodes occur in lesser degrees of abduction and external rotation, often requiring a powerful translation as the major deforming force. Although no clearly proven injury pattern has been identified that is unique to a HAGL lesion, Nicola proposed pure hyperabduction and maximum external rotation as the common mechanism for the HAGL lesion (8). The activities reported to have the highest incidence of HAGL lesions may be skewed on the basis of the prevalence of a particular sport; however, in the largest series, rugby was the most common pursuit, with ice hockey and wrestling (15), motocross (24,25), skiing and volleyball also described (7,24,25).

Taljanovic et al. (23) have postulated a specific injury pattern in female volleyball players leading to an APHAGL (axillary pouch HAGL) lesion. They proposed that the volleyball spike requires a higher release point, leading to greater abduction and external rotation to achieve such a posture. Repetitive hitting in this position leads to failure of the inferior capsule on a microtraumatic basis manifested by symptoms of pain and dysfunction rather than the typical complaints of shoulder instability.

HISTORY AND PHYSICAL EXAMINATION

Patients with HAGL lesions present with complaints similar to other patients with instability, and special athletic populations such as rugby or volleyball, should alert the examiner to the possibility of a HAGL phenomenon. Patients with a HAGL lesion can complain of significantly greater instability episodes with regard to duration and intensity and a crescendo pattern is not uncommon. George et al. (26) reported that anterior shoulder pain was more severe in those with HAGL lesions, and furthermore that those patients who had failed a prior stabilization procedure should be carefully scrutinized for a HAGL lesion (7,27).

On physical examination, there is no specific finding that is pathognomonic for a HAGL lesion. The typical findings associated with shoulder instability are often elicited during the physical examination. The principles of inspection, palpation, range of motion, and special testing remain cogent for all patients suspected of instability. In terms of specific testing, the apprehension test (28) is perhaps the most accurate test for anterior instability. It is performed either seated or supine, and the examiner takes the patient's arm into maximal external rotation with the shoulder at 90 degrees of abduction. Reproduction of the patient's symptoms is a reliable indicator of anterior instability (29). Another method of assessment for instability is the anterior load and shift test. This test is performed with the patient either seated or in the supine position and can also be undertaken with the patient in the lateral decubitus position. This latter position is helpful as the scapula can be controlled with one hand while the humerus is translated with the other. The humeral head is loaded axially to ensure it is centered, and then translated forward. The test is graded on the basis of how far the humeral head travels in relation to the glenoid (30): Grade 0, little movement of the humeral head; grade 1, the humeral head rides up to the glenoid labrum; grade 2, the humeral head is shifted off the glenoid but spontaneously reduces when pressure is removed; and grade 3, the humeral head is shifted off the glenoid and remains dislocated once the pressure is removed.

For posterior instability, a similar load and shift maneuver can be performed. A modification of this test, the push–pull test (31), can be effective in reproducing symptoms with posterior translation. This test is performed with the patient supine, and the arm is placed at 90-degree abduction in neutral rotation and 30-degree horizontal adduction. The examiner grasps around the patient's wrist with one hand (the pull), and posteriorly loads the humerus (the push). This places a fulcrum on the shoulder and enhances the examiner's ability to control subluxation. Finally, ligamentous laxity should be evaluated with the use of Beighton and Horan criteria (32). A prominent sulcus sign may indicate symptomatic multidirectional instability.

DIAGNOSTIC IMAGING

Rarely do routine radiographs reveal any diagnostic evidence regarding the actual capsular injury itself although secondary findings such as an associated Hill-Sachs lesion or glenoid bone loss can be detected. In the infrequent occurrence of a bony HAGL lesion,

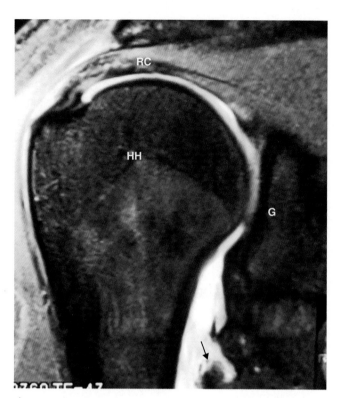

▲ **FIGURE 12-5:** Coronal MR image with contrast revealing "J" sign (*arrow*) with avulsion of the humeral attachment of the inferior glenohumeral ligament (HH, humeral head; G, glenoid; RC, rotator cuff).

plain radiographs may detect the avulsed medial bony humeral fragment adjacent to the attachment site of the IGHL, inferior to the lesser tuberosity anteriorly and to the greater tuberosity in posterior-based lesions. Scalloping along the medial neck of the humerus may also be an indication of a humeral-sided failure of the IGHL. Bokor et al. (7) noted that 7 of 41 documented HAGL lesions were detected on plain radiographs using the criteria described above. Because of overlapping bone on plain x-rays, these avulsions can be easily missed on routine films.

The imaging technique of choice when evaluating a potential HAGL lesion is the MR arthrogram (26) in which the typical finding confirming the HAGL lesion is the conversion of the "U" shaped inferior capsule into the "J" sign caused by the loss of integrity of the IGHL humeral attachment, best seen on the coronal view (Fig. 12-5). Extravasation of contrast on both the sagittal oblique and the coronal view (Fig. 12-6) also confirms the loss of IGHL integrity inferiorly.

Numerous authors have described the MR arthrographic findings, and the correlation between these findings and arthroscopic documentation has been robust (33,34). One report warned against the "over-reading" of MR arthrograms in the assessment of HAGL lesions. Melvin et al. (35) described four cases in which an MR arthrogram established a HAGL lesion by the criteria

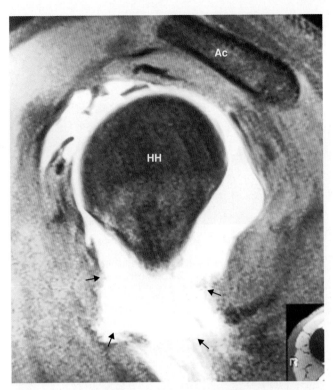

▲ **FIGURE 12-6:** Sagittal oblique image of the avulsed inferior capsular attachment with gross extravasation of contrast material (*arrows*) (HH, humeral head; Ac, acromion).

described, and at arthroscopy although inferior capsular pathology was noted, a detectable HAGL lesion was not confirmed. As with most lesions that are difficult to verify with diagnostic testing or from the physical examination, arthroscopic confirmation remains the gold standard prior to treatment being rendered.

TREATMENT ALTERNATIVES

Patients with symptomatic HAGL lesions present similarly to other patients with instability, and decisions regarding nonoperative versus operative management mirror those discussions. While it is unknown whether the HAGL lesion represents a different prognosis than the labral avulsion with regard to risk of recurrence, progression of bone loss, or risk for late arthritis, the pathology of the acute HAGL is much clearer than its chronic counterpart, and early intervention may be considered. Delayed presentation may result in ineffective scar that spans the gap to the humerus creating a functionally lengthened complex with inferior biomechanical properties compared to the native ligament. This scar can be indistinguishable from normal IGHL, and may make the surgery more technically difficult. We prefer an early approach to these lesions, especially in the young athlete or active laborer, as the anatomy is clearer and the repair is histologically more sound.

The surgical approach to the HAGL lesion is directed towards a primary repair of the capsular disruption. It is critical to determine the extent of this avulsion, as the severity of the disruption may determine the best surgical approach. For the anterior HAGL lesion, an anatomic repair can be accomplished either arthroscopically or through a mini-open anterior incision. Studies using both techniques have uniformly demonstrated satisfactory outcomes with regard to low recurrence rates and return to high-functioning levels (16,19,20,23,36,37). The open approach, which should always be preceded by a diagnostic evaluation to confirm the ligament tear and associated pathology, is achieved through a mini-incision through an axillary approach. Arciero and Mazzocca (36) and later Bhatia et al. (37) have described exposure through the inferior one-third of the subscapularis attachment, either via an "L" shaped takedown or upward retraction of the inferior subscapularis in the "sparing" technique described by Bhatia. The anterior HAGL lesion is easily identified with this approach although care must be taken not to obscure the tear by cutting through the subscapularis and the capsule at the same time, leaving in doubt whether the capsular defect was pathologic or iatrogenic in nature.

When utilizing an open approach in those cases with an associated glenohumeral ligament injury on the glenoid side, greater exposure will be required in order to view the glenoid attachment of the IGHL from the lateral aspect of the joint. Once the glenoid lesion is repaired, the humeral avulsion is repaired utilizing a suture anchor technique with closure and shifting of tissue to restore capsular integrity (20).

Arthroscopic repair of the anterior HAGL lesion is challenging. A perpendicular approach to the humeral head is often unavailable for anchor or instrument insertion due to the neurovascular structures inferiorly. Several techniques have been described, all of which require advanced arthroscopic skills. Wolf et al. (16) described an arthroscopic technique in which sutures were passed through the HAGL lesion which was then reapproximated to the humeral attachment site as the sutures were brought out via an accessory anterolateral portal and tied over the deltoid fascia. Richards and Burkhart (25) and later Kon et al. (24) were some of the first to pioneer an all-arthroscopic technique in which the sutures were passed and tied within the joint, using a 5-o'clock portal through the subscapularis. In his technique, Burkhart described suture passage through the HAGL lesion from a posterior approach while viewing from the anterior-superior portal.

When choosing an arthroscopic repair for an anterior–inferior HAGL lesion, visualization is of paramount importance. Using both the 30- and 70-degree lenses through multiple portals is mandatory for this

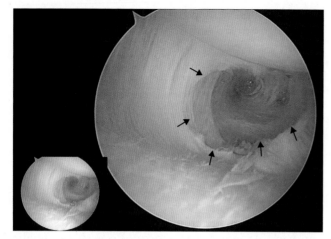

▲ **FIGURE 12-7:** Viewing from the anterior of a right shoulder portal, an inferior axillary HAGL lesion is identified (*arrows*).

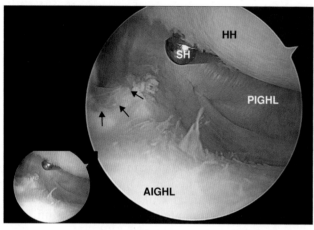

▲ **FIGURE 12-8:** Viewing from an anterior of a right shoulder portal, the humeral attachment is prepared with a shaving tool (SH) through a low anterior–inferior portal (*arrows* outline HAGL lesion) (HH, humeral head; AIGHL, anterior inferior glenohumeral ligament; PIGHL, posterior inferior glenohumeral ligament).

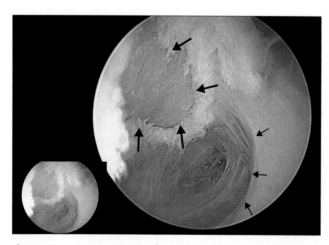

▲ **FIGURE 12-9:** Viewing from a low posterior portal, the prepared bony bed (*large arrows*) at the humeral attachment site is clearly visualized (*small arrows* outline axillary pouch HAGL lesion).

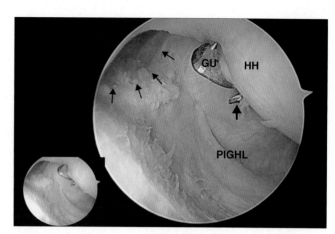

▲ **FIGURE 12-10:** Viewing from an anterior portal, a drill guide (GU) is seen at the inferior humeral head attachment site, facilitating transhumeral head drilling, beginning at the postero-lateral aspect of the greater tuberosity (HH, humeral head; drill pin (*large arrows*); APHAGL lesion (*small arrows*); AIGHL, anterior inferior glenohumeral ligament).

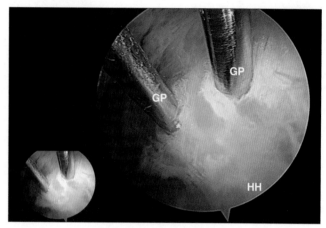

▲ **FIGURE 12-11:** Viewing from a lateral subacromial portal, two guide pins (GP) are placed through the humeral head into the inferior aspect of the humeral head (HH).

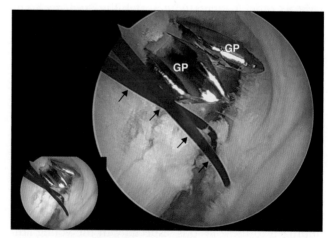

▲ **FIGURE 12-12:** Viewing from a low posterior portal, the two guide pins are seen exiting the prepared bony bed on the humeral neck (*arrows* outline the sutures passed through the HAGL lesion; GP, transhumeral head guide pins).

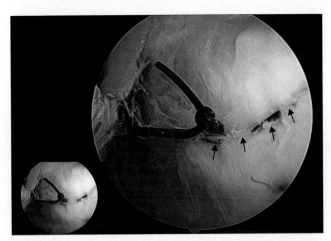

▲ **FIGURE 12-13:** Sutures passed through the HAGL lesion are in turn passed through the drill tunnels and tied over a bone bridge in the subacromial space, reapproximating the inferior glenohumeral ligament to the humeral attachment site (*arrows* outline sutures passed through transhumeral head tunnels and tied in the subacromial space).

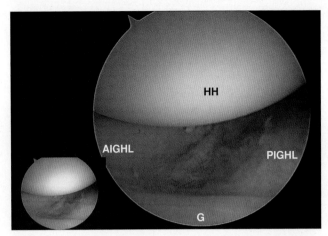

▲ **FIGURE 12-14:** Intra-articular view of the inferior HAGL lesion after reapproximation of the HAGL lesion to the humeral neck (HH, humeral head; G, glenoid; AIGHL, anterior inferior glenohumeral ligament; PIGHL, posterior inferior glenohumeral ligament).

demanding procedure. The primary steps involve creating a bony trough at the humeral attachment site for the IGHL, creating a working portal through the intra-articular tendinous portion of the subscapularis and passing sutures through the HAGL lesion using either a suture shuttling technique or a direct pass and retrieve maneuver. In those situations in which a Bankart lesion is encountered in addition to the HAGL lesion, the HAGL lesion is addressed first, followed by a standard suture anchor Bankart repair, making sure not to over-tension the final construct. It is critical to appreciate the inferior extent of the HAGL, as significant extension makes an all-arthroscopic approach through anterior portals potentially unsafe.

A recent surgical technique described by Taljanovic et al. (23) addresses this challenge by approaching distal fixation through a transhumeral head technique in which multiple sutures are passed through the free edge of the avulsed edge of the HAGL lesion and then brought through multiple bone tunnels drilled through the humeral head with the use of a guided system. The sutures are then tied over bone bridges along the posterior aspect of the greater tuberosity (Figs. 12-7–12-14).

The treatment of the posterior HAGL lesion is almost always approachable from an arthroscopic perspective. Although extracapsular repairs can also be accomplished, intra-articular anchor placement, suture passage and knot tying are relatively easier and more accessible. Much like the anterior HAGL lesion, arthroscopic treatment of the reverse HAGL lesion has been uniformly successful (17,18,38,39). If an open procedure is selected for posterior repair, we prefer a deltoid split in line with its fibers, followed by dissection between the infraspinatus and the teres minor to approach the posterior capsule. The capsular avulsion can be identified through this interval, and repaired

back after biologic preparation with suture anchors. This technique has been reported uncommonly, but with successful results (40,41).

POSTOPERATIVE REHABILITATION

The principles of postoperative rehabilitation after HAGL repair are protection with mobilization. The patient leaves the operating room in a sling, and this is worn full time, except during specific rehabilitative sessions, for 3 weeks. Range of motion limitations are dependent on the direction of the repair, but generally 30 degrees of rotational stretch is allowed beyond neutral (external rotation for an anterior repair, internal rotation for a posterior repair), and full rotation is allowed in the opposite direction. Abduction and elevation are limited for the first 6 weeks to 90 degrees, and may be limited further for axillary pouch repairs. Muscle strengthening is timed on the basis of the approach to the repair. In an all-arthroscopic repair or open repair which does not take down any muscle, we begin isometric and short chain mobilization and strengthening immediately to prevent disuse atrophy. In cases where the subscapularis is taken down anteriorly, resisted internal rotation is limited until healing of the tendon is assured, usually around the 8-week point postoperatively. Once tissue healing is assured, patients are placed in a return-to-sport program that emphasizes dynamic stabilization with an emphasis on scapular rhythm. Co-contraction exercises of the anterior and posterior rotator cuff as well as specific exercises to target the periscapular musculature are emphasized. If the patient is an athlete, return to sport may be considered once he or she regains dynamic strength and rhythm as well as endurance and confidence.

S U M M A R Y

Instability due to HAGL lesions can be a diagnostic and therapeutic challenge. Seven types of HAGL lesions have been reported in the literature, and care must be taken to ascertain an accurate diagnosis in order to optimize treatment. When HAGL lesions occur, trauma, either macro or repetitive, is the usual cause. Evaluations must include a thorough search for associated pathology. The diagnostic imaging of choice is the MR arthrogram with the "J" sign and extravasation along the medial humeral attachment representing the cardinal signs of capsular failure and a HAGL lesion. Although the possibility of HAGL lesions healing does exist, once a HAGL lesion is identified, a surgical repair is deemed the most appropriate solution. The anticipated surgical technique is based on the surgeon's experience, the degree of inferior capsular extension and the patient's choice after the merits of an open versus arthroscopic approach are discussed in detail. Published reports indicate that both open and arthroscopic techniques to treat HAGL lesions are largely successful and resumption of unrestricted activities can be anticipated.

References

1. Bankart AS. Recurrent or habitual dislocation of the shoulder-joint. *Br Med J.* 1923;2(3285):1132–1133.
2. Bigliani LU, Pollock RG, Soslowsky LJ, et al. Tensile properties of the inferior glenohumeral ligament. *J Orthop Res.* 1992;10(2):187–197.
3. Bottoni CR, Smith EL, Berkowitz MJ, et al. Arthroscopic versus open shoulder stabilization for recurrent anterior instability: A prospective randomized clinical trial. *Am J Sports Med.* 2006;34(11):1730–1737.
4. Owens BD, Duffey ML, Nelson BJ, et al. The incidence and characteristics of shoulder instability at the United States Military Academy. *Am J Sports Med.* 2007;35(7):1168–1173.
5. Taylor DC, Arciero RA. Pathologic changes associated with shoulder dislocations. Arthroscopic and physical examination findings in first-time, traumatic anterior dislocations. *Am J Sports Med.* 1997;25(3):306–311.
6. Bach BR, Warren RF, Fronek J. Disruption of the lateral capsule of the shoulder. A cause of recurrent dislocation. *J Bone Joint Surg Br.* 1988;70(2):274–276.
7. Bokor DJ, Conboy VB, Olson C. Anterior instability of the glenohumeral joint with humeral avulsion of the glenohumeral ligament. A review of 41 cases. *J Bone Joint Surg Br.* 1999;81(1):93–96.
8. Nicola T. Acute anterior dislocation of the shoulder. *J Bone Joint Surg Am.* 1949;31A(1):153–159.
9. Matsen FA 3rd, Chebli CM, Lippitt SB. Principles for the evaluation and management of shoulder instability. *Instr Course Lect.* 2007;56:23–34.
10. Pouliart N, Gagey O. Simulated humeral avulsion of the glenohumeral ligaments: A new instability model. *J Shoulder Elbow Surg.* 2006;15(6):728–735.
11. Ticker JB, Bigliani LU, Soslowsky LJ, et al. Inferior glenohumeral ligament: Geometric and strain-rate dependent properties. *J Shoulder Elbow Surg.* 1996; 5(4):269–279.
12. O'Brien SJ, Neves MC, Arnoczky SP, et al. The anatomy and histology of the inferior glenohumeral ligament complex of the shoulder. *Am J Sports Med.* 1990;18(5): 449–456.
13. Turkel SJ, Panio MW, Marshall JL, et al. Stabilizing mechanisms preventing anterior dislocation of the glenohumeral joint. *J Bone Joint Surg Am.* 1981;63(8): 1208–1217.
14. Stefko JM, Tibone JE, Cawley PW, et al. Strain of the anterior band of the inferior glenohumeral ligament during capsule failure. *J Shoulder Elbow Surg.* 1997;6(5): 473–479.
15. Bui-Mansfield LT, Banks KP, Taylor DC. Humeral avulsion of the glenohumeral ligaments: The HAGL lesion. *Am J Sports Med.* 2007;35(11):1960–1966.
16. Wolf EM, Cheng JC, Dickson K. Humeral avulsion of glenohumeral ligaments as a cause of anterior shoulder instability. *Arthroscopy.* 1995;11(5):600–607.
17. Abrams JS. Arthroscopic repair of posterior instability and reverse humeral glenohumeral ligament avulsion lesions. *Orthop Clin North Am.* 2003;34(4):475–483.
18. Castagna A, Snyder SJ, Conti M, et al. Posterior humeral avulsion of the glenohumeral ligament: A clinical review of 9 cases. *Arthroscopy.* 2007;23(8):809–815.
19. Warner JJ, Beim GM. Combined Bankart and HAGL lesion associated with anterior shoulder instability. *Arthroscopy.* 1997;13(6):749–752.
20. Field LD, Bokor DJ, Savoie FH 3rd. Humeral and glenoid detachment of the anterior inferior glenohumeral ligament: A cause of anterior shoulder instability. *J Shoulder Elbow Surg.* 1997;6(1):6–10.
21. Speer KP, Deng X, Borrero S, et al. Biomechanical evaluation of a simulated Bankart lesion. *J Bone Joint Surg Am.* 1994;76(12):1819–1826.
22. Neviaser RJ, Neviaser TJ, Neviaser JS. Anterior dislocation of the shoulder and rotator cuff rupture. *Clin Orthop Relat Res.* 1993;(291):103–106.
23. Taljanovic MS, Nisbet JK, Hunter TB, et al. Humeral avulsion of the inferior glenohumeral ligament in college female volleyball players caused by repetitive microtrauma. *Am J Sports Med.* 2011;39(5):1067–1076.
24. Kon Y, Shiozaki H, Sugaya H. Arthroscopic repair of a humeral avulsion of the glenohumeral ligament lesion. *Arthroscopy.* 2005;21(5):632.
25. Richards DP, Burkhart SS. Arthroscopic humeral avulsion of the glenohumeral ligaments (HAGL) repair. *Arthroscopy.* 2004;20(suppl 2):134–141.
26. George MS, Khazzam M, Kuhn JE. Humeral avulsion of glenohumeral ligaments. *J Am Acad Orthop Surg.* 2011; 19(3):127–133.

27. Schippinger G, Vasiu PS, Fankhauser F, et al. HAGL lesion occurring after successful arthroscopic Bankart repair. *Arthroscopy.* 2001;17(2):206–208.
28. Rowe CR, Zarins B. Recurrent transient subluxation of the shoulder. *J Bone Joint Surg Am.* 1981;63(6): 863–872.
29. Tzannes A, Paxinos A, Callanan M, et al. An assessment of the interexaminer reliability of tests for shoulder instability. *J Shoulder Elbow Surg.* 2004;13(1):18–23.
30. McFarland EG, Torpey BM, Curl LA. Evaluation of shoulder laxity. *Sports Med.* 1996;22(4):264–272.
31. Tokish J, Krishnan SG, Hawkins RJ. Clinical examination of the overhead athlete: The "differential-directed approach. In: Krishnan SG, Hawkins RJ, Warren RF, eds. *The Shoulder and the Overhead Athlete.* Philadelphia, PA: Lippincott Williams & Wilkins; 2004:23–49.
32. Beighton P, Horan F. Orthopaedic aspects of the Ehlers-Danlos syndrome. *J Bone Joint Surg Br.* 1969;51(3): 444–453.
33. Chung CB, Sorenson S, Dwek JR, et al. Humeral avulsion of the posterior band of the inferior glenohumeral ligament: MR arthrography and clinical correlation in 17 patients. *AJR Am J Roentgenol.* 2004;183(2): 355–359.
34. Hottya GA, Tirman PF, Bost FW, et al. Tear of the posterior shoulder stabilizers after posterior dislocation: MR imaging and MR arthrographic findings with arthroscopic correlation. *AJR Am J Roentgenol.* 1998; 171(3):763–768.
35. Melvin JS, Mackenzie JD, Nacke E, et al. MRI of HAGL lesions: Four arthroscopically confirmed cases of false-positive diagnosis. *AJR Am J Roentgenol.* 2008;191(3): 730–734.
36. Arciero RA, Mazzocca AD. Mini-open repair technique of HAGL (humeral avulsion of the glenohumeral ligament) lesion. *Arthroscopy.* 2005;21(9):1152.
37. Bhatia DN, DeBeer JF, van Rooyen KS. The "subscapularis-sparing" approach: A new mini-open technique to repair a humeral avulsion of the glenohumeral ligament lesion. *Arthroscopy.* 2009;25(6):686–690.
38. Bokor DJ, Fritsch BA. Posterior shoulder instability secondary to reverse humeral avulsion of the glenohumeral ligament. *J Shoulder Elbow Surg.* 2010;19(6):853–858.
39. Chhabra A, Diduch DR, Anderson M. Arthroscopic repair of a posterior humeral avulsion of the inferior glenohumeral ligament (HAGL) lesion. *Arthroscopy.* 2004;20(suppl 2):73–76.
40. Hasan SS, Fleckenstein C, Albright J. Open treatment of posterior humeral avulsion of the glenohumeral ligaments: A case report and review of the literature. *J Shoulder Elbow Surg.* 2007;16(4):e3–e5.
41. Weinberg J, McFarland EG. Posterior capsular avulsion in a college football player. *Am J Sports Med.* 1999;27(2): 235–237.

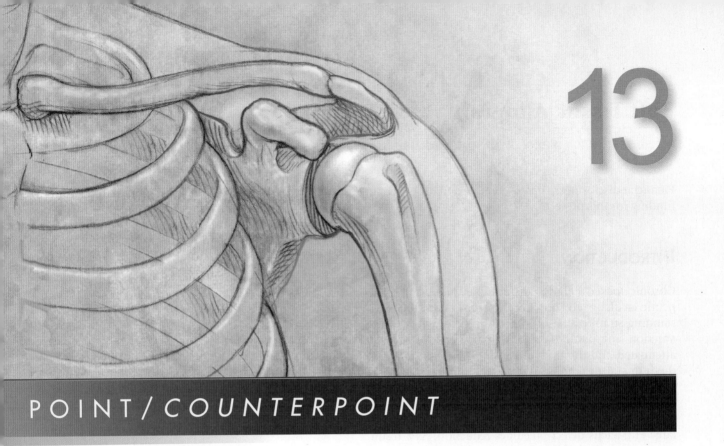

CHRONIC LOCKED ANTERIOR DISLOCATIONS

Chronic locked anterior dislocations present a therapeutic challenge to shoulder surgeons. As a result of the persistent stress on the anterior structures from the dislocated head, the anterior capsule can become compromised rendering a reconstruction difficult. However, arthroplasty in this population can also be a significant challenge. The damage to the surrounding soft tissues can compromise any arthroplasty procedure leading to instability and possibly infection. The following chapters will highlight each author's approach to this problem with two distinct treatment pathways: Allograft reconstruction versus arthroplasty.

Soft Tissue Allograft

Miguel A. Ramirez / Anand M. Murthi

Financial disclosures: There were no external sources of funding for this project.

INTRODUCTION

Chronic locked anterior dislocations present a therapeutic challenge to shoulder surgeons. Given the long-standing strain of the dislocated humeral head on the anterior soft tissues, the anterior capsule is usually attenuated and the inferior capsule is scarred down to the humeral neck (1). Via the same mechanism, these patients may often also have an attenuated or incompetent subscapularis tendon. Furthermore, the glenohumeral joint has often "filled" with scar tissue and a large Hill-Sachs defect precludes reduction. As a result, reconstruction of the anterior structures using local tissues is challenging given that the soft tissue quality is tenuous at best.

Because these are devastating but rare injuries, no large series of allograft reconstruction for deficient anterior capsulolabral structures have been reported. If open glenohumeral reduction is possible, soft tissue allograft is a reasonable option for anterior soft tissue reconstruction in patients with chronic anterior dislocations and attenuated soft tissues. Several allograft options have been described in the literature (2–6). In 1993, Moeckel used an Achilles tendon allograft in three patients who had persistent anterior instability after total shoulder replacement. The investigators reported that all three patients regained shoulder instability with no subsequent episodes of dislocation (5). Lazarus and Harzman (6) performed a semitendinosus allograft in 25 patients and reported a success rate of 70%. More recently, Iannotti et al. (4) used iliotibial band allograft and autograft in seven patients with capsular deficiency and noted no episodes of redislocation. Dewing et al. (3) reported a 45% success rate for stability after revision capsulolabral reconstruction with allograft. Alcid et al. (2) reported in their series of revision stabilization procedures with hamstring allograft that success may be achieved but with resultant shoulder stiffness.

Given these generally favorable results of allograft reconstruction and the reduced morbidity compared to autograft harvest, we prefer a soft tissue reconstruction as our procedure of choice in patients with chronic locked anterior dislocations. It is crucial for patients to understand that this is a salvage procedure, and as such, the functional outcomes in terms of range of motion are often limited. However, this procedure is highly successful when stability and pain relief are the essential goals. The allograft reconstruction provides a tenodesis effect to "contain" the humeral head versus a dynamic reconstruction, which we believe provides long-term stability for patients with chronic instability.

INDICATIONS

Glenohumeral tendon allograft is indicated in patients with chronic locked anterior dislocations and an intact or repairable subscapularis tendon. Preservation of an intact humeral head is a prerequisite for stabilization surgery.

PREOPERATIVE EVALUATION

A thorough history and physical examination is done before reconstruction. Important information includes how did the dislocation occur? How much time has passed since the injury? What if any treatment has occurred? For example, has a closed reduction been attempted? Are there any neurovascular symptoms in that extremity? It is important to establish why the patient has not had adequate treatment and now has a chronic dislocation. Are there social or psychiatric issues to consider that may preclude a complex operation with complex rehabilitation requiring patient compliance?

Physical Examination

Upon evaluation in the office, the main complaint of patients with chronic shoulder dislocations is loss of motion and associated pain. Presentation is typically a marked restriction of abduction and internal rotation. There may be an associated palsy of the axillary nerve, which is manifested as deltoid weakness and loss of sensation along the lateral shoulder. Disuse atrophy can also be substantial, especially in patients who have had significant delay in diagnosis.

For patients presenting to our office with the above symptoms and radiographs (Fig. 13-1) concerning for shoulder dislocation, CT scans with and without three-dimensional reconstruction are obtained (Fig. 13-2). CT scan can be an extremely helpful tool for preoperative planning because it can identify any glenoid bone loss as well as quantify the size of any existing Hill-Sachs lesion.

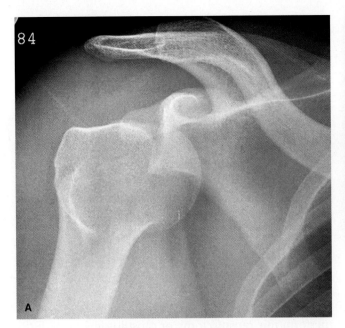

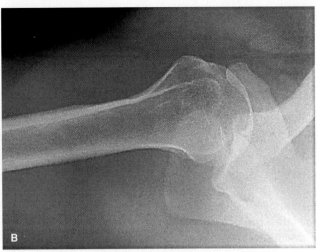

▲ **FIGURE 13-1:** Shoulder radiographs demonstrating a locked anterior dislocation. **A:** Anteroposterior view. **B:** Axillary view.

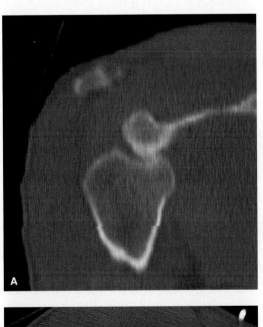

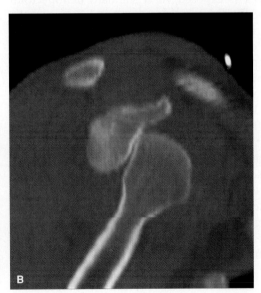

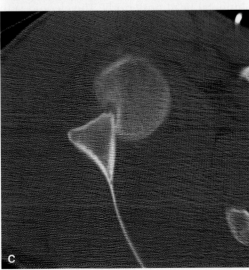

▲ **FIGURE 13-2:** Shoulder CT scan demonstrating an anterior shoulder dislocation with minimal Hill-Sachs lesion and an intact glenoid. **A:** Coronal view. **B:** Sagittal view. **C:** Axial view.

Procedure

Setup

General anesthesia is used in all patients. Interscalene block is an option for postoperative pain control and intraoperative muscular relaxation. Prophylactic antibiotics are infused during patient positioning and induction.

Patient positioning is typically in a beach chair position with the head secured to headrest. The head is subsequently elevated approximately 20 to 30 degrees. Care must be taken to allow the humeral head to drop posteriorly and not sit in a dislocated or anteriorly subluxed position. This will allow easier dissection through the subscapularis and underlying tissues. With chronic dislocations, the approach is often difficult because of the dynamic anterior fixed instability of the shoulder. The shoulder is draped in sterile fashion with arm draped free.

Exposure

The shoulder is exposed via a standard deltopectoral approach. Superficial incision is carried down to the deltopectoral fascia, where the cephalic vein is identified and protected. The deltopectoral interval is identified and expanded using blunt dissection. Care is taken to release adhesions in the subdeltoid and subacromial spaces. A large deltoid retractor is placed between the deltoid and the greater tuberosity to provide adequate exposure. The branches of the circumflex humeral artery and veins are identified and coagulated.

Scar tissue formation from chronic trauma is common, and soft tissue planes can be significantly scarred. The pectoralis and conjoined tendons are carefully identified and separated. The interval between the conjoined tendon and the subscapularis is also released. One to 2 cm of the proximal pectoralis tendon is released from the humerus to enhance exposure.

If the subscapularis tendon is intact, it is released from the proximal humerus. A vertical incision is used, starting 1 cm medial to its attachment to the lesser tuberosity. The incision is carried through the tendinous proximal two-thirds of the tendon. Tagging traction sutures are placed. If possible, the underlying capsule is dissected off the subscapularis tendon. The inferior one-third of the subscapularis muscle is then carefully dissected off any remaining inferior capsule. This tissue may be atrophic or absent.

Mobilizing the subscapularis is crucial to prevent internal rotation contracture postoperatively. Release from the anterior capsule is then carried out bluntly at first, and then any remaining adhesions can be freed with Mayo scissors. It is important to identify and protect the axillary nerve before releasing the subscapularis with scissors. The remaining anterior and inferior capsule is released from the head and neck of the humerus. Care must be taken to release posteriorly past the 6-o'clock position to reduce capsular redundancy and obliterate the capsular pouch. This capsule may be imbricated with the allograft reconstruction either superficial or deep to the allograft weave.

Glenohumeral Reduction

Reduction of the dislocation is then carried out. It is important to verify with the anesthesiologist that there is complete paralysis before attempting reduction. The shoulder is reduced first by adduction and external rotation to free the glenoid from the defect in the humeral head. Retaining the humeral head is usually possible with less than a 25% humeral head defect. With chronic dislocations, avascular necrosis and head collapse may occur. In our experience, chronic dislocations over 3 months often have unsalvageable humeral heads. Essentially a complete inferior and posterior capsular release is necessary to allow reduction. A combination of scissors and long-handled scalpels are used to perform this capsulectomy or capsulotomy posteriorly. The glenohumeral joint is often blocked with scar tissue preventing adequate reduction. Lateral distraction is applied to the humerus. The head is then located by directing it posteriorly with the arm in flexion and internal rotation.

Glenohumeral Inspection

Once the shoulder is located, the humeral head in carefully inspected. We carefully internally and externally rotate the arm to see whether the humeral head defect engages with the glenoid. The amount of humeral head defect is quantified. If there is greater than 33% bone loss of the humeral head, we elect for prosthetic replacement. In many chronic cases the humeral head undergoes subchondral collapse due to osteonecrosis of dislocation. If at the time of surgery significant head collapse with avascular necrosis is identified, arthroplasty is then considered.

A Fukuda retractor is inserted to displace the humeral head posteriorly. The glenoid is then carefully inspected for evidence of bone loss or wear. Significant arthritic changes, especially in older patients, are an indication for prosthetic replacement. The labrum is inspected. In some instances, a Bankart labral lesion is identified. This is often associated with complete capsular stripping off the front of the glenoid. If possible, the medial capsule is repaired to the anterior glenoid with suture anchors to assist with stability. This long-standing capsular disruption often precludes any capsular shift or repair to either the glenoid or lateral humerus.

Allograft Site Preparation and Insertion

The anterior glenoid rim is usually devoid of soft tissue including capsule or redundant labral tissue. A small diameter burr is then used to decorticate the anterior glenoid rim down to bleeding cancellous bone. Labral type

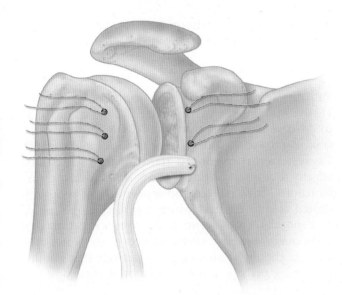

▲ **FIGURE 13-3:** Allograft fixation to the glenoid. Three suture anchors are placed at the inferior, middle, and superior thirds of the glenoid. Allograft is secured to inferior glenoid anchor.

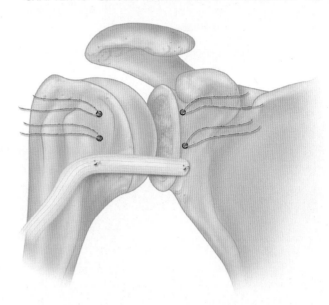

▲ **FIGURE 13-4:** Allograft is passed across the glenohumeral joint and secured to the humerus using a suture anchor placed at the subscapularis footprint—0.5–1 cm medial to the bicipital groove at the level of the lesser tuberosity.

suture anchors are placed along the anterior–inferior glenoid rim with adequate spacing to place the allograft weave. In our practice, we prefer to use single-loaded PEEK or biocomposite anchors with a no. 2 Fiberwire (Arthrex, Naples, FL) (Fig. 13-3).

Attention is then directed to the humeral side, where two rotator cuff type anchors are placed on the proximal humerus at the subscapularis footprint. Alternatively, the allograft may be affixed using interference type screws into the humerus. Optimal location is 0.5 to 1 cm medial to the bicipital groove at the level of the lesser tuberosity. Any remaining anterior or inferior capsule is secured to the humeral neck using these anchors but leaving the suture tails intact to incorporate the allograft weave. The arm is optimally positioned in approximately 30 degrees of abduction, 30 degrees of external rotation during the reconstruction. Where there is chronic instability, it may be necessary to maintain shoulder in a more internally rotated, flexed position to maintain reduction.

Soft Tissue Allograft Selection and Preparation

Although several soft tissue allograft options have been described (2–4,6), we prefer semitendinosus or anterior tibialis tendon allograft. These are often robust quality allografts. We prefer this tissue for allografts because the diameter of the graft allows for better coverage of the joint. Thinner allografts require multiple zigzag passes across the joint to cover the joint appropriately. The graft is then placed in a warm saline bath during the case to allow the tendon to fully thaw prior to insertion.

Once suture anchors are placed, the allograft is removed from the saline bath. The allograft is carefully inspected and frayed or friable fibrils are excised.

Allograft Fixation Technique

Once the allograft is prepared, sutures from the inferior glenoid anchors are passed through one end of the allograft using a Mason-Allen suture technique. The allograft is subsequently brought to the humeral anchors (Fig. 13-4). During this process, care is taken to ensure that the glenohumeral joint is adequately reduced. The arm is placed in 10 degrees of flexion, 30 degrees of abduction, and 30 degrees of external rotation to assure optimal graft tension across the glenohumeral joint. The graft is secured to the humerus using the previously placed suture anchors. Care is taken to affix the graft in a tensioned state without laxity.

The arm is then positioned at 20 degrees of abduction and 20 degrees of external rotation. The graft is folded over itself across the glenohumeral joint and sutured to the superior glenoid anchors. The final construct should yield four passes of allograft across the glenohumeral joint spanning its entire superior/inferior dimensions. This pattern recreates the anterior labrum and the middle glenohumeral ligament and the anterior band of the inferior glenohumeral ligament.

Finally, the two ends of the graft are sutured together. The superior limb is attached to the leading edge of the supraspinatus, and the inferior limb is sutured to any remaining inferior capsule. Excess superior graft may be run through the rotator interval and to the coracoid to recreate the superior glenohumeral and coracohumeral ligaments (Fig. 13-5). This may assist in diminishing any chronic inferior instability.

The subscapularis tendon is then identified. In cases of chronic anterior dislocations, the subscapularis

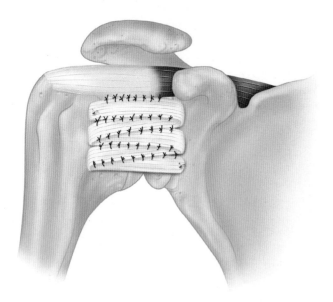

▲ **FIGURE 13-5:** Final construct. Allograft is passed across the glenohumeral joint a total of four times and secured to the anchors. Running sutures are placed to close the rotator interval and to secure the graft limbs to each other.

tendon may be frayed, thin, or torn. An effort is made to identify all remaining tendon and circumferentially release it. Once this is done, the tendon is advanced to the lesser tuberosity. The subscapularis tendon is repaired to the stump on the lesser tuberosity and may be reinforced using bone tunnels or suture anchors. We avoid repairing the subscapularis tendon to the allograft itself.

Wound Closure

Once the capsule and the subscapularis tendon are repaired, the biceps is evaluated. Evidence of fraying or instability of the tendon is an indication for tenodesis.

The wound is irrigated thoroughly. The incision is closed over a drain according to surgeon preference.

Postoperative Care

Patients are placed in a shoulder orthosis for 6 weeks. Passive motion is started at their first follow-up visit 10 to 14 days after the procedure. Passive forward elevation is allowed to 120 degrees in the scapular plane. Passive external rotation is started 4 to 6 weeks after surgery to protect the subscapularis and capsular reconstruction. Active-assisted and active range of motion is started at 6 to 8 weeks. Strengthening may be started at 4 months. Proprioception exercises are instituted at 3 months. These are often limited goals procedures. Patients should be advised preoperatively that stability is the goal, perhaps at the risk of motion loss.

Complications

Potential complications include infection, subscapularis failure, recurrent instability, hardware failure, posttraumatic arthritis, and profound stiffness. Because these are complex cases, patients must be aware of these issues and the often necessary secondary operations.

CONCLUSIONS

Chronic locked anterior shoulder dislocations remain one of the most challenging reconstructions to achieve a satisfactory outcome. Careful preoperative evaluation is necessary to evaluate both the bony architecture and soft tissue injuries about the shoulder. An in-depth understanding of the surgical approach and allograft application will help provide for a stable shoulder. Patients must be counseled on appropriate expectations of shoulder stability with likely loss of motion.

Arthroplasty

Clay Riley / T. Bradley Edwards

INTRODUCTION

Chronic locked anterior shoulder dislocations are not commonly encountered and pose a treatment dilemma. These dislocations usually occur within two distinct patient subsets. Younger patients (<60 years) may present with a chronically dislocated shoulder because the diagnosis was missed, most often as a result of these patients sustaining multiple traumatic injuries simultaneously and the shoulder dislocation not being recognized until concomitant injuries have been stabilized.

A second subset, and the one that we will be focusing on in this section, includes older patients that have dislocated their shoulder and usually have sustained a massive rotator cuff tear that contributes to the instability. These become chronic locked dislocations as a result of a delay in seeking treatment or after having actually been reduced in a timely manner but recurring with the shoulder remaining dislocated for an indeterminate amount of time. In addition to the massive rotator cuff tear often sustained by the elderly patient, rapidly developing osteoarthritis may occur with or without significant glenoid erosion or large Hill-Sachs lesion. The following chapter will outline why and how these older patients with chronic locked anterior dislocations should be treated with a reverse shoulder arthroplasty.

INDICATIONS

Chronic locked anterior dislocations can have a myriad of associated injury components. This varied presentation and lack of distinctly superior treatment options make these dislocations difficult to manage. Although the length of time necessary to define a dislocation as chronic has ranged from several days to 6 months, we generally use 3 weeks as a guide (7). Once the shoulder has been dislocated for a prolonged period of time, closed reduction attempts will rarely be successful and can actually cause further damage such as fracture.

In younger patients, treatment is almost always surgical and options are directed at the underlying pathology. Open reduction alone with appropriate postoperative immobilization may be all that is necessary if no significant injuries are identified that will compromise stability. However, additional procedures are generally necessary to ensure stability and rely on repair

or reconstruction to return functionality to the glenohumeral joint.

An older patient may present without discomfort, and if his or her functional demands are limited or they are not a candidate for surgery due to medical comorbidities, nonoperative management can be considered. As with any clinical evaluation, thorough neurologic examination is important. Specifically with chronic anterior dislocations there is an increased risk of axillary nerve injury, so sensory and motor function should be evaluated. While this distinction is important with most shoulder problems, deltoid function is paramount for function and stability in a reverse shoulder arthroplasty. We consider this as a contraindication and surgery should be delayed until the neuropraxia resolves.

If surgical intervention is the best option, while many of the same procedures employed in younger patients can be utilized in a select group of older patients, most will require prosthetic replacement. The older population tends to present with a longer duration of dislocation, which leads to the rapid appearance of significant articular cartilage degeneration. Massive rotator cuff tears frequently accompany the dislocation and severe bone loss of the glenoid and/or humerus may also occur (8).

Heroic efforts to repair and restore normal anatomy in these patients might fail for many reasons. Diminished healing potential in patients with medical comorbidities can increase the likelihood of an unsuccessful outcome. Even if healing occurs, prolonged immobilization and limited rehabilitation potential could render the joint with little functionality. Another scenario is that everything goes perfectly, with healing of all repairs and function returning appropriately, only to soon see the rapid onset of degenerative joint disease as mentioned earlier. Although articular cartilage may appear normal at the time of surgery, the cumulative effects of damage occurring at the initial trauma, repetitive injury due to abnormal articulation and loss of normal cartilage loading and metabolism can result in cartilage cell death and its precipitous disappearance. All of these problems in isolation could prevent a successful outcome, but the looming possibility of recurrent instability is also a major concern independent of these other factors (Fig. 13-6).

With these concerns in mind, along with other indications for arthroplasty such as age and activity level, prosthetic replacement becomes the clear choice

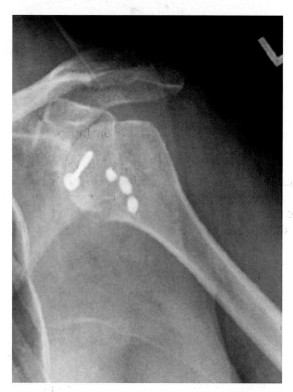

▲ **FIGURE 13-6:** Radiograph of a chronic anterior dislocation with recurrent instability despite undergoing multiple surgical procedures.

for older patients. Prosthetic options include hemiarthroplasty, unconstrained total shoulder arthroplasty, or reverse shoulder arthroplasty. It has been our experience that unconstrained shoulder arthroplasty leads to a high rate of recurrent instability (9). This recurrent instability, the frequent presence of massive rotator cuff tears (including increased incidence of subscapularis tears in chronic anterior dislocations) and the occasional need for glenoid bone grafting has made reverse shoulder arthroplasty our treatment of choice for chronic anterior dislocations in this population of patients (10).

SURGICAL TECHNIQUE

We use a standard operating table with the patient positioned sufficiently to the operative side to allow extension of the arm. The patient is placed in the modified beach chair position, with the back of the table elevated approximately 45 to 60 degrees. A standard deltopectoral approach is used for exposure. With chronic anterior dislocations there can be significant subcoracoid, subdeltoid, and subacromial adhesions (11). It is important to release these adhesions in order to allow adequate exposure, implant stability, and postoperative function. Also there may be fibrous tissue that has formed overlying the glenoid that will have to be excised. Often normal anatomy is distorted, and the humeral head can be underneath the conjoined tendon. Clearly identifying

the subscapularis tendon is important for making a tenotomy in the desired location, which we do 1 cm from its insertion to allow later repair. Identification of the biceps tendon should aid in locating the subscapularis and we always tenotomize the biceps tendon, with or without suture tenodesis. The joint is now exposed and implantation of a reverse shoulder arthroplasty is performed using standard technique, except when glenoid bone grafting is required, which is described below.

GLENOID BONE GRAFTING

Since chronic anterior shoulder dislocations in older patients often result in anterior glenoid erosion, assessing the glenoid is a top priority. This can be done preoperatively with x-ray and preferably a CT scan (Fig. 13-7). If glenoid bone grafting is a possibility, the contralateral iliac crest should be prepped out for harvesting. Alternatively the humeral head can be a local source for autograft bone harvest, but often the bone has become too osteoporotic from its chronic disuse to permit usage in these situations. Intraoperatively, if no native glenoid can be seen under the anterior base plate screw hole, anterior glenoid reconstruction with iliac crest bone is required. A tricortical segment of iliac crest bone graft is harvested and shaped with a small oscillating saw to fill the glenoid defect. The bone graft is positioned anteriorly and fixed with two or three guide pins for 4-mm cannulated screws. Make sure that the pins are placed so that they will not interfere with the post of the glenoid base plate. Partially threaded 4-mm cannulated screws with washers are inserted after overdrilling the guide pins. After restoration of the glenoid bone stock with the bone graft, the glenoid is prepared as usual and the glenoid component is inserted (Fig. 13-8).

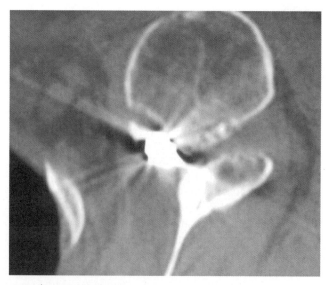

▲ **FIGURE 13-7:** CT scan of the same shoulder as the previous x-ray which demonstrates significant anterior glenoid bone loss.

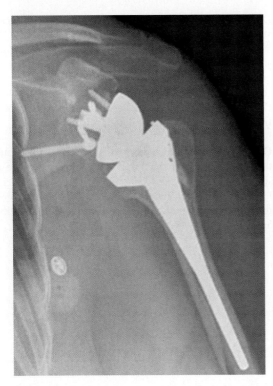

▲ **FIGURE 13-8:** Postoperative radiograph of the same shoulder after iliac crest reconstruction of the glenoid and reverse shoulder arthroplasty.

When glenoid reconstruction with iliac crest bone graft is necessary, it is desirable to have a portion of the central post of the base plate placed in native glenoid bone. Some companies manufacture base plates with a longer central post to address this problem. If the central post cannot be placed within the native glenoid bone or if the glenoid component does not seem securely fixed, staged arthroplasty should be performed. In staged arthroplasty, the glenoid component is inserted, and the humerus, after the head has been reamed for the humeral component, is left without a humeral implant for 6 months to allow the glenoid bone graft to consolidate without being subjected to normal loads and stresses. Although function will be limited, after the initial immobilization period the patient is allowed to use the arm as tolerated. After 6 months, the second stage is completed by inserting the humeral component.

REHABILITATION

All patients are instructed in hand, wrist, and elbow mobility exercises on postoperative day one. For the first 3 weeks, the patient is protected in a shoulder sling immobilizer and no shoulder motion is allowed during this time. At 3 weeks passive and active motions are started. We prefer an aquatic physical therapy protocol if a pool is available (12). We do not advise a strengthening program and allow them to regain strength through normal activities. By 3 months, the patients should be rehabilitating on their own and are released without restrictions at 6 months. The only restriction we have is no contact sports, which rarely is an issue in this subset of older patients.

PEARLS AND PITFALLS

1. Always obtain appropriate preoperative imaging. A CT scan is most helpful to assess bone loss for both the humerus and the glenoid. MRI is most helpful in assessing the rotator cuff, but a CT arthrogram may be sufficient to allow evaluation of the rotator cuff.
2. Use the preoperative imaging studies to establish a surgical plan. The surgeon should be fairly certain of which procedure is to be performed preoperatively.
3. Heroic efforts at closed reduction should be avoided. Closed reduction is rarely successful in dealing with chronic shoulder dislocations and may actually cause more damage such as fracture.
4. Always be prepared to perform a generous release of soft tissue contractures. These long-standing dislocations usually have a large amount of scar tissue present that must be addressed at the time of surgery.
5. Have a plan for dealing with bone loss. The patient must be informed about the possible necessity of using an autogenous iliac crest bone graft and the harvest site on the contralateral hip should be prepped out in advance.
6. Older patients with chronic dislocations usually have complete glenohumeral chondrolysis. The articular surfaces in older patients do not tolerate prolonged dislocation. It is difficult to evaluate the articular surfaces preoperatively because the joint space cannot be assessed, as the articular surfaces are not opposed. Always be prepared to perform an arthroplasty in these cases.

References

1. Hejna WF, Fossier CH, Goldstein TB, et al. Ancient anterior dislocation of the shoulder. *J Bone Joint Surg Am.* 1969;51:1030–1031.
2. Alcid JG, Powell SE, Tibone JE. Revision anterior capsular shoulder stabilization using hamstring tendon autograft and tibialis tendon allograft reinforcement: Minimum two-year follow-up. *J Shoulder Elbow Surg.* 2007;16(3):268–272.
3. Dewing CB, Horan MP, Millett PJ. Two-year outcomes of open shoulder anterior capsular reconstruction for instability from severe capsular deficiency. *Arthroscopy.* 2012;28(1):43–51.
4. Iannotti JP, Antoniou J, Williams GR, et al. Iliotibial band reconstruction for treatment of glenohumeral

instability associated with irreparable capsular deficiency. *J Shoulder Elbow Surg.* 2002;11(6):618–623.

5. Moeckel BH, Altchek DW, Warren RF, et al. Instability of the shoulder after arthroplasty. *J Bone Joint Surg Am.* 1993;75(4):492–497.

6. Lazarus M, Harzman D. Open repairs for anterior instability. In: Warner J, Iannotti J, Gerber C, eds. *Complex and Revision Problems in Shoulder Surgery.* Philadelphia, PA: Lippincott Raven, 1997:129–139.

7. Sahajpal DT, Zuckerman JD. Chronic glenohumeral dislocation. *J Am Acad Orthop Surg.* 2008;16(7): 385–398.

8. Griggs SM, Holloway B, Williams GR. Treatment of locked anterior and posterior dislocations of the shoulder. In: Iannotti JP, Williams GR, eds. *Disorders of the Shoulder: Diagnosis and Management.* Philadelphia, PA: Lippincott Williams & Wilkins; 1999:335–359.

9. Matsoukis J, Tabib W, Guiffault P, et al. Primary unconstrained shoulder arthroplasty in patients with a fixed anterior glenohumeral dislocation: Results of a multicenter study. *J Bone Joint Surg Am.* 2006;88(3):547–552.

10. Gartsman GM, Edwards TB. Results and complications. In: *Shoulder Arthroplasty.* Philadelphia, PA: Saunders Elsevier; 2008:305–321.

11. Oyston JK. Unreduced posterior dislocation of the shoulder treated by open reduction and transposition of the subscapularis tendon. *J Bone Joint Surg Br.* 1964;46:256–259.

12. Liotard JP, Edwards TB, Padey A, et al. Hydrotherapy rehabilitation after shoulder surgery. *Tech Shoulder Elbow Surg.* 2003;4:44–49.

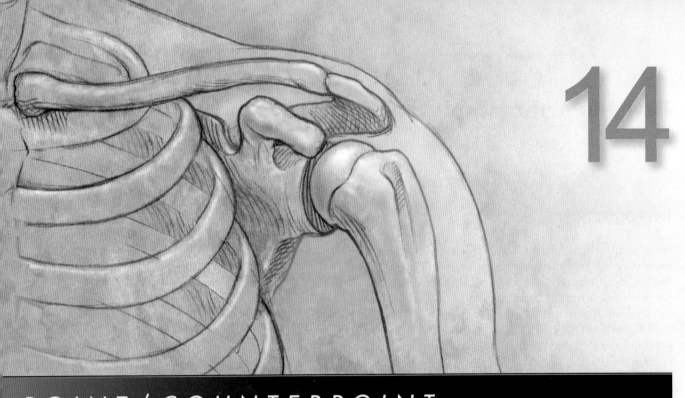

RECURRENT INSTABILITY AFTER ARTHROSCOPIC STABILIZATION

*T*he treatment of recurrent instability really depends on the indication for revision. Previous open surgery is not a contraindication to revision arthroscopic stabilization; however, a thorough, preoperative patient workup needs to be completed to ascertain whether or not the patient is an appropriate candidate. The following chapters will discuss the methods used to determine which revision stabilization technique is most appropriate for a given patient. Surgical pearls will be highlighted to achieve the best outcomes in these difficult cases.

Revision Arthroscopic Stabilization

Albert O. Gee / Asheesh Bedi /
Answorth A. Allen

INTRODUCTION

Arthroscopic shoulder stabilization for anterior shoulder instability has become more common recently as techniques, instrumentation, and implants have improved. Despite these advances, recurrence after surgical fixation ranges from 4% to 18% (1–8). When revision surgery is indicated, whether to perform another arthroscopic procedure or to convert to an open procedure remains a controversial and difficult decision.

There are few randomized prospective studies that advocate an arthroscopic approach for revision shoulder stabilization. In this chapter, we will present our rationale for the arthroscopic approach for revision anterior stabilization.

BENEFITS OF ARTHROSCOPIC SHOULDER STABILIZATION

The benefits of arthroscopic treatment of shoulder instability include less surgical morbidity, improved visualization, and the ability to address concomitant intra-articular pathology. Most importantly, the arthroscopic approach limits the violation of the normal intra-articular structures such as the subscapularis tendon.

Advances in instrumentation and innovative surgical techniques have seen arthroscopy become the mainstay for the treatment of intra-articular shoulder pathology. Several studies comparing arthroscopic repair of Bankart and anterior instability with the more conventional open approach have shown similar outcomes in terms of patient satisfaction, function, and recurrence rates (4,7).

CAUSES OF FAILURE AFTER INITIAL ARTHROSCOPIC REPAIR

It is imperative to understand the cause of failure for the index procedure before prescribing any treatment or remedy. This can be accomplished by identifying factors that led to initial repair failure and whether these factors can be addressed with an arthroscopic approach. This crucial step in patient selection will determine the likelihood of success after arthroscopic revision.

IDENTIFYING FACTORS FOR FAILURE OF PREVIOUS SURGERY

Evaluation should begin with a comprehensive history and physical examination. In addition, the clinician must get an understanding of the patient's expectations for shoulder function, taking into account factors such as age, hand dominance, activity level, comorbid conditions, and desired return to sports and recreational levels.

Most important, this evaluation should be aimed at identifying the mechanism of failure of the index procedure. If the etiology of failure is not recognized and corrected at the revision surgery, then the patient is at risk for subsequent poor outcomes and potential recurrence of symptomatic instability.

We classify failure mechanisms into three categories which are centered about the previous surgery.

a. Preoperative etiologies
b. Intraoperative causes
c. Postoperative failures

Preoperative Etiologies

One of the major issues in failure of the index arthroscopic stabilization is poor patient selection. Factors such as multidirectional instability (MDI) or global ligament laxity owing to collagen abnormality such as the spectrum of Ehlers–Danlos disease can lead to early failure after arthroscopic treatment. Previous studies involving these patients have shown that they have a higher failure rate after arthroscopic Bankart repair compared to open stabilization (2,9–17). The surgeon should seek this out by asking about developmental and family history as it relates to generalized ligamentous laxity and look for signs on examination such as hyperextension at the elbow, thumb-to-forearm test, hands flat on the floor test, and sulcus sign at the shoulder. If excess capsule laxity is not addressed at the index procedure, then initial containment of the humeral head in the glenoid socket will not be achieved and the procedure is bound to fail.

Under appreciation of bone loss at the time of initial anterior stabilization is another common etiology of arthroscopic failure. This applies to defects involving the glenoid bone, humeral head bone, or a combination of both.

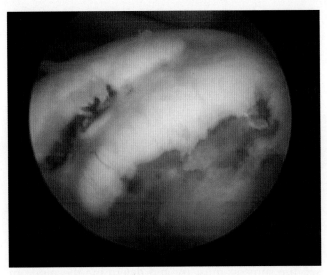

▲ **FIGURE 14-1:** Large Hill–Sachs lesion visualized at the time of arthroscopy.

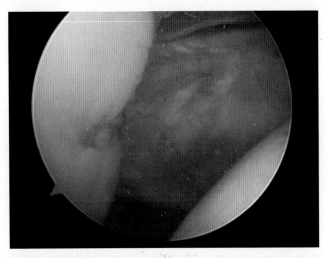

▲ **FIGURE 14-2:** An arthroscopic image of an anterior labrum periosteal sleeve avulsion (ALPSA) lesion. The normal anterior-inferior labrum is not visualized adjacent to the glenoid articular surface when viewing from the posterior portal as the labrum has been stripped and healed medially on the glenoid neck.

Glenoid bone loss after shoulder dislocation has been studied extensively and shown to be a factor in failed instability surgery (2,18–21). The inverted pear glenoid morphology from anterior-inferior glenoid bone loss was first described by Burkhart (22,23), and has been shown to be associated with an increased arthroscopic failure rate. Cadaveric studies of glenoid bone loss have also demonstrated that 20% to 30% loss of the anterior–posterior diameter of the inferior glenoid approaches the limit at which a bone reconstituting procedure may be required to re-establish the anatomic integrity of the glenoid (24,25).

Bone loss on the humeral head (engaging Hill–Sachs lesions) is another potential factor in failed arthroscopic repair (Fig. 14-1). Engaging Hill–Sachs lesions decrease the stable arc of motion of the humerus on the glenoid and several studies have demonstrated that patients with large Hill–Sachs lesions have a lower recurrence rate when stabilization surgery is performed open (2,19,22). Again, these findings are important and should be taken into consideration when planning revision surgery.

Intraoperative Causes

This refers to problems with surgical technique at the time of the index arthroscopic anterior stabilization. These are another class of factors which have been shown to be associated with recurrence of instability. The goal of any anterior stabilization procedure is to repair the torn labrum to its anatomic location and in so doing return the capsule and anterior inferior glenohumeral ligament (IGHL) complex to its normal tension and length profile. In essence, the goal is containment of the humeral head within the glenoid socket. Any issues

in achieving this goal will put the repaired shoulder at increased risk for recurrent instability.

In order to achieve appropriate reduction and repair of the capsulolabral structures, adequate mobilization of the Bankart lesion is paramount. Often times after the dislocation event, the labrum will scar down to the periosteum of the medial neck of the glenoid in what has become well established as an anterior labrum periosteal sleeve avulsion (ALPSA) lesion (Fig. 14-2). This lesion must be adequately released off the medial neck of the glenoid so that it can be restored to its proper position on the anterior articular margin. When this is not accomplished, there is an increase in potential failure rate as the IGHL will be improperly tensioned, the bumper effect of the anterior labrum will be lacking and loss of concavity compression of a concentric reduction of the humeral head on the center of the glenoid is not achieved (2).

Another intraoperative factor is inadequate tissue tensioning. Often the labrum and the capsular tissue are adequately elevated from the medial glenoid neck but are not appropriately tensioned. Plastic deformation of the capsuloligamentous complex at the time of injury will require that the ligament complex be retensioned at the time of the index repair. In order to achieve this, the tissue must be advanced from inferior to superior up the face of the glenoid. Failure to do so may lead to healing in a lengthened position and will not provide the adequate restraint to humeral head translation.

Hardware failure or poor anchor placement are additional causes of failed repair. In order to reduce the labrum and retension the anterior inferior capsuloligamentous complex, arthroscopic anchors must be able to maintain strength and fixation of the tissue until biologic healing occurs. Placement of anchors requires accurate positioning in the medial–lateral plane as well as superior–inferior (often described as time along the clockface of the circular glenoid). Anchors should be placed just off the articular face of the glenoid in order to bring the labrum into apposition with the articular surface and restore its mechanical bumper effect. Anchor placement must also be inferior enough to capture the injured inferior ligamentous structures. Visualization and access down to the 6-o'clock position inferiorly is necessary to achieve appropriate repair.

Failure to recognize bone loss at the time of surgery is another intraoperative factor that affects success after initial arthroscopic repair. Advanced imaging modalities (computed tomography [CT] and magnetic resonance imaging [MRI]) allow the surgeon to evaluate for this possibility prior to surgery, but this should be reassessed intraoperatively. The inverted pear glenoid viewed from the anterior-superior portal is a sign of significant anterior-inferior bone loss. Another intraoperative method to evaluate glenoid bone deficiency is to measure from the bare area as this represents the midpoint of the circle that encompasses the lower most circular portion of the glenoid. This being the case, the anterior and posterior radii should normally equal one another.

Moreover, failure to recognize associated intra-articular injury can be a mechanism for failure. This includes injury to the rotator cuff that may compromise the dynamic concavity-compression stability, tears of the capsule elsewhere in the shoulder including posterior-inferior labral tears and superior labral tears. Humeral avulsion of the glenohumeral ligament (HAGL) lesions should also be sought out. This injury can often be subtle on preoperative MRI and has been documented as a potential cause of recurrent instability (26,27). Occasionally, they can occur concomitantly with a Bankart tear and if the HAGL lesion is not addressed the repair will usually fail (28,29).

Postoperative Failures

Postoperative failures are often overlooked but can be associated with initial arthroscopic stabilization failure. The surgeon must elicit a good history of the rehabilitation protocol after the initial arthroscopic repair and whether the patient was compliant with immobilization and physical therapy.

Most surgeons will recommend immobilization for 4 to 6 weeks after initial arthroscopic stabilization to ensure healing of the labrum. Initiating postoperative motion too early after surgery is a factor associated with failure of arthroscopic repair (2,3). Conversely, prolonged immobilization can lead to loss of motion and poor patient outcomes as well. Like all sound postoperative rehabilitation programs, there must be a balance between protection of surgical repair to allow healing and the prevention of stiffness and loss of motion.

Despite a technically proficient repair in the appropriately selected patient with appropriate rehabilitation and healing after surgery, recurrence of instability can occur in the setting of new traumatic injury. Especially in patients who are involved in high-risk activities such as contact sports (American football, rugby, wrestling, etc.) this may be an unavoidable consequence.

APPROACH TO THE PATIENT WITH FAILED ARTHROSCOPIC REPAIR

The evaluation of the patient with a failed arthroscopic stabilization is a systematic process starting with history and thorough physical examination. From the outset, the surgeon must try and determine the mode of failure. History should attempt to elicit the timeline of events—did the patient progress through a full rehabilitation process and return to full activities prior to the recurrence of instability? Was this instigated by a new traumatic injury? When does the patient feel instability or apprehension? How many and/or how often do subluxations or dislocations occur? During the history, the surgeon is also assessing the patient's expectations for return of normal shoulder function, the desired level of return to activities or sports participation.

A complete shoulder examination should be performed. This begins with inspection, evaluating previous surgical scars, muscle atrophy and asymmetry between the two shoulders. Next, palpation of the involved shoulder is performed looking for reproducible pain especially over the acromioclavicular joint and the biceps tendon in the intertubercular groove of the humerus. Comparison of shoulder range of motion, strength testing, degree of instability, and the pattern of instability between the injured side and the uninvolved shoulder should be crucial in attempting to identify an etiology. Special attention is paid to in order to rule out MDI patterns, looking for positive sulcus sign, posterior instability and evidence of generalized ligamentous laxity, and hypermobility at other joints. Apprehension and relocation tests are performed. Load and shift examination should evaluate direction of instability as on occasion patients may have new onset unidirectional posterior instability after previous anterior stabilization surgery.

Initial imaging studies include a complete orthogonal shoulder series including Axillary and Stryker-Notch views. Plain radiographs can give the surgeon an initial overview of the shoulder, diagnose arthritis and evaluate for potential bone loss patterns. In addition, if previous surgical fixation involved radio-opaque anchors, their location can be ascertained from these images.

MRI can be helpful in the evaluation of a failed repair. An MR arthrogram may increase the sensitivity of the study in visualizing a new tear and evaluating the quality of the residual labral tissue (30). From the x-ray and MRI evaluation, if there is any concern for glenoid or humeral bone loss, a CT scan can be considered to better evaluate this possibility and calculate the extent of the bone deficits.

Recently CT scans which include three-dimensional reconstructions of the humerus and the glenoid have the ability to provide more detailed understanding of bone and bone loss. These may be helpful especially in the revision setting and for preoperative planning.

Again, patient selection is paramount when considering arthroscopic revision repair. The surgeon must go through the thought-process outlined above and determine which factors played the most significant role in the failure of the initial repair. If the failure is believed to be due to preoperative factors such as bone loss, MDI or generalized ligamentous laxity, then arthroscopic revision surgery may be contraindicated for revision stabilization. If intraoperative factors involving poor surgical technique are believed to be the etiology of failure, arthroscopic revision may be a reasonable option.

Despite the etiology of failure, the anterior capsulolabral tissue will no longer be in its virgin state and will undoubtedly be of lesser quality than at the time of the index procedure. This should be carefully considered when deciding to perform arthroscopic versus open revision.

SURGICAL TECHNIQUE

Once the decision is made to perform an arthroscopic revision surgery, the risks and benefits as well as rehabilitation process and duration are discussed with the patient. Once in the operating room, we use a combination of interscalene nerve blockade in addition to general anesthesia as this allows for optimal soft tissue relaxation and glenohumeral joint distraction during surgery.

After the induction of anesthesia, we prefer the beach chair position with a sterile arm-positioning device attached to the operating table. Others prefer the lateral decubitus position—either position is fine and is up to the individual surgeon's preference and comfort level.

A thorough examination under anesthesia is performed. From the history and physical examination performed preoperatively the direction of instability has already been established. However, muscle guarding in the awake patient can make instability testing difficult and subtle instability patterns may be missed in the office. Evaluation of laxity in all directions should be performed and compared with the contralateral shoulder.

Once the arm is prepped and draped, previous portal incisions are marked out and used if they are appropriately located. If this is not the case, then we make separate portal incisions in the appropriate location in order to achieve adequate visualization and allow access for instrumentation.

Arthroscopy is initiated using a standard posterior viewing portal. We make two anterior portals using a spinal needle to localize position and trajectory. One portal is made just above the subscapularis tendon (anterior-inferior portal) in the rotator interval and the second is made just inferior to the anterior edge of the supraspinatus tendon superior and far lateral in the rotator interval (anterior-superior portal). The anterior-inferior portal we use as a working portal and place a large 8-mm cannula while the anterior-superior portal requires a smaller 5-mm cannula which will accept the arthroscope and graspers as needed for visualization and suture passage. We attempt to maximize the distance between these two portals to avoid cannula crowding during later instrumentation and visualization.

A thorough diagnostic arthroscopy is performed which includes evaluation of the cartilage surfaces, superior labrum and biceps anchor, posterior labrum, and the integrity of the rotator cuff. The capsular attachment on the humeral side must be thoroughly evaluated so as not to miss a HAGL lesion.

While viewing from the standard posterior portal, the previous repair is inspected for tissue quality, previous anchor placement, and potential glenoid bone loss. If there is a concern for glenoid bone loss anteriorly, we move the arthroscope to look from the anterior-superior portal for the "inverted pear" glenoid morphology. Another option is to use a 70-degree arthroscope, which can provide a panoramic view of the anterior-medial aspect of the glenoid around the front of the glenoid even from the posterior portal.

If significant glenoid bone loss is identified, we perform arthroscopic measurement of the degree of bone loss by using the bare area as the center point of the glenoid and comparing the posterior and anterior radii using an arthroscopic probe. If glenoid bone loss is greater than 25% then we will abandon arthroscopic revision and convert to an open stabilization with the consideration of a bone restoration procedure.

Once the decision is made to proceed with an arthroscopic revision, we begin by performing a comprehensive mobilization of the labrum and the capsular tissue. Time must be spent achieving full mobilization of the torn labrum and the capsule off the anterior glenoid and free it from the most inferior point at the 6-o'clock position up superiorly along the glenoid. This is performed using an arthroscopic periosteal elevator from the anterior-inferior working portal (Fig. 14-3). Sufficient mobilization has occurred when the subscapularis muscle belly can be easily visualized underlying the elevated labrum and the capsule (Fig. 14-4). This can be done through both of the anterior portals while viewing from the posterior portal. Once again we will often utilize a 70-degree arthroscope for visualization during this portion of the procedure. If access to a 70-degree objective is not an option, the arthroscope is placed into

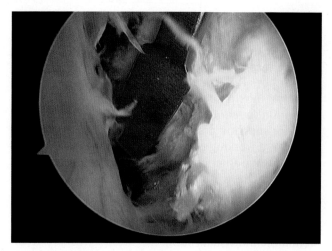

▲ **FIGURE 14-3:** Periosteal elevator being used to fully mobilize the labrum and the capsule off the glenoid neck in preparation for revision repair.

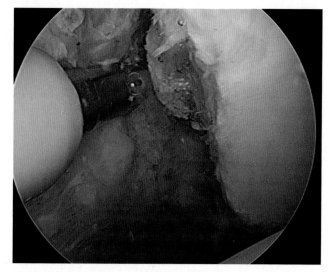

▲ **FIGURE 14-5:** Preparation of the glenoid to a bleeding bone bed using an arthroscopic burr prior to repair.

the anterior-superior cannula to gain visualization of the entire anterior aspect of the glenoid while working from the anterior-inferior cannula.

Next we use an arthroscopic bone-cutting shaver to prepare the entire glenoid articular margin from inferior to superior to a bleeding bone bed for labral repair (Fig. 14-5). Suture anchors are then placed juxta-articular on the glenoid starting with the most inferior anchor (Fig. 14-6). For the first suture anchor, we attempt to place it just superior to the 6-o'clock position. We use small glenoid suture anchors and space the anchors approximately 2 mm apart as we move superiorly up the glenoid. An angled arthroscopic suture-passing device is used to pass a shuttle suture through the mobilized Bankart lesion, with the first pass occurring virtually at the 6-o'clock position such that this tissue can be advanced up the face of

the glenoid superiorly. The capsulolabral complex should be advanced from inferior to superior with each anchor in order to retension the IGHL and diminish the capsular volume anteriorly. We use a minimum of three anchors in the revision setting and tie our knots with our post limb more medial such that the knot sits off the articular face of the glenoid to avoid any abrasion between the glenoid and the humeral head with range of motion.

Simple suture configuration can be used to tie arthroscopic knots over a medial post to keep the knots off the glenoid surface (Fig. 14-7). Another option for repair is to utilize a double-row anchor configuration. In this method, suture anchors are placed more medially on the neck of the glenoid than usual and then passed through the capsule and the labrum as in the standard repair technique. These sutures are then secured using a second row

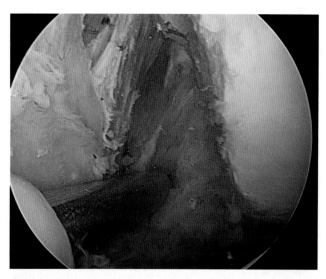

▲ **FIGURE 14-4:** Visualization of the subscapularis muscle fibers (identified by the probe) signifying complete mobilization of the labrum and the capsule off the neck of the glenoid.

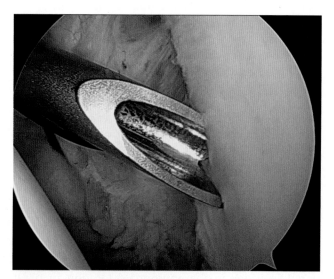

▲ **FIGURE 14-6:** Drill sleeve in place at the edge of the articular surface of the glenoid demonstrating appropriate position for drilling and placement of suture anchors.

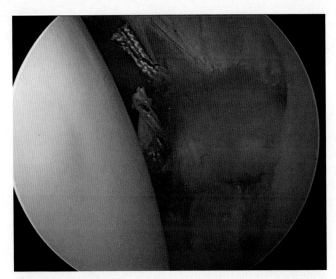

▲ **FIGURE 14-7:** Simple suture configuration for anterior stabilization demonstrating that the knots are tied medially off of the glenoid. The bumper effect of the labrum has been successfully recreated.

of knotless anchors which are impacted into the glenoid on the articular margin—creating a "double-row" repair.

OUTCOMES

Multiple studies have shown reasonable outcomes after arthroscopic revision stabilization (31–35). These studies have consistently demonstrated that appropriate patient selection is the key to successful arthroscopic revision. Although all studies are relatively small case series, the authors have shown success after minimum 2-year follow-up in patient satisfaction scores and recurrence rates.

Most recently, Arce et al. (31) reported on a retrospective review of 16 patients who underwent revision arthroscopic anterior shoulder stabilization. They excluded patients with significant glenoid or humeral head bone loss and also excluded patients who were attempting to return to contact sports. Final surgical approach was determined after their examination under anesthesia. In patients with 3+ laxity anterior-inferior and a Hill–Sachs lesion, they converted to an open stabilization. Otherwise, a diagnostic arthroscopy was performed and if they noted good quality capsulolabral tissue, they went ahead and performed the repair arthroscopically using suture anchors. They reported improvement in patient-reported outcome scores and reported a recurrence in 3 of 16 patients at an average follow-up of 31 months (18.8% recurrence rate).

Bartl et al. (32) in a recent case series evaluated 56 patients that underwent arthroscopic revision anterior stabilization after a previous open or arthroscopic repair. They excluded patients with findings consistent with MDI at the time of surgery and any case of glenoid bone loss greater than 20% or an engaging Hill–Sachs

lesion. Repairs were performed with a minimum of three suture anchors and their surgical technique included a separate 5:30 clock portal to ensure inferior anchor placement on the glenoid. They reported an 11% recurrent instability rate in their series with significant improvement in Rowe, Constant, and SST scores after surgery.

Another recent study by Barnes et al. (33) looked at arthroscopic revision anterior stabilizations after failed surgery performed either open or arthroscopically. In a series of 18 patients who underwent arthroscopic revision using suture anchors and found only one recurrence in this group (94% success rate). At an average follow-up of 38 months, the average Rowe score was 84 and 13 of the 18 patients reported good-to-excellent outcomes by this scale.

Krueger et al. (34) recently published a case-control study comparing revision arthroscopic stabilization with primary arthroscopic repair. They evaluated 20 patients who had an arthroscopic revision and compared them to a matched cohort of patients who underwent primary arthroscopic stabilization. Patients were matched by age, gender, and hand dominance. They reported two recurrent cases of instability in the revision group compared to no failures in the primary group. The investigators noted no significant difference between primary and revision groups on the Rowe Scale, but found significantly poorer outcomes using the Walch-Duplay, Melbourne Instability, the Western Ontario Shoulder Instability Score, and Subjective Shoulder Value scoring systems.

Neri et al. (35) showed in a small series of 12 patients that underwent arthroscopic revision stabilization after a previously failed open or arthroscopic surgery that there 73% of patients reported good-to-excellent results by Rowe and UCLA scores. They did, however, had a rate of 27% recurrence of instability. They excluded patients with significant bone loss and all patients had unidirectional instability.

CONCLUSION

Successful anterior stabilization of the shoulder can be achieved arthroscopically after failure of an initial attempt at stabilization if the correct patient is selected. In the revision setting, the surgeon must attempt to identify mechanisms of failure for the index procedure. In our clinical approach to these patients, we find it helpful to classify the failure mechanisms into three categories: Preoperative, Intraoperative, and Postoperative factors. We cannot overemphasize the importance of appropriate patient selection based on a thorough evaluation that identifies why the index procedure failed. Being systematic allows the surgeon to identify the patient with the appropriate patho-anatomy that can be corrected arthroscopically. If the ideal patient is selected excellent results can be expected after revision arthroscopic stabilization.

Revision with Open Stabilization

Travis G. Maak / Robert T. Burks

CHAPTER OVERVIEW

Albert Einstein has stated, "The definition of insanity is doing the same thing over and over again and expecting a different result." At times one may be able to apply this to arthroscopic anterior shoulder stabilization that has failed. In some circumstances, the treating surgeon may attribute the failure to previous suboptimal surgery including insufficient suture anchors, poor capsulolabral reduction, inadequate postoperative rehabilitation, among others, and proceed with revision arthroscopic surgery. However, the truth may lie in the fact that the indications for arthroscopic surgery may be flawed, and the patient would be more effectively treated with open stabilization. Richard Hawkins has previously stated, "If one is confronted with failure, the next time do something different." This statement may be a sage advice regarding revision of a failed arthroscopic stabilization.

Open treatment of failed anterior shoulder instability has been the gold standard for many decades with good functional results. The advent of arthroscopic surgery resulted in attempts at treating failed anterior shoulder instability, often with resultant increased rates of recurrent instability, as compared to open techniques (36–40). For this reason, many authors suggested open treatment for failed anterior shoulder instability. However, recent data have suggested that newer arthroscopic techniques and implants may produce recurrence rates that are comparable with open surgery with the added potential benefits of arthroscopic surgery including smaller incisions and reduced postoperative pain (41–44). Unfortunately, however, studies continue to document unacceptably high rates of recurrence with arthroscopic techniques.

This chapter will attempt to analyze the available published data in combination with the current authors' experience in an attempt to produce a management algorithm aimed at one fundamental goal: To maximize postoperative shoulder function and motion and minimize the risk of recurrent instability. Many authors and proponents of arthroscopic stabilization tout the many benefits of this approach including: Minimally invasive surgery with small incisions, increased postoperative range of motion without loss of external rotation, and rapid postoperative recovery. While these benefits may have some merit, they should not overshadow the underlying goal of stabilization, which is to prevent recurrent instability.

BIOMECHANICS

Glenohumeral biomechanics can be significantly altered by traumatic or atraumatic injury, with the specifics of the injury frequently dictating the subsequent biomechanical dysfunction. Anterior instability frequently occurs following failure of the anterior labrum due to a Bankart lesion, intrasubstance capsular tearing, and/or possible HAGL. An engaging Hill–Sachs lesion and anterior glenoid bone loss may also contribute to subsequent instability. Notably, an isolated Bankart lesion is not sufficient to produce recurrent instability according to cadaveric studies. Capsular deformation or tearing of some degree is a necessary component of biomechanical instability. Glenoid- and humeral-based bone loss is also a key contributor to increased instability (24,39,45). Careful evaluation and management of all components of this injury including capsular laxity is crucial to minimize recurrent instability (46).

NATURAL HISTORY

The recurrence rate following an anterior shoulder instability episode is largely proportional to activity level and inversely proportional to age at the time of initial dislocation. Hovelius et al. (47) evaluated 245 patients treated nonoperatively with sling immobilization and documented no recurrent dislocation in 52% of the patients; however, a 70% recurrence rate was documented in the subset of patients less than 23 years of age. Burkhead et al. (48) documented 80% good-to-excellent results following nonoperative treatment of atraumatic shoulder subluxations, as compared to 16% for traumatic subluxations. These data were further substantiated in a prospective study that documented a 90% recurrence rate following nonoperative treatment of young athletes less than 24 years old with first-time dislocations (49). Arciero et al. (50) evaluated surgical outcomes following transglenoid suture repair in a West Point cadet population. This study documented 80% recurrent instability following nonoperative treatment, as compared to a 14% recurrence following surgical stabilization. These studies demonstrated the importance of patient-based factors on management outcomes.

Evaluation of the effects of age on recurrent dislocation risk also demonstrated important trends. Prior data have documented a 62% anterior instability recurrence rate following nonoperative management of patients younger than 30 years of age, as compared to a 9% recurrence rate observed for patients older than 30 years of age (47). A recent systematic review using a decision analysis model suggested arthroscopic stabilization should be utilized for primary anterior glenohumeral dislocation in most circumstances; however, age and activity level were not subdivided in this review (51).

"FAILED" ANTERIOR SHOULDER INSTABILITY

Specific criteria must be detailed to allow a consistent analysis and comparison of published or personal outcome data regarding failed anterior shoulder instability. Significant variability exists regarding the definition of "failure" in studies that document postoperative outcomes following open or anterior stabilization. In the current authors' opinion the physician should have a very low threshold for defining failure, as an excellent management outcome must be defined as a stable, symptom-free shoulder. Using this definition, postoperative failure includes recurrent dislocation or subluxation and persistent symptoms including pain, loss of motion, or failure to return-to-normal activities. This last criterion is particularly difficult to define as "normal activity" broadly ranges from normal daily function to elite sports participation including collision athletics. For the current analysis regarding open and arthroscopic stabilization, we define return-to-normal activities as a return to the level of activity that was present prior to the instability episode. Therefore, an inability to return to play at the previous level of participation is defined as a failure.

CAUSES OF FAILED ANTERIOR STABILIZATION

Many studies have evaluated the contributing risk factors for recurrent instability following nonoperative and operative treatments of anterior shoulder instability. Recurrent instability is the most frequently reported complication following open and arthroscopic shoulder stabilization procedures and may be secondary to a new traumatic or atraumatic event (52,53). There are many different potential causes for this instability including incorrect preoperative diagnosis, technical failure, glenoid bony deficiency, and patient-related factors. Careful, accurate preoperative diagnosis is crucial to ensure an appropriate surgical plan and should include evaluation of posterior or MDI patterns, voluntary instability, unrecognized subacromial impingement and glenohumeral osteoarthritis (54,55). Technical failures have also been associated with failed stabilizations due to subscapularis rupture, residual Bankart lesions, under corrected capsular redundancy, and

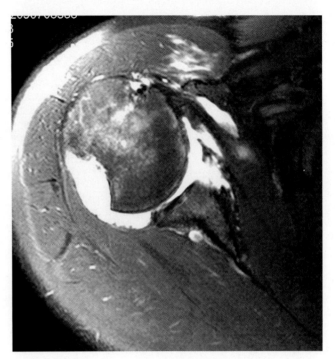

▲ **FIGURE 14-8:** Axial T2 MRI demonstrating a large Hill–Sachs lesion with concomitant anterior bony Bankart.

unrecognized rotator interval laxity or HAGL (39,56). Anterior glenoid bone deficiency or a large posterior Hill–Sachs lesion should also be adequately evaluated as unrecognized and untreated bone loss may significantly increase postoperative recurrent instability (Fig. 14-8) (22,57). Patient factors have also been shown to affect recurrence rates including young age (47,50), participation in contact or collision sports, and new, recurrent trauma (22,42,55–58). Recurrent instability following new trauma to the stabilized shoulder has been associated with improved postoperative outcomes following revision surgery (53). Nontraumatic causes for recurrent instability, however, do not share this improved result. Lastly, increased recurrent instability has also been associated with the number of prior ipsilateral shoulder surgeries (Fig. 14-9). Levine et al. (53) analyzed the outcomes following revision open stabilization and documented a 17% recurrence rate following a single prior stabilization, as compared to a 44% rate following multiple prior surgeries.

While these many diagnostic factors have been suggested as contributing to failure following anterior shoulder stabilization, of particular importance is the contribution of bone loss. Milano et al. (58) utilized CT scanning in patients with anterior instability. These authors documented identifiable bone loss in 72% of cases and 20% or greater bone loss in 8% of cases (Fig. 14-10). A preoperative 20% bone loss threshold was suggested as the crucial amount that, if left unaddressed, would lead to an increased risk for recurrent dislocation. Itoi et al. (24) have also suggested this threshold as a 21% defect. However, it is often very difficult to identify where

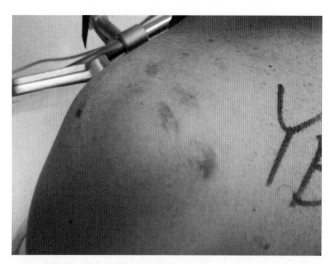

▲ **FIGURE 14-9:** Preoperative patient image of the anterior right shoulder demonstrating multiple prior arthroscopic portal scars due to multiple arthroscopic stabilization procedures. Definitive open stabilization was conducted in this patient.

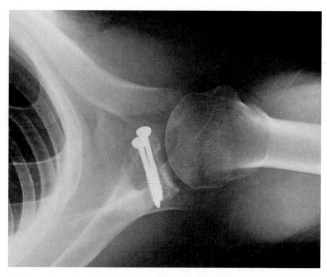

▲ **FIGURE 14-11:** Axillary plain radiograph following Latarjet procedure in a patient with significant anterior glenoid osseous deficiency.

the specific threshold may exist for a single patient—do we draw the line at 19%, 20%, or 21%? Should concomitant injuries, patient-specific factors or surgeon preference contribute to this decision? Pessimistically, it may be possible in some circumstances that a busy orthopedic surgeon may potentially convince him or herself that the degree of bone loss and tissue laxity may be slightly less than the "threshold" for open stabilization if he or she is more comfortable with arthroscopic surgery. This tempta-

tion is significant and may place unacceptable bias toward arthroscopic stabilization in the setting of necessary open surgery such as an open capsulorrhaphy, Bristow, or Latarjet (Fig. 14-11). Unfortunately, in these circumstances, the outcome of recurrence and failure is predetermined.

OPEN VERSUS ARTHROSCOPIC ANTERIOR STABILIZATION: COMPARING APPLES TO APPLES

Many of the aforementioned causes of instability may be eliminated with careful preoperative evaluation including history, physical examination, and diagnostic imaging. Other factors are more difficult or impossible to control such as patient participation in collision sports and unexpected new trauma to the operative extremity. In order to appropriately compare open and arthroscopic revision stabilization outcome studies, one must take into account the underlying cause of failure. For example, if a significant glenoid bone deficit is unrecognized and unaddressed, the open versus arthroscopic surgical approach becomes less relevant (Fig. 14-12). Moreover, surgical treatment of MDI is significantly different than treatment of traumatic unidirectional instability and thus outcomes following open treatment of MDI cannot be compared to outcomes following arthroscopic treatment of traumatic unidirectional instability. Unfortunately, many studies combine these patient populations when discussing outcome data and thus retrospective comparisons among these studies is difficult. Nevertheless, recent studies have attempted to produce more homogeneous patient populations that allow a more clearer data comparison between open and arthroscopic management.

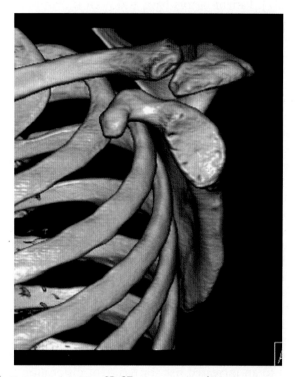

▲ **FIGURE 14-10:** 3D CT reconstruction demonstrating anterior glenoid deficiency and evidence of prior arthroscopic stabilization with bone tunnels along the anterior glenoid face.

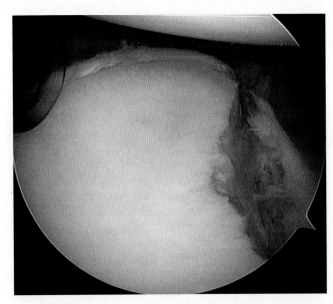

▲ FIGURE 14-12: Arthroscopic image demonstrating significant anterior glenoid osseous deficiency following a prior traumatic anterior dislocation. Definitive stabilization with a Latarjet procedure was conducted in this patient.

OPEN VERSUS ARTHROSCOPIC STABILIZATION: GETTING IT RIGHT THE FIRST TIME

The preferred method for surgical management of anterior glenohumeral instability between open and arthroscopic stabilization has been controversial from the beginning of arthroscopic shoulder surgery. Questions continue to be raised regarding which method produces the optimal postoperative outcomes, maximal range of motion, and lowest recurrence rates. Many studies have been conducted in an attempt to resolve this controversy.

Initial data suggested arthroscopic anterior stabilization was less predictable than open techniques. In 1996, Guanche et al. (59) compared open and arthroscopic stabilizations of Bankart lesions in patients with traumatic, unidirectional anterior glenohumeral instability. Patient follow-up of up to 42 months demonstrated a recurrent instability rate of 8% (1/12) in open stabilizations, as compared to 33% (5/15) in the arthroscopic group. In addition, the arthroscopic group had worse results in stability, apprehension, loss of forward flexion, and patient satisfaction. These results were further substantiated by a study by Geiger et al. (60), which documented an 83% good-to-excellent result with no recurrent instability in patients treated with an open Bankart procedure, as compared to 50% good-to-excellent results and 44% recurrent instability with arthroscopic management. Further data continued to support open stabilization, although the three- to four-fold differences in recurrence rates declined as arthroscopic techniques and instrumentation improved. In 2000, Cole et al. (16) followed 63 patients

with recurrent anterior instability treated with either open or arthroscopic stabilization. Two- to 6-year follow-up demonstrated 16% recurrence in patients treated arthroscopically, as compared to 9% treated with open stabilization. Again, the fundamental goal of stabilization is more effectively addressed with open stabilization. Recurrent instability following arthroscopic stabilization far overshadows the aforementioned secondary benefits that may be present with this minimally invasive approach.

OPEN VERSUS ARTHROSCOPIC STABILIZATION

Initial comparison of open and arthroscopic stabilization should include the evaluation of the surgical outcomes following a "best case scenario"—a patient with a primary surgical indication including isolated traumatic anterior shoulder instability with a soft tissue Bankart lesion (Fig. 14-13). A review of the literature paints a sobering reality in this regard, especially in the setting of the young population less than 20 years of age. Multiple authors have documented recurrence rates from 20% to 40% in patients under 20 years old following arthroscopic stabilization (3,5,61,62). Porcellini et al. (63) documented a two-fold recurrence following arthroscopic stabilization in patients under 22 years old. In yet another study by Mohtadi et al. (64) of ideal patients for arthroscopic stabilization, arthroscopic stabilization led to a recurrence rate of 23%, as compared to 11% following open surgery. A recent study by Netto et al. (65) evaluated 42 patients less than 40 years of age with this exact scenario in a

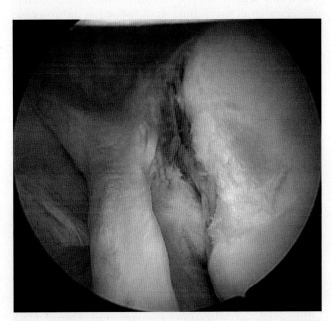

▲ FIGURE 14-13: Arthroscopic image of the anterior glenoid demonstrating full-thickness anteroinferior labral tear with minimal osseous involvement of the anterior glenoid.

randomized controlled trial with 37.5-month follow-up. This study concluded that open and arthroscopic techniques were both effective and lower functional limitations may be associated with arthroscopically treated patients as assessed by the DASH score. Careful analysis of this study, however, revealed an interesting result. According to the study by the authors, "two cases of failure were present in the arthroscopic group and none in the open technique group. These two patients reported symptoms of anterior instability with a new traumatic episode of shoulder dislocation that required additional surgical intervention, with and open technique." Thus, if shoulder stability with reduced recurrence is the principal fundamental goal of surgical management, the conclusion from the study could be that open stabilization is superior.

Nevertheless, the frequency of arthroscopic stabilization continues to increase despite the continued increased recurrent instability rates. Owens et al. (66) analyzed the practice patterns of recently trained orthopedic surgeons during the board collections period. Interestingly, 2003 to 2005 documented a 71.2% incidence of arthroscopic stabilization, as compared with 87.7% between 2006 and 2008. Given the aforementioned outcome data demonstrating the clear increased risk of recurrence following arthroscopic stabilization, one must ask the question, "Why does the incidence of arthroscopic surgery continue to increase?" The answer to this question may directly relate to surgical training, experience, and surgeon comfort. In other words, recently trained surgeons may be more comfortable with arthroscopic surgery and thus default to this treatment method—even if an open stabilization may be a better treatment option. This reality is particularly concerning when one considers the aforementioned failure rates following arthroscopic stabilization.

COLLISION AND CONTACT SPORTS: A CASE FOR OPEN SURGERY?

At this point, this chapter has detailed the benefit of open stabilization in the best case scenario. However, further evaluation of higher-risk patients including contact and collision athletes and revision stabilizations is warranted. Careful analysis of patients participating in contact or collision sports demonstrated a potential increased risk for recurrent anterior instability following operative management. This subgroup of patients primarily includes football, wrestling, rugby, hockey, and soccer. These high recurrence rates have inspired significant controversy regarding the optimal surgical management of this high-risk group, specifically open versus arthroscopic stabilization. Pagnani and Dome (14) further substantiated these data in 2008 in contact athletes with a 2% failure rate following open stabilization.

Mazzocca et al. (10) documented an 11% (2/18) recurrence following arthroscopic stabilization in contact and collision athletes younger than 20 years old. Cole et al. (16) documented a 16% recurrence rate following arthroscopic stabilization, as compared to a 9% recurrence rate following open stabilization, with all recurrences occurring in contact athletes. Again, the ultimate purpose of surgical stabilization is to limit the potential for recurrent instability.

These data prompted a direct comparison of arthroscopic and open management in this high-risk group. Rhee et al. (67) compared the results of arthroscopic versus open stabilization in young collision athletes. Forty-eight shoulders were compared with a mean patient age of 20 years old and mean follow-up of 72 months. These authors documented a total instability recurrence rate of 16.5%, with a 25% recurrence following arthroscopic stabilization and 13% following open stabilization. For this reason, these authors concluded that open stabilization might be a more reliable method for the treatment of anterior shoulder instability in collision athletes. These mean recurrence rates suggest that the specific athletic activity plays a significant role in recurrence in addition to the method of stabilization. Again one must ask the question: Why would open stabilization produce a more reliable result in a high risk, collision sports setting if arthroscopic and open techniques are otherwise equal? The answer to this question is clear and the same—despite some claims to the contrary, these two methods are not equal.

REVISION STABILIZATION

Minimizing the need for revision stabilization is of paramount importance as multiple revision stabilization procedures have been associated with an increased risk for recurrent instability (53). Careful identification of the underlying cause of failure among the aforementioned contributing factors is of paramount importance in guiding subsequent management including the decision between open and arthroscopic stabilization.

Failure due to glenoid- or humeral-based osseous deficiency is a clear indication for open surgical management. While anterior instability in the setting of significant bone loss is not the primary aim of this chapter, frequently humeral bone loss, or a Hill–Sachs lesion, exists without significant glenoid bone loss (68). In this setting, the question remains if an isolated Bankart repair—either open or arthroscopic is sufficient to produce an optimal postoperative result. In addition, will an open approach in this setting produce a more reliable outcome than an arthroscopic approach. The current authors maintain that an open approach will produce a more reliable result in any case in which factors exist that may predispose to recurrent instability, including a large Hill–Sachs lesion. The decision regarding when and how to address a potentially "engaging Hill–Sachs lesion" remains uncertain. Yamamoto et al. (69) suggested that an engaging Hill–Sachs only occurs when the lesion extends medially from an inferomedial to a superolateral position on the posterior humeral head. Treatment for this engaging lesion may include tenodesis of the infraspinatus into the humeral lesion (remplissage) or direct bone grafting of the lesion. Boileau et al. (45) recently documented 98% stability following concomitant Bankart repair and remplissage in 47 patients with recurrent instability secondary to large humeral lesions. Notably, 90% of patients returned to sports and 68% of these returned at a preinjury activity level. On the other hand, other data documented no differences between patients with recurrent instability treated with Bankart repair with or without remplissage. Notably, almost 33% of the patients in the concomitant

remplissage group experienced posterior superior shoulder pain (70). These data suggest that remplissage may be an attractive addition to decrease recurrence rates in the setting of a primary arthroscopic Bankart repair with a significant (20% to 25%) Hill–Sachs lesion. However, these results mainly pertain to primary surgery when the defect has been appreciated. These results may not universally extend to patients in the revision setting. The current authors recommend utilization of the remplissage only in the setting of a primary repair with a large Hill–Sachs lesion involving at least 20% to 25% of the posterior humeral head. In the setting of revision surgery for recurrent instability secondary to a large Hill–Sachs Lesion, the current authors recommend open surgical treatment with a Latarjet procedure. Notably, in some exceptional cases in which the Hill–Sachs lesion is particularly extreme, consideration should be given to concomitant bone grafting of the lesion.

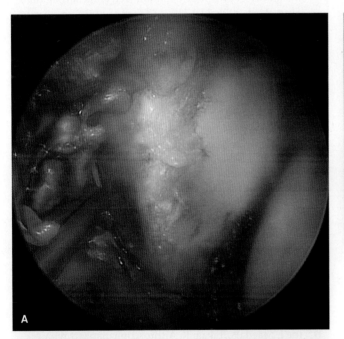

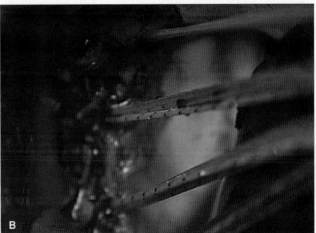

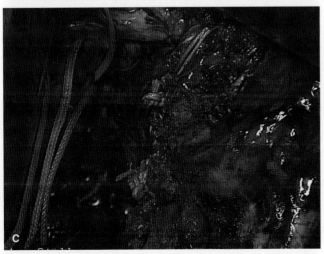

▲ **FIGURE 14-14:** **A:** Arthroscopic camera image taken through an open approach prior to revision open stabilization. Note the suture material medial to the anterior glenoid as remnants of the prior failed stabilization. Arthroscopic stabilization failure occurred despite the minimal glenoid bone loss. **B:** Anterior glenoid suture anchors placed prior to final stabilization. **C:** Completion of the open stabilization procedure with final suture security.

Failure due to new trauma or technical error, however, is more controversial. Notably, the term "technical error" should be applied very carefully as this suggests that the revision surgeon can identify a clear cause for failure due to a prior poor surgical performance including inadequately addressed pathology or incorrect diagnosis. In the current authors' opinion, this can be a slippery slope. A traumatic etiology for failure, on the other hand, represents an opportunity for either arthroscopic or open revision stabilization. Comparisons, however, are difficult due to the heterogeneity of the populations, confounding variables, and clear selection biases, and further studies are necessary to substantiate these results. In many cases, however, the authors recommend open stabilization in most revision cases and utilization of arthroscopic stabilization only in specifically selected populations (Fig. 14-14A–C). One must ask why this is the case if the two techniques are equivalent in the setting of revision stabilization (8,71,72). The answer to this question in the revision setting is identical to the high risk, collision population, and need not be repeated.

CONCLUSIONS: TO SCOPE OR NOT TO SCOPE

Recent advances and innovation in shoulder arthroscopy have broadened the application of arthroscopic anterior shoulder stabilization techniques. The increased utilization of minimally invasive surgery due to reduced morbidity and improved aesthetics have similarly improved the appeal of arthroscopy. While these aspects of arthroscopic stabilization are important and appealing, the fundamental purpose of the surgical indication—shoulder stability—should not be compromised. The aforementioned studies have documented similar outcomes following arthroscopic and open stabilization for soft tissue primary Bankart repair. However, many authors prefer open stabilization techniques for revision stabilization, stabilization in the high-risk population of collision and contact athletes, and HAGL lesions. Open management is also indicated in the setting of humeral head defects and significant glenoid osseous deficiency—the amount of this deficiency that necessitates augmentation remains controversial. In addition, many authors prefer open stabilization without bone augmentation in the setting of moderate glenoid erosion.

There is no question that multiple articles exist in the literature that can be interpreted such that arthroscopic revision of failed anterior instability in high-risk populations is a reasonable option. However, it would seem that the failure rate in many studies with technically proficient surgeons is higher than we might prefer to acknowledge. This sobering reality is particularly true for high-risk populations and young patients. The current authors believe that if selection bias is removed and the two techniques are compared in a failed prior stabilization group, the answer to this question is clear—open stabilization produces better outcomes than arthroscopic techniques.

References

1. Mauro CS, Voos JE, Hammoud S, et al. Failed anterior shoulder stabilization. *J Shoulder Elbow Surg.* 2011;20: 1340–1350.
2. Bedi A, Ryu RK. Revision arthroscopic Bankart repair. *Sports Med Arthrosc.* 2010;18:130–139.
3. Boileau P, Villalba M, Héry J, et al. Risk factors for recurrence of shoulder instability after arthroscopic Bankart repair. *J Bone Joint Surg Am.* 2006;88(8):1755–1763.
4. Bottoni C, Smith E, Berkowitz M, et al. Arthroscopic versus open shoulder stabilization for recurrent anterior instability: A prospective randomized clinical trial. *Am J Sports Med.* 2006;34:1730–1737.
5. Voos JE, Livermore RW, Feeley BT, et al. Prospective evaluation of arthroscopic bankart repairs for anterior instability. *Am J Sports Med.* 2010;38(2):302–307.
6. Carreira DS, Mazzocca AD, Oryhon J, et al. A prospective outcome evaluation of arthroscopic Bankart repairs: Minimum 2-year follow-up. *Am J Sports Med.* 2006;34:771–777.
7. Fabbriciani C, Milano G, Demontis A, et al. Arthroscopic versus open treatment of Bankart lesion of the shoulder: A prospective randomized study. *Arthroscopy.* 2004;20:456–462.
8. Kim SH, Ha KI, Cho YB, et al. Arthroscopic anterior stabilization of the shoulder: Two to six-year follow-up. *J Bone Joint Surg Am.* 2003;85-A(8):1511–1518.
9. Kirkley A, Griffin S, Richards C, et al. Prospective randomized clinical trial comparing the effectiveness of immediate arthroscopic stabilization versus immobilization and rehabilitation in first traumatic anterior dislocations of the shoulder. *Arthroscopy.* 1999;15:507–514.
10. Mazzocca AD, Brown FM Jr, Carreira DS, et al. Arthroscopic anterior shoulder stabilization of collision and contact athletes. *Am J Sports Med.* 2005;33(1):52–60.
11. Ide J, Maeda S, Takagi K. Arthroscopic Bankart repair using suture anchors in athletes: Patient selection and postoperative sports activity. *Am J Sports Med.* 2004;32: 1899–1905.
12. Habermeyer P, Gleyze P, Rickert M. Evolution of lesions of the labrum-ligament complex in posttraumatic anterior shoulder instability: A prospective study. *J Shoulder Elbow Surg.* 1999;8:66–74.
13. Hayashida K, Yoneda M, Nakagawa S, et al. Arthroscopic Bankart suture repair for traumatic anterior shoulder instability: Analysis of the causes of a recurrence. *Arthroscopy.* 1998;14:295–301.
14. Pagnani MJ, Dome DC. Surgical treatment of traumatic anterior shoulder instability in american football players. *J Bone Joint Surg Am.* 2002;84-A(5):711–715.
15. Kim SH, Ha KI. Bankart repair in traumatic anterior shoulder instability: Open versus arthroscopic technique. *Arthroscopy.* 2002;18:755–763.

16. Cole BJ, L'Insalata J, Irrgang J, et al. Comparison of arthroscopic and open anterior shoulder stabilization. A two to six-year follow-up study. *J Bone Joint Surg Am.* 2000;82-A(8):1108–1114.

17. Bacilla P, Field LD, Savoie FH 3rd. Arthroscopic Bankart repair in a high demand patient population. *Arthroscopy.* 1997;13:51–60.

18. Piasecki DP, Verma NN, Romeo AA, et al. Glenoid bone deficiency in recurrent anterior shoulder instability: Diagnosis and management. *J Am Acad Orthop Surg.* 2009;17:482–493.

19. Chen AL, Hunt SA, Hawkins RJ, et al. Management of bone loss associated with recurrent anterior glenohumeral instability. *Am J Sports Med.* 2005;33:912–925.

20. Mologne TS, Provencher MT, Menzel KA, et al. Arthroscopic stabilization in patients with an inverted pear glenoid: Results in patients with bone loss of the anterior glenoid. *Am J Sports Med.* 2007;35:1276–1283.

21. Lynch JR, Clinton JM, Dewing CB, et al. Treatment of osseous defects associated with anterior shoulder instability. *J Shoulder Elbow Surg.* 2009;18:317–328.

22. Burkhart SS, De Beer JF. Traumatic glenohumeral bone defects and their relationship to failure of arthroscopic Bankart repairs: Significance of the inverted-pear glenoid and the humeral engaging Hill-Sachs lesion. *Arthroscopy.* 2000;16(7):677–694.

23. Lo IK, Parten PM, Burkhart SS. The inverted pear glenoid: An indicator of significant glenoid bone loss. *Arthroscopy.* 2004;20:169–174.

24. Itoi E, Lee SB, Berglund LJ, et al. The effect of a glenoid defect on anteroinferior stability of the shoulder after Bankart repair: A cadaveric study. *J Bone Joint Surg Am.* 2000(1);82:35–46.

25. Greis PE, Scuderi MG, Mohr A, et al. Glenohumeral articular contact areas and pressures following labral and osseous injury to the anteroinferior quadrant of the glenoid. *J Shoulder Elbow Surg.* 2002;11:442–451.

26. Bach BR, Warren RF, Fronek J. Disruption of the lateral capsule of the shoulder. A cause of recurrent dislocation. *J Bone Joint Surg Br.* 1988;70:274–276.

27. Bokor DJ, Conboy VB, Olson C. Anterior instability of the glenohumeral joint with humeral avulsion of the glenohumeral ligament. A review of 41 cases. *J Bone Joint Surg Br.* 1999;81:93–96.

28. Warner JJ, Beim GM. Combined Bankart and HAGL lesion associated with anterior shoulder instability. *Arthroscopy.* 1997;13:749–752.

29. Field LD, Bokor DJ, Savoie FH 3rd. Humeral and glenoid detachment of the anterior inferior glenohumeral ligament: A cause of anterior shoulder instability. *J Shoulder Elbow Surg.* 1997;6:6–10.

30. Major NM, Browne J, Domzalski T, et al. Evaluation of the glenoid labrum with 3-T MRI: Is intraarticular contrast necessary? *AJR Am J Roentgenol.* 2011;196:1139–1144.

31. Arce G, Arcuri F, Ferro D, et al. Is selective arthroscopic revision beneficial for treating recurrent anterior shoulder instability? *Clin Orthop Relat Res.* 2012;470:965–971.

32. Bartl C, Schumann K, Paul J, et al. Arthroscopic capsulolabral revision repair for recurrent anterior shoulder instability. *Am J Sports Med.* 2011;39:511–518.

33. Barnes CJ, Getelman MH, Snyder SJ. Results of arthroscopic revision anterior shoulder reconstruction. *Am J Sports Med.* 2009;37:715–719.

34. Krueger D, Kraus N, Pauly S, et al. Subjective and objective outcome after revision arthroscopic stabilization for recurrent anterior instability versus initial shoulder stabilization. *Am J Sports Med.* 2011;39:71–77.

35. Neri BR, Tuckman DV, Bravman JT, et al. Arthroscopic revision of Bankart repair. *J Shoulder Elbow Surg.* 2007;16:419–424.

36. Cho NS, Yi JW, Lee BG, et al. Revision open Bankart surgery after arthroscopic repair for traumatic anterior shoulder instability. *Am J Sports Med.* 2009;37(11):2158–2164.

37. Fehringer EV, Buck DC, Puumala SE, et al. Open anterior repair without routine capsulorrhaphy for traumatic anterior shoulder instability in a community setting. *Orthopedics.* 2008;31(4):365.

38. Lai D, Ma HL, Hung SC, et al. Open Bankart repair with suture anchors for traumatic recurrent anterior shoulder instability: Comparison of results between small and large Bankart lesions. *Knee Surg Sports Traumatol Arthrosc.* 2006;14(1):82–87.

39. Tauber M, Resch H, Forstner R, et al. Reasons for failure after surgical repair of anterior shoulder instability. *J Shoulder Elbow Surg.* 2004;13(3):279–285.

40. Zabinski SJ, Callaway GH, Cohen S, et al. Revision shoulder stabilization: 2- to 10-year results. *J Shoulder Elbow Surg.* 1999;8(1):58–65.

41. Bottoni CR, Wilckens JH, DeBerardino TM, et al. A prospective, randomized evaluation of arthroscopic stabilization versus nonoperative treatment in patients with acute, traumatic, first-time shoulder dislocations. *Am J Sports Med.* 2002;30(4):576–580.

42. Millar NL, Murrell GA. The effectiveness of arthroscopic stabilisation for failed open shoulder instability surgery. *J Bone Joint Surg Br.* 2008;90(6):745–750.

43. Franceschi F, Longo UG, Ruzzini L, et al. Arthroscopic salvage of failed arthroscopic Bankart repair: A prospective study with a minimum follow-up of 4 years. *Am J Sports Med.* 2008;36(7):1330–1336.

44. Freedman KB, Smith AP, Romeo AA, et al. Open Bankart repair versus arthroscopic repair with transglenoid sutures or bioabsorbable tacks for Recurrent Anterior instability of the shoulder: A meta-analysis. *Am J Sports Med.* 2004;32(6):1520–1527.

45. Boileau P, O'Shea K, Vargas P, et al. Anatomical and functional results after arthroscopic Hill-Sachs remplissage. *J Bone Joint Surg Am.* 2012;94(7):618–626.

46. Speer KP, Deng X, Borrero S, et al. Biomechanical evaluation of a simulated Bankart lesion. *J Bone Joint Surg Am.* 1994;76(12):1819–1826.

47. Hovelius L, Augustini BG, Fredin H, et al. Primary anterior dislocation of the shoulder in young patients. A ten-year prospective study. *J Bone Joint Surg Am.* 1996;78(11):1677–1684.

48. Burkhead WZ Jr., Rockwood CA Jr. Treatment of instability of the shoulder with an exercise program. *J Bone Joint Surg Am.* 1992;74(6):890–896.

49. Taylor DC, Arciero RA. Pathologic changes associated with shoulder dislocations. Arthroscopic and physical

examination findings in first-time, traumatic anterior dislocations. *Am J Sports Med.* 1997;25(3):306–311.

50. Arciero RA, Wheeler JH, Ryan JB, et al. Arthroscopic Bankart repair versus nonoperative treatment for acute, initial anterior shoulder dislocations. *Am J Sports Med.* 1994;22(5):589–594.

51. Bishop JA, Crall TS, Kocher MS. Operative versus nonoperative treatment after primary traumatic anterior glenohumeral dislocation: Expected-value decision analysis. *J Shoulder Elbow Surg.* 2011;20(7):1087–1094.

52. Youssef JA, Carr CF, Walther CE, et al. Arthroscopic Bankart suture repair for recurrent traumatic unidirectional anterior shoulder dislocations. *Arthroscopy.* 1995;11(5):561–563.

53. Levine WN, Arroyo JS, Pollock RG, et al. Open revision stabilization surgery for recurrent anterior glenohumeral instability. *Am J Sports Med.* 2000; 28(2):156–160.

54. Hawkins RH, Hawkins RJ. Failed anterior reconstruction for shoulder instability. *J Bone Joint Surg Br.* 1985;67(5): 709–714.

55. Rowe CR, Pierce DS, Clark JG. Voluntary dislocation of the shoulder. A preliminary report on a clinical, electromyographic, and psychiatric study of twenty-six patients. *J Bone Joint Surg Am.* 1973;55(3):445–460.

56. Rowe CR, Zarins B, Ciullo JV. Recurrent anterior dislocation of the shoulder after surgical repair. Apparent causes of failure and treatment. *J Bone Joint Surg Am.* 1984;66(2):159–168.

57. Weber BG, Simpson LA, Hardegger F. Rotational humeral osteotomy for recurrent anterior dislocation of the shoulder associated with a large Hill-Sachs lesion. *J Bone Joint Surg Am.* 1984;66(9):1443–1450.

58. Milano G, Grasso A, Russo A, et al. Analysis of risk factors for glenoid bone defect in anterior shoulder instability. *Am J Sports Med.* 2011;39(9):1870–1876.

59. Guanche CA, Quick DC, Sodergren KM, et al. Arthroscopic versus open reconstruction of the shoulder in patients with isolated Bankart lesions. *Am J Sports Med.* 1996;24(2):144–148.

60. Geiger DF, Hurley JA, Tovey JA, et al. Results of arthroscopic versus open Bankart suture repair. *Clin Orthop Relat Res.* 1997(337):111–117.

61. Balg F, Boileau P. The instability severity index score. A simple pre-operative score to select patients for arthroscopic or open shoulder stabilisation. *J Bone Joint Surg Br.* 2007;89(11):1470–1477.

62. Imhoff AB, Ansah P, Tischer T, et al. Arthroscopic repair of anterior-inferior glenohumeral instability using a portal at the 5:30-o'clock position: Analysis of the effects of age, fixation method, and concomitant shoulder injury on surgical outcomes. *Am J Sports Med.* 2010;38(9):1795–1803.

63. Porcellini G, Campi F, Pegreffi F, et al. Predisposing factors for recurrent shoulder dislocation after arthroscopic treatment. *J Bone Joint Surg Am.* 2009;91(11):2537–2542.

64. Mohtadi NG, Bitar IJ, Sasyniuk TM, et al. Arthroscopic versus open repair for traumatic anterior shoulder instability: A meta-analysis. *Arthroscopy.* 2005;21(6):652–658.

65. Netto NNA, Tamaoki MJSM, Lenza MM, et al. Treatment of bankart lesions in traumatic anterior instability of the shoulder: A randomized controlled trial comparing arthroscopy and open techniques. *Arthroscopy.* 2012;28(7):900–908.

66. Owens BD, Harrast JJ, Hurwitz SR, et al. Surgical trends in Bankart repair: An analysis of data from the American Board of Orthopaedic Surgery certification examination. *Am J Sports Med.* 2011;39(9):1865–1869.

67. Rhee YG, Ha JH, Cho NS. Anterior shoulder stabilization in collision athletes: Arthroscopic versus open Bankart repair. *Am J Sports Med.* 2006;34(6):979–985.

68. Hill H. The groove defect of the humeral head. A frequently unrecognized complication of dislocations of the shoulder joint. *Radiology.* 1940;35:690–700.

69. Yamamoto N, Itoi E, Abe H, et al. Contact between the glenoid and the humeral head in abduction, external rotation, and horizontal extension: A new concept of glenoid track. *J Shoulder Elbow Surg.* 2007; 16(5):649–656.

70. Nourissat G, Kilinc AS, Werther JR, et al. A prospective, comparative, radiological, and clinical study of the influence of the "remplissage" procedure on shoulder range of motion after stabilization by arthroscopic Bankart repair. *Am J Sports Med.* 2011;39(10): 2147–2152.

71. Kim SH, Ha KI, Kim YM. Arthroscopic revision Bankart repair: A prospective outcome study. *Arthroscopy.* 2002;18(5):469–482.

72. Meehan RE, Petersen SA. Results and factors affecting outcome of revision surgery for shoulder instability. *J Shoulder Elbow Surg.* 2005;14(1):31–37.

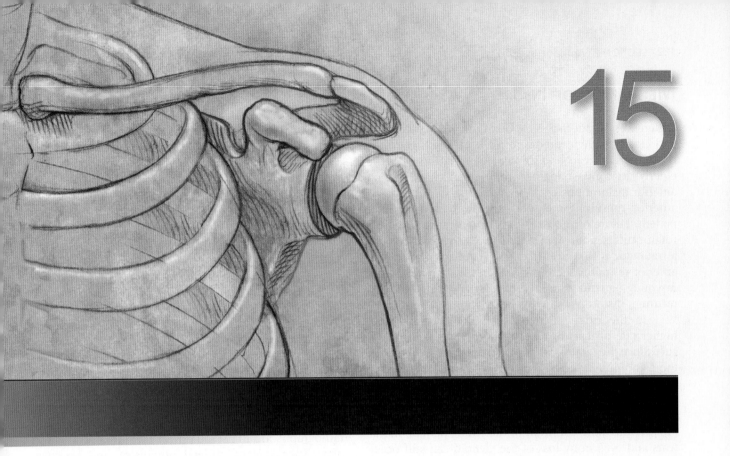

15

TREATMENT OF RECURRENT ANTERIOR INSTABILITY IN THE ELDERLY: WHEN AND WHY

Thomas O'Hagan / Steven Cohen

INTRODUCTION

Anterior instability of the shoulder is commonly associated with the young active patient. Despite reports that the incidence of dislocations is similar between the young and elderly populations, there is a relatively small amount of literature focusing on dislocations and instability specifically in those over the age of 40 (1,2). Of note, the prevalence of traumatic anterior shoulder dislocations in the elderly has increased in recent years, possibly due to greater participation in sports and increased life expectancy (3).

The mechanism of injury, rate of recurrence, and concomitant injuries are all quite different in the elderly patient. Dislocations in the elderly are often the result of low energy injuries with recurrence rates being much lower than seen in the younger patient (4–7). Yet, rotator cuff injuries and neurovascular injuries are much more prevalent in this population after a dislocation (8–11). It is important to consider these factors when evaluating and treating primary and recurrent instability in the elderly patient.

MECHANISM OF INJURY

Differences in mechanisms of injury between young and elderly patients are responsible for the higher rate of rotator cuff tears and lower rate of instability in the elderly. In contrast to the proposed mechanism that anterior dislocations result in a disruption of the static anterior capsuloligamentous structures in the young patient, failure of the weakened degenerative posterior rotator cuff is more often seen in the elderly patient with a traumatic dislocation (12,13). The disruption of the anterior restraints such as labral and ligamentous tears in young patients accounts for the higher incidence of recurrent dislocations in this population.

In the elderly patient, dislocations result in a higher rate of tears of the already degenerated rotator cuff. Since the rotator cuff acts as a dynamic stabilizer of the glenohumeral joint, this can also lead to recurrent instability. However, some studies have reported that the anterior structures can be injured and contribute to recurrent instability in the older population as well (14). While more common in the young patient, labral tears and even bony loss of the glenoid can still occur in older patients after dislocation. This necessitates a thorough evaluation in order to identify the pathology responsible for recurrent instability as well as any other associated injuries.

PATIENT EVALUATION

Evaluation of an elderly individual with shoulder instability requires careful review of the patient's history. The clinician must determine the initial cause, how often dislocations occur, and what inciting factors have led to current symptoms. Careful review of pre- and post-injury activity level can lead to clues regarding the integrity of the rotator cuff. The number of dislocation episodes and circumstances surrounding these can also help direct evaluation and treatment plan.

Physical examination should involve both shoulders with the goal of evaluating joint stability, range of motion, strength, and neurologic status. Inspection should look for gross deformity or atrophy of the rotator cuff muscles. Obvious deformity of the shoulder may be present indicating a chronically dislocated shoulder in the elderly patient. Range of motion should be assessed both passively and actively in order to provide information regarding stability, joint stiffness, and rotator cuff integrity. Deficits in motion or strength can be an indicator of rotator cuff deficits or potential nerve palsies. In the elderly patient, each muscle of the rotator cuff should be carefully examined. A belly or lift-off test is utilized to test the integrity of the subscapularis while resisted abduction with the thumb down assesses the supraspinatus (15). Resisted external rotation in adduction and again at 90 degrees of abduction evaluates the infraspinatus and teres minor, respectively (3).

Provocative maneuvers and apprehension signs should be utilized to determine the direction of instability. The Jobe relocation test can screen for potential anterior labral pathology while the jerk test and load and shift tests can determine possible posterior labral pathology. Finally, a neurovascular examination should be performed with special attention to the axillary nerve. This can be tested by assessing sensation on the lateral aspect of the shoulder and checking for deltoid function. Brachial plexus injury can also be assessed by a thorough neurologic examination focused distally in the arm.

IMAGING STUDIES

When concern for a shoulder dislocation is present, a standard radiographic trauma series should be obtained which consists of a true anteroposterior (AP) of the shoulder, an axillary view, and a scapular Y view. Plain radiographs are the standard for the initial evaluation of a suspected glenohumeral joint dislocation; however, play a limited role in further evaluation of concomitant soft tissue pathology or recurrent instability. An axillary view is critical to confirm that a chronic dislocation is not present. MRI has become the preferred modality to assess associated soft tissue and bony shoulder injury after primary or recurrent glenohumeral dislocation.

Various reports have suggested timing of further imaging evaluation after a primary acute dislocation in the elderly (11,16–18). If pain or disabling symptoms persist after a short period of immobilization, MRI is warranted to further assess for associated injuries. Shin et al. (17) looked at patients over the age of 60 following a dislocation event and found that 21 of 25 patients who had continuous pain after 2 to 4 weeks of immobilization were found to have an associated shoulder injury. Some would argue that due to the high percentage of concomitant injury in this population MRI is warranted at initial presentation to the orthopedic office. At minimum, the threshold for further imaging should be low. We have found that physical examination in this group to be difficult in the setting of acute shoulder dislocation and routinely obtain an MRI scan early to define the specific structural injury and allow the initiation of physical therapy.

ROTATOR CUFF INVOLVEMENT

The most commonly associated injury after dislocation of the shoulder in the elderly is a tear of the rotator cuff (17). The rate of associated rotator cuff tears after glenohumeral dislocations in patients over the age of 40

TABLE 15-1 Prevalence of Concomitant Rotator Cuff Tears in the Elderly After Shoulder Dislocation

Investigator	Number of Patients	Patient Age	Incidence of Associated RTC Tears
Gumina and Postacchini (19)	58	>60	61%
Hawkins et al. (11)	39	>40	90%
Neviaser et al. (8)	21	>40	86%
Pevny et al. (16)	52	>40	35%
Toolanen et al. (9)	63	>40	38%
Shin et al. (17)	67	>60	49%
Simank et al. (20)	87	>40	54%

ranges from 35% to 90% (Table 15-1) (9,11,16–21). Debate remains as to whether a tear of the rotator cuff is the result of, or rather contributes to instability of the shoulder in the elderly (13,14,20,22).

Several studies have shown that the rotator cuff is a dynamic stabilizer of the shoulder, and tears after dislocation in the elderly can lead to both recurrence and loss of function (8,18,23). Utilizing EMG, Day et al. (24) showed that the rotator cuff muscles demonstrate preactivation in response to external forces demonstrating a feed forward muscle activation pattern contributing to stability. Tardo et al. (25) also utilized EMG to assess the role of the rotator cuff with varying external rotation exercises and found that in varying positions, it does indeed contribute to stability.

Because it serves as a stabilizer of the shoulder, degeneration of the rotator cuff may disturb the coordinated balance between the deltoid, glenohumeral ligaments, and rotator cuff itself (23). There is still debate as to whether shoulder dislocations are the cause of cuff tears which lead to instability, or whether pre-existing rotator cuff tears lead to abnormal, uncoordinated shoulder motion and related instability in cases of even low energy trauma (14). In general, for most patients who have normal shoulder function prior to an instability event, it can be presumed that rotator cuff function was close to normal. As such, any subsequent tear identified is believed to have been caused by the traumatic injury.

RECURRENT INSTABILITY

While recurrent instability of the glenohumeral joint following a dislocation is primarily associated with the younger population, it can be associated with the elderly patient as well. It remains difficult to confirm the exact mechanism of recurrent instability in the elderly; however, it appears to correlate with associated rotator cuff pathology. The actual rate of recurrence after primary dislocation in older patients reported in the literature varies widely.

Pevny et al. (16) reported a recurrence rate of 4% of 52 in patients over 40 years of age. Rowe (1) reported a recurrence rate of 14% in his cohort of patients over the age of 40. Gumina and Postacchini (19) found 22% of patients reported recurrent instability in patients 60 years and older. Hawkins et al. (11) noted only 4 of 39 patients (10%) over the age of 40 experiencing recurrence after dislocation despite 35 of those patients demonstrating clinical evidence of rotator cuff tear.

Several explanations as to the pathophysiology of recurrence have been theorized. The "posterior mechanism" postulates that the destabilizing effect of a torn rotator cuff can lead to recurrent instability (12,13). Several studies have shown that the rotator cuff plays a role in stabilization of the shoulder (24,25). When torn, the normal recruitment and firing of individual muscle units is disrupted which inhibits the rotator cuff's role as a dynamic stabilizer of the shoulder (25).

However, some studies report the disruption of the anterior ligamentous structures can occur in this older population as well leading to instability (14). As in the younger dislocator, labral tears and bony Bankart injuries can also lead to recurrent instability in the elderly. Therefore, appropriate evaluation and treatment for recurrent glenohumeral instability in the older population must carefully assess both the rotator cuff as well as the anterior static structures of the shoulder and management of both problems may be necessary.

MANAGEMENT AND TREATMENT

Appropriate treatment of primary shoulder dislocations, recurrent instability, and associated injuries is debated. However, some guidelines and treatment algorithms can be drawn from the current literature. Initial immobilization for 2 to 4 weeks is appropriate for primary dislocations of the glenohumeral joint. Thorough patient examination should be conducted following a dislocation to assess for possible associated injury. For those patients who exhibit resolution of pain and no significant or focal deficit, rehabilitation may begin early. For patients who exhibit pain or disability beyond 2 to 4 weeks, further imaging evaluation with MRI (with or without arthrogram) is indicated. At this point, significant associated pathology should be treated early for optimal outcome.

Because large rotator cuff tears alone can lead to instability, several authors agree that isolated repair is warranted in acceptable surgical candidates. In these patients, Bankart repair may be deferred to avoid capsular tightening and loss of motion depending on the size of the rotator cuff tear and degree of instability. Good results with low recurrent dislocation have been reported after repairing larger full thickness tears in isolation (8,11,16,26,27).

Several studies have demonstrated that associated rotator cuff pathology is a major factor determining functional outcome after first time dislocation in the elderly. Pevny et al. (16) found that in a cohort of patients 40 years and older, those with an isolated cuff tear had good to excellent outcomes 50% of the time when treated nonoperatively compared to 84% good to excellent in those who had a repair.

In patients with combined rotator cuff and anterior capsuloligamentous injury, the surgeon should consider repair of both with a focus on minimal capsular shift to prevent stiffness. While recurrent instability in the absence of rotator cuff pathology in the elderly is rare, Bankart pathology can be responsible for instability in this patient population (28). Outcomes after Bankart repair are less predictable in the older patient and should be confined to patients who have recurrent instability with isolated labral pathology (2,11,28).

Maier et al. (3) compared outcomes of Bankart repair between patients older and younger than 40 years of age and found poorer Constant, Rowe, and visual analogue (VAS) scores in the older cohort. Therefore, the indication for Bankart repair in the older patient should be reserved for patients who clearly demonstrate labral injury as the source for their instability.

AUTHOR'S PREFERRED MANAGEMENT

Glenohumeral dislocations in the elderly population are treated with initial closed reduction and follow-up in the orthopedic office within 7 to 10 days. If the dislocation was treated and reduced at an outside hospital, we perform x-rays in the office with a required axillary view. For patients over age 60 or any history of osteoporosis,

x-rays are assessed for obvious or occult fracture. We recommend an MRI examination (with arthrogram when possible) on all patients over the age of 50 at their initial evaluation. In our experience, this aggressive approach to soft tissue imaging helps ensure early and appropriate treatment of associated pathology, specifically the rotator cuff. Treatment plans for concomitant pathology such as labral or rotator cuff injury are based on patient activity level and extent of the associated injury.

When partial rotator cuff tears are identified, we establish a focused physical therapy program directed at rotator cuff strengthening, range of motion, and stabilization exercises. For symptomatic, full thickness rotator cuff tears we recommend early arthroscopic or open surgical repair. Delayed surgical treatment in these patients can result in recurrent instability, propagation of the tear, and loss of function.

When an isolated labral tear is discovered on MRI, we advise an initial conservative approach, as it is our experience that labral pathology in this cohort of patients does not necessarily lead to recurrent instability. We, therefore, begin focused physical therapy and only when recurrent instability occurs do we consider labral repair in this population (Fig. 15-1). When repair is necessary, we avoid a capsular shift when repairing the labrum in the elderly as this can lead to over tightening and loss of motion. Larger engaging Hill-Sachs (Fig. 15-2) lesions or bony Bankart lesions as in the younger population may also need to be addressed.

Isolated supraspinatus tears are repaired arthroscopically using standard anchor techniques (Figs. 15-3 and 15-4). For acute subscapularis tears, either open or arthroscopic techniques are used for acute repair. Following rotator cuff repair, patients are maintained in a sling for 4 to 6 weeks with passive ROM only. After sling removal, active ROM is initiated and strengthening exercises are not begun until 8 to 10 weeks

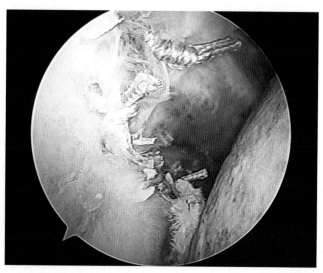

▲ FIGURE 15-1: Labral repair.

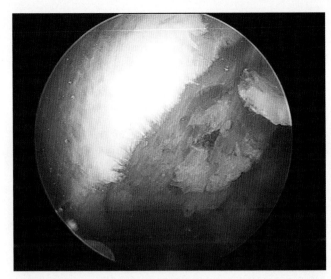

▲ FIGURE 15-2: Hill-Sachs lesion.

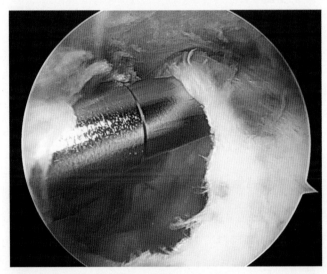

▲ FIGURE 15-3: Rotator cuff tear.

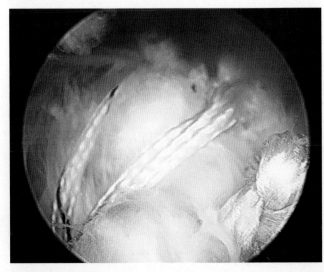

▲ FIGURE 15-4: Rotator cuff repair.

after surgery. Return to full function and activities is allowed at 4 to 6 months.

CONCLUSION

In conclusion, appropriate treatment of instability of the glenohumeral joint in the elderly hinges upon prompt and accurate diagnosis of the primary dislocation and associated injuries. While some debate remains as to timing of further imaging after dislocation, persistent pain or disability after primary dislocation warrants further imaging evaluation such as MRI to look for associated injuries. A detailed history and physical examination can aid in decision making on the need for immediate imaging and hence dictate a treatment plan. Elderly who demonstrate recurrent instability episodes warrant imaging to identify pathology and early treatment to avoid continued instability and restore function. Whether conservative or operative, treatment must address underlying rotator cuff tears or capsuloligamentous injuries in order to stabilize the joint and provide the best chance for good functional outcomes.

References

1. Rowe CR. Prognosis in dislocations of the shoulder. *J Bone Joint Surg Am.* 1956;38:957–977.
2. Murthi AM, Ramirez MA. Shoulder dislocation in the older patient. *J Am Acad Orthop Surg.* 2012;20:615–622.
3. Maier M, Geiger EV, Ilius C, et al. Midterm results after operatively stabilized shoulder dislocations in elderly patients. *Int Orthop.* 2009;33:719–723.
4. Araghi A, Prasarn M, St Clair S, et al. Recurrent anterior glenohumeral instability with onset after forty years of age. *Bull Hosp Jt Dis.* 2005;62:99–101.
5. Hovelius L, Lind B, Thorling J. Primary dislocation of the shoulder: Factors affecting 2-year prognosis. *Clin Orthop.* 1983;176:181–185.
6. Hovelius L, Eriksson GK, Fredin FH, et al. Recurrences after initial dislocation of the shoulder: Results of prospective study of treatment. *J Bone Joint Surg Am.* 1983;65:343–349.
7. Hoelen MA, Burgers AM, Rozing PM. Prognosis of primary anterior shoulder dislocation in young adults. *Arch Orthop Trauma Surg.* 1990;110:51–54.
8. Neviaser RJ, Neviaser TJ, Neviaser JS. Concurrent rupture of the rotator cuff and anterior dislocation of the shoulder in the older patient. *J Bone Joint Surg Am.* 1988;70:1308–1311.
9. Toolanen G, Hildingsson C, Hedlund T, et al. Early complications after anterior dislocation of the shoulder in patients over 40 years. *Acta Orthop Scand.* 1993;64(5): 549–552.
10. Travlos J, Goldberg I, Boome RS. Brachial plexus lesions associated with dislocated shoulders. *J Bone Joint Surg Br.* 1990;72:68–71.

11. Hawkins RJ, Bell RH, Hawkins RH, et al. Anterior dislocation of the shoulder in the older patient. *Clin Orthop.* 1986;206:192–195.

12. McLaughlin H. Injuries of the shoulder and arm. In: McLaughlin H, Harrison L, eds. *Trauma.* Philadelphia, PA: W.B. Saunders; 1959:233–296.

13. Craig EV. The posterior mechanism of acute anterior shoulder dislocations. *Clin Orthop.* 1984;190:212–216.

14. Porcellini G, Paladini P, Campi F, et al. Shoulder instability and related rotator cuff tears: Arthroscopic findings and treatment in patients aged 40 to 60 years. *Arthroscopy.* 2006;22:270–276.

15. Gerber C, Krushell RJ. Isolated rupture of the tendon of the subscapularis muscle: Clinical features in 16 cases. *J Bone Joint Surg Br.* 1991;73:389–394.

16. Pevny T, Hunter RE, Freeman JR. Primary traumatic anterior shoulder dislocations in patients 40 years of age and older. *Arthroscopy.* 1998;14:289–294.

17. Shin SJ, Yun YH, Kim DJ, et al. Treatment of traumatic anterior shoulder dislocation in patients older than 60 years. *Am J Sports Med.* 2012;40:822–827.

18. Neviaser RJ, Neviaser TJ, Neviaser JS. Anterior dislocation of the shoulder and rotator cuff rupture. *Clin Orthop Relat Res.* 1993;291:103–106.

19. Gumina S, Postacchini F. Anterior dislocation of the shoulder in elderly patients. *J Bone Joint Surg Br.* 1997;79:540–543.

20. Simank HG, Dauer G, Schneider S, et al. Incidence of rotator cuff tears in shoulder dislocations and results of therapy in older patients. *Arch Orthop Trauma Surg.* 2006;126:235–240.

21. Stayner LR, Cummings J, Andersen J, et al. Shoulder dislocations in patients older than 40 years of age. *Orthop Clin North Am.* 2000;31:231–239.

22. Loehr JF, Helmig P, Sojbjerg JO, et al. Shoulder instability caused by rotator cuff lesions: An in vitro study. *Clin Orthop Relat Res.* 1994;304:84–90.

23. Itoi E, Newman SR, Kuechle DK, et al. Dynamic anterior stabilizers of the shoulder with the arm in abduction. *J Bone Joint Surg Br.* 1994;76:834–836.

24. Day A, Taylor NF, Green RA. The stabilizing role of the rotator cuff at the shoulder – responses to external perturbations. *Clin Biomech.* 2012;27:551–556.

25. Tardo DT, Halaki M, Cathers I, et al. Rotator cuff muscles perform different functional roles during shoulder external rotation exercises. *Clin Anat.* 2013;26:236–243.

26. Bassett RW, Cofield RH. Acute tears of the rotator cuff: The timing of surgical repair. *Clin Orthop Relat Res.* 1983;175:18–24.

27. Sonnabend DH. Treatment of primary anterior shoulder dislocation in patients older than 40 years of age: Conservative versus operative. *Clin Orthop Relat Res.* 1998;304:74–77.

28. Sperling JW, Duncan SF, Torchia ME, et al. Bankart repair in patients aged fifty years or greater: Results of arthroscopic and open repairs. *J Shoulder Elbow Surg.* 2005;14:111–113.

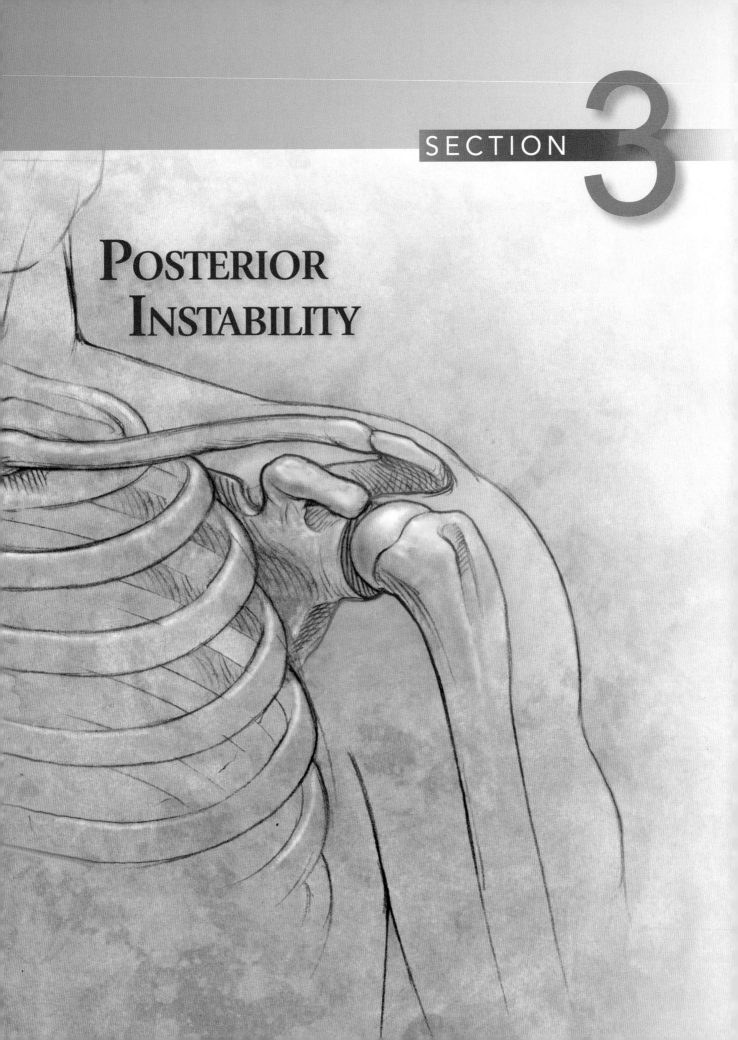

POSTERIOR INSTABILITY

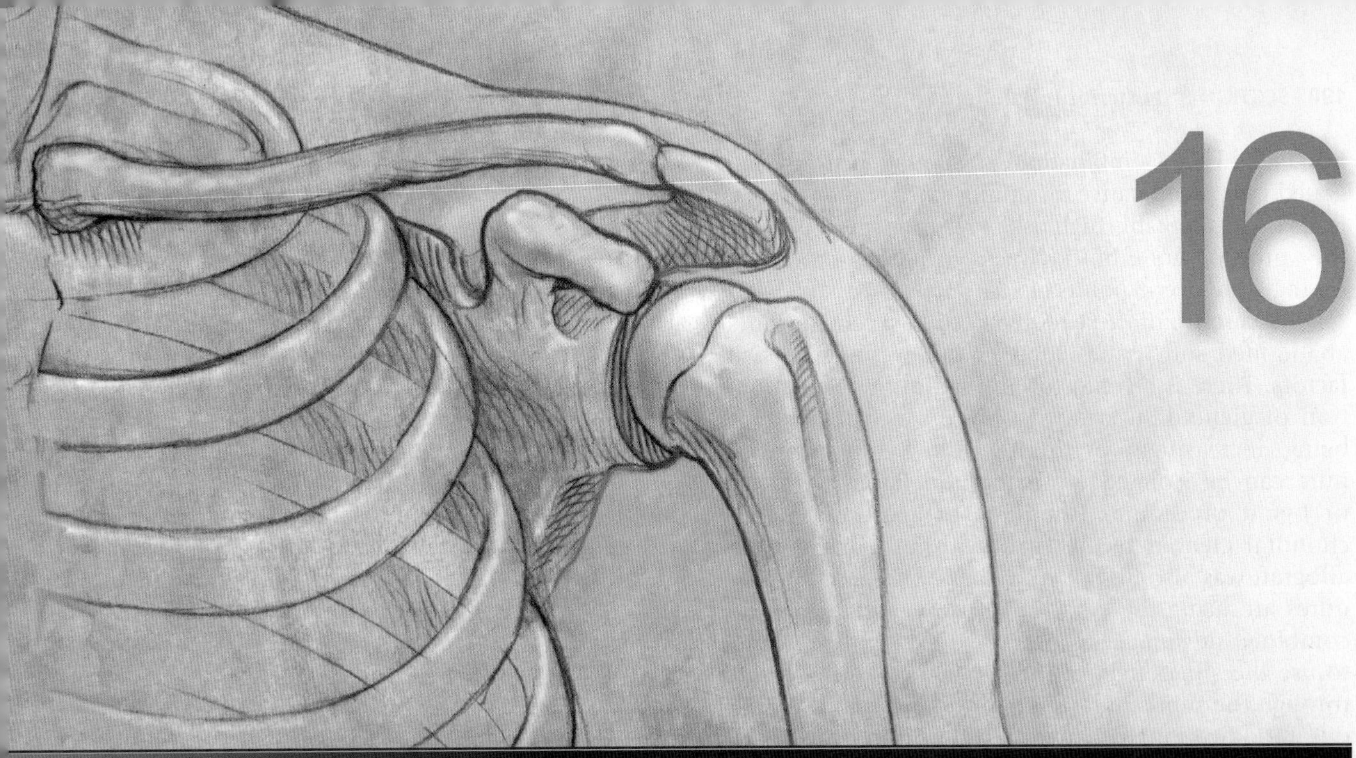

16

Treating Complications of Bone Block Procedures

Laurent Lafosse / Antonios Giannakos / Daniel G. Schwartz

Introduction

Either arthroscopic or open Bankart stabilization surgery remains nowadays the mostly used technique for treating posttraumatic anterior shoulder instability. Despite the success of this surgery, recurrence of instability remains the most frequent complication. When other, more extensive soft tissue injuries exist, such as irreparable complex labral disruptions, or humeral avulsion of glenohumeral ligament (HAGL) lesions, this technique may not be sufficient to stabilize the shoulder. Currently glenoid and humeral head bone deficiency is an increasingly recognized cause of failure. Performing arthroscopic Bankart repair in the presence of bone loss (either glenoid or humeral) may lead to a high failure rate and unpredictable outcomes. Reported of unacceptable failure rate of 67% in patients where soft tissue repair was performed in the presence of anterior glenoid bone defect >25% of the width of the glenoid, with or without engaging Hill-Sachs lesion; contrary to failure rate of 4.9% if bone loss was not present. These findings are also supported by cadaveric studies of Itoi et al. and Yamamoto et al. showing that bone loss of anterior glenoid comprising approximately 21%, or 19%, respectively, of glenoid length is the critical size of defect for soft tissue repair.

Balg and Boileau defined risk factors for failure of the Bankart procedure for anterior instability. The most important were age less than 20 years, involvement in competitive or contact sports, bone loss on the glenoid, and bone loss on the humeral head. Combination of several factors, integrated into preoperative instability severity index score, leads to unacceptably high risk of recurrence of 70% and they propose bone block (Bristow-Latarjet) procedure for the score over 6 points of 10.

As a result of these recent studies, several authors abandoned soft tissue repair in the presence of risk factors. There is a trend toward anatomic reconstruction of glenoid surface with bone block techniques being increasingly performed. Bone block procedure can be isolated reconstruction Eden-Hybinette or J-graft procedure. Technique of anatomic osteochondral glenoid reconstruction using a distal tibia allograft was also described. Other bone block procedures are using the coracoid process, which has the combined advantage to better expose the joint and to use the sling effect of the conjoint tendon passed through the subscapularis. The most popular are various modifications of open Bristow modified Helfet using the coracoid on an up ride position with one screw and the Latarjet which consist on a double screw fixation of the coracoid process placed in a laying position.

More recently, arthroscopic bone block procedures are introduced. Several authors describe various techniques of arthroscopic Bristow or arthroscopic Latarjet (8), Eden-Hybinette procedure using iliac crest bone graft or osteochondral allograft, or even J-graft technique.

Long-term studies of the Bristow or Latarjet procedure have confirmed its efficacy and lasting benefits. Subsequent revision surgery after failed Bristow or Latarjet surgery; however, is a challenging surgical problem. The use of screws close to the articular surface, changed anatomical conditions—as the absence of coracoid or often deteriorated subscapularis muscle–tendon unit or scar tissue formation around neurovascular structures (axillary nerve, musculocutaneous nerve) can make this surgery a complex and demanding procedure. The reasons of failure after Bristow-Latarjet surgery may be caused by trauma (the breakage of coracoid-screw construct), technical failure, such as malposition of coracoid graft, malposition of screws, graft resorption or graft nonunion, which may lead to construct failure. Other potentially serious complications of Bristow-Latarjet procedure include glenohumeral arthrosis, posterior instability, neurologic or vascular complications, or infection.

SHORT-TERM COMPLICATIONS

Early complication within the 6 postoperative weeks as malposition or avulsion may be treated by revision surgery using the same coracoid process, by an open or arthroscopic manner.

Different types of complication are described according to the position of the graft and the screws.

According to the Graft Position

The graft can be too high, too low, too medial, or too proud. On our experience, permanent instability can be due to a too medial and/or too inferior graft. When the graft is too high, the range of motion is limited in external rotation, even more if the split on the subscapularis tendon is too high. In case the graft is too proud, this always leads to a humeral head impingement and arthritis. In that case it is urgent to revise the patient and to reduce the surface of the graft with eventual hardware removal if the graft is already healed.

According to the Screw(s) Position

The location of the screw is related to the position of the graft. In case the graft is too low, the inferior screw may be out of the glenoid and not correctly fixed to the bone. In that case, the bad feeling of the screwdriver is obvious during the surgery and the bone graft must be replaced higher.

Out of the location, the direction of the screws is crucial. Screws must be parallel to the glenoid and in case of excessive obliquity that can lead to very bad humeral head damage. Crepitation during mobilization and more specifically during internal rotation is very symptomatic of this problem, which must be evaluated by accurate axillary profile or better a 3D CT scan. Early revision is necessary to remove the hardware and to replace it in case it is an early stage revision.

The length of the screw must be excessive and create an impingement with the infraspinatus muscle. The examiner in the infraspinatus fossae between the tip of the screw and the muscle can feel crepitation during external rotation. Revision is necessary to remove or to shorten the screws.

Early Detachment of the Graft

Most of the time due to a bad fixation, the graft can be detached from the glenoid. Three cases are possible for each screw.

- The screws are detached from the glenoid (Fig. 16-1)
- The screws are intact and still in the glenoid
- The screws are broken, one part in the glenoid, the other in the coracoid (Fig. 16-2)

It is necessary to remove the hardware as much as possible and to reinsert the coracoid with bigger screw providing stronger fixation. When the screws are broken, the glenoid part cannot be removed without bone damage and it is better to keep them in without creating any conflict with the new screws.

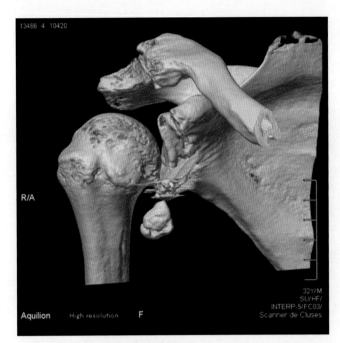

▲ **FIGURE 16-1:** 3D CT screw detached with the bone graft.

LONG-TERM COMPLICATIONS

As for short-term complications, same problems can happen but as soon as they happen latter after surgery, the symptoms are not always evident to understand.

Ideally, the bone graft should totally heal along the glenoid, keep its initial size and create a perfect continuity. Unfortunately, it is common that a part of the graft gets more or less resorbed or that there is a non-union between the graft and the glenoid. Symptoms are not necessarily recurrence of dislocations; it can be only apprehension, pain, and/or weakness. The constant factor is that it happens when the shoulder is placed in abduction external rotation. The exact assessment of the reason of these symptoms is the 3D CT scan which gives the exact dimension and statue of the bone graft.

Nonunion

The potential of healing of the graft is obviously linked to its surface of contact on the glenoid. A plane surface should be obtained on both sides to provide a good healing. Sometimes, due to bad contact area, the fusion is not obtained and some nonunion will lead to long-term complication. In cases of recurrent trauma, as the loading forces are only managed by the screws, they can bent after dislocation (Fig. 16-3).

Bony Resorption

Some resorption of the bone graft always happen after some months, but partially and more specifically at the upper part of the graft, certainly due to the unloaded part of it. More resorption can happen and it is unfortunately not exceptional that some bone graft has totally disappeared after a few years.

In these chronic cases, there is no option to use the coracoid process again because most of the bone is resorbed and has lost its potential of healing. The Eden-Hybinette procedure is an ideal way to restore long-term reconstruction for failed Bristow or Latarjet procedure.

We describe here how to use this technique arthroscopically for failed bone block reconstruction.

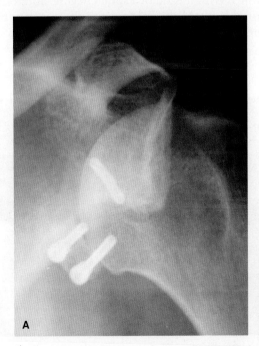
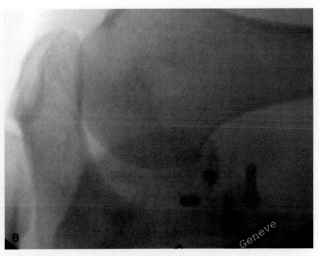

▲ **FIGURE 16-2:** X-ray of a screw broken **(A)** during dislocation and **(B)** after reduction.

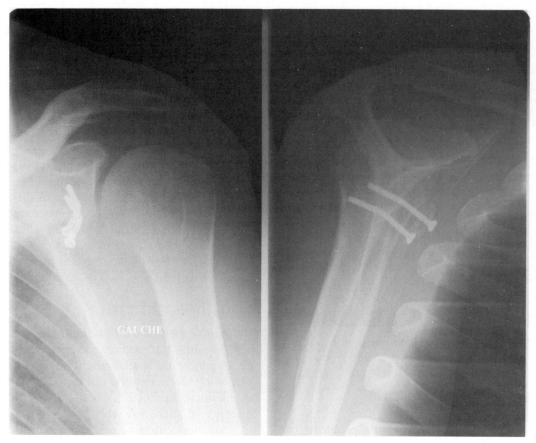

▲ **FIGURE 16-3:** Screws bent.

SURGICAL TECHNIQUE OF ARTHROSCOPIC EDEN-HYBINETTE FOR FAILED BONE BLOCK PROCEDURE

General Setting

The procedure is performed under general anesthesia with associated interscalene block, in beach chair position without the use of traction, the arm being freely draped, ensuring good mobility. The arthroscopic technique resembles to the published arthroscopic Latarjet procedure (1). Same portal are used (Fig. 16-4) except of the H portal used for the coracoid graft preparation.

Diagnostic Arthroscopy

First, standard diagnostic arthroscopy is performed, using posterior "soft spot" or A portal for visualization and anterior E portal for instrumentation. This enables to assess the status of soft tissues (glenohumeral ligaments, glenoidal labrum, articular cartilage, capsule, rotator cuff, long head of the biceps tendon), as well as osseous defects (Hill-Sachs lesion, glenoid bone loss) and previous coracoid graft appearance, if visible (graft position, graft resorption, nonunion, or fracture). With the aid of a spinal needle, antero-lateral D portal is established along with the superior border of the tendon of subscapularis muscle. As soon as the indication is confirmed, the next step is to harvest the iliac crest.

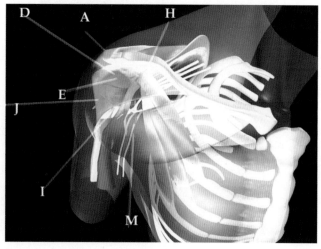

▲ **FIGURE 16-4:** Portals.

Graft Harvesting

The autologous iliac crest bicortical bone graft is harvested, with the use of double-barrel cannula from the standardized Bristow-Latarjet instability shoulder system (DePuy Mitek, Inc., Raynham, MA, USA), using two top-hat washers. Fixing the graft to the double-barrel cannula before harvesting allows full control of the graft and enables the correct graft positioning on the glenoid later, during the arthroscopic procedure (Fig. 16-5).

Glenoid Preparation

After iliac crest closure, the final step is the shoulder arthroscopy. Antero-lateral D portal is used for visualization through the rotator interval and the antero-inferior margin of glenoid is prepared with the use of radiofrequency system (VAPR 3, DePuy Mitek, Inc., Raynham, MA, USA) and motorized shaver and burr (FMS Tornado, DePuy Mitek, Inc., Raynham, MA, USA), detaching the soft tissue, preserving anterior portion of inferior glenohumeral ligament if present. After removing the soft tissue, glenoid neck is exposed, to evaluate the previous coracoid graft positioning and status (Fig. 16-6).

Arthrolysis and subscapularis muscle release are important part of the intra-articular procedure. The extra-articular step is often a difficult part of the technique as the soft tissues are very difficult to release and because there is no landmark due to the missing coracoid process and conjoint tendon.

With the use of radiofrequency system and shaver, release of the subscapularis muscle is performed, removing all the adhesions and scarring, enabling good external rotation. On the posterior surface, the subscapularis muscle is released from the scapula, on the anterior surface the release is performed with special focus on

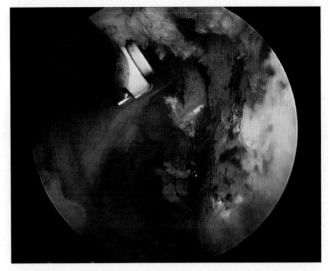

▲ **FIGURE 16-6:** Anterior glenoid exposure.

releasing the brachial plexus, often scarred down to the subscapularis muscle after previous open Latarjet procedure, and visualizing axillary nerve to avoid damaging it (Fig. 16-7). When stiff shoulder is present as a part of clinical appearance preoperatively, further arthrolysis is performed, both intra- and extra-articular until a full range of motion is obtained.

Subscapularis Split and Hardware Removal

With J portal used for visualization, subscapularis muscle is split with the use of radiofrequency system. The extent of the split; however, is smaller than in Latarjet procedure, only big enough to allow removal of the hardware and passage of the graft. If possible, all previous hardware is removed, using either antero-inferior I portal, or

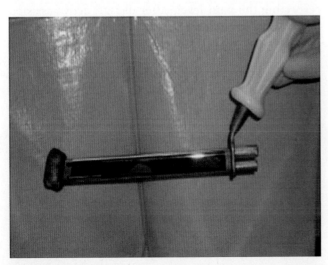

▲ **FIGURE 16-5:** Graft on cannula.

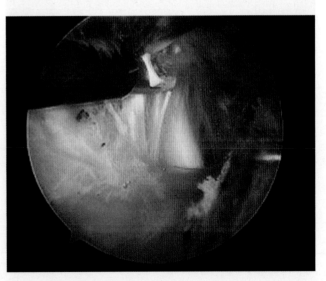

▲ **FIGURE 16-7:** Axillary nerve.

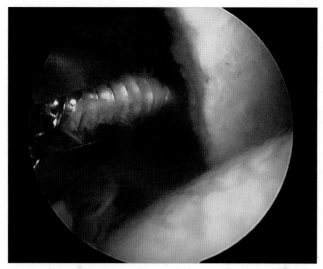

▲ **FIGURE 16-8:** Hardware removal.

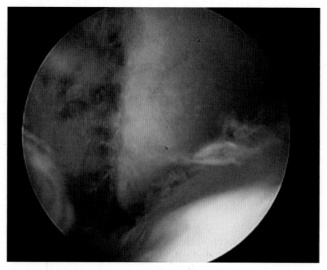

▲ **FIGURE 16-10:** Graft fixed.

medial M portal for instrumentation. This is often a demanding part of surgery, both time wise and technically (Fig. 16-8). Then, remnants of the coracoid graft are, if not interfering with the planned position of bone block, left in place, or removed with the use of a burr.

Graft Passage and Fixation

Graft, fixed on the double cannula, is then introduced through the medial M portal and passed through subscapularis split, avoiding neurovascular structures which absolutely need to be located before performing the M portal. Graft is positioned, under direct visual control from at least two angles, using switching-stick inserted through the posterior A portal to help control the graft position, ensuring it is aligned with glenoid surface, ide-

ally placing the graft few millimeters medially to the glenoid cartilage level, between 3'o-clock and 5'o-clock positions. Graft is then fixed temporary with two Kirschner wires (1.5 × 350 mm), position is verified and after drilling, final fixation with two cannulated titanium lag screws is performed (Fig. 16-9). If necessary, final adjustment of the graft with the use of a burr is possible. In this technique, capsule is not reattached to the glenoid (Fig. 16-10).

POSTOPERATIVE TREATMENT

After surgery, patient's arm is immobilized on an abduction pillow for 3 weeks at all times, then for another 3 weeks only during the night. From the postoperative day one, active-assisted exercises of the elbow, wrist and hand is allowed, passive motion of the shoulder was started at the postoperative day two, respecting the pain level. After day 21, active-assisted exercises of the shoulder were allowed, without limitation of the shoulder motion. Active rehabilitation of the shoulder, together with strengthening exercises began 6 weeks postoperatively, after verifying the graft position on x-rays in both true antero-posterior and lateral scapular view (Fig. 16-11). Return to sport activities, including contact- and high-risk sports was allowed 3 months after surgery.

SERIES

We used this technique in 18 shoulders to treat persistent instability after failed Latarjet surgery, between 2007 and 2011. Twelve of 18 patients (nine men, three

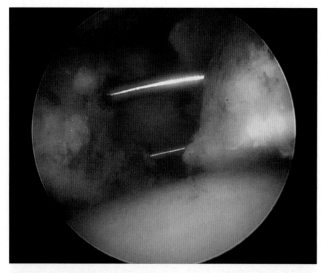

▲ **FIGURE 16-9:** K-wire fixation.

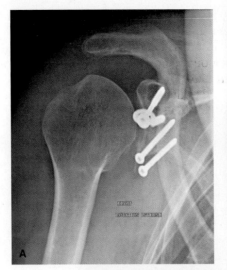
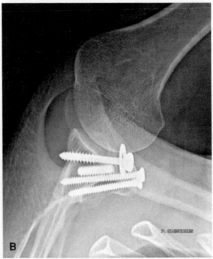
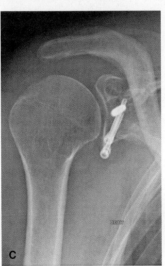
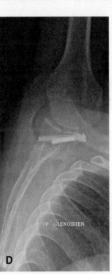

▶ **FIGURE 16-11:** X-ray **(A)** before and **(B)** after open Latarjet followed by **(C)** open Eden-Hybinette revised by **(D)** arthroscopic Eden-Hybinette.

women) were available for review. Average follow-up was 28.8 months (range 15 to 60 months). Latarjet surgery was performed as an index surgery in 10 patients (83%), 2 patients (17%) had a previous arthroscopic Bankart repair. There were no new observed neurologic deficits after revision surgery. There was no case of infection, or vascular complication related to the revision surgery.

No recurrence occurred, although two patients (16.67%) described persisting subluxations and five patients (41.67%) described persisting apprehension. Four patients (33%) had to be revised because of a conflict between the humeral head and a screw.

A good and excellent result was reported by eight patients (67%), whereas four patients (33%) described a fair or poor result. Seven patients (58%) returned to sport activities. A positive apprehension persisted in five patients (42%) including two patients (17%) with recurrent subluxations. The Rowe score increased

from 30 to 78.33 points ($p < 0.0001$). The Walch-Duplay score increased from 11.67 to 76.67 points ($p < 0.0001$). The WOSI score showed a good result of 28.71% (603 patients). Average anterior flexion was 176 degrees (150 to 180 degrees) and respectively 66 degrees (0 to 90 degrees) for external rotation. Two patients (16.67%) showed a progression for osteoarthritis, raising one stage in the classification of Samilson-Prieto. All four patients (33%) with a fair or poor result show a nonunion in the postoperative CT scan.

CONCLUSION

Many complications may happen during or after bone block procedure. For most of long-term complications, all-arthroscopic technique of Eden-Hybinette operation, as a revision procedure, although technically demanding, is a safe and reproducible surgery. Offering

all advantages of arthroscopic surgery, it allows reconstruction of glenoid defects and restores shoulder stability after failed Bristow-Latarjet surgery. In our hands, it
yields excellent and good results with subjective satisfaction in 75% of the patients and is correlated to the bony
healing of the iliac crest graft.

Reference

1. Cerciello S, Edwards TB, Walch G. Chronic anterior
glenohumeral instability in soccer players: Results for a
series of 28 shoulders treated with the Latarjet procedure.
J Orthop Traumatol. 2012;13(4):197–202.

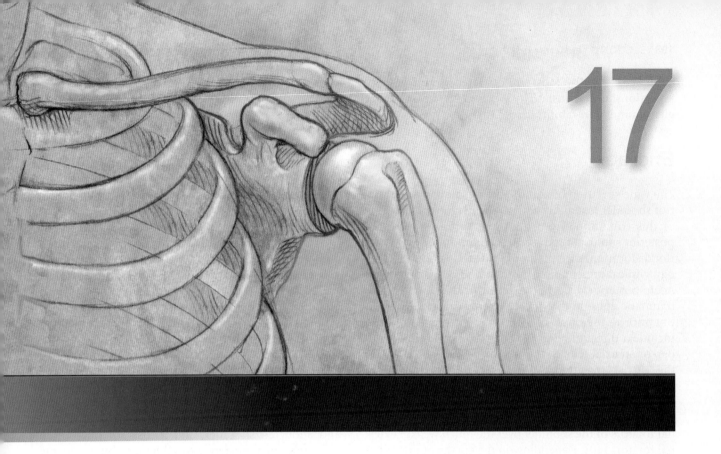

NATURAL HISTORY OF POSTERIOR SHOULDER INSTABILITY

James P. Leonard / John E. Kuhn

EPIDEMIOLOGY OF POSTERIOR SHOULDER INSTABILITY

Glenohumeral instability is a relatively common pathologic process of the shoulder, affecting approximately 2% of the general population (1). Most of these cases are categorized as anterior instability, most commonly due to a traumatic event leading to an anterior shoulder dislocation that may or may not recur. Conversely, posterior dislocations are far less common, representing only 4% of all shoulder dislocations (2,3). Unlike the traumatic etiology of most anterior instability cases, posterior instability presents with a much more insidious onset. Although about 50% of patients report a discrete injury to the shoulder, less than 25% have a documented dislocation (3,4).

Rather than an acute dislocation event, most instances of posterior shoulder instability result from repetitive microtrauma commonly seen during specific sporting activities. Consequently, posterior shoulder instability is often unrecognized, leading to incorrect diagnosis, delays in diagnosis, and even missed diagnosis (5). The early literature on posterior shoulder instability reported an incidence of 2% to 4% of all shoulder instability cases (3). As our knowledge of this condition has increased, so has our ability to diagnose patients. A prospective cohort study of United States Military Academy students found a 10.3% incidence of posterior instability following a traumatic event (6). Wolf and Eakin (7) report that 11.6% of all patients having surgery for long-term shoulder instability have recurrent posterior shoulder instability. Most authors agree the incidence of posterior shoulder instability is between 4% and 12% of glenohumeral instability cases (4,6–9).

ETIOLOGY

The wide spectrum of pathologies encompassing posterior shoulder instability adds to the diagnostic difficulty of this condition. From the more common recurrent posterior subluxation to the less common locked posterior dislocation, each of these entities has a unique etiology, clinical presentation, and method of management. Acute posterior dislocations result from a high-energy, traumatic episode that most patients can readily identify prior to the onset of their symptoms. Such injuries include a direct blow to the anterior part of the shoulder, or an axial load to the arm while the shoulder is in the "at risk" position of forward elevation, adduction, and internal rotation. In addition, seizures and electrical shocks can indirectly cause posterior shoulder dislocations by causing a violent contracture of the strong internal rotators of the shoulder over the much weaker external rotators (10). Depending on the energy of the initial injury, the resultant posteriorly directed force on the humeral head can result in a subluxation, dislocation that either spontaneously reduces or requires reduction, or a locked dislocation with a large impaction fracture about the anteromedial humeral head, referred to as a reverse Hill-Sachs lesion (Fig. 17-1). The quality of a patient's bone will have an impact on the size of the

reverse Hill-Sachs lesion, but may also lead to an associated proximal humerus fracture in osteoporotic bone.

A prospective cohort of patients with an acute traumatic posterior dislocation found 67% of dislocations were produced by a traumatic accident, while the remainder was due to seizures (11). The prevalence was highest in men between 20 and 49 years of age, with a secondary peak noticed in elderly patients affecting both sexes equally. The risk of recurrent posterior instability was 19.2%, with 17.7% occurring within 1 year of the traumatic event. Risk factors for recurrence include an age less than 40 years, dislocation during a seizure, and a large reverse Hill-Sachs lesion measuring greater than 1.3 cm^3. Despite these risk factors, the overall risk of posterior shoulder dislocation recurrence following a traumatic injury is substantially lower than that for patients with anterior dislocation (11–14).

The most frequent etiology of recurrent posterior instability involves repetitive, minor injuries to the shoulder while in the "at risk position." There are several different mechanisms common in athletic activities that place the arm in the flexed, internally rotated, and adducted shoulder, and at risk for microtrauma and subsequent posterior shoulder instability. The most common and most direct mechanism involves repetitive, posteriorly directed loads applied to the front of the body. The most common example of this mechanism is blocking offensive lineman in football, but other susceptible activities include lacrosse, rowing, push-ups, and weight lifting. However, there are other indirect actions that have been implicated as a source for posterior instability. Overhead activities such as throwing in baseball/softball, the volleyball serve, or the tennis serve generate a tremendous posteriorly directed force to decelerate the shoulder during the follow-through phase of throwing (15). Similarly, the pull-through phase of the freestyle and butterfly strokes in swimmers places the shoulder in an adducted, flexed, and internally rotated position at risk for developing posterior shoulder instability (16,17). Other provocative sport maneuvers that repeatedly place the shoulder in the "at risk position" include the backswing of golf, the backhand in tennis, and the baseball swing. Each action alone produces a minute insult to the posterior structures of the shoulder and is essentially insignificant. However, over time the accumulation of microtrauma generates damage to the shoulder that may eventually become symptomatic. Thus, most patients with recurrent posterior instability cannot recall a specific injury episode; rather they describe an insidious onset of symptoms.

Some early classifications of posterior shoulder instability considered repetitive microtrauma to be an atraumatic injury because there was no acute dislocation event. However, a true atraumatic history of posterior shoulder instability should alert the clinician to the possibility of an underlying collagen disease or bony abnormality.

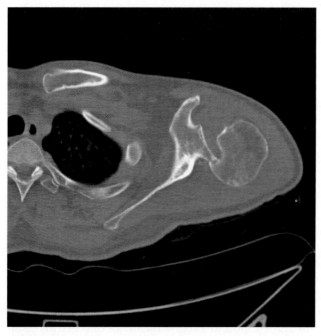

▲ **FIGURE 17-1:** Axial CT showing an impaction fracture to the anteromedial aspect of the humeral head which remains dislocated following a seizure-induced posterior shoulder dislocation.

Most of these patterns of instability are part of a more complex bidirectional instability with both posterior and inferior components, or multidirectional instability with posterior, inferior, and anterior components (12,18).

PATHOANATOMY

Most mechanisms of injury in posterior shoulder instability implicate the posterior capsule as the key functional structure. However, given the multitude of static and dynamic stabilizers associated with shoulder instability, it is unlikely that posterior capsular injury alone creates posterior shoulder instability (19). Rather, this process is multifactorial involving both static and dynamic stabilizers of the shoulder.

Static Stabilizers

The posterior capsule is defined as the area superior to the posterior band of the inferior glenohumeral ligament (IGHL) and inferior to the insertion of the long head of the biceps. Compared to the anterior capsule, the posterior capsule, which lacks ligamentous thickenings, is thinner and has a lower failure strain (20,21). The thinnest and weakest portion of the capsule appears to be the inferior posterior capsule. During a posterior insult to the shoulder, the posteroinferior aspect of the capsule can either be torn in the case of a dislocation or undergo plastic formation leading to redundancy and increased joint volume (Fig. 17-2) (7,14,17,18,22). A

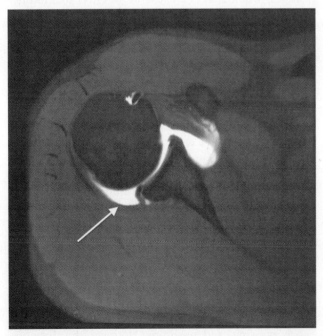

▲ **FIGURE 17-2:** T$_1$-weighted magnetic resonance arthrogram of a lax posteroinferior aspect of the capsule (*arrow*) in a patient with recurrent posterior instability. Note the posterior Bankart lesion.

biomechanical study evaluating the restraints to posterior dislocation reported the posterior capsule was damaged in 100% of cases (23). However, given its frailty, concomitant injuries to other shoulder stabilizers would need to occur to initiate instability.

The glenohumeral ligaments are capsular thickenings that function at the end ranges of motion when they are tensioned to provide stability to the shoulder. Most biomechanical studies have found the IGHL to be the most important ligamentous structure with respect to posterior shoulder instability (22,24–26). A cadaveric biomechanical study reported the IGHL and the posteroinferior capsule to be the primary static restraint to posterior translation with the shoulder in 90 degrees of abduction (27). The posterior band of the IGHL became increasingly important as the arm was forward flexed, while the anterior band of the IGHL became increasingly important as the arm was extended back. Internal rotation of the shoulder moves the posterior band of the IGHL into an anteroposterior (AP) orientation, increasing its importance as a posterior stabilizer (24,25,27,28). Sports involving the arm in front of the body places the posterior band of the IGHL under tension, risking potential injury and subsequent posterior shoulder instability (19,29).

Most activities implicated in posterior shoulder instability do not occur at the end ranges of motion; rather they occur with the shoulder in the midrange of motion when ligaments are not fully taut. Thus, capsular and ligamentous injury alone cannot fully explain posterior shoulder instability (30). Several biomechanical studies have conveyed the importance of the rotator interval and its contents. The rotator interval is bordered by the supraspinatus superiorly, subscapularis inferiorly, coracoid medially, and the biceps and humerus laterally. Its contents include the intra-articular portion of the biceps tendon, the superior glenohumeral ligament (SGHL), the coracohumeral ligament (CHL), and the middle glenohumeral ligament (MGHL). With the arm in the "at risk" position of flexion, adduction, and internal rotation, a cadaveric study of static restraints failed to produce a posterior dislocation after excision of the posterior rotator cuff and the entire posterior capsule. Subsequent excision of the anterosuperior capsule, including the SGHL, did result in posterior dislocation. The study also emphasized the role of the CHL in posterior instability (31). Another group found that the rotator interval limits inferior and posterior joint translation with the arm in an adducted position (32). This adducted position puts the SGHL under tension, and likely has a secondary role in opposing posterior translation in the "at risk" position (27).

Another soft tissue restraint to posterior translation is the labrum. Despite providing resistance to posterior translation, the posterior labrum is less of a factor in stability compared to the anterior labrum. An important role of the labrum is to anchor the posterior capsule and ligaments to the glenoid. Unlike the anterior labrum, the posterior labrum is only loosely attached to the surrounding capsule, with less ligamentous reinforcement (12,20,30). Thus, the mere presence of a posterior labral tear does not necessarily lead to recurrent posterior shoulder instability. A biomechanical study evaluating the restraints to posterior dislocation reported the posterior labrum was damaged in 70% of cases (23).

Nevertheless, the labrum still functions to increase the depth and surface area of the glenoid cavity, effectively decreasing the amount of lateral humeral displacement necessary for subluxation (33,34). A biomechanical study found that labral excision decreases the depth of the shoulder socket by 50% and reduces the resistance to shoulder instability by 20% (35).

Although only one-third of the humeral head articulates with the glenoid, the bony anatomy of the shoulder also contributes to static stabilization (36). Bony anatomic deformities that have been implicated in posterior shoulder instability include humeral head retroversion, glenoid hypoplasia, glenoid retroversion, posterior glenoid erosion, and an engaging anterior humeral head defect (14,37,38). Several case control studies comparing recurrent posterior instability shoulders with normal shoulders found unstable shoulders to have flatter glenoids (34,39) with increased retroversion (34,37,38,40). Localized erosion to the posteroinferior glenoid has been documented with recurrent subluxations; however, it is unclear if the bony erosion is the cause or effect of repeat posterior subluxations (22,41). One study found 94% of shoulders with recurrent posterior shoulder instability had a deficiency of the posteroinferior glenoid rim (40). Following a traumatic posterior dislocation, the presence of a reverse Hill-Sachs lesion increases the chances for further instability episodes by engaging the posterior part of the glenoid rim as the arm is internally rotated. As Robinson et al. (11) showed in their prospective cohort of traumatic posterior dislocations, a large reverse Hill-Sachs lesion greater than 1.5 cm^3 was a risk factor for recurrent instability. Although not likely to be the primary factor for posterior instability, the bony anatomy is a contributing factor that should be evaluated in all atraumatic and recurrent posterior instability patients.

Dynamic Stabilizers

In addition to the static factors, two important dynamic mechanisms maintain shoulder stability as well, the concavity-compression mechanism and scapulohumeral balance (42). The concavity-compression mechanism relies on both static and dynamic components to maintain shoulder stability. This process relies on the rotator cuff, deltoid, and biceps providing a compression force

on the humeral head into the glenoid fossa. Important to this process is the glenoid maintaining a sufficient depth based on its bone morphology and maintenance of a labrum. As mentioned previously, a hypoplastic or flat glenoid increased the risk of recurrent posterior shoulder instability. Of all the muscles, the subscapularis has been shown to provide the greatest force against subluxation (24). In their biomechanical study, Blasier et al. (24) postulated that the redirection of the subscapularis tendon as it turns around the glenoid rim yields a more anteriorly directed force. However, more important than any individual muscle strength or weakness is the maintenance of an equivalent force coupling between external and internal rotations, so that the humeral head can remain centered within the glenoid fossa.

Preserving the dynamic relationship between scapular motion and humeral motion is another important factor in shoulder stability. Similar to a sea lion balancing a ball on its nose, the ability of the scapula to move to keep the humeral head centered on the glenoid fossa is important in stabilizing the glenohumeral joint. Although disturbances in scapulothoracic motion may be apparent in patients in posterior shoulder instability (43), the pathogenesis is not well understood. Serratus anterior weakness with subsequent medial scapular winging has been implicated as the cause of posterior shoulder instability in elite golfers (44,45). However, other studies have demonstrated scapular winging as a compensatory mechanism for posterior instability, with winging resulting in increased glenoid anteversion and increased bony stability (46). The importance of scapulothoracic motion in shoulder stability is definite; however, whether it is a cause or an effect to shoulder instability is still uncertain.

CLINICAL EVALUATION FOR POSTERIOR SHOULDER INSTABILITY

The lack of an acute, traumatic dislocation event in a majority of patients with posterior shoulder instability can make its diagnosis challenging. Several studies have shown 60% to 80% of cases of posterior shoulder instability are missed when they initially seek medical consultation for the injury (5,47). For the most part, the signs and symptoms are subtle, so a high index of suspicion is required to make the appropriate diagnosis. For patients without a dislocation event, patients will be younger than 35 years old, most commonly male, participating in activities in which the arm is positioned in front of the body in flexion and internal rotation. Such activities include a football offensive lineman, lacrosse, rowing, bench pressing, and push-ups. However, the diagnosis should also be expected in overhead throwing because of being in the "at risk" position in follow-through;

swimming in the butterfly and freestyle strokes during pull-through; and swinging activities such as baseball, golf, and tennis during the backswing.

Patient History

The clinical evaluation of posterior shoulder instability should begin with a determination of the type and mechanism of the event that originally caused the instability. The first step is to inquire about a history of trauma. For patients who recall a specific, traumatic episode, the direction of the applied force and the position of the arm should be inquired. A posteriorly directed force; an injury with the arm in the "at risk" position of shoulder forward flexion, internal rotation, and adduction; and an electrical shock or seizure support the diagnosis of a posterior shoulder dislocation. The severity of the event should be determined from a subluxation to a dislocation that required a formal reduction. In addition, the number and severity of subsequent episodes of instability should be ascertained.

Patients without a history of trauma typically complain of pain rather than instability as their primary complaint. However, this pain usually occurs during episodes of instability. The specific characteristics of this pain are often unclear; however, most commonly it is described as a deep, posterior shoulder pain (48,49) or more rarely as a vague anterior pain. These symptoms are brought on with specific activities associated with the "at risk" position of shoulder forward flexion, internal rotation, and adduction. It is important to evaluate which specific activity and position the shoulder is in during these pain occurrences. With careful questioning, the direction, frequency, and severity of the patient's symptoms can be established.

Physical Examination

The physical examination of a shoulder begins with inspection, evaluating for atrophy or asymmetry. Patients with a posterior shoulder dislocation may have a prominent humeral head posteriorly, as well as flattening of the anterior contour and prominence of the coracoid. However, these findings are often quite subtle and obliterated by swelling or a large deltoid muscle mass (50). Often times, even with a posterior dislocation, the shoulders will appear normal and symmetric.

Tenderness to palpation may be present along the posterior joint line, with one study reporting approximately two-thirds of patients experienced posterior joint line tenderness (16). They proposed the joint line tenderness was due to synovitis from recurrent instability. Superolateral tenderness of the affected shoulder may also be present, and is thought to represent stress-related changes in the rotator cuff. Finally, crepitus may be palpated as the arm is internally rotated (51).

Glenohumeral motion of the shoulder, both active and passive, are typically normal in patients with recurrent posterior shoulder instability (41). Classically, external rotation is limited in a locked posterior shoulder dislocation while the arm is held in adduction and internal rotation. In addition to evaluating glenohumeral motion, scapulothoracic motion should also be evaluated. Scapulohumeral rhythm and scapulothoracic mechanics should be assessed to exclude the possibility of scapular winging, which is frequently confused with posterior instability (46).

Testing for overall ligamentous laxity should first be evaluated. The sulcus sign is recognized as an increase in the distance between the acromion and greater tuberosity with inferior distraction of the humerus. A measurement greater than 2 cm is pathognomonic for multidirectional instability, but pain and symptoms of inferior instability must also be present for this diagnosis. The incidence of a positive sulcus sign in the setting of posterior instability has been shown to range from 7% to 75% (8,16). The contralateral shoulder should be evaluated as a comparison, as well as hyperextension of the knees and elbows, and the ability to oppose the thumb to the forearm.

Provocative tests specific for posterior shoulder instability focus on replicating the symptoms of pain and/or instability in the "at risk" position. The posterior stress test positions the arm in 90 degrees forward elevation and internal rotation while a posterior force is directed onto the humerus (Fig. 17-3). A positive test occurs when the humeral head subluxes over the glenoid rim by either observation or palpation. Likewise,

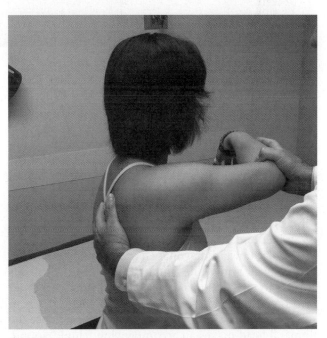

▲ **FIGURE 17-3:** Posterior stress test. Evaluation for posterior humeral head subluxation or dislocation of forward flexion and internal rotation.

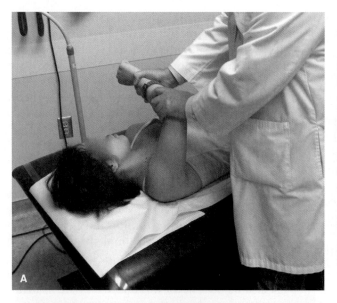

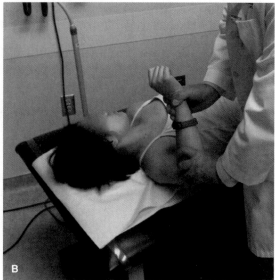

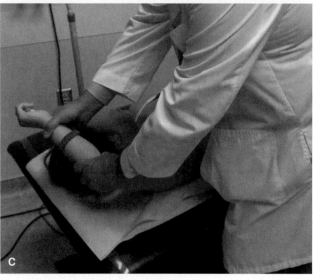

▲ **FIGURE 17-4:** Jerk test. **A:** Adduction, forward flexion, and internal rotation results in posterior subluxation or dislocation. **B:** Abduction of the shoulder results in the unstable shoulder reducing back into the glenoid. **C:** A modified test will reduce the shoulder in forward elevation.

the jerk test subluxes or dislocates the shoulder with a similar maneuver, but then extends the arm to allow the glenohumeral joint to reduce (Fig. 17-4). Evaluation of the jerk test found that nonsurgical treatment was more than 90% likely to be successful in patients with a painless positive jerk test, whereas more than 80% of those with a painful jerk test fail to respond to nonsurgical treatment (52).

A completely different maneuver described by Kim et al. (52) is performed with the arm in 90 degrees of abduction. A simultaneous axial loading force and 45 degrees upward diagonal elevation are then applied to the distal arm while inferior and posterior force is applied to the proximal arm (Fig. 17-5). A sudden onset of posterior shoulder pain with this maneuver is considered a positive test result, regardless of whether the humeral head makes an accompanying "clunk" sound. This Kim test was found to be more sensitive than the jerk test in revealing inferior labral lesions, whereas the jerk test was more sensitive in revealing posterior labral

tears. When the two tests were combined, the overall sensitivity in detecting a posteroinferior labral tear was 97%.

Diagnostic Imaging

Initial imaging on any potential shoulder instability patient is the standard trauma series of the shoulder, which consists of a true AP view, a trans-scapular "Y" view, and an axillary view. Often times this series may appear normal; however, the addition of an axillary view or a Velpeau view prevents a missed posterior dislocation (Fig. 17-6). Other than identifying a current dislocation, radiographs are useful for the evaluation of bony abnormalities such as a reverse Hill-Sachs lesion, a posterior bony Bankart lesion, a fracture of the lesser tuberosity, glenoid retroversion, or glenoid hypoplasia. A CT scan can provide more detailed, multiplanar information about glenoid version and bone loss (53). MRI evaluation detects pathologies to many of the static and

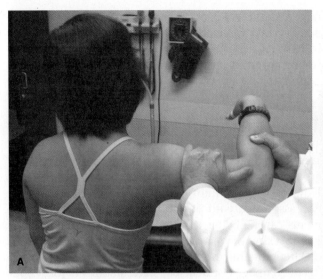
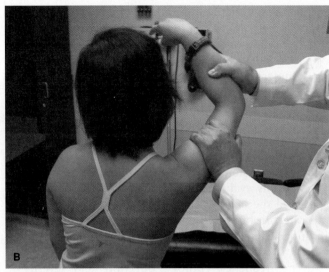

▲ **FIGURE 17-5:** Kim test. Posterior and inferior forces applied to the proximal arm simultaneously with axial force and upward elevation. **A:** Beginning posision. **B:** Ending position.

dynamic restraints of shoulder stability, such as labral tears, capsular injury, and rotator cuff tears (54).

CLASSIFICATION

The wide range of pathologies, mechanisms of injury, and clinical presentation of posterior shoulder instability have made its classification difficult. Early studies did not account for differences between dislocations and subluxations, traumatic versus atraumatic causes, unidirectional versus multidirectional conditions, or voluntary versus involuntary stability (3,7,36). Thus early classification schemes of posterior shoulder instability did not account for the broad continuum of disease, with subsequent surgical results of this heterogeneous population being less consistent with higher failure rates and various complications reported (16,17,22,36,41). With

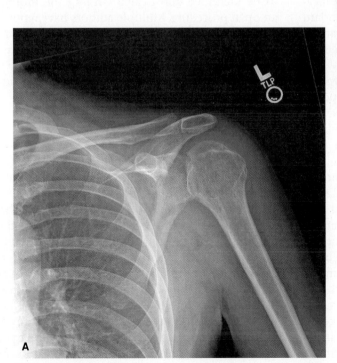
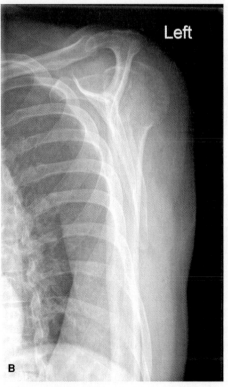

▲ **FIGURE 17-6:** Standard shoulder radiographic trauma series. **A:** Scapular AP view demonstrating posterior dislocation. This view shows the characteristic "light bulb sign" which can only occur with extremes of internal rotation of the humerus. **B:** Scapular "Y" view of a posterior dislocation. Axillary view or CT should be obtained in all patients with suspected posterior dislocation (see Fig. 17-1. Axial CT of the same patient).

an increasing understanding of the pathoanatomy and clinical presentation, improved classification schemes have been developed that better identify the key etiologic factors that can better direct treatment.

Numerous classification systems have been developed for shoulder instability, but none are completely satisfactory (14). A study comparing four different classification systems for instability found great variability, particularly with regards to the diagnostic criteria of instability (55). In an attempt to develop a standardized classification system for shoulder instability, Kuhn (56) systematically evaluated each classification system and developed the FEDS system. This system relies on the four categories most commonly used in all other classifications, namely frequency, etiology, direction, and severity.

The frequency, etiology, direction, and severity (FEDS) system defines instability as patients with discomfort and a sense of looseness, slipping, or the shoulder "going out." Frequency is categorized as solitary if there is only one subluxation or dislocation episode over the course of 1 year, occasional is two to five episodes, and frequent is more than five episodes per year. Etiology is defined as either a specific traumatic episode that causes instability or atraumatic. In the cases of athletes with repetitive microtrauma, this system would classify their etiology as atraumatic because of the lack of a specific episode of trauma. The primary direction of instability is labeled as anterior, posterior, or inferior, and is confirmed with physical examination maneuvers. Severity is graded as either a subluxation or a dislocation. The goal of this system is to provide a standard classification scheme across the literature, so that the natural history and treatment of different pathologies can be evaluated and compared.

One important factor left out of the FEDS system is the concept of volition (14,51). Involuntary posterior instability typically results from a traumatic event, either acute or repetitive, and manifests as mild subluxation. As defined, these symptoms do not occur willfully and usually are not controllable. Conversely, voluntary posterior instability occurs when a patient can willfully dislocate or sublux the shoulder. Muscular, or habitual, voluntary posterior instability is defined by a muscular imbalance that allows voluntary subluxation/ dislocation of the shoulder with the arm in adduction (57,58). These patients often develop instability during adolescence for secondary gain, and are poor surgical candidates. Another category of posterior instability, positional posterior instability, has been identified as both voluntary and involuntary, with a lack of agreement between authors (14,51). This pattern of instability occurs when the arm is placed in the unstable position of flexion, adduction, and internal rotation; however, patients tend to avoid this position (57,58). The actual subluxation event is considered an involun-tary event; however, the decision to place the arm in this position is completely voluntary, thus controversy exists in its categorization. Either way, these patients tend to respond well to surgery provided they do not have any underlying psychiatric or secondary gain issues.

TREATMENT OPTIONS

Treatment outcomes for posterior shoulder instability are far less predictable than anterior instability (19). However, with an improved recognition of the pathologies associated with posterior instability, specific treatments can be better tailored to the individual patient. The first line of treatment is physical therapy, focusing on strengthening the dynamic stabilizers to compensate for the damaged or deficient static stabilizers (59). Specifically, the focus is on strengthening the posterior deltoid, external rotators, and periscapular muscles, with a success rate for posterior instability of 65% to 80% of cases (38,59). Patients who respond to physical therapy typically have a history of atraumatic or repetitive microtrauma, rather than a history of trauma.

Surgical treatment focuses on identifying and repairing static structures that are injured in patients not responding to physical therapy. Historically, open treatment has been unsatisfactory, with successful results ranging from 30% to 70% and fraught with complications, technical difficulty, and unpredictable outcomes. The advent of arthroscopy allows specific injury patterns to be identified and treated without the morbidity of an open procedure. Multiple authors have reported success rate exceeding 90% with good subjectively assessed outcomes and low recurrence rates of instability (48,60–64). However, no randomized control studies have been published comparing open techniques to arthroscopic techniques.

CONCLUSION

Posterior shoulder instability is a complex, multifactorial syndrome that often goes misdiagnosed or undiagnosed on initial evaluation. Many different mechanisms can initiate this pathologic process, from a high-energy trauma to normal athletic activities such as blocking in football, pitching in baseball, or swinging in golf. Regardless of the mechanism, several structures involved in shoulder stability, both static and dynamic, must be injured or abnormal to result in posterior shoulder instability. Even then, most patients complain of pain rather than instability when the arm is placed in the provocative position of shoulder forward flexion, internal rotation, and adduction. To make the correct diagnosis, a high index of suspicion is necessary during the clinical evaluation to identify specific sporting maneuvers that place patients at risk, assess signs and symptoms, and perform the appropriate diagnostic examinations and tests. The advent of arthroscopy has only improved our understanding of the pathoanatomy behind posterior shoulder instability, while also enabling these structures to be repaired without concurrent injury to the rest of the shoulder. As our knowledge of the natural history of posterior shoulder instability continues to improve, so will our ability to treat it.

References

1. Hovelius L. Incidence of shoulder dislocation in Sweden. *Clin Orthop Relat Res.* 1982;166:127–131.
2. Kroner K, Lind T, Jensen J. The epidemiology of shoulder dislocations. *Arch Orthop Trauma Surg.* 1989;108:288–290.
3. McLaughlin HJ. Posterior dislocation of the shoulder. *J Bone Joint Surg.* 1952;24:584–590.
4. Arciero RA, Robert A, Mazzocca AD. Traumatic posterior shoulder dislocation with labral injury: Suture anchor technique. *TSES.* 2004;5:13–24.
5. Hawkins RJ. Unrecognized dislocations of the shoulder. *Instr Course Lect.* 1985;34:258–263.
6. Owens BD, Duffey ML, Nelson BJ, et al. The incidence and characteristics of shoulder instability at the United States Military Academy. *Am J Sports Med.* 2007;35:1168–1173.
7. Wolf EM, Eakin CL. Arthroscopic capsular plication for posterior shoulder instability. *Arthroscopy.* 1998;14:153–163.
8. Bradley JP, Forsythe B, Mascarenhas R. Arthroscopic management of posterior shoulder instability: Diagnosis, indications, and technique. *Clin Sports Med.* 2008;27:649–670.
9. Escobedo EM, Richardson ML, Schulz YB, et al. Increased risk of posterior glenoid labrum tears in football players. *AJR Am J Roentgenol.* 2007;188:193–197.
10. Buhler M, Gerber C. Shoulder instability related to epileptic seizures. *J Shoulder Elbow Surg.* 2002;11:339–344.
11. Robinson CM, Seah M, Akhtar MA. The epidemiology, risk of recurrence, and functional outcome after an acute traumatic posterior dislocation of the shoulder. *J Bone Joint Surg.* 2011;93:1605–1613.
12. Provencher MT, Romeo AA. Posterior and multidirectional instability of the shoulder: Challenges associated with diagnosis and management. *Instr Course Lect.* 2008;57:133–152.
13. Robinson CM, Aderinto J. Posterior shoulder dislocations and fracture-dislocations. *J Bone Joint Surg Am.* 2005;87:639–650.
14. Robinson CM, Aderinto J. Recurrent posterior shoulder instability. *J Bone Joint Surg Am.* 2005;87:883–892.
15. Fleisig GS, Andrews JR, Dillman CJ, et al. Kinetics of baseball pitching with implications about injury mechanisms. *Am J Sports Med.* 1995;23:233–239.
16. Pollock RG, Bigliani LU. Recurrent posterior shoulder instability. Diagnosis and treatment. *Clin Orthop Relat Res.* 1993;291:85–96.
17. Tibone JE, Bradley JP. The treatment of posterior subluxation in athletes. *Clin Orthop Relat Res.* 1993;291:124–137.
18. Antoniou J, Duckworth DT, Harryman DT 2nd. Capsulolabral augmentation for the management of posteroinferior instability of the shoulder. *J Bone Joint Surg Am.* 2000;82:1220–1230.
19. Yanke A, Van Thiel G, LeClere L et al. Diagnosis and arthroscopic management of posterior shoulder instability. *OKOJ* 2011;9:1–8.
20. Bey MJ, Hunter SA, Kilambi N, et al. Structural and mechanical properties of the glenohumeral joint posterior capsule. *J Shoulder Elbow Surg.* 2005;14:201–206.
21. Ciccone WJ 2nd, Hunt TJ, Lieber R, et al. Multiquadrant digital analysis of shoulder capsular thickness. *Arthroscopy.* 2000;16:457–461.
22. Schwartz E, Warren RF, O'Brien SJ, et al. Posterior shoulder instability. *Orthop Clin North Am.* 1987;18:409–419.
23. Weber SC, Caspari RB. A biochemical evaluation of the restraints to posterior shoulder dislocation. *Arthroscopy.* 1989;5:115–121.
24. Blasier RB, Soslowsky LJ, Malicky DM, et al. Posterior glenohumeral subluxation: Active and passive stabilization in a biomechanical model. *J Bone Joint Surg Am.* 1997;79:433–440.
25. Bowen MK, Warren RF. Ligamentous control of shoulder stability based on selective cutting and static translation experiments. *Clin Sports Med.* 1991;10:757–782.
26. O'Brien SJ, Neves MC, Arnoczky SP, et al. The anatomy and histology of the inferior glenohumeral ligament complex of the shoulder. *Am J Sports Med.* 1990;18:449–456.
27. O'Brien SJ, Schwartz RS, Warren RF, et al. Capsular restraints to anterior-posterior motion of the abducted shoulder: A biomechanical study. *J Shoulder Elbow Surg.* 1995;4:298–308.
28. Pagnani MJ, Warren RF. Stabilizers of the glenohumeral joint. *J Shoulder Elbow Surg.* 1994;3:173–190.
29. Mair SD, Zarzour RH, Speer KP. Posterior labral injury in contact athletes. *Am J Sports Med.* 1998;26:753–758.
30. Antoniou J, Harryman DT 2nd. Posterior instability. *Op Tech Sports Med.* 2000;8:225–233.
31. Warren RF, Kornblatt I, Marchand R. Static factors affecting posterior shoulder stability. *Orthop Trans.* 1984;8:89.
32. Harryman DT 2nd, Sidles JA, Harris SL, et al. The role of the rotator interval capsule in passive motion and stability of the shoulder. *J Bone Joint Surg Am.* 1992;74:53–66.
33. Lazarus MD, Sidles JA, Harryman DT 2nd, et al. Effect of a chondral-labral defect on glenoid concavity and glenohumeral stability. A cadaveric model. *J Bone Joint Surg Am.* 1996;78:94–102.
34. Kim SH, Noh KC, Park JS, et al. Loss of chondrolabral containment of the glenohumeral joint in atraumatic posteroinferior multidirectional instability. *J Bone Joint Surg Am.* 2005;87:92–98.
35. Lippitt SB, Vanderhooft JE, Harris SL, et al. Glenohumeral stability from concavity-compression: A quantitative analysis. *J Shoulder Elbow Surg.* 1993;2:27–35.
36. Hawkins RJ, Koppert G, Johnston G. Recurrent posterior instability (subluxation) of the shoulder. *J Bone Joint Surg Am.* 1984;66:169–174.

37. Brewer BJ, Wubben RC, Carrera GF. Excessive retroversion of the glenoid cavity. A cause of non-traumatic posterior instability of the shoulder. *J Bone Joint Surg.* 1986;68:724–731.

38. Hurley JA, Anderson TE, Dear W, et al. Posterior shoulder instability. Surgical versus conservative results with evaluation of glenoid version. *Am J Sports Med.* 1992;20: 396–400.

39. Inui H, Sugamoto K, Miyamoto T, et al. Glenoid shape in atraumatic posterior instability of the shoulder. *Clin Orthop Relat Res.* 2002;403:87–92.

40. Weishaupt D, Zanetti M, Nyffeler RW, et al. Posterior glenoid rim deficiency in recurrent (atraumatic) posterior shoulder instability. *Skeletal Radiol.* 2000;29:204–210.

41. Fronek J, Warren RF, Bowen M. Posterior subluxation of the glenohumeral joint. *J Bone Joint Surg Am.* 1989;71: 205–216.

42. Lippitt S, Matsen F. Mechanisms of glenohumeral joint stability. *Clin Orthop Relat Res.* 1993;291:20–28.

43. Warner JJ, Micheli LJ, Arslanian LE, et al. Scapulothoracic motion in normal shoulders and shoulders with glenohumeral instability and impingement syndrome. A study using Moire topographic analysis. *Clin Orthop Relat Res.* 1992;285:191–199.

44. Kao JT, Pink M, Jobe FW, et al. Electromyographic analysis of the scapular muscles during a golf swing. *Am J Sports Med.* 1995;23:19–23.

45. Hovis WD, Dean MT, Mallon WJ, et al. Posterior instability of the shoulder with secondary impingement in elite golfers. *Am J Sports Med.* 2002;30:886–890.

46. Warner JJ, Navarro RA. Serratus anterior dysfunction. Recognition and treatment. *Clin Ortho Rel Res.* 1998;349: 139–148.

47. Rowe CR, Zarins B. Chronic unreduced dislocations of the shoulder. *J Bone Joint Surg Am.* 1982;64:494–505.

48. Provencher MT, Bell SJ, Menzel KA, et al. Arthroscopic treatment of posterior shoulder instability: Results in 33 patients. *Am J Sports Med.* 2005;33:1463–1471.

49. Yeargan SA 3rd, Briggs KK, Horan MP, et al. Determinants of patient satisfaction following surgery for multidirectional instability. *Orthopedics.* 2008;31:647.

50. Dimon JH 3rd. Posterior dislocation and posterior fracture dislocation of the shoulder: A report of 25 cases. *South Med J.* 1967;60:661–666.

51. Millett PJ, Clavert P, Hatch GF 3rd, et al. Recurrent posterior shoulder instability. *J Am Acad Orthop Surg.* 2006;14:464–476.

52. Kim SH, Park JS, Jeong WK, et al. The Kim test: A novel test for posteroinferior labral lesion of the shoulder–a comparison to the jerk test. *Am J Sports Med.* 2005;33: 1188–1192.

53. Harish S, Nagar A, Moro J, et al. Imaging findings in posterior instability of the shoulder. *Skeletal Radiol.* 2008;37:693–707.

54. Oh CH, Schweitzer ME, Spettell CM. Internal derangements of the shoulder: Decision tree and cost-effectiveness analysis of conventional arthrography, conventional MRI, and MR arthrography. *Skeletal Radiol.* 1999;28: 670–678.

55. McFarland EG, Kim TK, Park HB, et al. The effect of variation in definition on the diagnosis of multidirectional instability of the shoulder. *J Bone Joint Surg Am.* 2003;85:2138–2144.

56. Kuhn JE. A new classification system for shoulder instability. *Br J Sports Med.* 2010;44:341–346.

57. Rowe CR, Pierce DS, Clark JG. Voluntary dislocation of the shoulder. A preliminary report on a clinical, electromyographic, and psychiatric study of twenty-six patients. *J Bone Joint Surg Am.* 1973;55:445–460.

58. Pande P, Hawkins R, Peat M. Electromyography in voluntary posterior instability of the shoulder. *Am J Sports Med.* 1989;17:644–648.

59. Burkhead WZ Jr., Rockwood CA Jr. Treatment of instability of the shoulder with an exercise program. *J Bone Joint Surg Am.* 1992;74:890–896.

60. Bradley JP, Baker CL 3rd, Kline AJ, et al. Arthroscopic capsulolabral reconstruction for posterior instability of the shoulder: A prospective study of 100 shoulders. *Am J Sports Med.* 2006;34:1061–1071.

61. Cheatham SA, Mair SD. Arthroscopic technique for the evaluation and treatment of posterior shoulder instability. *Orthopedics.* 2009;32:194.

62. Kim SH, Ha KI, Park JH, et al. Arthroscopic posterior labral repair and capsular shift for traumatic unidirectional recurrent posterior subluxation of the shoulder. *J Bone Joint Surg Am.* 2003;85:1479–1487.

63. McIntyre LF, Caspari RB, Savoie FH 3rd. The arthroscopic treatment of posterior shoulder instability: Two-year results of a multiple suture technique. *Arthroscopy.* 1997; 13:426–432.

64. Misamore GW, Facibene WA. Posterior capsulorrhaphy for the treatment of traumatic recurrent posterior subluxations of the shoulder in athletes. *J Shoulder Elbow Surg.* 2000;9:403–408.

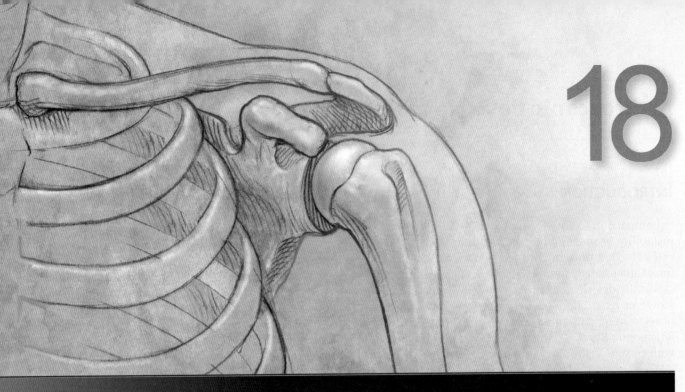

TECHNIQUE FOR POSTERIOR STABILIZATION

Although much less common than its anterior counterpart, posterior instability of the shoulder can be a disabling condition in the athletic population. It also typically has a much more subtle presentation when compared to anterior instability. Patients with posterior instability often present with diffuse pain and without distinct injury as opposed to patients with anterior instability who will complain of frank instability or the shoulder popping out of the joint. Despite modern advances in arthroscopic shoulder surgery, there are still indications to perform open procedures for recurrent posterior instability, particularly when associated with bony pathology. The following chapters will address both arthroscopic and open techniques for the treatment of recurrent posterior instability, including the indications, techniques, and results.

Arthroscopic Posterior Stabilization

James P. Bradley / Sam G. Tejwani

Introduction

In comparison to anterior shoulder instability, posterior instability is uncommon, occurring in 2% to 10% of cases (1–5). A posteriorly directed blow to an adducted, internally rotated, and forward flexed upper extremity is classically described as the sentinel traumatic event (6). However, recurrent or locked posterior shoulder dislocations from macrotrauma are exceedingly rare in the athletic population (2,7). Instead, athletes typically present with posterior shoulder instability secondary to repeti-tive microtrauma, which can occur in multiple arm positions and under a variety of loading conditions. In 1952, McLaughlin (2) first acknowledged the existence of a wide clinical spectrum of posterior shoulder insta-bility, ranging from locked posterior dislocation to the often subclinical recurrent posterior subluxation (RPS).

In athletics, RPS has been observed in weight lift-ers, football lineman, golfers, tennis players, butterfly and freestyle swimmers, overhead throwers and base-ball hitters, among others (8–10). The etiology of RPS is repetitive microtrauma, most commonly leading to posterior capsular attenuation and labral tear (Fig. 18-1).

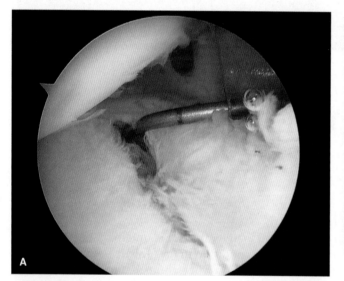

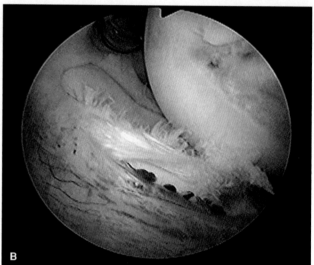

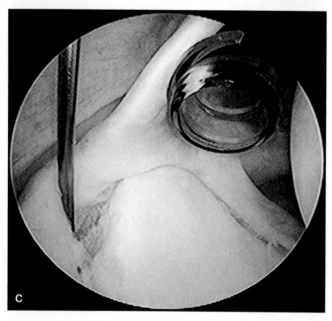

▲ **Figure 18-1:** Labral tears. **A:** Posterior labral tear from the glenoid (right shoulder, viewed from the anterior portal). **B:** Posterior labral splitting and tear (right shoulder, viewed from the posterior portal). Placing the patient in the lateral decubitus position facilitates posterior labral visualization and repair. **C:** Com-plete detachment of the posterosuperior labrum from the glenoid in an overhead thrower, as localized by the spinal needle (right shoulder, viewed from the posterior portal).

Regardless of the sport, athletes with RPS often present with ambiguous complaints of diffuse pain and shoulder fatigue, without distinct injury, often making it challenging to elucidate the underlying pathology and diagnosis.

A thorough history and physical examination, coupled with specific imaging studies, are required to determine the exact pathogenesis of and appropriate treatment options for RPS. With increased clinical awareness, imaging advances such as the magnetic resonance arthrogram (MRA), and the development of specific provocative physical examination tests, the identification of RPS in the athletic population is improving. Several variables which must be considered during the workup include mechanism of injury (true posterior traumatic dislocation vs. repetitive microtrauma vs. an acute or chronic subluxation), specific direction of instability (posterior vs. posteroinferior or posterosuperior), and the pattern of instability (unidirectional or multidirectional), as these factors will ultimately affect treatment and outcome (11).

Successful treatment of RPS begins with thorough identification of all of the structural abnormalities present in the affected shoulder, which can include any combination of the labrum, capsule, supporting ligaments, and rotator cuff. Over time, posterior glenohumeral stabilization has evolved from various open procedures to an anatomic-based arthroscopic approach, which allows for enhanced identification and repair of intra-articular pathology including posterior capsular laxity, complete or incomplete detachment of the posterior capsulolabral complex, and inferior capsular tears (12). While postoperative results are generally good to excellent after stabilization for RPS, there is room for improvement. Accordingly, research continues on both the biomechanical and clinical fronts to further refine our diagnostic and treatment approaches to RPS.

HISTORY AND PHYSICAL EXAMINATION

Thorough knowledge of an athlete's sport, position, and training regimen is critical in deducing the pathogenesis and specific pathology associated with RPS. Based on this information, treatment options may ultimately include labral debridement, labral repair, posterior capsular release, or posterior capsular plication. Pollock and Bigliani (13) noted that two-thirds of athletes who ultimately required surgery presented with complaints of difficulty using the shoulder outside of sports, particularly with arm above the horizontal. An inquiry should also be made regarding mechanical symptoms, as one study found that 90% of patients with symptomatic RPS noted clicking or crepitation with motion (14). Often times this crepitus can be reproduced during examination, and is due to discrete posterior capsulolabral pathology.

Physical examination of a shoulder suspected of RPS begins with inspection, focusing on asymmetry, scapular dysrhythmia, and muscular atrophy. A skin dimple over the posteromedial deltoid of both shoulders has been found to be 62% sensitive and 92% specific in correlating with posterior instability (15). Tenderness to palpation as a result of inflammation is next assessed at the posterior glenohumeral joint line, greater tuberosity, and biceps tendon. A majority of patients with posterior instability have been found to have posterior joint line tenderness, likely due to posterior synovitis or posterior rotator cuff tendinosis secondary to multiple episodes of instability (13).

Standard range of motion (ROM) of both shoulders is assessed, measuring forward elevation, abduction in the scapular plane, external rotation with the arm at the side and internal rotation behind the back to the highest vertebral level. With the patient supine, the arm is abducted 90 degrees, the scapula stabilized, and internal and external glenohumeral rotations are measured. These supine measurements are compared to the contralateral shoulder and are used to calculate total arc of rotation and glenohumeral internal rotation deficit (GIRD).

Strength testing is performed bilaterally, with a focus on the rotator cuff musculature. Glenohumeral stability is assessed on both shoulders with the patient supine, and the differences between the two are documented. The "Load and Shift" maneuver is performed with the arm held in 90 degrees of abduction and neutral rotation (16). In this position, a moderate axial load is applied to the glenohumeral joint in combination first with an anterior force in an attempt to translate the humeral head over the anterior glenoid rim. The test is repeated with a posterior-directed force (Fig. 18-2). Anterior and posterior laxity is quantified as 0 for a humeral head that does not translate to the glenoid rim, 1+ for a humeral head that translates to but does not

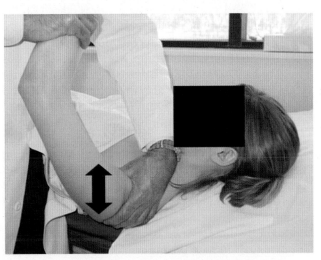

▲ **FIGURE 18-2:** The "load and shift" test is performed to assess anterior and posterior glenohumeral stabilities.

translate over the glenoid rim, 2+ for a humeral head that translates over the glenoid rim, but spontaneously reduces, and 3+ for a humeral head that translates over the glenoid rim and does not spontaneously reduce.

To assess for excessive inferior laxity, a "sulcus" test is performed by applying longitudinal traction with the arm adducted and in neutral rotation, with the patient seated. The test is repeated in 30 degrees of external rotation. Laxity is quantified as 1+ for an acromiohumeral distance <1 cm, 2+ for an acromiohumeral distance between 1 and 2 cm, or 3+ for an acromiohumeral distance >2 cm. A 3+ "sulcus sign" that remains 2+ or greater in 30 degrees of external rotation is considered pathognomonic for multidirectional instability (MDI). The implications of a patient who has RPS and concomitant MDI pertain to the potential need to address the rotator interval and superior glenohumeral ligament, as well as the posterior capsulolabral complex, for successful glenohumeral stabilization. Generalized ligamentous laxity may also contribute to MDI and thus should be graded on the 9-point Beighton scale, with a score of 5 or higher indicating ligamentous laxity (17).

A number of specialized tests have been devised to further elucidate capsulolabral pathology in the shoulder. The Jerk test is used to assess posterior stability in the seated position. The medial border of the scapula is stabilized with one hand, and the other hand applies a posteriorly directed force to the 90 degree forward flexed, adducted, and internally rotated arm. The test is positive if posterior subluxation or dislocation of the humeral head occurs while simultaneously reproducing the symptoms of pain and apprehension; variable sensitivity of the Jerk test has been reported (7,18,19).

The Kim test can also aid in the diagnosis of posterior and posteroinferior shoulder instability (20). With the patient seated, the arm is placed 90 degrees of abduction in the scapular plane and an axial load is applied. The arm is subsequently forward elevated an additional 45 degrees, and a posteroinferior vector is placed on the glenohumeral joint. Kim et al. concluded the test is positive with a sudden onset of posterior subluxation with pain. This test, in combination with the Jerk test, was found to be 97% sensitive in detecting a posteroinferior labral lesion. The authors also found that patients who experienced pain with the Kim test were more likely to require operative intervention to alleviate their symptoms than those who did not experience pain.

The Circumduction test is particularly useful in higher grades of chronic posterior instability, and is performed with the patient seated. With the elbow in full extension, the arm is brought into 90 degrees of forward elevation and slight adduction. Similar to the Jerk test, a posteriorly directed load is applied, which subluxates, or possibly dislocates, the humeral head posteriorly. The arm is then circumducted with a combination of abduction and extension until the head reduces into the glenoid. A positive test is a palpable, and typically audible, clunk as the posteriorly displaced head reduces into the glenoid. In patients with chronic posterior instability this test can often be performed without pain or muscle guarding.

In some cases of RPS, particularly involving overhead throwers, a posterior labral tear is associated with a superior labral tear, resulting in the Type VIII Superior Labrum Anterior to Posterior (SLAP) tear (21). Accordingly, when examining a shoulder suspected of RPS, the Obrien's test for superior labral pathology should also be performed. For this test, the patient is seated and the arm is forward elevated 90 degrees, adducted 10 degrees, and internally rotated with the elbow extended. A downward force is placed on the arm. A positive test is confirmed when pain elicited in this position does not occur in the same position with the arm externally rotated and the same force applied.

Impingement signs may also be positive in patients with RPS, and should be sought during physical examination. It is believed that the stress-related changes that can occur in the posterior rotator cuff can manifest as a secondary impingement syndrome in some cases, if severe enough, potentially warranting treatment.

IMAGING

Three radiographs of the shoulder are routinely obtained for the workup of RPS: (1) an anteroposterior (AP) view in the plane of the scapula, (2) an axillary view, and (3) a scapular Y lateral view. In most patients with RPS radiographic images are normal, although in some cases a posterior glenoid lesion or impaction of anterior humeral head (Reverse Hill–Sachs lesion) can be visualized. In rare instances, a fracture of the lesser tuberosity will give evidence to a previous posterior dislocation (22). In addition, the West Point radiographic view can be useful for detecting fractures of the glenoid rim or subtle ectopic bone formation around the glenoid (23,24).

MRA is the most sensitive diagnostic test for identifying lesions of the posterior labrum and capsule (25). Specific MRA findings indicative of posterior shoulder instability include posterior translation of the humeral head relative to the glenoid, posterior labrocapsular avulsion, posterior labral tear or splitting, discrete posterior capsular tears or rents, reverse humeral avulsion of the glenohumeral ligaments (HAGL), posterior labrum periosteal sleeve avulsion (POLPSA), and subscapularis tendon avulsion (Fig. 18-3) (26,27). The Kim classification is used to specifically describe posterior labral tear morphology: Type I, incomplete detachment; Type II (the "Kim Lesion"), a concealed complete detachment; Type III, chondrolabral erosion; and Type IV, flap tear of the posteroinferior labrum (Fig. 18-4) (28). The Kim lesion appears arthroscopically as a crack at the junction of the posteroinferior glenoid articular cartilage and labrum, through which a complete detachment of the

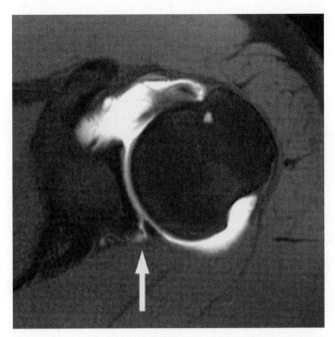

▲ **FIGURE 18-3:** Axial MRI arthrogram image (left shoulder) demonstrating a posterior capsulolabral avulsion from the glenoid with associated posterior translation of the humeral head relative to the glenoid (*arrow*).

deeper labrum from the glenoid rim can be identified (Fig. 18-4B).

In a further work by Kim et al. (29), 33 shoulders with atraumatic posterior instability were studied with MRA to examine chondrolabral changes. In comparison to age-matched normal shoulders, the affected shoulders had a glenoid that was shallower, with more osseous and chondrolabral retroversions present in the middle and inferior glenoids (Fig. 18-5). The study was not able to determine whether these changes were etiologic or pathologic, but nonetheless they should be sought when diagnosing posterior instability of the shoulder. Similar findings were presented in a 2006 study by Bradley et al., in which MRA of 48 shoulders with RPS revealed increased chondrolabral retroversion (10.7 degrees vs. 5.5 degrees) and increased glenoid bony retroversion (7.1 degrees vs. 3.5 degrees) in comparison to controls (8). More recent data by Bradley et al. has revealed that 16 baseball pitchers with RPS examined with MRA had even higher chondrolabral retroversion (11.5 degrees) and glenoid bony retroversion (8.4 degrees) (30). In addition, Tung and Hou (25) found that in 24 patients with RPS, MRA revealed more posterior humeral head

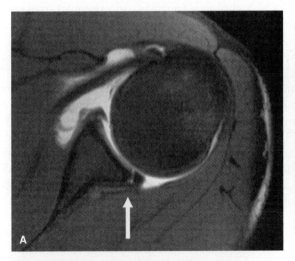

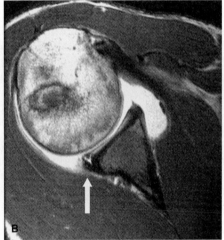

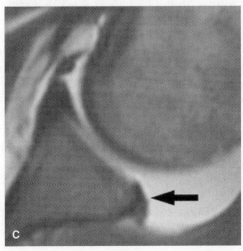

▲ **FIGURE 18-4:** Kim Lesions. **A:** Axial MRI arthrogram image (left shoulder) demonstrating a Type I Kim Lesion: Posterior chondrolabral fissure without displacement (*arrow*). **B:** Axial MRI arthrogram image (right shoulder) demonstrating a Type II Kim Lesion: A concealed complete detachment of the posterior labrum from the glenoid (*arrow*). **C:** Axial MRI arthrogram image (left shoulder) demonstrating a Type III Kim Lesion: Posterior chondrolabral erosion with loss of contour (*arrow*).

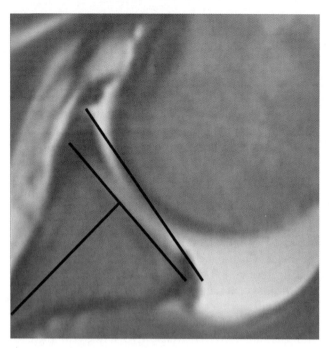

▲ **FIGURE 18-5:** Axial MRI arthrogram image (left shoulder) demonstrating the technique used to measure the degree of chondrolabral retroversion, which can be increased in patients with recurrent posterior subluxation of the shoulder.

translation, posterior labral tears, and posterior labrocapsular avulsions when compared to normal controls.

As a supplementary test, dynamic MRA can be performed to demonstrate labral "peel back" in the ABER position, which is consistent with posterosuperior labral tear (31). This finding has been most commonly seen in the overhead thrower, who often presents with concomitant posterior and superior labral tears in the Type VIII SLAP morphology. Last, in our practice the use of CT is limited to cases where a significant amount of bony glenoid retroversion is suspected, and an accurate measurement is desired when considering operative intervention.

NONOPERATIVE TREATMENT

A variety of operative and nonoperative treatment methods for posterior shoulder instability have been described. Rehabilitation with an emphasis on strengthening the rotator cuff, posterior deltoid, and periscapular muscles is frequently the first line of treatment and may allow an athlete to return to the preinjury level of sport (7,13,32–36). It is recommended to maintain this physical therapy protocol for a minimum of 6 months in order to decrease an athlete's functional disability. Previous studies have reported subjective improvement in up to 70% of athletes with this protocol. Objectively, the RPS is typically not completely eliminated, but the functional disability during athletics is improved sufficiently to allow participation in sport without signifi-

cant problem. If an athlete is not able to return to the preinjury level of competition, operative treatment is a reasonable option (37,38). Therapy has traditionally been more effective in those patients who have an atraumatic cause of RPS, as opposed to those with generalized ligamentous laxity or who have suffered a discrete traumatic event (32,34).

SURGICAL TREATMENT

Many operative procedures have been described for the treatment of posterior instability. Overall, the results of surgical treatment of posterior instability have been less consistent compared with those for anterior instability, particularly in the overhead thrower (37,39,40). While in general there is a relative paucity of clinical data on attempted posterior shoulder stabilization, the last decade has produced multiple noteworthy studies. Overall, there has been a trend from open to arthroscopic repair, and from nonanatomic to anatomic reconstruction. However, there are multiple confounding variables that make the literature difficult to compare, including differing causes of instability (RPS vs. traumatic dislocation), patterns of instability (unidirectional posterior vs. MDI), surgical techniques (open vs. arthroscopic), patient populations (athletic vs. nonathletic, throwers vs. nonthrowers), postoperative rehabilitation protocols, postoperative functional demands (return to work, sport, or neither), and definitions of clinical success and failure.

Historically, multiple open procedures for posterior shoulder stabilization have been performed, involving patients of wide demographics, variable patterns of instability, and differing levels of athletic competition. These have included the reverse Putti–Platt procedure, biceps tendon transfer, subscapularis transfer, infraspinatus advancement, posterior opening glenoid wedge osteotomy, proximal humeral rotational osteotomy, bone block augmentation of the posterior glenoid or acromion, posterior staple capsulorrhaphy, allograft reconstruction, capsulolabral reconstruction, and open capsular shift (2,32,36,37,40–52). Results have been variable and morbidity can be notable depending on the procedure and surgical exposure.

Due to interest in minimizing iatrogenic surgical trauma, arthroscopic techniques have been implemented with gaining popularity for the treatment of shoulder instability. Arthroscopic thermal capsulorrhaphy has been used in the treatment of shoulder instability with mixed results. Bisson (53) presented results of 14 shoulders with unidirectional posterior instability without labral detachment, which were treated with thermal capsulorrhaphy; 3 patients (21%) were found to have failure at 2-year follow-up. D'Alessandro et al. (54) found that 37% of patients who underwent thermal capsulorrhaphy for anterior, anteroinferior, or multidirectional shoulder instability had unsatisfactory results based on American Shoulder and Elbow Surgeons (ASES) scores, at 2- to 5-year follow-up, lending additional skepticism to the reliability of this surgical technique. Miniaci and McBirnie (55) presented similar disappointing results in another study of 19 shoulders with MDI treated with thermal capsulorrhaphy, in which 9 patients (47%) had recurrent instability at an average of 9 months postoperative, 5 patients (26%) had stiffness, and 4 patients (21%) had neurologic complications. Accordingly, we presently do not advocate thermal capsulorrhaphy for the treatment of RPS, due to the variable response patients have demonstrated to thermal energy.

Over time there has been an evolution to arthroscopic capsulolabral repair for RPS, which is an anatomic and minimally invasive procedure, and our preferred method of treatment. Our indications for surgery include failure of 6 or more months of physical therapy, large labral tear on MRA, chondrolabral retroversion of greater than 10 degrees, reverse HAGL or discrete posterior capsular tear, or an inability to return to sport or activity at preinjury level.

ARTHROSCOPIC POSTERIOR SHOULDER STABILIZATION: SURGICAL TECHNIQUE

Setup and Examination Under Anesthesia

Arthroscopic posterior shoulder stabilization is performed under general anesthesia, with an optional interscalene block performed perioperatively to optimize postoperative pain control. After intubation, examination under anesthesia (EUA) is performed on the affected and contralateral shoulder with the patient in the supine position on the operating table. Particular attention is paid to measurements of anterior, posterior, and inferior glenohumeral translations utilizing the "Load and Shift" and "sulcus" tests, as previously described. Our preference is then to place the patient on a beanbag in the lateral decubitus position, with the affected shoulder oriented superior. The operative shoulder is placed in 4.53 kg (10 lb) of longitudinal traction with a shoulder holder and positioned in 45 degrees of abduction and 20 degrees of forward flexion. This position displaces the humeral head anteriorly and inferiorly, bringing the posterior labrum into clear, unobstructed view (Fig. 18-1B).

Portal Creation and Diagnostic Arthroscopy

Arthroscopic posterior labral repair is performed using a two-portal technique. Sterile saline is injected into the joint to facilitate safe insertion of the arthroscope cannula and blunt trochar.

Location of the posterior portal for posterior stabilization is critical in order to properly establish access to the posterior glenoid rim for labral preparation and repair. The posterior portal is created in a "modified" location, approximately 1 cm distal and 1 cm lateral to a standard posterior portal; this allows an advantageous trajectory of instruments toward the posterior glenoid rim. Difficulty in the placement of suture anchors and the use of suture passers can be encountered if the posterior portal is located too far superior or medial in the posterior capsule. The conventional posterior portal is located near the 10-o'clock position on the right glenoid, which makes approach to the posteroinferior glenoid difficult for the placement of suture anchors. A spinal needle is used to localize the modified posterior portal at the 7-o'clock position on the glenoid rim in a right shoulder, approximately 1 to 2 cm lateral to the glenoid rim. Cadaveric study has shown the 7-o'clock portal to be located at a safe distance from the axillary nerve and posterior humeral circumflex artery (39 ± 4 mm), and the suprascapular nerve and artery (29 ± 3 mm) (56). In the event that the posterior portal has been made too far superior or medial, a supplementary posterior portal is made further inferior and lateral to the existing posterior portal.

A 30-degree arthroscope is introduced into the glenohumeral joint via the posterior portal and systematic diagnostic arthroscopy is performed. To best visualize and address the posterior structures the arthroscope is switched to the anterior portal. Typical pathology associated with posterior instability includes posterior labral fraying and splitting, posterior labral detachment from the glenoid rim, a patulous posterior capsule, discrete posterior capsular tear, undersurface partial-thickness rotator cuff tears, and widening of the rotator interval (Fig. 18-6). The surgeon must also be cognizant of the

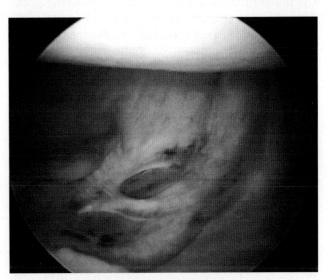

▲ **FIGURE 18-6:** A discrete posterior capsular tear in an athlete with recurrent posterior subluxation of the shoulder (right shoulder, viewed from the anterior portal).

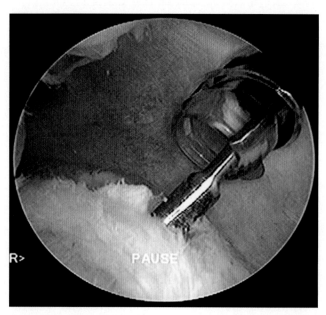

▲ **FIGURE 18-7:** An arthroscopic chisel used to elevate the torn labrum, which is scarred medially, away from the glenoid rim. In this case, a split in the labrum is used to access the scarred tissue (right shoulder, viewed from the anterior portal).

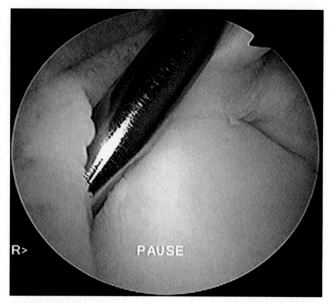

▲ **FIGURE 18-8:** A motorized shaver is used at the posterosuperior extent of the labral tear to decorticate the glenoid rim and abrade the labral undersurface (right shoulder, viewed from the posterior portal). To complete the abrasion posteroinferiorly, the shaver is switched to the posterior portal and the arthroscope is placed in the anterior portal.

subtle "Kim Lesion"—a concealed incomplete detachment of the posterior labrum (28).

A switching stick is used to replace the posterior metallic arthroscope cannula with an 8.25-mm diameter threaded clear plastic cannula (Arthrex Inc., Naples, FL), in either 7- or 9-cm lengths, depending on the musculature girth of the patient. This cannula allows unobstructed passage of the required arthroscopic drill guide and 45-degree angled or curved suture passers for work on the labrum and the capsule.

Labral Preparation

The posterior labrum is visualized from both the posterior and anterior portals to appreciate the full extent of the tear. The arthroscope then remains in the anterior portal and the posterior portal serves as the working portal for the repair. An arthroscopic chisel is first used to elevate the torn labrum, which is often scarred medially, away from the glenoid rim, throughout the entire extent of the tear (Fig. 18-7). An angled rasp or motorized shaver is then used to decorticate the glenoid rim and abrade the labral undersurface in order to remove scar tissue and achieve a vascularized surface for healing (Fig. 18-8). Debridement of the labrum with an arthroscopic shaver is limited to only those portions involving free flaps of tissue or extensive fraying, as the goal is to preserve as much tissue as possible for incorporation into the repair.

Labral Repair

The posterior labrum is repaired to the glenoid rim with suture anchors. We typically use the 2.4-mm Biocomposite Suture-Tak anchor (Arthrex Inc., Naples, FL),

which is single loaded with a no. 2 FiberWire suture and has been found to have equivalent pull-out strength to the 3- and 3.7-mm anchors with the same design. Multiple similar anchors are commercially available. The anchors should be placed on the chondral rim of the glenoid, as opposed to on the glenoid neck, thereby enabling labral tissue to be repaired in an anatomic position on the glenoid face. An offset drill guide for this specific purpose is commercially available (Arthrex Inc., Naples, FL), and allows the guide to be securely positioned on the rim of the glenoid while simultaneously directing the drill onto the chondral surface (Fig. 18-9). During placement of the suture anchor, care must be taken to avoid inadvertent injury to the articular cartilage; this typically occurs with a low, tangential drilling angle (<30 degrees) and can be avoided by a properly placed posterior portal which allows a higher angle (>30 degrees) of approach to the glenoid rim. Suture anchors are placed along the posterior glenoid rim in an inferior-to-superior direction, and the labrum is secured to the articular margin to restore the length–tension relationship of the posterior band of the inferior glenohumeral ligament (IGHL).

The number of suture anchors utilized is dependent on the size of the labral tear. The o'clock nomenclature is used to describe the location and the extent of labral tear. For example, a posterior labral tear extending from the 6-o'clock to the 9-o'clock position in a right shoulder is typically repaired with suture anchors at the 6:30, 7:30, 8:30, and 9:30 positions. The first anchor is typically placed more superiorly than the inferior extent of the tear, in order to perform a superior shift of the

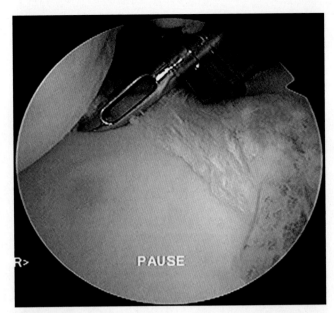

▲ **FIGURE 18-9:** An offset drill guide is used to place the suture anchor directly on the border of glenoid face (right shoulder, viewed from the anterior portal). The most inferior anchor is placed first. The advantageous position of the 7-o'clock portal and working cannula is appreciated in relation to the location of the posterior labral tear and the required approach to the repair.

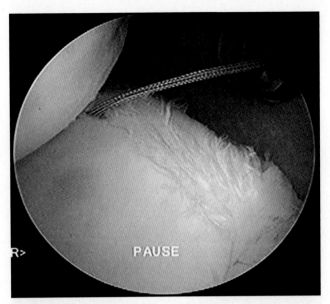

▲ **FIGURE 18-10:** The first suture anchor is placed on the glenoid face. The two suture limbs are visualized exiting the anchor (right shoulder, viewed from the anterior portal).

capsulolabral complex concomitantly. Thus, in this scenario the first anchor would be placed at the 6:30 position to advance the labral tissue from the 6-o'clock position. Advancing the suture passer in this fashion restores tension in the posterior band of the IGHL, which is necessary to restore posterior stability.

Upon insertion, the suture anchor is rotated to orient the sutures perpendicular to the glenoid rim to facilitate passage of the most posterior suture through the torn labrum; this suture will be used as the post for the arthroscopic knot to be tied later, thus allowing the knot to be positioned away from the chondral surfaces of the glenoid and the humeral head (Fig. 18-10). This knot position is selected in an attempt to minimize postoperative iatrogenic chondral injury from knot abrasion.

Following placement of the first suture anchor, one of a number of commercially available suture passers can be used to shuttle one limb of the no. 2 FiberWire suture around the labrum to be repaired (Fig. 18-11). The suture passer is passed through the labral tissue beginning posteriorly and exits at the edge of the glenoid articular surface at the level of the suture anchor.

When using the Spectrum, the PDS is then fed into the glenohumeral joint and the suture passer is withdrawn through the posterior cannula. While withdrawing the suture passer from the posterior cannula, additional suture is advanced into the joint to prevent inadvertently pulling the PDS back through the torn edge of the labrum. An arthroscopic suture grasper is used to withdraw both the most posterior no. 2 Fiber-Wire suture from the suture anchor and the end of the

PDS suture that has been advanced through the torn labrum. The PDS is then fashioned into a single loop and tightly tied over the FiberWire, approximately 5 cm from the end. By pulling on the other end of the PDS suture, the more posterior FiberWire suture from the suture anchor is shuttled behind the labral tear. At this point, with one suture limb on either side of the torn labrum, our preference is to tie a sliding–locking arthroscopic Weston knot to begin the repair; multiple alternative knots can be utilized. Of utmost importance is the surgeon's familiarity and proficiency with the

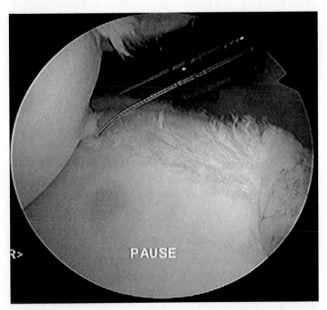

▲ **FIGURE 18-11:** Using a suture passing technique, one limb of the suture from the suture anchor is shuttled around the posterior labrum (right shoulder, viewed from the anterior portal). Additional anchors are placed superiorly to complete the repair.

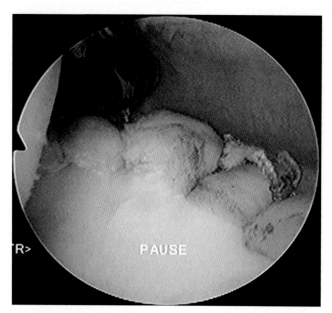

▲ **FIGURE 18-12:** Completed repair of the posterior labrum (right shoulder, viewed from the anterior portal).

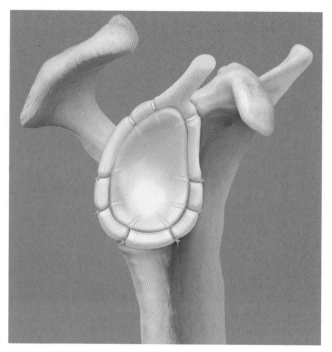

▲ **FIGURE 18-13:** Knotless anchors used for labral repair above the "horizontal equator" of the glenoid (right shoulder), to minimize irritation of the biceps tendon from knot abrasion. Traditional suture anchors are used below the horizontal equator. [Courtesy of Arthrex Inc., Naples, FL]

knot technique, whichever selected. The posterior suture limb serves as the post, which in effect will advance the labrum to the glenoid rim when the knot is tightened. As stated, an emphasis should be made to secure the knot posteriorly and not on the rim of the glenoid to prevent humeral head abrasion from the knot.

Additional suture anchors are then placed in similar fashion to complete the labral repair. The labral tear at the 7-o'clock position is advanced to the 7:30 suture anchor, the 8-o'clock labral tear position is advanced to the 8:30 suture anchor, and the labral tear at 9-o'clock labral tear position is advanced to the 9:30 suture anchor (Fig. 18-12). In the case of the Type VIII SLAP tear, additional anchors are incrementally placed superiorly, up to the 12-o'clock or 1-o'clock position as indicated, in order to repair the associated superior labral tear (21). Recently, we have elected to use knotless anchors for labral repair above the "horizontal equator", or midpoint of the glenoid. This is done to minimize postoperative irritation of the biceps complex from knot abrasion, which can occur during circumduction and overhead activity (Fig. 18-13).

Upon completion of the capsulolabral repair, an arthroscopic awl is used to penetrate the bare area of the humeral head, under the infraspinatus tendon, in an effort to allow egress of stem cells and marrow elements into the intra-articular space to augment the healing response (21). Finally, the posterior capsular portal incision is closed by partially withdrawing the arthroscopic cannula, and passing a PDS suture through one side of the portal site with a crescent Spectrum suture passer and retrieving the suture through the other side of the portal with an arthroscopic penetrating suture grasper. Varying the distance that the penetrator is passed from

the border of the portal incision allows titration of the capsulorrhaphy performed with the closure. The PDS is then tied over the capsule, with care to taken to avoid incorporating the overlying musculature into the knot.

Labral Repair with Capsular Plication

The clinical history, EUA, MRA images, and arthroscopic findings regarding posterior capsular pathology dictate the specific type of capsular procedure performed in addition to the labral repair. Patients with acute injuries and minimal evidence of capsular stretching do not require the same degree of capsular advancement as those with more chronic instability or MDI. Based on these factors, the surgeon may consider capsular plication at the time of labral repair, or immediately after the labrum has been repaired.

When a patulous posterior capsule is observed at the onset of the procedure, this tissue is also abraded in preparation for a concomitant capsular plication using the sutures from the suture anchors. We have found this technique to have superior clinical results in comparison to the placement of independent plication sutures in the posterior capsule without suture anchors (8). Care should be taken in the use of the motorized shaver when abrading the posterior capsule, which is thin and can be easily penetrated with an overly aggressive technique; we typically favor the rasp for this purpose. In the setting of a labral tear with excessive posterior capsular laxity, the suture passer is advanced through the posterior capsule approximately 1 cm lateral to the edge of the labral tear and then is advanced as described previously, underneath the labral tear, to the edge of the articular cartilage, creating a "pleat stitch". Placing as many of these pleat stitches as necessary in the face of a patulous shoulder capsule will reduce the associated capsular redundancy while simultaneously repairing the torn labrum.

If the labrum has been repaired in isolated fashion initially, and then it is determined that the capsule requires further tension, suture capsulorrhaphy can be performed in the intervals between the suture anchors directly to the newly secured labrum. Knots are tied following passage of each suture approximately 1 cm lateral to the edge of the labral border. This allows continued assessment of the repair and the degree of the capsular shift achieved by each suture. Care must be taken with the sharp Spectrum suture passer tip to avoid cutting or placing undue tension on previously tied sutures from the suture anchors.

Isolated Capsular Plication

In some instances, patients with unidirectional posterior instability or primary posterior MDI do not have a posterior labral tear, but rather display only significant capsular laxity and capaciousness at arthroscopy. In this setting, an isolated posterior capsulorrhaphy is performed with suture anchors in a similar fashion as described above. For example, in a right shoulder suture anchors are typically placed beginning inferior (6:30), and progressing superior (9:30) incrementally, as indicated. Depending on the degree of capsular laxity present, the 1 cm 6-o'clock capsular pleat suture is typically advanced to the 6:30 position on the glenoid. This suture is tied, as described previously, and the reduction in capsular volume is assessed. Restoring adequate tension in the posterior band of the IGHL and capsule is critical to the success of the reconstruction. If necessary, a second 1-cm capsulorrhaphy pleat suture is placed at the 7-o'clock position on the capsule and advanced to the 7:30 position on the glenoid. Likewise, if indicated additional sutures are then placed at the 8-o'clock and 9-o'clock positions on the capsule, advancing to the 8:30 and 9:30 positions on the glenoid, respectively (8).

Labral Repair with Posterior Capsular Release

It has been observed, as previously discussed, that some overhead throwers such as baseball pitchers develop GIRD, which is associated with a posterior capsular contracture, in conjunction with a posterosuperior, or isolated posterior, labral tear. Accordingly, both elements of this pathology need to be addressed for alleviation of symptoms. Initially, we treat the GIRD with preoperative "Sleeper Stretches." In a majority of throwers this is successful; however, in rare cases the GIRD is recalci-

trant to stretching. In these scenarios, we first perform an arthroscopic posterior labral repair as described previously. Next, to treat the posterior capsular contracture and associated GIRD, we proceed with a limited arthroscopic posterior capsular release. This is performed with a thermal device, which is used to create a full-thickness incision in the posterior capsular tissue. The posterior capsular release is performed through a viewing portal anteriorly in the rotator interval, while working through the posterior portal. We begin approximately 5 mm away from the glenoid rim, at the 7-o'clock position (right shoulder), and progress superiorly with the thermal device to the 8-o'clock position, thereby incising the contracted posterior band of the IGHL. On rare occasion, we will extend this release slightly more superiorly, as indicated, based on the extent of the contracture.

Rotator Interval Closure

Biomechanical study has demonstrated that in the setting of unidirectional posterior shoulder instability, the rotator interval need not be addressed with closure to restore glenohumeral stability (57). However, in the setting of MDI with a primary posterior component, the rotator interval requires closure to restore stability. These patients are defined preoperatively by having a 2+ or greater sulcus sign that does not decrease in 30 degrees of external rotation. Rotator interval closure is performed through a working portal anteriorly in the rotator interval, viewed from an arthroscope in the posterior portal. The goal is to plicate the tissue between the supraspinatus and subscapularis tendons. Specifically, this requires suturing the anterior capsule, superior tissue of the rotator interval, and superior glenohumeral ligament (SGHL) to the anterior capsule and middle glenohumeral ligament (MGHL). The closure begins medially and is performed with a number-0 PDS suture, which is passed through the superior tissue with a Spectrum suture passer and retrieved with an arthroscopic penetrating grasper passed through the inferior tissue. A Weston knot is tied through the anterior cannula. Additional interrupted plication sutures are placed in a similar fashion progressing laterally, as needed, to complete the closure.

Postoperative Rehabilitation

At the conclusion of surgery the shoulder is placed in an Ultrasling (DonJoy, Carlsbad, CA) with an abduction pillow, which immobilizes the shoulder in 30 degrees of abduction and prevents internal rotation. A cryotherapy device is utilized for the first 3 postoperative days to minimize swelling and pain. The day after surgery, patients begin active ROM of the elbow, wrist, and fingers. At 1-week postoperative formal physical therapy for the shoulder is initiated, beginning with passive forward flexion and abduction in the scapular plane to 90 degrees. Over the subsequent 5 weeks, full passive ROM is achieved. At 6 weeks postoperative, the sling is discontinued and active-assisted ROM begins, progressing to full active ROM as able. Full active ROM should be achieved by 3 months postoperative. Strengthening of the rotator cuff, deltoid, and periscapular muscles begins at 2 to 3 months postoperative.

Once patients are able to achieve 80% of the strength of their contralateral shoulders, as measured by isokinetic testing, a sport-specific rehabilitation protocol is initiated. This typically takes place between 4 and 6 months postoperative. Athletes are cleared to return to sport when they demonstrate full ROM and strength, along with restoration of glenohumeral stability, typically between 6 and 9 months postoperative.

Throwing athletes require special consideration, and follow a specific protocol designed to monitor their throwing distance and speed, which is slowly advanced over 2 to 3 months. Initially, at 6 months postoperative, an easy tossing program is commenced at a distance of 6.09 m (20 ft), without a windup. Before each session, stretching and heat application is performed to increase circulation and improve ROM. At 7 months, light throwing with an easy windup at a distance of 9.14 m (30 ft) is allowed for 2 to 3 days per week, for 10 minutes per session. Easy throws from 45.72 to 60.96 m (from 150 to 200 ft) are permitted at 9 months postoperatively and stronger throws from the same distance are allowed at 10 months. Pitchers can throw half to three-quarters speed from the mound, with an emphasis on accuracy and technique, at 11 months. At 12 months, pitchers can throw at three-quarters to full speed. Throwers are released to full competition when they are able to throw at full speed without discomfort for 2 weeks, typically between 9 and 12 months postoperative.

Clinical Outcome

With expanding interested in minimally invasive surgical techniques, the 1990s produced the first successful accounts of arthroscopic posterior glenohumeral stabilization (58–60). In 1998, Wolf and Eakin (58) reported on 14 patients who had arthroscopic posterior capsular plication for unidirectional posterior instability; at 33-month follow-up 86% had good or excellent results and 93% had restoration of stability. With improvement in arthroscopic techniques and surgical implants, research has led to the evolution of suture-anchor-based arthroscopic posterior glenohumeral stabilization. Multiple recent studies have revealed a majority of good or excellent results, fueling interest in these methods.

Of specific interest are studies presenting data on arthroscopic stabilization for unidirectional posterior glenohumeral instability. Williams et al. (12) retrospectively reported on 27 shoulders with symptomatic

posterior capsulolabral complex detachment from the posterior glenoid rim, with minimal posterior capsular laxity, after a distinct traumatic event. Isolated arthroscopic posterior capsulolabral repair was performed with bioabsorbable tack fixation in all patients. Subjective instability and pain were eliminated in 92% of patients, with all of these patients returning to unlimited athletic activity by 6 months. Kim et al. (28) prospectively reported on 27 athletes with traumatic unidirectional RPS treated with arthroscopic posterior labral repair and capsular shift; all patients had a labral lesion, and 81% also had stretching of the posterior band of the IGHL. The posterior capsule was shifted superiorly in all cases. All complete labral lesions were repaired directly and incomplete labral lesions were converted to complete tears and then repaired. The mean ASES scores improved from 51.2 to 96.5. All but one patient had restoration of stability and was able to return to previous athletic activities with little or no limitations. Multiple additional studies between 12 and 34 shoulders have presented similar successful results for arthroscopic posterior stabilization, with recurrence rates between 0% and 12% at a minimum mean follow-up of 3 years (6,8,61–65).

In 2006, Bradley et al. (8) presented a prospective study on 91 athletes (100 shoulders) treated with arthroscopic capsulolabral reconstruction for posterior instability. At 27-month mean follow-up the mean ASES scores improved from 50.4 to 85.7, with 89% returning to sport and 67% returning to their same level as preoperative. Several potential reasons elucidated for the 11 failures included undiagnosed MDI, inadequate capsular shift due to unappreciated capsular laxity, inadequate recognition of poor capsular tissue quality in those patients referred after thermal capsulorrhaphy, and capsular plication performed in an isolated fashion without suture anchors. These conclusions led to further refinement of the surgical approach to posterior instability.

In 2008, Radkowski et al. (61) reported on arthroscopic capsulolabral repair for posterior shoulder instability in throwing athletes compared to nonthrowing athletes. At mean 27-month follow-up, there were no differences in the ASES score or scores for stability, ROM, strength, pain, and function between the 27 throwing shoulders and the 80 nonthrowing shoulders, with both groups showing significant improvement in all categories. Excellent or good results were achieved in 89% of throwers and 93% of nonthrowers. However, throwing athletes were less likely to return to the pre-injury level of sport (55%) compared to nonthrowing athletes (71%). Due to the relatively small patient population in this study, the authors had difficulty elucidating the reasoning for the lower rate of return to sport in throwers, although it was found that all of the three throwers who failed underwent capsulolabral repair without suture anchors. Based on the findings of this study, the authors presently advocate repair with suture anchors uniformly. Also, within the thrower group there were more athletes unable to return to their previous levels of sport than there were failures based on the subjective instability scale, suggesting it is possible that some of these athletes had lower levels of subjective instability but enough to keep them from returning the same high level of competition and the unique demands required from the shoulder during throwing activities.

In 2012, Lenart et al. reported 100% return to previous level of athletic activity for 34 shoulders which underwent arthroscopic repair for posterior shoulder instability. The majority (78%) had a traumatic event, but only 2 (6%) a frank dislocation, consistent with a population of RPS. Suture anchor repair was performed in 30 patients (88%) and capsular plication to an intact labrum in 4 (12%) (64). Wanich et al. (65), recently presented the results of arthroscopic treatment of posterior capsulolabral lesions in "Batter's shoulder," defined as posterior subluxation of the lead shoulder during a baseball swing. Eleven of twelve (92%) surgically treated patients returned to their previous level of batting at an average of 5.9 months after surgery, with no detectable ROM deficit compared to preoperatively.

In a continuation of their index study, Bradley et al. (8) recently presented novel prospective Level II data on 200 shoulders in athletes treated with arthroscopic capsulolabral repair for posterior instability, the largest such cohort to date in the literature (66). There were 99 contact athletes and 101 noncontact athletes included in the study. All patients had unidirectional posterior instability and failed a course of nonoperative management. Arthroscopy with suture anchor repair was the most common procedure performed ($n = 119$), followed by suture-only repair without anchors ($n = 44$) and suture anchor repair with supplementary plication sutures ($n = 37$). For 123 shoulders that were evaluated at a minimum follow-up of 2 years, mean ASES scores increased from 47 to 85.4. For the entire cohort of 200 shoulders, mean ASES scores increased from 46 to 85.1. Overall rate of return to sport was 90%, with shoulders treated with capsulolabral repair with suture anchors faring slightly better than shoulders treated with sutures only.

SUMMARY

Posterior shoulder instability poses significant challenges both diagnostically and therapeutically. It is a broad clinical entity, ranging from RPS to locked posterior dislocations. The pathogenesis varies tremendously, based upon the stressed placed on the involved shoulder. As opposed to a singular traumatic event, athletes with RPS typically suffer from chronic, repetitive microtrauma which leads to posterior labral tear, posterior capsular laxity, and symptoms. Overhead throwers are a unique patient population, often with a varied presentation which can include posterior capsular contracture and the Type VIII SLAP tear. Extensive basic science and clinical research is ongoing to elucidate a biomechanical explanation of the pathogenesis of RPS in throwers. Increased clinical awareness, as well as advances in imaging and physical examination techniques has improved diagnosis in athletes and patients from wide demographic presentations. Multiple distinct pathologic lesions can be identified on MRA in patients with RPS; these should be sought carefully during the workup of symptomatic patients. Likewise, specific provocative physical examination tests have been found to be useful in making the diagnosis of posterior shoulder instability.

Successful outcomes can be achieved with physical therapy, although many patients still require surgical intervention to alleviate symptoms and return to sport at their preinjury level. The transition from open to arthroscopic surgical techniques has facilitated more comprehensive identification and treatment of coexisting structural pathologies in RPS. For patients with unidirectional posterior instability, an arthroscopic repair of the capsulolabral complex is recommended. When a patulous posterior capsule or a posteroinferior component of instability is also present, an arthroscopic superiorly directed capsular shift and capsular plication is added. In throwers with RPS and a posterior labral tear, we advocate repairing the posterior labrum only, while treating excessive GIRD, if present, initially with preoperative "Sleeper Stretches," and, if recalcitrant, with a limited posterior capsular release at the time of surgery. In regard to addressing capsular pathology, we generally tend toward overtightening contact athletes and those with significant capsular laxity, and undertightening overhead throwers.

At midterm follow-up, promising success rates between 90% and 100% have been achieved with arthroscopic repair techniques, with generally lower results in throwers. Longer-term studies are necessary to evaluate the durability of arthroscopic techniques in the treatment of posterior glenohumeral instability. Further work is also needed to elucidate the complex mechanics of the elite thrower's shoulder, and the best path to alleviating the symptoms of RPS while simultaneously allowing return to sport at a preinjury level.

Open Posterior Stabilization

Corinne VanBeek / Matthew L. Ramsey

INTRODUCTION

Posterior glenohumeral instability manifesting as a dislocation or recurrent subluxation is a rare occurrence relative to its anterior counterpart. RPS is the most common form of posterior instability and represents the focus of this discussion. The pathoanatomy associated with recurrent posterior instability may involve the labrum, capsule, rotator interval, or the bony anatomy of the shoulder. If a nonoperative program does not improve the symptoms of instability, surgical intervention is considered. Numerous open and arthroscopic procedures have been described to address recurrent posterior instability, with satisfactory short- and medium-term outcomes (7,12,38,39,63,67). Despite modern advances in arthroscopic shoulder surgery, there are still indications to perform open procedures for recurrent posterior instability, particularly when associated with bony pathology. In this chapter, we present the techniques for open treatment of recurrent posterior instability, including the indications, techniques, and results.

PREOPERATIVE EVALUATION

Successful management of symptomatic recurrent posterior instability requires an accurate diagnosis established through a careful history, physical examination, and imaging studies. A thorough yet focused physical examination should aim to reproduce the patient's symptoms and define the character of instability. The patient's shoulder girdle should be inspected from the front and back, examining for atrophy, gross deformity, and dynamic abnormalities. A standard shoulder examination should include evaluation of active and passive ranges of motion, rotator cuff strength, and scapulothoracic kinematics. A careful neurovascular examination should look for abnormalities in circulation and any focal neurologic deficits that might contribute to instability. In addition, the cervical spine should be examined for its possible contribution to nerve-related abnormalities.

IMAGING STUDIES

Standard radiographs of the shoulder should be obtained and include a true AP view taken in the plane of the scapula, a lateral (scapular Y) view, and an axillary view. Attention should be directed at the axillary radiograph to determine the relationship of the humeral head to the glenoid vault. The radiographs should be further evaluated for evidence of calcification of the posterior capsule, fracture, or erosion of the posterior glenoid or reverse Hill–Sachs defects on the humeral head.

Advanced imaging studies need not be routinely used, but should be considered when the underlying pathologic lesion is in question. Magnetic resonance imaging (MRI) should be considered for documentation of any capsulolabral pathology (Fig. 18-14). MR arthrography is highly sensitive and specific for defining capsulolabral lesions and is preferred over standard MRI. Computed tomography (CT) is very useful for evaluating the osseous anatomy and is used to supplement plain radiographs (Fig. 18-15).

Advanced imaging affords more precise definition of bone and soft tissue pathologies. However, the clinician should be cautious not to use advanced imaging as a screening tool for poorly defined pathology. The history and physical examination must support the findings of advanced imaging modalities.

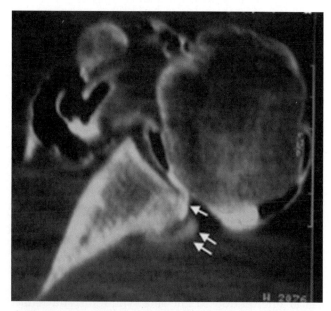

▲ **FIGURE 18-14:** Magnetic resonance arthrogram (MRA) demonstrating a posterior labral tear (*single arrow*) with associated bony fragment and calcification of the stripped posterior capsule (*double arrow*).

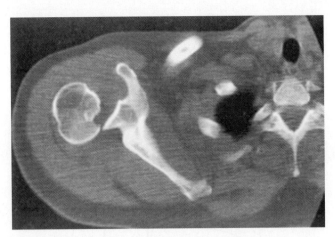

▲ FIGURE 18-15: A computed tomography (CT) scan image demonstrating a posterior glenohumeral dislocation associated with a large reverse Hill–Sachs lesion.

OPERATIVE MANAGEMENT: OVERVIEW

A variety of surgical procedures have been described for posterior instability. These procedures include posterior capsulorrhaphy with or without a bone block, posterior bone block alone, glenoid osteotomy, posterior infraspinatus capsular tenodesis, and posteroinferior capsular shift (47,48,51,68–75). Outcomes following these procedures have historically been very disappointing, with recurrence rates approaching 50% with high complication rates (7,76). These failures are, in part, due to the lack of recognition and understanding of the true pathologic lesion underlying the instability. Improved understanding of the pathologic lesions leading to posterior instability and the introduction of techniques that restore normal anatomy have led to improved results (32,77). It is imperative that the surgical procedure performed be dictated by the preoperatively defined etiology of the posterior instability, including both bony and soft tissue lesions.

In general, soft tissue contributions to posterior instability, such as an incompetent capsule or labrum, are better addressed arthroscopically. Arthroscopic treatment of posterior instability provides a global view of the glenohumeral joint, enabling anterior joint pathology to be identified and concomitantly treated, if necessary. Despite increasing enthusiasm in using the arthroscope to treat shoulder pathology, there still remains a role for open surgical reconstruction for posterior instability. Bony involvement frequently necessitates open surgical approaches to adequately manage the pathology and some consider it to be a contraindication to arthroscopic management. Since the mandate of this chapter is to discuss open surgical reconstruction, arthroscopic treatment will not be discussed further.

Acquired RPS is most often secondary to soft tissue incompetency, posterior glenoid deficiency, or scapulothoracic dyskinesis. A redundant posterior capsule is the primary pathologic lesion in the majority of cases. In the presence of a reverse Bankart lesion with a patulous posterior capsule, a combined repair of the reverse Bankart and posterior capsular plication or shift is necessary. When both posterior capsular redundancy and bony glenoid abnormalities (i.e., posterior glenoid erosion/fracture, increased glenoid retroversion) coexist, then posterior capsular plication must be combined with posterior glenoid bone grafting or posterior opening wedge osteotomy, respectively. In some instances posterior bone block may be indicated for failed capsular procedures, even in the absence of abnormalities of glenoid architecture.

In determining the appropriate surgical procedure, knowledge of the primary direction of instability is imperative. Patients with isolated posterior instability should have the associated patulous posterior capsule addressed. Frequently posterior subluxation is accompanied by some degree of inferior translation or MDI. In cases of posteroinferior subluxation with a competent rotator interval, a posteroinferior capsular shift from a posterior approach is necessary. When instability is multidirectional, the primary location of symptoms determines the surgical approach. If symptoms are focused to the posterior aspect of the shoulder, we prefer to approach these posteriorly and perform a posteroinferior capsular shift. If anterior symptoms predominate, then an anteroinferior capsular shift is performed. Combined anterior and posterior capsular procedures are necessary in the rare patient with true MDI with anterior and posterior symptoms.

Although outside the realm of this chapter, functional and pathologic abnormalities of scapulothoracic mechanics play a critical role in posterior instability. It is critical that scapulothoracic dyskinesia be treated before posterior instability is addressed surgically. Failure to do so will result in unsuccessful surgical management, whether performed open or arthroscopically. In the presence of scapular winging caused by long thoracic nerve injury, pectoralis major transfer possibly along with posterior capsulorrhaphy, may be indicated (78). Determining the need for a capsulorrhaphy in these situations is often difficult, but in most cases, muscle transfer alone is sufficient to alleviate the posterior instability symptoms.

Dysplasia of the glenoid or humerus are uncommon causes of recurrent posterior instability. In cases of glenoid hypoplasia or increased glenoid retroversion, a glenoid osteotomy may be appropriate (47). Humeral rotational osteotomy is performed only when abnormal humeral retrotorsion is the underlying cause of posterior instability (46). Shoulders with significant anteromedial humeral head defects (reverse Hill–Sachs lesion) may be indicated for a subscapularis transfer into the defect, bone grafting of the lesion, or humeral head replacement for defects greater than 30% to 40% the size of the humeral head articular surface (54,79). While eradicating the lesion with bone graft or replacement avoids further engagement of the glenoid with the lesion, a subscapularis transfer fills the lesion and also limits shoulder ROM to prevent contact with the glenoid.

OPERATIVE MANAGEMENT: OPEN SURGICAL TECHNIQUE

Patient Positioning

The lateral decubitus position is favored for this approach, with the patient secured with a beanbag and anterior and posterior body posts. The head and neck are stabilized in neutral position, and the hips and knees kept flexed. All bony prominences are padded, especially at the knees and ankles. Impervious drapes block out the surgical field, with one at the base of the neck and another around the axilla, medial to the vertebral border of the scapula and a minimum of 6 cm medial to the anterior axillary crease (Fig. 18-16). The arm is prepared and draped free, although an arm positioner (McConnell Orthopedic Manufacturing Co.; Greenville, TX) or Mayo stand may be used as supportive devices.

Surgical Approach

The incision begins at the spine of the scapula and extends distally to the posterior axillary fold (Fig. 18-17). Subcutaneous dissection is carried out to the inferior border of the posterior deltoid medially and laterally to the acromion. The posterior deltoid fibers are split in the portion of the deltoid overlying the posterior glenohumeral joint line, from the scapular spine distally for 4

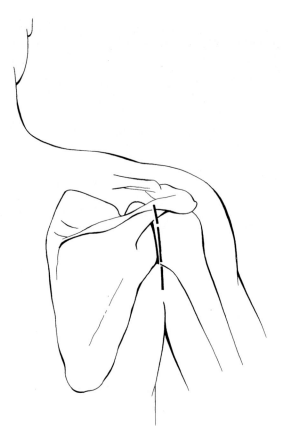

▲ **FIGURE 18-17:** The posterior approach to the shoulder uses a vertical incision extending from the spine of the scapula to the posterior axillary crease. (From Iannotti JP, Williams GR. *Disorders of the Shoulders.* 2nd ed. Philadelphia, PA: Lippincott Williams & Wilkins 2007, with permission.)

to 5 cm. With blunt dissection, the underlying infraspinatus and teres minor muscles are exposed (Fig. 18-18). Alternatively, the posterior deltoid can be elevated along its inferior margin to expose the infraspinatus and teres minor muscles (Fig. 18-19).

> **Technique Pearls:** Dissection to the subdeltoid space and abduction of the shoulder facilitate superior retraction of the posterior deltoid. Remain cognizant of the inferior border of the teres minor, as the quadrangular space containing the axillary nerve and posterior humeral circumflex vessels lie immediately inferior.

To obtain exposure to the posterior capsule, dissection occurs within the posterior fat stripe that separates the upper and lower portions of the infraspinatus muscle at the midequator of the glenohumeral joint (80,81).

> **Technique Pearls:** Use of the infraspinatus fat stripe places the operative field more central within the joint and thus facilitates better exposure of the superior portion of the joint. The infraspinatus insertion need not be detached during posterior capsulorrhaphy through this interval, and it is our preferred technique.

Once the capsule is reached, deep retractors are placed to facilitate exposure (Fig. 18-20). Dissection

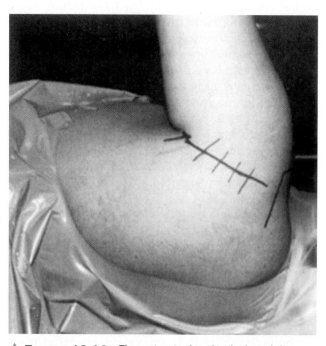

▲ **FIGURE 18-16:** The patient is placed in the lateral decubitus position and the shoulder is draped widely to permit sterile palpation and visualization of surrounding anatomic landmarks.

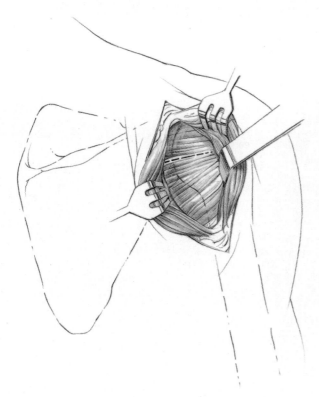

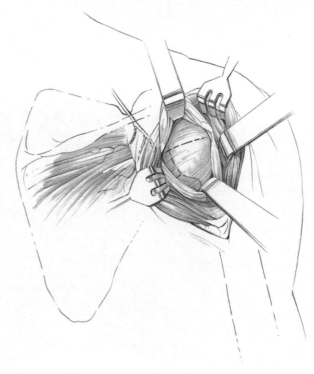

▲ **FIGURE 18-18:** The posterior deltoid is split longitudinally over the center of the glenohumeral joint, revealing the infraspinatus and teres minor muscles beneath it. (From Iannotti JP, Williams GR. *Disorders of the Shoulders.* 2nd ed. Philadelphia, PA: Lippincott Williams & Wilkins 2007, with permission.)

▲ **FIGURE 18-20:** Dissection through a fat stripe between the upper and lower portions of the infraspinatus allows access to the posterior glenohumeral capsule. The inferior branch of the suprascapular nerve limits medial dissection to 1.5 cm medial to the glenoid rim. (From Iannotti JP, Williams GR. *Disorders of the Shoulders.* 2nd ed. Philadelphia, PA: Lippincott Williams & Wilkins 2007, with permission.)

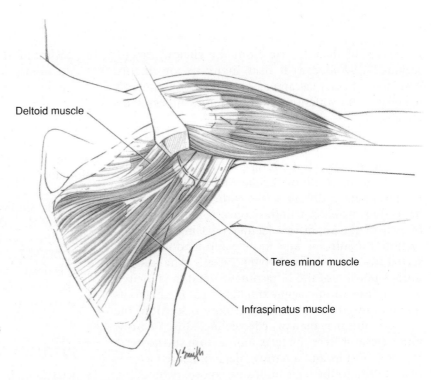

Deltoid muscle

Teres minor muscle

Infraspinatus muscle

▶ **FIGURE 18-19:** The deltoid may be superiorly retracted with the arm at 90 degrees or more of elevation to expose the muscles below in order to avoid splitting the deltoid during the approach. (From Iannotti JP, Williams GR. *Disorders of the Shoulders.* 2nd ed. Philadelphia, PA: Lippincott Williams & Wilkins 2007, with permission.)

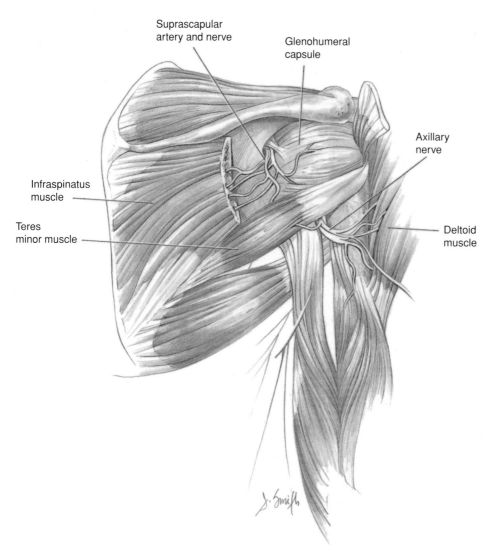

Suprascapular
artery and nerve

Glenohumeral
capsule

Axillary
nerve

Infraspinatus
muscle

Teres
minor muscle

Deltoid
muscle

◀ **FIGURE 18-21:** The interval between the infraspinatus and teres minor may be used to access the posterior capsule. Aggressive medial retraction of the infraspinatus must be avoided during this approach to avoid injury to the suprascapular nerve. (From Iannotti JP, Williams GR. *Disorders of the Shoulders.* 2nd ed. Philadelphia, PA: Lippincott Williams & Wilkins 2007, with permission.)

more medial than 1.5 cm from the glenoid margin should be avoided as it risks injury to the inferior branch of the suprascapular nerve and consequently denervates the inferior portion of the infraspinatus muscle.

When a more extensive exposure to the posterior capsule is desired, dissection is carried out in the interval between the infraspinatus (suprascapular nerve) and teres minor (axillary nerve) (Fig. 18-21). An advantage of this approach is the ability to extend dissection medially without concern for the inferior branch of the suprascapular nerve. Using blunt dissection, the infraspinatus muscle and tendon are dissected free from the underlying capsule. The midtendinous portion of the infraspinatus tendon is incised down to the capsule, approximately 1 cm medial to its humeral insertion. After further blunt dissection, the infraspinatus may then be reflected medially. A narrow blunt elevator frees the teres minor from the posteroinferior capsule, and a narrow, deep blunt retractor is placed deep to the teres minor to expose the underlying capsule.

Technique Pearl: Care should be used in retracting the infraspinatus medially to avoid excessive traction on the suprascapular nerve at the spinoglenoid notch.

All of the following surgical techniques utilize the same method of patient positioning and exposure as described above. Closure routinely involves return of the retracted muscles back to their normal resting position and reapproximation of the fascia and subcutaneous tissue and then skin with absorbable and nonabsorbable sutures, respectively. A drain inserted in the depth of the wound helps with hematoma evacuation. Once the wound is dressed, the arm is positioned in a prefabricated prefitted thoracobrachial orthosis. The arm is positioned slightly posterior to the coronal plane of the thorax in 20 degrees of abduction and 10 degrees of external rotation.

Posterior Capsulorrhaphy

Once exposed, the capsule is incised in a medial to lateral direction in the middle of the glenohumeral joint

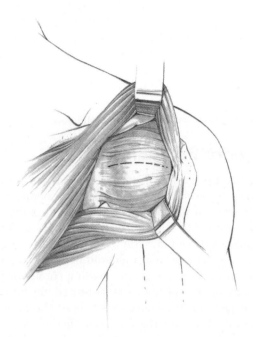

▲ **FIGURE 18-22:** A horizontal capsulotomy at the midequator of the joint enables intra-articular visualization. The vertical limb of the capsulotomy should be placed 5 mm medial to the lateral humeral capsular attachment when no posterior labral pathology is suspected, to avoid iatrogenic injury. (From Iannotti JP, Williams GR. *Disorders of the Shoulders.* 2nd ed. Philadelphia, PA: Lippincott Williams & Wilkins 2007, with permission.)

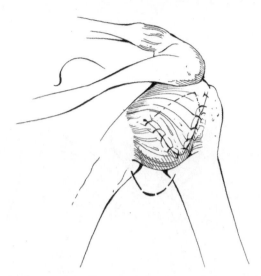

▲ **FIGURE 18-23:** Illustration of a posteroinferior capsular shift, with the inferior leaflet shifted superiorly and the superior leaflet shifted inferiorly. The arm should be positioned in approximately 45 degrees of abduction and neutral to slight external rotation when tensioning the shifted tissue. (From Iannotti JP, Williams GR. *Disorders of the Shoulders.* 2nd ed. Philadelphia, PA: Lippincott Williams & Wilkins 2007, with permission.)

(Fig. 18-22). Traction sutures placed in the superior and inferior portions of the capsule help facilitate exposure of the joint. A humeral head retractor is inserted, and the glenoid rim is evaluated. When a capsular avulsion is not evident, then a vertical capsulotomy is made 5 mm medial to the humeral insertion site of the capsule. While the proximal extent of the capsular incision is superior to the posterior insertion of the supraspinatus tendon, the distal extent depends on the degree of inferior capsular redundancy and usually reaches the 6-o'clock position. The arm is then positioned in the scapular plane in 45 degrees of abduction and neutral rotation to approximately 15 degrees of external rotation. The inferior capsular leaflet is then advanced superiorly under slight tension to obliterate the inferior capsular pouch. The superior capsular flap is shifted inferiorly, maintaining slight tissue tension. Nonabsorbable sutures close the capsule laterally and additional sutures close the interval between the superior and inferior leaflets (Fig. 18-23).

If the infraspinatus tendon was cut during exposure, it must be sutured back to its humeral stump with slight overlap. The fascia is closed with absorbable sutures, and the muscles retracted during exposure are allowed to return to normal position. The remainder of the closure and bracing is performed as discussed in the foregoing section.

Technique Pearl: Traction sutures placed in the capsular leaflets greatly help with joint exposure.

Posterior Labral Repair

Once the patient is positioned and posterior capsule exposed as previously described, a horizontal capsulotomy is performed. With the humeral head retractor in place, the joint is inspected for lesions. Identification of a reverse Bankart lesion requires the scapular neck to be prepared and the capsule reattached to the glenoid rim. First, the capsulolabral tissue of the reverse Bankart lesion must be mobilized and reflected from the glenoid margin. The posterior glenoid and scapular neck are decorticated with a curette or power burr. Finally, with the use of suture anchors or transosseous tunnels, the labrum is reattached to the articular margin of the posterior glenoid (Fig. 18-24).

Consideration must be given to performing a posteroinferior capsular shift, in addition to reverse Bankart repair, if excessive posteroinferior capsular redundancy exists. The capsule may be advanced on the glenoid side when the labrum is repaired or on the humeral side after the labrum is repaired. When performing the shift on the glenoid side, the capsulolabral tissue is cut at the midglenoid creating a superior and an inferior flap. The inferior leaflet is advanced superiorly and repaired under slight tension to the glenoid margin with suture anchors. The inferior capsular redundancy should be obliterated with this shift. The superior leaflet is subsequently shifted inferiorly under slight tissue tension, and the sutures used to repair the inferior leaflet to the glenoid are used to secure the superior leaflet. Closure and bracing are completed as outlined above (Fig. 18-25).

Technique Pearls: Caution should be used to avoid overtightening the capsule. The author's recommend

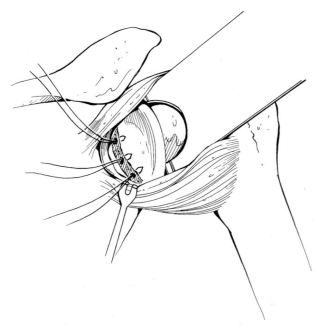

▲ **FIGURE 18-24:** Illustration of a posterior labral repair. The humeral head is retracted to expose the posterior glenoid. Suture anchors or transosseous sutures are placed along the glenoid margin. Then the sutures are passed through the detached labrum and tied to re-establish the normal anatomy. (From Iannotti JP, Williams GR. *Disorders of the Shoulders.* 2nd ed. Philadelphia, PA: Lippincott Williams & Wilkins 2007, with permission.)

positioning the humerus in less external rotation (10 degrees) during the capsular shift.

Our preferred technique for performing a capsular shift in the presence of a reverse Bankart lesion involves advancing the capsule on the humeral side instead of

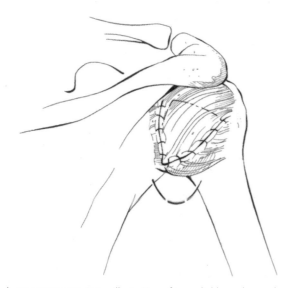

▲ **FIGURE 18-25:** Illustration of a medial-based capsular shift. The inferior capsular leaflet and labrum are shifting superiorly to place slight tension on the tissue with the arm at 45 degrees of abduction and neutral to slight external rotation. A shift of the superior capsular leaflet and labrum in the inferior direction then follows. (From Iannotti JP, Williams GR. *Disorders of the Shoulders.* 2nd ed. Philadelphia, PA: Lippincott Williams & Wilkins 2007, with permission.)

the glenoid. The horizontal capsulotomy is made at the midglenoid level to, but not through, the labrum. The labrum is repaired anatomically to the glenoid margin. Then, the capsule is cut vertically 5 mm medial to its humeral insertion. The posteroinferior capsular shift is performed with the arm in 45 degrees abduction and neutral to 10 degrees of external rotation.

Posterior Bone Block

Once the posterior capsule is exposed as described above, it is incised in the medial lateral direction at the midlevel of the glenoid and the joint is inspected. A 2 × 2 cm, 7- to 10-mm thick bone graft is obtained from the posterior iliac crest or posterior scapular spine (Fig. 18-26). The posterior glenoid neck is exposed and the inferior half is decorticated with a curette or power burr. Leaving the capsulolabral complex attached to the inferior glenoid, the cancellous side of the bone graft is positioned against the posterior glenoid neck along the posterior glenoid rim, but not beyond the rim (Fig. 18-27). One or two partially threaded cancellous screws secure the bone graft in place. Closure proceeds as described above. If a capsular plication or shift is subsequently performed after the bone block procedure, and a reverse Bankart lesion is not evident, then a humeral sided vertical capsulotomy is performed and the capsule is advanced as previously discussed.

> **Technique Pearls:** Every attempt should be made to avoid advancing the bone graft beyond the glenoid rim to avoid joint incongruity. A burr may be used to contour the graft in areas that extend beyond the glenoid rim.

Posterior Opening Wedge Glenoid Osteotomy

To perform a posterior opening wedge glenoid osteotomy, exposure is executed as previously described. The capsular incision extends in a superior-to-inferior direction at the midlevel of the capsule and the joint is evaluated. A straight, flat instrument (e.g., an osteotome) is placed along the surface of the glenoid fossa. The osteotomy cut parallels the glenoid face 10 mm medial to the posterior glenoid rim. The cut must not breach the anterior glenoid cortex, but rather just reach it to maintain stability of the osteotomy. The osteotomy is then wedged open and a cortical bone graft harvested from the scapular spine is inserted (Fig. 18-28). Frequently, internal fixation is unnecessary but a small staple or bridging plate to secure the osteotomy may be utilized. In the presence of a patulous capsule, a horizontal capsular incision in the medial to lateral direction is made and a medial-based capsular shift is performed. Closure follows, as previously described.

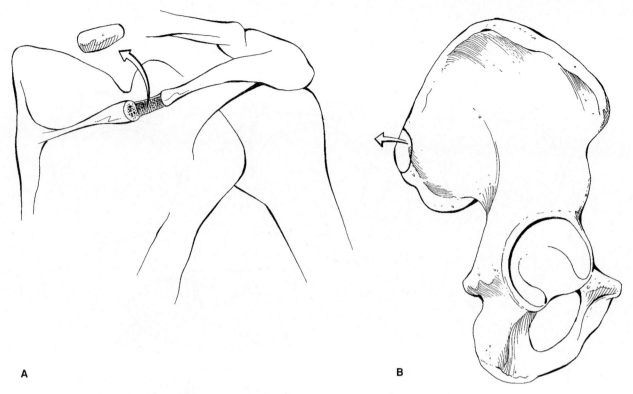

A   B

▲ **FIGURE 18-26:** Autogenous bone graft may be harvested from the scapular spine or posterior iliac crest. (From Iannotti JP, Williams GR. *Disorders of the Shoulders.* 2nd ed. Philadelphia, PA:
Lippincott Williams & Wilkins 2007, with permission.)

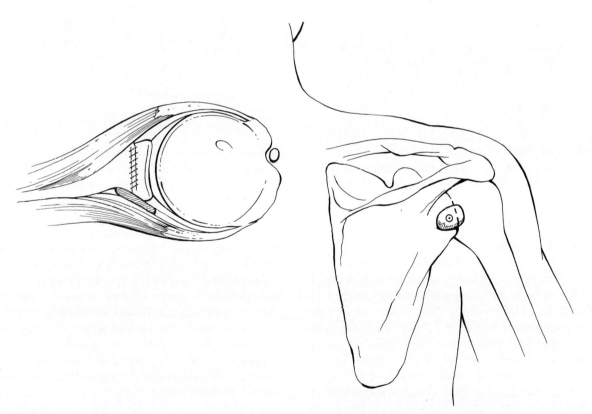

▲ **FIGURE 18-27:** Illustration of a posterior bone block. The bone graft is positioned just below
the equator of the posterior glenoid not extending beyond the arc of the glenoid vault. (From Iannotti JP, Williams GR. *Disorders of the Shoulders.* 2nd ed. Philadelphia, PA: Lippincott Williams &
Wilkins 2007, with permission.)

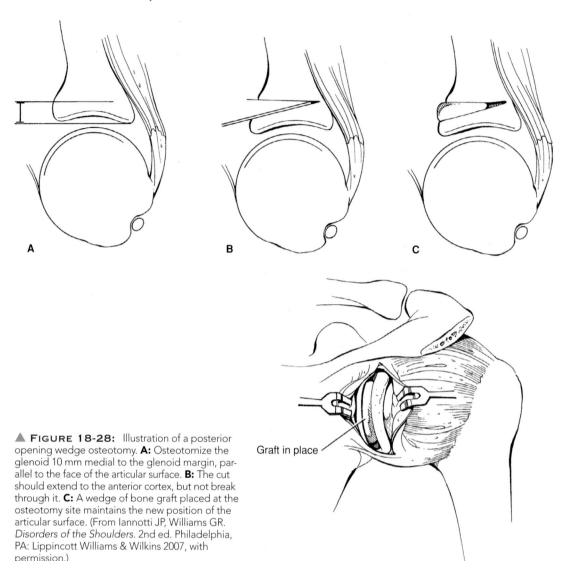

▲ FIGURE 18-28: Illustration of a posterior opening wedge osteotomy. **A:** Osteotomize the glenoid 10 mm medial to the glenoid margin, parallel to the face of the articular surface. **B:** The cut should extend to the anterior cortex, but not break through it. **C:** A wedge of bone graft placed at the osteotomy site maintains the new position of the articular surface. (From Iannotti JP, Williams GR. *Disorders of the Shoulders*. 2nd ed. Philadelphia, PA: Lippincott Williams & Wilkins 2007, with permission.)

Graft in place

Technique Pearl: Surgeons must heed the warning to not breach the anterior glenoid cortex, as doing so makes the osteotomy unstable and predisposes to graft dislocation.

REHABILITATION

Open or arthroscopic posterior shoulder surgery necessitates the use of a thoracobrachial orthosis or external rotation brace postoperatively. Patients are fitted for the brace preoperatively, and then it is applied in the operating room at the conclusion of the surgery. Initially, the brace is removed only for therapy. Active-assisted external rotation with the elbow tucked at the side is begun immediately, as is elbow flexion and extension and shoulder shrugs. Immobilization in the brace continues for 4 to 6 weeks. The exact time period depends on the degree of passive motion at 4 weeks postoperatively. Stiffness with an inability to internally rotate past neutral is reason to discontinue the brace at 4 weeks. A sling is used for an additional 2 weeks, at which time the patient starts a gentle exercise program. Patients with known ligament laxity are kept in the brace for 6 weeks.

Once the brace is discontinued, active-assisted supine forward flexion, external rotation, and internal rotation are begun. Seated and standing exercises are permitted once full forward flexion is achieved in the supine position with the scapula stabilized. At 8 weeks postoperatively, gentle external rotation resistive exercises and scapular stabilizing exercises may be initiated.

Functional and sports-specific training may be started at 3 to 4 months with an anticipated return to noncontact sports at 4 months and contact sports at 6 months. Training should continue until full ROM and normal strength return. Patients with sedentary careers may return to work in the brace when comfortable if transportation is available. Jobs involving strenuous activities must be avoided for 8 to 16 weeks postoperatively, depending on the nature of the job.

RESULTS

Despite the abundance of published literature reporting results of treatment of posterior shoulder instability, the outcomes are difficult to interpret. Numerous confounding variables make objective comparison near impossible. Furthermore, superficial evaluation of the results of surgical treatment of RPS led some authors to conclude that it should not be treated surgically as the results are discouraging (7). However, more thorough examination of the literature should allow one to be cautiously optimistic.

As emphasized earlier, the most common finding in patients with RPS is a patulous posterior capsule. All anatomic repairs of this pathology emphasize rebalancing of this redundant capsule to restore glenohumeral stability. Fronek et al. (32) published a 91% success rate with posterior capsulorrhaphy on 24 patients with isolated posterior subluxation. Similarly, Hawkins and McCormack (82) reported an 85% success rate with posterior capsulorrhaphy when reinforced with infraspinatus tendon. Bigliani reported the early results of the inferior capsular shift for patients with posteroinferior instability in 25 patients, with 88% satisfactory results (18). Pollock and Bigliani (13) offered longer-term follow-up of this same procedure, with a satisfactory rate approximating 80%. The majority of the failures associated with this procedure occurred in patients with revision surgery, and exclusion of these cases reveals a success rate of 96%.

While not a common finding, posterior labral detachment (reverse Bankart) in patients with RPS can be successfully treated with an anatomic labral repair that resolves the subluxation. Rowe and Yee (83) reported successful repairs of reverse Bankart lesions on two patients with no recurrence of instability.

Several nonanatomic procedures have been described with mixed results. McLaughlin (2) described subscapularis advancement into the anterior humeral head defect for patients with recurrent posterior shoulder instability and locked posterior dislocations. This procedure has been utilized for treatment of reverse Hill–Sachs lesions with posterior instability although with mixed results (79). The reverse Putti–Platt procedure with infraspinatus tenodesis has also been used to treat recurrent posterior instability; however, a high rate of recurrent instability has been associated with this operation (7,38). Hawkins et al. (7) reported good results in his patients after performing a reverse Putti–Platt but further noted a recurrence rate of 83% in patients who were originally operated on by other surgeons. This suggests that outcomes following this operation may depend on surgeon's experience. In addition, Boyd and Sisk (3) described subdeltoid transfer of the long head of the biceps tendon to the posterior glenoid with mixed results.

Besides soft tissue repairs, reconstruction of bony pathology has also been addressed in the literature. Scott (47) initially described a posterior opening wedge osteotomy of the glenoid neck with bone graft interposition and succeeded in two of his three patients. However, subsequent attempts at this procedure by other surgeons revealed a high rate of complication and recurrence (75). In one study, three patients (16%) continued to experience isolated posterior instability, four patients (21%) developed isolated anterior instability, and two patients (12%) had MDI in the postoperative period (75). There has been a spectrum of anterior instabilities reported following glenoid osteotomy that ranges from coracoid impingement to anterior dislocation (47,75). Given the technically demanding nature of this operation and the associated complication rate, caution should be taken when performing glenoplasty.

Several authors have reported outcomes following the use of posterior bone block procedures that buttress the posterior glenoid for recurrent posterior instability (48,68). The bone graft harvest sites include the iliac crest or scapular spine. Ahlgren et al. (68) reported recurrent posterior instability in three of their five patients treated with posterior bone block. More frequently, posterior bone block buttressing is combined with a posterior capsulorrhaphy or performed for failed posterior soft tissue procedures (48,84).

Rotational osteotomy of the humerus has been used to treat RPS due to increased proximal humeral retrotorsion. By limiting internal rotation through a rotational osteotomy, posterior instability should theoretically subside. Surin et al. (46) described an external rotation osteotomy and reported good or excellent results in 10 of his 12 patients, with one nonunion and one recurrence of instability. Most patients had significant restriction of external rotation postoperatively.

CONCLUSIONS

While less common than its anterior counterpart, posterior glenohumeral instability has received much attention in the literature and a variety of surgical procedures have been described. A thorough understanding of the underlying pathology should dictate treatment. Despite initial mixed results following surgical treatment, improved recognition of the underlying pathology combined with more anatomic surgical techniques have yielded improved results. Even with recent advances in arthroscopic shoulder stabilization procedures, a few scenarios still remain in which open techniques are preferred. With appropriate patient selection based on history, physical examination, and imaging, open treatment of posterior instability is an excellent option for patients with posterior instability.

References

1. Antoniou J, Duckworth DT, Harryman DT II. Capsulolabral augmentation for the management of posteroinferior instability of the shoulder. *J Bone Joint Surg Am.* 2000;82(9):1220–1230.

2. McLaughlin H. Posterior dislocation of the shoulder. *J Bone Joint Surg Am.* 1952;24-A-3:584–590.

3. Boyd HB, Sisk TD. Recurrent posterior dislocation of the shoulder. *J Bone Joint Surg Am.* 1972;54(4):779–786.

4. Robinson CM, Aderinto J. Recurrent posterior shoulder instability. *J Bone Joint Surg Am.* 2005;87(4):883–892.

5. Arciero RA, Mazzocca AD. Traumatic posterior shoulder subluxation with labral injury: Suture anchor-technique. *Tech Shoulder Elbow Surg.* 2004;5:13–24.

6. Bottoni CR, Franks BR, Moore JH, et al. Operative stabilization of posterior shoulder instability. *Am J Sports Med.* 2005;33(7):996–1002.

7. Hawkins RJ, Koppert G, Johnston G. Recurrent posterior instability (subluxation) of the shoulder. *J Bone Joint Surg Am.* 1984;66(2):169–174.

8. Bradley JP, Baker CL III, Kline AJ, et al. Arthroscopic capsulolabral reconstruction for posterior instability of the shoulder: A prospective study of 100 shoulders. *Am J Sports Med.* 2006;34(7):1061–1071.

9. Kaplan LD, Flanigan DC, Norwig J, et al. Prevalence and variance of shoulder injuries in elite collegiate football players. *Am J Sports Med.* 2005;33(8):1142–1146.

10. Mair SD, Zarzour RH, Speer KP. Posterior labral injury in contact athletes. *Am J Sports Med.* 1998;26(6):753–758.

11. Fuchs B, Jost B, Gerber C. Posterior-inferior capsular shift for the treatment of recurrent voluntary posterior subluxation of the shoulder. *J Bone Joint Surg Am.* 2000;82(1):16–25.

12. Williams RJ III, Strickland S, Cohen M, et al. Arthroscopic repair for traumatic posterior shoulder instability. *Am J Sports Med.* 2003;31(2):203–209.

13. Pollock RG, Bigliani LU. Recurrent posterior shoulder instability. Diagnosis and treatment. *Clin Orthop Rel Res.* 1993;291:85–96.

14. Cyprien JM, Vasey HM, Burdet A, et al. Humeral retrotorsion and glenohumeral relationship in the normal shoulder and in recurrent anterior dislocation (scapulometry). *Clin Orthop Rel Res.* 1983;175:8–17.

15. Von Raebrox A, Campbell B, Ramesh R, et al. The association of subacromial dimples with recurrent posterior dislocation of the shoulder. *J Shoulder Elbow Surg.* 2006;15(5):591–593.

16. Murrell GA, Warren RF. The surgical treatment of posterior shoulder instability. *Clin Sports Med.* 1995;14(4):903–915.

17. Beighton P, Solomon L, Soskolne CL. Articular mobility in an African population. *Ann Rheum Dis.* 1973;32(5):413–418.

18. Bigliani LU, Endrizzi DP, McIlveon SJ. Operative management of posterior shoulder instability. *Orthop Trans.* 1989;13:232.

19. Hernandez A, Drez D. Operative treatment of posterior shoulder dislocations by posterior glenoidplasty, capsulorrhaphy and infraspinatus advancement. *Am J Sports Med.* 1986;14(3):187–191.

20. Kim SH, Park JS, Jeong WK, et al. The Kim test: A novel test for posteroinferior labral lesion of the shoulder—a comparison to the jerk test. *Am J Sports Med.* 2005;33(8):1188–1192.

21. Seroyer S, Tejwani SG, Bradley JP. Arthroscopic capsulolabral reconstruction of the type VIII superior labrum anterior posterior lesion: Mean 2-year follow-up on 13 shoulders. *Am J Sports Med.* 2007;35(9):1477–1483.

22. Pagnani MJ, Warren RF. Instability of the shoulder. In: Nicholas JA, Hershman EB, eds. *The Upper Extremity and Spine in Sports Medicine.* Philadelphia, PA: J.B. Lippincott; 1994:173.

23. Engebretsen L, Craig EV. Radiologic features of shoulder instability. *Clin Orthop Rel Res.* 1993;291:29–44.

24. Pavlov H, Warren RF. Weiss CB Jr. et al. The roentgenographic evaluation of anterior shoulder instability. *Clin Orthop Rel Res.* 1985;194:153–158.

25. Tung GA, Hou DD. MR arthrography of the posterior labrocapsular complex: Relationship with glenohumeral joint alignment and clinical posterior instability. *Am J Roentgenol.* 2003;180(2):369–375.

26. Safran O, Defranco MJ, Hatem S, et al. Posterior humeral avulsion of the glenohumeral ligament as a case of posterior shoulder instability. A case report. *J Bone Joint Surg Am.* 2004;86-A(12):2732–2736.

27. Yu JS, Ashman CJ, Jones G. The POLPSA lesion: MR imaging findings with arthroscopic correlation in patients with posterior instability. *Skeletal Radiol.* 2002;31(7):396–399.

28. Kim SH, Ha KI, Park JH, et al. Arthroscopic posterior labral repair and capsular shift for traumatic unidirectional recurrent posterior subluxation of the shoulder. *J Bone Joint Surg Am.* 2003;85-A(8):1479–1487.

29. Kim SH, Noh KC, Park JS, et al. Loss of chondrolabral containment of the glenohumeral joint in atraumatic posteroinferior multidirectional instability. *J Bone Joint Surg Am.* 2005;87(1):92–98.

30. Bradley JP, Lesniak BP, McClincy M. Arthroscopic capsulolabral reconstruction for posterior shoulder instability in athletes: A prospective study of 161 shoulders. Presented at the annual closed meeting of the American Shoulder and Elbow Society, New York, NY, 2009.

31. Borrero CG, Casagranda BU, Towers JD, et al. Magnetic resonance appearance of posterosuperior labral peel back during humeral abduction and external rotation. *Skel Radiol.* 2010;39(1):19–26.

32. Fronek J, Warren RF, Bowen M. Posterior subluxation of the glenohumeral joint. *J Bone Joint Surg Am.* 1989;71(2):205–216.

33. Bell RH, Noble JS. An appreciation of posterior instability of the shoulder. *Clin Sports Med.* 1991;10(4):887–899.

34. Burkhead WZ Jr, Rockwood CA Jr. Treatment of instability of the shoulder with an exercise program. *J Bone Joint Surg Am.* 1992;74:890–896.

35. Hawkins RJ, Janda DH. Posterior instability of the glenohumeral joint: A technique of repair. *Am J Sports Med.* 1996;24(3):275–278.

36. Misamore GW, Facibene WA. Posterior capsulorrhaphy for the treatment of traumatic recurrent posterior subluxations of the shoulder in athletes. *J Shoulder Elbow Surg.* 2000;9(5):403–408.

37. Tibone JE, Bradley JP. The treatment of posterior subluxation in athletes. *Clin Orthop Rel Res.* 1993;291:124–137.

38. Hurley JA, Anderson TE, Dear W, et al. Posterior shoulder instability. Surgical versus conservative results with evaluation of glenoid version. *Am J Sports Med.* 1992; 20(4):396–400.

39. Tibone JE, Preitto C, Jobe FW, et al. Staple capsulorrhaphy for recurrent posterior shoulder dislocation. *Am J Sports Med.* 1981;9(3):135–139.

40. Schwartz E, Warren RF, O'Brien SJ, et al. Posterior shoulder instability. *Orthop Clin North Am.* 1987;18(3):409–419.

41. Bigliani LU, Pollock RG, McIlveen SJ, et al. Shift of the posteroinferior aspect of the capsule for recurrent posterior glenohumeral instability. *J Bone Joint Surg Am.* 1995;77(7):1011–1020.

42. Hawkins RJ, Belle RM. Posterior instability of the shoulder. *Instr Course Lect.* 1989;38:211–215.

43. Wolf BR, Strickland S, Williams RJ, et al. Open posterior shoulder stabilization for recurrent posterior glenohumeral instability. *J Shoulder Elbow Surg.* 2005;14(2):157–164.

44. Rhee YG, Lee DH, Lim CT. Posterior capsulolabral reconstruction in posterior shoulder instability: Deltoid saving. *J Shoulder Elbow Surg.* 2005;14(4):355–360.

45. Chaudhuri GK, Sengupta A, Saha AK. Rotation osteotomy of the shaft of the humerus for recurrent dislocation of the shoulder: Anterior and posterior. *Acta Orthop Scand.* 1974;45(2):193–198.

46. Surin V, Blåder S, Markhede G, et al. Rotational osteotomy of the humerus for posterior instability of the shoulder. *J Bone Joint Surg Am.* 1990;72(2):181–186.

47. Scott DJ Jr. Treatment of recurrent posterior dislocations of the shoulder by glenoidplasty. Report of three cases. *J Bone Joint Surg Am.* 1967;49(3):471–476.

48. Jones V. Recurrent posterior dislocation of the shoulder: Report of a case treated by posterior bone block. *J Bone Joint Surg Br.* 1958;40-B(2):203–207.

49. Scapinelli R. Posterior addition acromioplasty in the treatment of recurrent posterior instability of the shoulder. *J Shoulder Elbow Surg.* 2006;15(4):424–431.

50. Severin A. Anterior and posterior recurrent dislocation of the shoulder: The Putti-Platt operation. *Acta Orthop Scand.* 1953;23:14–22.

51. Neer CS II, Foster CR. Inferior capsular shift for involuntary inferior and multidirectional instability of the shoulder. A preliminary report. *J Bone Joint Surg Am.* 1980;62(6):897–908.

52. Gerber C, Lambert SM. Allograft reconstruction of segmental defects of the humeral head for treatment of chronic locked posterior dislocation of the shoulder. *J Bone Joint Surg Am.* 1996;78(3):376–382.

53. Bisson LJ. Thermal capsulorrhaphy for isolated posterior instability of the glenohumeral joint without labral detachment. *Am J Sports Med.* 2005;33:1898–1904.

54. D'Alessandro DF, Bradley JP, Fleischli JE, et al. Prospective evaluation of thermal capsulorrhaphy for shoulder instability: Indications and results, two- to five-year follow-up. *Am J Sports Med.* 2004;32(1):21–33.

55. Miniaci A, McBirnie J. Thermal capsular shrinkage for treatment of multidirectional instability of the shoulder. *J Bone Joint Surg Am.* 2003;85-A(12):2283–2287.

56. Davidson PA, Rivenburgh DW. The 7-o'clock posteroinferior portal for shoulder arthroscopy. *Am J Sports Med.* 2002;30(5):693–696.

57. Provencher MT, Mologne TS, Hongo M, et al. Arthroscopic rotator interval closure: Effect on glenohumeral translation and range of motion in an anterior and posterior stabilization model. Presented at the American Orthopaedic Society for Sports Medicine, Annual Meeting, Calgary, Alberta, 2007.

58. Wolf EM, Eakin CL. Arthroscopic capsular plication for posterior shoulder instability. *Arthroscopy.* 1998;14(2): 153–163.

59. Papendick LW, Savoie FH III. Anatomy-specific repair techniques for posterior shoulder instability. *J South Orthop Assoc.* 1995;4:169–176.

60. McIntyre LF, Caspari RB, Savoie FH III. The arthroscopic treatment of posterior shoulder instability: Two-year results of a multiple suture technique. *Arthroscopy.* 1997; 13(4):426–432.

61. Radkowski CA, Chhabra A, Baker CL III, et al. Arthroscopic capsulolabral repair for posterior shoulder instability in throwing athletes compared with non-throwing athletes. *Am J Sports Med.* 2008;36(4):693–699.

62. Goubier JN, Iserin A, Duranthon LD, et al. A 4 portal arthroscopic stabilization in posterior shoulder instability. *J Shoulder Elbow Surg.* 2003;12(4):337–341.

63. Provencher MT, Bell SJ, Menzel KA, et al. Arthroscopic treatment of posterior shoulder instability: Results in 33 patients. *Am J Sports Med.* 2005;33(10):1463–1471.

64. Lenart BA, Sherman SL, Mall NA, et al. Arthroscopic repair for posterior shoulder instability. *Arthroscopy.* 2012;28(10):1337–1343.

65. Wanich T, Dines J, Dines D, et al. 'Batter's shoulder': Can athletes return to play at the same level after operative treatment. *Clin Orthop Rel Res.* 2012;470(6):1565–1570.

66. McClincy M, Arner J, Tejwani SG, et al. Arthroscopic repair of posterior shoulder instability: A prospective study of 200 shoulders. Poster Presentation, American Orthopaedic Society for Sports Medicine, Annual Meeting, Baltimore, MD, 2012.

67. Millett PJ, Clavert P, Warner JJ. Arthroscopic management of anterior, posterior, and multidirectional shoulder instability: Pearls and pitfalls. *Arthroscopy.* 2003;19(suppl 1): 86–93.

68. Ahlgren SA, Hedlund T, Nistor L. Idiopathic posterior instability of the shoulder joint. Results of operation with posterior bone graft. *Acta Orthop Scand.* 1978;49: 600–603.

69. Brewer BJ, Wubben RC, Carrera GF. Excessive retroversion of the glenoid cavity. A cause of non-traumatic posterior instability of the shoulder. *J Bone Joint Surg Am.* 1986;68:724–731 [Erratum : *J Bone Joint Surg Am.* 1986; 68(7):1128].

70. Fried A. Habitual posterior dislocation of the shoulder joint: A case report on 5 operated cases. *Acta Orthop Scand.* 1949;18(3):329–345.

71. Kretzler H. Scapular osteotomy for posterior shoulder dislocation. *J Bone Joint Surg Am.* 1974;56:197.

72. McLaughlin H. Follow-up notes on articles previously published in the journal-posterior dislocation of the shoulder. *J Bone Joint Surg Am.* 1972;44:1477.

73. Mowery C, Garfin S, Booth R, et al. Recurrent posterior dislocation of the shoulder: Treatment using a bone block. *J Bone Joint Surg Am.* 1985;67: 777–781.

74. Nobel W. Posterior traumatic dislocation of the shoulder. *J Bone Joint Surg.* 1962;44 A:523–538.

75. Norwood LA, Terry G. Shoulder posterior subluxation. *Am J Sports Med.* 1984;12:25–30.

76. Tibone J, Ting A. Capsulorrhaphy with a staple for recurrent posterior subluxation of the shoulder. *J Bone Joint Surg Am.* 1990;72:999–1002.

77. Bigliani L, Pollock R, Endrizzi D, et al. Surgical repair of posterior instability of the shoulder: Long term results. 9th Combined Meeting of the Orthopaedic Association of the English-Speaking Worlds. Toronto: 1992.

78. Post M. Pectoralis major transfer for winging of the scapula. *J Shoulder Elbow Surg.* 1995;4:1–9.

79. Loebenberg MI, Cuomo F. The treatment of chronic anterior and posterior dislocations of the glenohumeral joint and associated articular surface defects. *Orthop Clin North Am.* 2000;31:23–34.

80. Shaffer BS, Conway J, Jobe FW, et al. Infraspinatus muscle-splitting incision in posterior shoulder surgery. An anatomic and electromyographic study. *Am J Sports Med.* 1994;22:113–120.

81. Wirth MA, Butters KP, Rockwood CA Jr. The posterior deltoid-splitting approach to the shoulder. *Clin Orthop.* 1993;92–98.

82. Hawkins RJ, McCormack RG. Posterior shoulder instability. *Orthopedics.* 1988;11:101–107.

83. Rowe CR, Yee LBK. A posterior approach to the shoulder joint. *J Bone Joint Surg.* 1944;26:580–584.

84. Toumey JW. Posterior recurrent dislocation of the shoulder treated by capsulorrhaphy and iliac bone block. *Lahey Clin Bull.* 1948;5:197–201.

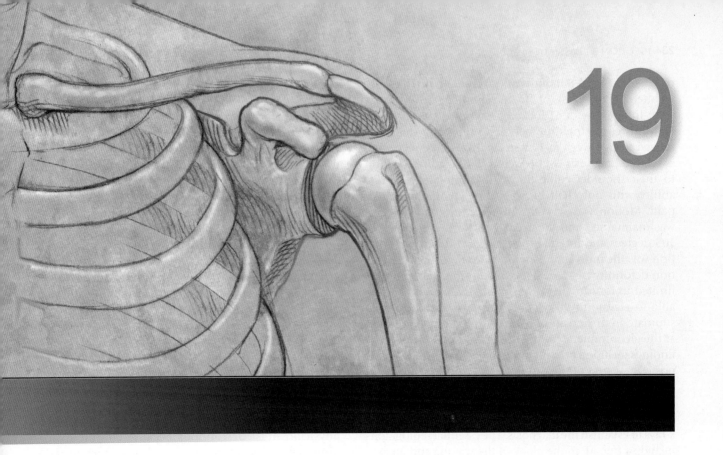

19

POSTERIOR LOCKED SHOULDER DISLOCATION: TREATMENT OPTIONS

Andrew L. Merritt / Russell F. Warren

INTRODUCTION

Locked posterior shoulder dislocations represent the far end of the spectrum of posterior shoulder instability. A feature of these dislocations is the humeral head being incarcerated on the posterior glenoid with an associated articular impaction fracture. The pathologic articulation of the posterior glenoid with the humeral head can be irreducible and stable in the dislocated position and is termed a "locked" posterior dislocation. This injury pattern can be difficult to diagnose and is difficult to treat. Over the last three decades many advances have been made that make it possible to deal with both the soft tissue and bony deficiencies in this complex injury. In this chapter, we aim to discuss the current treatment strategies that exist for locked posterior dislocations.

PRESENTATION AND DIAGNOSIS

The first step in treatment of a locked posterior shoulder dislocation is to obtain an accurate diagnosis. Historically these injuries have been missed on initial presentation about 50% to 79% of the time because of benign patient presentation and incomplete evaluation (1–4). The time between injury and diagnosis has been reported between 8 months and 1 year and often carries an alternate diagnosis of "frozen shoulder" (5–7).

In a review of 41 locked posterior dislocations by Hawkins et al., the time between injury and diagnosis ranged from 1 week to 10 years with 25 patients having a delayed diagnosis over 6 weeks (5,8). At presentation to their shoulder clinic the main complaint was disability with only half of the patients complaining of pain. Motion was severely limited but some function was maintained and the average forward elevation was 105 degrees and internal rotation to T12. External rotation was the most limited with an average internal rotation deformity of 40 degrees. In addition, supination is limited in forward elevation. While the patient is often able to elevate to 90 degrees, they are unable to fully supinate in this position because that requires rotation at the glenohumeral joint. Other common examination findings include a prominent coracoid and fullness in the posterior aspect of the shoulder.

It is clear that while the shoulder does not function normally, patients often present with minimal pain and in a delayed fashion, so it is critical to get appropriate x-rays to establish the diagnosis. The essential radiographs include a true AP in the plane of the scapula and an axillary view. A scapular "Y" view is also recommended. The axillary x-ray is essential and can accurately diagnose the dislocation, but it can be difficult to obtain if abduction is painful (1,5). In this situation, pain medication can be given in order to obtain the needed abduction or a modified axillary must be obtained. The most common modified axillary is the Velpeau axillary that can be completed with the shoulder adducted in a sling (5,8,9). Another technique is to use a curved cassette in the axilla with the x-ray beam directed cranial to caudal but this is often not possible with modern PACS cassettes (1,10).

Properly done x-rays can establish the diagnosis and the axillary can demonstrate the extent of the humeral head impaction fracture. This articular impaction fracture is the hallmark of locked posterior dislocations and has been titled the "reverse Hill-Sachs lesion." Evaluation and quantification of the fracture and understanding the bony contribution to shoulder instability is essential for determining the appropriate treatment. As a result, a CT scan of the shoulder is usually done to better evaluate the extent of the fracture and the morphology of the glenoid. Additionally, a CT is required if there are any fracture lines seen on the x-rays as displaced humeral head fractures have occurred during the reduction attempt.

REDUCTION OF THE DISLOCATION

Appropriate x-rays will diagnose the locked posterior dislocation and can also help to identify any associated fractures of the surgical neck or tuberosities. A closed reduction can be considered if there is a small impaction fracture and no associated fractures. In cases of a chronic dislocation with a large engaging reverse Hill-Sachs lesion, a closed reduction may be contraindicated. It has been recommended that closed reduction not be done if the humeral head defect is greater than 20% of the articular surface because these patients have a high chance of redislocation (5,11).

If a closed reduction is appropriate the patient should be sedated with sufficient muscle relaxation to prevent the ability to fight the reduction and possibly cause a humeral head fracture. Hawkins et al. described a reduction attempt by "flexion and adduction of the shoulder, traction on the affected extremity, and direct pressure from behind in an effort to push the humeral head anteriorly into the socket" (5,12). More recently, a case report by Godry et al. described a four step reduction technique that included: (1) constant traction to the injured arm, (2) internal rotation of the arm, and (3) and (4) simultaneous leverage to lateralize and ventralize the shoulder (7,13).

Regardless of the reduction technique used, the physician must be cautious because chronic dislocations can be incarcerated with a bony block to reduction. Fractures can occur during reduction and many require open reduction, Figure 19-2. Once reduced and while the patient is still sedated, the stability of the shoulder should be evaluated. The adducted and internally rotated shoulder position should be checked because this is the position of instability for posterior dislocations. As discussed below, if the shoulder is stable after reduction nonoperative treatment should be considered.

If the shoulder is unable to be reduced then an open reduction should be planned if the patient is healthy and can tolerate the procedure. In patients with minimal discomfort and low demands or patients with poor health, or who are not considered surgical candidates the shoulder can be left dislocated.

TREATMENT OPTIONS

The determination of appropriate treatment depends on four main factors: (1) the disability of the shoulder and health of the patient, (2) the duration of time that the shoulder has been locked in a dislocated position, (3) the stability of the shoulder after reduction, and (4) the bony defect of the humeral head and glenoid. This assessment starts with investigation into the initial dislocation. The etiology is important because if the trauma was the result of a seizure it is important that the seizure disorder be well controlled prior to consideration of treatment. A seizure early in the postoperative course will place catastrophic stress on the surgical fixation and lead to failure.

The time between the index dislocation and treatment is important because prolonged dislocation makes the impaction fracture larger and can injure the remaining articular cartilage. Schliemann et al. reported worse results with delayed diagnosis compared to acute treatment (1,5,14). Patients diagnosed within 1 month of the trauma had a Constant score of 80 at follow-up and 60% to 78% returned to previous work and sports. This is compared to patients diagnosed over 3 months from the index trauma who had a follow-up Constant score of 59 with only 44% returning to work and sports.

The age of the patient also plays a critical role in determining treatment as the choice is made between joint preservation versus arthroplasty. Finally, the size of the humeral head defect has been cited as the most important determinant of treatment option. The treatment options detailed in the remainder of the chapter discuss the indicated humeral head defect size and take into account the chronicity of the dislocation.

Closed Reduction and Nonoperative Management

After closed reduction, the shoulder should be evaluated for stability in the adducted and internally rotated position. The majority of stable reductions reported in the literature involve a small reverse Hill-Sachs lesion (less than 20% of the articular surface) and a short duration of dislocation (1 to 4 weeks) (5,14,15). At 2 to 5 years follow-up the shoulders were stable, painless, and had full range of motion and function.

Checchia et al. reported successfully treating these injuries with closed reduction if the defect was less than 20% of the articular surface and the time since dislocation was less than 4 weeks (8,15). At an average of 22 months follow-up all nine patients had excellent results with no difference in range of motion between the injured and the nonaffected shoulder with 160 degrees of elevation, 54 degrees of external rotation, and internal rotation to T7.

The results of nonoperative management are excellent if the shoulder has been dislocated for less than 1 month. Schliemann et al. reported on one patient with bilateral dislocations who was reduced and treated nonoperatively after 1 year of a locked dislocation. She was able to do daily activities but had only fair function of the shoulders (1,16).

There is no consensus on the appropriate immobilization of a stable shoulder after reduction. Historically, most patients were immobilized in an adducted and externally rotated position. Hawkins et al. initially advocated for the position of adduction with 20 degrees of external rotation and Checchia et al. recommended 20 degrees of abduction and 30 degrees of external rotation (5,8,14).

Recently Schliemann et al. have recommended immobilization of the shoulder in internal rotation and gone against the previous literature. They base this recommendation on recent studies that recommend anterior shoulder dislocations be immobilized in external rotation. Therefore they hypothesize the opposite is true and there will be more anatomic healing of the posteroinferior capsulolabral structures if immobilized in internal rotation.

In one reported case, a loose body was identified on CT and thought to be contributing to the shoulder instability by interposition of the fragment between the glenoid fossa and the humeral head (10,17). In this case, the loose body was arthroscopically removed with no other repair and then 4 weeks of external rotation immobilization. At 2 years, the patient had no recurrent instability and the authors concluded that this is a viable treatment option if the loose body was thought to be contributing to the instability.

In general, conservative management is successful for acute locked dislocations with small humeral head defects (<15% to 20% of the articular surface) that are stable after reduction.

Soft Tissue Repair

Posterior Capsulolabral Repair

Much like anterior dislocations, posterior dislocations can stretch the posteroinferior capsule and detach the adjacent labrum. This injury, in combination with the humeral head impaction fracture, can cause recurrent instability. In cases where the impaction fracture is small (20% of the articular surface or less) but the shoulder remains grossly unstable, isolated treatment of the posterior capsulolabral complex has been reported. Romeo et al. obtained excellent results in one patient at 4 years who underwent an arthroscopic reduction and repair of a locked posterior dislocation (1,11). The bony defect was 20% of the articular surface in the one case they reported. The authors suggest that this technique can be used on small- or moderate-sized bony defects.

Treatment of the Humeral Impaction Fracture

The hallmark of the posterior dislocation is a humeral head impaction fracture. The size is variable and is related to the initial trauma and the chronicity of the dislocation. The size of the bony defect can be measured on the axillary x-ray or, more commonly, on a CT. The size of the defect is described as a percentage of the projected total articular surface (12,18). If the shoulder is unstable after reduction and the humeral head defect needs to be addressed (>20% of the articular surface), there are many techniques that have been described. Transfer of the subscapularis tendon into the defect is a nonanatomic solution that prevents engagement of the defect and has been described and presented by multiple authors. More recently, authors have advocated for an anatomic solution utilizing disimpaction of the fracture or allograft reconstruction.

Transfer of the Subscapularis Tendon

Humeral head impaction fractures that involve around one-quarter of the humeral head are often unstable and redislocate because the defect can engage the posterior glenoid. Treatment options for these smaller defects have been aimed at preventing this impaction from engaging the glenoid. McLaughlin described a transfer of the subscapularis tendon into the anterior bony defect as a way to prevent engagement (7,19). This procedure has been modified to include transfer of the entire lesser tuberosity into the defect (Hawkins et al.) and plication of the subscapularis without detachment (Charalambous et al.), Figure 19-1 (1,5,14).

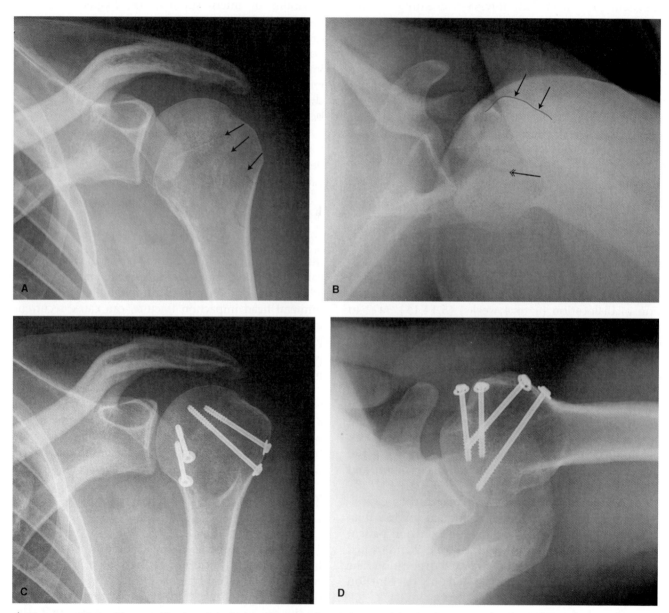

▲ **FIGURE 19-1:** Neer modification of the McLaughlin procedure. A 41-year-old male who fell off his bicycle and sustained a posterior fracture dislocation of his left shoulder. **A:** AP view of the shoulder demonstrating the difficulty in diagnosing the dislocation for this view alone. Also the patient has a greater tuberosity fracture outlines with black single arrows. **B:** Axillary view of the shoulder clearly demonstrating the dislocation. The greater tuberosity fracture is outlined in gray and identified with single arrows. There is also a fracture line of the impaction fracture extending into the head. **C,D:** Postoperative views with two screws used to secure the greater tuberosity and two screws to secure the lesser tuberosity transfer. At 1-year follow-up the patient had full strength with some limitation of motion. Internal rotation at the side was to L1 versus T10 and internal rotation at 90 degrees was 20 versus 60. External rotation was 60 versus 80.

These three techniques all aim to fill the bony defect with the soft tissue of the subscapularis to prevent engagement of the bony defect and the resultant instability. The procedures are done open and utilize the deltopectoral approach to the shoulder. Through this approach, an open reduction can be performed and the humeral head defect can be exposed completely. The original McLaughlin technique detached the subscapularis off of the humerus and placed it into a bone tunnel made in the humeral head defect. In an attempt to provide more secure fixation for the subscapularis, Neer described a lesser tuberosity osteotomy and transfer into the bony defect in the humeral head. He attached the lesser tuberosity to the humeral head using bone screws. The postoperative rehabilitation was slow with Neer's modification and they were kept in 20 degrees of external rotation shoulder spica for 4 weeks.

Two papers have performed an open approach and used suture anchors to plicate the subscapularis into the bony defect without detaching the subscapularis insertion (14,15,19). This technique does not change the length of the muscle-tendon unit and the authors hypothesize that this will lead to greater maintenance of subscapularis strength. In addition, because the subscapularis was not detached, Charalambous et al. allowed a more aggressive rehabilitation schedule of 1 week in a simple sling followed by active mobilization guided by pain. Spencer et al. used a more conservative rehabilitation schedule with 4 weeks of external rotation sling to allow the posterior capsule to heal (15,20).

The outcomes of subscapularis transfer procedures have been good in correctly selected patients. Hawkins and Neer reported on five failures referred to them and found two common causes for the failure: Too large of a humeral head defect for the procedure (2 patients) or nonviable articular cartilage causing pain and loss of function (3 patients). In properly selected patients with the defect between 20% and 45% of the articular surface they reported successful outcome in all four patients undergoing lesser tuberosity osteotomy and transfer. The patients had grade 5 strength and range of motion of 165 degrees of elevation, 40 degrees of external rotation, and internal rotation to T12 at 2 to 9 years. Their results with transfer of the subscapularis were similar with the exception of some patients having grade 4 strength at 2 to 8 years. Schliemann et al. reported on five patients using either the McLaughlin procedure or Neer modification and noted a Constant score of 62 at follow-up. They noted the results of their series were worse compared with the results of anatomic reconstruction techniques.

McLaughlin stressed the importance of patient selection and avoided the subscapularis transfer if the joint was "beyond any hope of useful function." He performed the procedure in three patients and reported good results with some loss of motion but no recurrent instability or pain. Walch et al. reported on 10 patients with subscapularis transfer and reported 3 excellent, 1 good, 5 fair, and 1 poor result (16,21).

Good results have been reported without detaching the subscapularis and filling the defect with the use of suture anchors. Charalambous et al. published a case report using his technique with 6-month follow-up and symmetric strength and range of motion (14,22,23). Spencer et al. reported on two cases with no recurrent instability, slightly decreased range of motion, but no pain and patient satisfaction. It is noted that they had strict patient criteria with less than 30% humeral head defect and less than 8 weeks of dislocation.

As noted previously, results are related to the duration of the locked dislocation. Excellent results have been reported when a subscapularis transfer was performed in acute locked posterior dislocation. Banerjee et al. reported on seven male patients with reverse Hill-Sachs lesions between 25% and 45% treated within 3 weeks after injury and had excellent results. At an average of 41 months (range 27 to 54 months) the patients had an average Constant score of 92 with normal range of motion in all planes except external rotation at the side. They believe that despite being a nonanatomic procedure, the McLaughlin procedure can provide excellent results in the acute setting.

Soft tissue transfer procedures demonstrate good results in unstable shoulders with impaction defects of 20% to 45% of the articular surface. In these patients, near normal range of motion and strength has been reported with better results reported when done within 4 weeks of injury. The failures that have been reported have been because the defect was too large for this procedure or the articular cartilage had already been damaged beyond the utility of a joint preservation procedure.

Disimpaction and Bone Grafting

In an attempt for anatomic reconstruction, a few authors have described disimpacting the depressed fracture to reform the articular surface. The techniques are variable but most authors agree that the patient selection is important. Most recommend younger patients with medium-sized defects (20% to 45% of the articular surface) who have been dislocated less than 3 months. Assom et al. suggests a dislocated time of less than 4 weeks but others have reported on patients with 6 months of locked dislocation (17,23).

Elevation of the impaction fracture has been described through various techniques. Most commonly, the deltopectoral approach is used and the subscapularis is released to expose the impaction fracture. An attempt is made to elevate the articular and cancellous fragments as one piece, but this is often not possible in larger defects or chronic dislocations. Schliemann et al. (1) described 11 cases of elevating the impaction and supporting the defect with autograft, allograft, or Norian SRS cement (DePuy Synthes). Khayal et al. (18) described a case report with a similar technique but the chondral surface was in multiple pieces that were refixed using absorbable pins.

Bock et al. described elevation of the fragment and placement of suture anchors loaded with absorbable sutures in the bottom of the defect. The defect is then filled with a combination of iliac crest cancellous autograft and cancellous allograft. The absorbable sutures from the anchor are then tied over the graft material (19).

Assom et al. described a technique without detachment of the subscapularis that utilized a cortical window opposite the fracture to disimpact the segment. The rotator interval was used for direct visualization and the disimpacted fragment was supported by a bioabsorbable interference screw. The screw was introduced perpendicular to the fracture and from the opposite side. One advantage of this technique is that the screw can be advanced incrementally and the impaction slowly reduced. In addition, the screw provides a strong structural support. They advocate using this technique only in patients with acute lesions (3 to 4 weeks).

The results of disimpaction and bone grafting are encouraging. Schliemann et al. reported on 11 cases that involved disimpaction and bone grafting. At 5 years follow-up they reported an average Constant score of 88.5 (no range reported) (1). Bock et al. (19) reported on six patients with 5-year follow-up (range 18 to 95 months) using their technique and reported an average Constant score of 88.2 (range 83 to 98) with two patients having an excellent result and four patients with a good result. Subjectively, two patients were very satisfied while four were satisfied. The range of motion was asymmetric compared to the other side with most patients loosing 10 to 20 degrees of flexion, abduction, and external rotation compared to the contralateral shoulder. They noted maintenance of the articular contour on follow-up and no avascular necrosis, but one patient had asymptomatic progression of osteoarthrosis.

Assom et al. (17) presented two cases using the opposite side disimpaction technique and they reported excellent results at an average of 26 months. The Constant scores were 90 and 95 with no decrease in internal rotation. It is noted that although the defects were large (40% and 50% of the articular surface), these were acute injuries treated within 4 weeks of the dislocation. The acuity of the injury might allow for larger defects to still be successfully managed with anatomic joint preserving techniques.

Disimpaction and bone grafting is an option for younger patients with medium-sized defects when the goal is anatomic articular reconstruction. Most authors advocate for this treatment in the acute or subacute settings, but it has been successful up to 6 months. Good to excellent outcomes have been reported at 5 years with some slight global decrease in range of motion. As with other techniques, better outcomes can be expected with more acute treatment.

Allograft Articular Reconstruction of the Humerus

Reconstruction of the humeral head articular surface can be done using osteochondral allografts fixed into the defect. This technique is suitable for younger patient with a medium to large size engaging defect (25% to 50% of the articular surface) when anatomic reconstruction is desired. One additional advantage over the subscapularis transfer is maintenance of the normal humeral anatomy if a later arthroplasty is needed.

Gerber and Lambert (20) were the first to report on using bulk allograft structural grafts to fill the anteromedial humeral head defect. They reported on four patients with defects measuring 40% to 55% of the articular surface. The presentation, allograft material, and comorbidities were heterogeneous making interpretation difficult, but they found that range of motion, pain, and subjective evaluation to be consistent with the reported outcomes of the McLaughlin procedure. One patient who also abused alcohol developed osteonecrosis 6 years after the procedure and had worse results. They did caution using the technique in larger defects or osteopenic or avascular bone of the residual head.

Diklic et al. (21) reported on a case series of 13 patients with defects measuring between 25% and 50% of the articular surface who had been dislocated for an average of 4 months (range 2 to 9 months). They described using a deltopectoral approach with a subscapularis tenotomy giving access to the humeral head. In two patients they repaired the posterior capsulolabral structures because they had been avulsed off of the glenoid. In the remaining 11 patients the posterior capsule was stretched but not avulsed or separated and the posterior aspect of the rim was decorticated to assist in healing, but was not directly repaired. The allograft used in most cases was fresh frozen. The dimensions of the defect were measured on the humeral head and a corresponding cut was made on the allograft and then was secured using two or three cancellous screws.

Postoperatively the patients were immobilized for 6 weeks in slight abduction and external rotation but started therapy immediately after surgery with passive forward elevation and external rotation. At a minimum of 41 months follow-up most were free of pain and the average Constant score was 87 (range 43 to 98). There was incorporation of all of the allografts except for one patient who developed avascular necrosis and graft collapse. There was some flattening of the grafts in seven patients.

Martinez et al. reported on six patients at 5- and 10-year follow-up time points (22,23). The six patients were treated with a similar surgical technique as described above but postoperatively they were immobilized for 4 weeks in neutral rotation before starting motion. Three of the patients had excellent results with Constant scores of 90 to 100. One patient had excellent results until 8 years after surgery when he developed osteoarthritis with pain and stiffness and had to undergo an arthroplasty. Two patients had collapse of the graft evident at 4 years and developed early osteoarthritis and both underwent revision to arthroplasty at 8 years.

This procedure is attractive because it can provide a stable joint and restore the articular contour without the need to transfer the subscapularis and disrupt the native anatomy. Early reports demonstrate satisfactory results up to 5 years, but in the one long-term follow-up published, 50% of the patients required revision to arthroplasty by 10 years (23). It is again noted that the acuity of the injury plays an important role and might lead to better results because the remaining humeral head is strong enough to support the allograft and the remaining cartilage is less damaged.

Rotational Osteotomy of the Humerus

Humeral head impaction fractures decrease the articular arc of motion that the shoulder can tolerate. Anterior impaction fractures that occur with locked posterior dislocations can engage the posterior glenoid and cause shoulder instability. The vulnerable position of the shoulder in posterior instability is adduction and internal rotation and this is a common position during normal activity in life. A rotational humeral osteotomy has been used to change the position of engagement of the impaction fracture with the posterior glenoid. This technique does not change the articular arc of motion, but changes the position of the shoulder when engagement happens and allows for more functional motion without instability. The result is increased internal rotation before shoulder instability but the consequence is decreased external rotation.

The rotational osteotomy was first reported by Chaudhuri and was described for both anterior and posterior dislocations (1–4,24). This was followed up by a case report that used this technique as an alternative for arthroplasty or arthrodesis in a young patient with a 40% articular impaction defect (5–7,25). After reduction of the dislocation, the osteotomy was performed at the level of the surgical neck. The amount of correction was determined by placing the margin of the defect in the posterior third of the glenoid. Then the arm, flexed at the elbow, was rotated to the abdomen and fixed in this position with a wire loop. This change in rotation allows functional internal rotation to the abdomen without instability and the ability to do activities of daily living without recurrent dislocation. The case was reported with good results with the only consequence being limited external rotation to 20 degrees. Porteous and Miller reported two more cases using a modification of this technique with fair and good results (5,26). They recommended this approach for large defects when the alternatives are excision or replacement of the humeral head.

In a series of ten patients treated with a rotational osteotomy, Keppler et al. reported one excellent, five good, two fair, and two poor results. Both of the patients with poor results had been dislocated for 9 to 13 months compared to the other patients with better results who had been dislocated less than 9 months. They felt the poor results were due to advanced degenerative changes in the shoulder and recommended against a rotational osteotomy in these cases. The impaction fracture was less than 40% of the articular surface in all patients and they considered larger defects to be a contraindication to osteotomy and recommended arthroplasty.

While avascular necrosis remains a cited concern for this technique, no patients have been reported to have this complication in the setting of posterior instability. The primary disadvantages of this nonanatomic technique are nonunion or delayed union, malrotation and subsequent recurrent instability, the need for a large surgical dissection, and loss of external rotation. Overall authors report generally good results for defects measuring 30% to 40% of the humeral head in younger patients without degenerative wear of the shoulder. It is an alternative to arthroplasty in younger patients where arthroplasty is not a long lasting solution.

Arthroplasty

Large humeral head defects have been treated with hemiarthroplasty, total shoulder arthroplasty, humeral surface replacement, and reverse total shoulder replacement. The decision between the different joint replacement techniques depends on the existing bone quality of the remaining humerus, associated soft tissue injuries, and demands of the patient.

The use of humeral surface replacement has been published in one case report by Kappe et al. (5,27). They used a cemented humeral cap because there was no glenoid injury, the remaining humeral bone stock was adequate, and the authors felt that adjusting the retroversion was easier than with a stemmed arthroplasty. Short-term results were excellent.

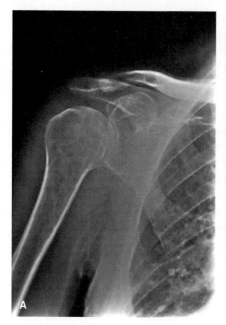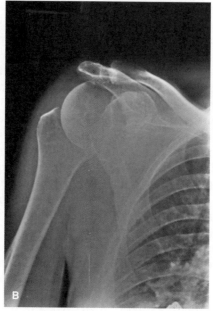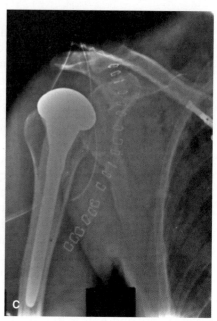

▲ **FIGURE 19-2:** Hemiarthroplasty after fracture of the humeral head during reduction of a posterior dislocation. **A:** Presentation in the emergency room with a posterior dislocation of the shoulder. **B:** A closed reduction was attempted and, despite appropriate sedation, a humeral head fracture occurred. **C:** The fracture was then treated with a hemiarthroplasty.

Hemiarthroplasty has long been used for treatment of locked posterior dislocations with large defects, Figure 19-2. Hawkins et al. reported on nine shoulders treated with hemiarthroplasty (5,9). Three patients had glenoid articular injury at surgery but at the time there was no total shoulder arthroplasty available. These three were revised to total shoulder arthroplasty with good results. The other six patients treated with hemiarthroplasty had good results with no or minimal pain, good motion, and no limitations in activities of daily living. Hemiarthroplasty is used for large defects of the humeral head with minimal glenoid damage, chronic dislocations with humeral articular cartilage damage, or dislocations associated with osteonecrosis or poor remaining bone stock making other treatments not feasible.

Hawkins et al. also reported on the use of total shoulder replacements for this condition (1,5). When used as a primary treatment for locked posterior dislocations, five of six patients had minimal or no pain and good results. One patient had a dislocation in the immediate postoperative period. In this early failure, the humeral component had been inserted in 20 degrees of retroversion and they subsequently modified their technique to decrease the retroversion when doing a total shoulder replacement for posterior instability. They recommend determining the amount of version by using trial components, but also note that the longer the shoulder has been dislocated the more the retroversion should be reduced.

Decreasing the humeral retroversion is advocated in this setting, but the efficacy of this modification has not been proven. Ionnotti studied the effect of antever-sion of the humeral component in the setting of glenoid retroversion and found no increase in the stability of the shoulder replacement. Another technique that can be used is posterior capsule plication at the time of arthroplasty. In the setting of a chronic dislocation and patulous posterior capsule, this can tension the posterior structures and increase stability of the arthroplasty.

Total shoulder arthroplasty can be technically difficult for this condition. Checchia et al. reported on four failures out of five patients (5,8). One patient developed detachment of the tuberosities after surgery, one had an anterior dislocation and required resection arthroplasty, and two noncompliant patients had poor results. These results stress the importance of patient selection in treating these complex injuries. In addition, the author notes that difficulty increases with increased time of dislocation and chronic dislocations should be handled by experience surgeons if arthroplasty is performed. To prevent recurrent instability, it is recommended that less retroversion be used for arthroplasty in posterior instability with most authors recommending between 10 and 20 degrees of retroversion (5,8,28,29).

General guidelines for this technique are similar to hemiarthroplasty except that glenoid erosion or articular injury necessitates a total replacement. Results have been poor in some patients, but many patients experience improvement of pain, ability to do activities of daily living, and rare recurrent instability (5,8,13,28,29). If the tuberosities are incompetent or there is associated rotator cuff insufficiency, a reverse total shoulder replacement can be performed for the treatment of locked posterior instability.

Author's Preferred Technique

Treatment of these injuries begins with appropriate history, examination, and imaging. Any patient with limited external rotation must be fully evaluated for a posterior dislocation with an axillary view. This is a routine view for all shoulder patients in the clinic. If there is any concern for a humeral head fracture or proximal humerus fracture, then a CT must be obtained and no reduction attempted. If the dislocation is acute and no fracture is present, a reduction is attempted under full sedation. If there is any concern for adjacent fracture or the dislocation is chronic, an open reduction is attempted. Open reduction can be difficult in chronic cases and we recommend levering the head from behind the glenoid using an elevator or a Darrach retractor. This can be done through the rotator interval or after taking down the subscapularis.

The senior author has typically used a lesser tuberosity transfer for small defects up to 25% of the humeral head, allograft for medium defects involving up to 50% of the head, and hemiarthroplasty for larger lesions or elderly patients instead of an allograft. Using an allograft to reconstruct the articular surface has promise and has been successful in our patients. The difficulty with this surgery is obtaining a graft but if they are available the indication can be expanded to smaller lesions in younger patients.

Chronic dislocations can present with small- or medium-sized impaction defects but have diffuse chondral thinning of the remaining head. Some have recommended arthroplasty if global chondral thinning, but we have not found these patients to develop end-stage arthritis out to 10 years. We will still attempt articular reconstruction and joint salvage in younger patients with chronic dislocations up to 1 year.

CONCLUSION

Locked posterior shoulder dislocations are difficult orthopedic problems to diagnose and treat. The diagnosis requires careful inspection and an appropriate work-up that includes an axillary x-ray. Once diagnosed, the treatment is determined by many factors that include duration of dislocation, age and function of the patient, and size of the humeral impaction fracture. Smaller lesions can be treated without surgery or with a tissue transfer into the impaction fracture to stabilize the joint and prevent engagement of the fracture. This has proven to be a reliable and successful technique for small impaction fractures.

Larger impaction fractures require a more complex approach that includes either articular reconstruction or arthroplasty. The decision to save the joint versus replace the joint is based on patient related factors and

the quality of the remaining cartilage. In a chronic dislocation, the adjacent cartilage is often damaged and the bone at the site of the impaction is poor and both of these factors make articular salvage less reliable. Arthroplasty is used for large lesions in older patients.

References

1. Schliemann B, Muder D, Gessmann J, et al. Locked posterior shoulder dislocation: Treatment options and clinical outcomes. *Arch Orthop Trauma Surg.* 2011;131(8):1127–1134.
2. Dorgan JA. Posterior dislocation of the shoulder. *Am J Surg.* 1955;89(4):890–900.
3. Rowe CR, Zarins B. Chronic unreduced dislocations of the shoulder. *J Bone Joint Surg Am.* 1982;64(4):494–505.
4. Schulz TJ, Jacobs B. Unrecognized dislocations of the shoulder. *J Trauma.* 1969;9(12):1009–10023.
5. Hawkins RJ, Neer CS, Pianta RM, et al. Locked posterior dislocation of the shoulder. *J Bone Joint Surg Am.* 1987;69(1):9–18.
6. Hill NA, McLaughlin HL. Locked posterior dislocation simulating a 'frozen shoulder'. *J Trauma.* 1963;3:225–234.
7. McLaughlin HL. Posterior dislocation of the shoulder. *J Bone Joint Surg Am.* 1952;24-A-3:584–590.
8. Checchia SL, Santos PD, Miyazaki AN. Surgical treatment of acute and chronic posterior fracture-dislocation of the shoulder. *J Shoulder Elbow Surg.* 1998;7(1):53–65.
9. Bloom MH, Obata WG. Diagnosis of posterior dislocation of the shoulder with use of Velpeau axillary and angle-up roentgenographic views. *J Bone Joint Surg Am.* 1967;49(5):943–949.
10. Alamo GG, Cimiano FJ, Suarez GG, et al. Locked posterior dislocation of the shoulder: Treatment using arthroscopic removal of a loose body. *Arthroscopy.* 1996;12(1):109–111.
11. Verma NN, Sellards RA, Romeo AA. Arthroscopic reduction and repair of a locked posterior shoulder dislocation. *Arthroscopy.* 2006;22(11):1252.e1–e5.
12. Tongel A, Karelse A, Berghs B, et al. Posterior shoulder instability: Current concepts review. *Knee Surg Sports Traumatol Arthrosc.* 2010;19(9):1547–1553.
13. Godry H, Citak M, Königshausen M, et al. Eine neue Repositionstechnik für die verhakte hintere Schulterluxation. *Unfallchirurg.* 2011;115(8):754–758.
14. Charalambous CP, Gullett TK, Ravenscroft MJ. A modification of the McLaughlin procedure for persistent posterior shoulder instability: Technical note. *Arch Orthop Trauma Surg.* 2009;129(6):753–755.
15. Spencer EE, Brems JJ. A simple technique for management of locked posterior shoulder dislocations: Report of two cases. *J Shoulder Elbow Surg.* 2005;14(6):650–652.
16. Walch G, Boileau P, Martin B, et al. [Unreduced posterior luxations and fractures-luxations of the shoulder. Apropos of 30 cases]. *Rev Chir Orthop Reparatrice Appar Mot.* 1990;76(8):546–558.
17. Assom M, Castoldi F, Rossi R, et al. Humeral head impression fracture in acute posterior shoulder dislocation: New surgical technique. *Knee Surg Sports Traumatol Arthrosc.* 2006.

18. Khayal T, Wild M, Windolf J. Reconstruction of the articular surface of the humeral head after locked posterior shoulder dislocation: A case report. *Arch Orthop Trauma Surg.* 2008;129(4):515–519.

19. Bock P, Kluger R, Hintermann B. Anatomical reconstruction for Reverse Hill-Sachs lesions after posterior locked shoulder dislocation fracture: A case series of six patients. *Arch Orthop Trauma Surg.* 2007;127(7):543–548.

20. Gerber C, Lambert SM. Allograft reconstruction of segmental defects of the humeral head for the treatment of chronic locked posterior dislocation of the shoulder. *J Bone Joint Surg Am.* 1996;78(3):376–382.

21. Diklic ID, Ganic ZD, Blagojevic ZD, et al. Treatment of locked chronic posterior dislocation of the shoulder by reconstruction of the defect in the humeral head with an allograft. *J Bone Joint Surg Br.* 2010;92(1):71–76.

22. Martinez AA, Calvo A, Domingo J, et al. Allograft reconstruction of segmental defects of the humeral head associated with posterior dislocations of the shoulder. *Injury.* 2008;39(3):319–322.

23. Martinez AA, Navarro E, Iglesias D, et al. Long-term follow-up of allograft reconstruction of segmental defects of the humeral head associated with posterior dislocation of the shoulder. *Injury.* 2012;44(4):488–491.

24. Chaudhuri GK, Sengupta A, Saha AK. Rotation osteotomy of the shaft of the humerus for recurrent dislocation of the shoulder: Anterior and posterior. *Acta Orthop Scand.* 1974;45(2):193–198.

25. Vukov V. Posterior dislocation of the shoulder with a large anteromedial defect of the head of the humerus. A case report. *Int Orthop.* 1985;9(1):37–40.

26. Porteous MJ, Miller AJ. Humeral rotation osteotomy for chronic posterior dislocation of the shoulder. *J Bone Joint Surg Br.* 1990;72(3):468–469.

27. Kappe T, Elsharkawi M, Reichel H, et al. Cemented humeral surface replacement for a locked posterior fracture-dislocation: A case report. *J Orthop Trauma.* 2011;25(9):e90–93.

28. Cicak N. Posterior dislocation of the shoulder. *J Bone Joint Sur Br.* 2004;86(3):324–332.

29. Cheng SL, Mackay MB, Richards RR. Treatment of locked posterior fracture-dislocations of the shoulder by total shoulder arthroplasty. *J Shoulder Elbow Surg.* 1997;6(1):11–17.

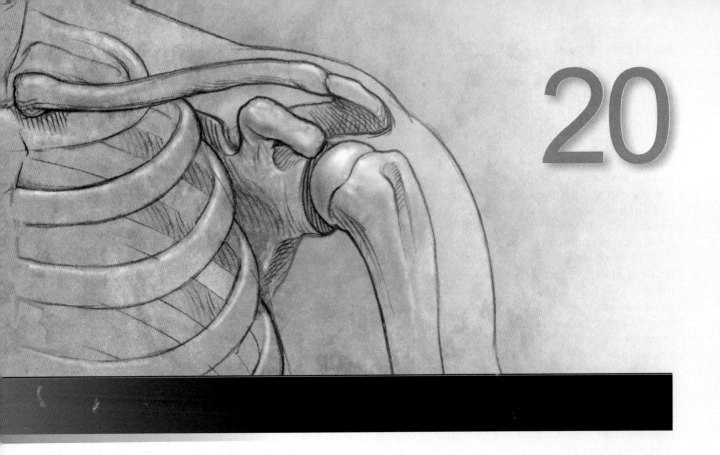

POSTERIOR FRACTURE-DISLOCATIONS OF THE SHOULDER: SPECTRUM OF PATHOLOGY AND TREATMENT OPTIONS

Bashar Alolabi / Eric T. Ricchetti

INTRODUCTION AND EPIDEMIOLOGY

The shoulder is the most commonly dislocated joint in the body, yet posterior dislocations are rare, accounting for <3% of all shoulder dislocations (1–6). The rarity of this injury is likely related to anatomical features. Although the humeral head and the glenoid are both retroverted relative to their long axes, the protraction of the scapula on the chest wall protects the shoulder from posterior dislocations by providing a buttressing effect of the posterior glenoid (2,7,8). The posterior capsulolabral complex, posterior band of the inferior glenohumeral ligament, rotator interval capsule, superior and middle glenohumeral ligaments, and coracohumeral ligament offer further static stability, while the rotator cuff and shoulder girdle muscles offer dynamic stability (9–15). Nevertheless, sustained contraction of the internal rotators during a seizure or axial forces applied to the shoulder while in the unstable position of internal rotation, forward elevation, and adduction can lead to traumatic posterior dislocations (16,17). Although these posterior dislocations often lead to the typical osteochondral impression lesion (known as the *ecoche* or reverse

Hill-Sachs lesion), severe forces, osteopenia, or osteoporosis can lead to fracture-dislocations of the humeral head or the proximal humerus.

Posterior fracture-dislocations are quite uncommon (18,19), representing 0.9% of over 1,500 shoulder fractures and dislocations reviewed by Neer (20) and 0.6 per 100,000 population per year in the study by Robinson et al. (21). The latter study, however, excluded isolated lesser tuberosity fractures. In fact, the true prevalence of this injury is unknown (2) since up to 60% of these injuries can be overlooked (22,23).

Most posterior fracture-dislocations occur as a result of epileptic seizures, high-energy trauma, sports injuries, falls from a height, alcohol-related injuries, or electrical shocks (such as those associated with electrocution or electroconvulsive therapy) (24–29). Bilateral posterior fracture-dislocations are pathognomonic of a seizure (4,20,30). In the study by Robinson et al. (21), of the 26 patients with posterior fracture-dislocations, 46% were the result of falls, generally from a height >182.88 cm (6 ft); 42% were the result of a seizure (secondary to epilepsy, alcohol or drug withdrawal, hypoglycemia or hypoxia); and 12% occurred as a consequence of motor vehicle accidents (2).

The majority of patients with posterior fracture-dislocations are middle-aged men, especially between the ages of 40 and 60 (2,21). The higher male prevalence is likely related to the fact that males are more commonly involved in motor vehicle accident and sports injuries. Moreover, the more muscular habitus of males may be a predisposing risk factor for shoulder injuries during seizures (2).

The spectrum of fractures associated with posterior shoulder fracture-dislocations includes lesser tuberosity, greater tuberosity, surgical neck, anatomic neck, and head-splitting fractures, or any combination of these fractures (5,18,25–29,31–34). Anatomic neck fractures are especially common in posterior fracture-dislocations. Scapular fractures and posterior glenoid rim fractures have also been reported (35–37).

Although isolated lesser tuberosity fractures are rare (38), they are commonly associated with posterior shoulder fracture-dislocations, similar to the association between greater tuberosity fractures and anterior shoulder dislocations (3,15,20,24,39).

The mechanism of four-part posterior fracture-dislocations as a result of seizures has been described by Shaw (40) as an extension of a posterior dislocation. When the humeral head is forced superiorly and posteriorly over the glenoid rim, the humeral head becomes lodged behind the glenoid and develops a depression medial to the lesser tuberosity. If the convulsive forces continue, however, the glenoid edge shears off the humeral head with an associated avulsion of the tuberosities as a result of spasm of the subscapularis and infraspinatus. Forced contraction of the triceps, coraco-

brachialis, biceps, and deltoid results in further comminution as the humeral shaft thrusts upward toward the acromion, separating the shaft from the head and resulting in a four-part fracture-dislocation. Robinson et al. (21) also proposed a mechanism for posterior shoulder fracture-dislocations, whereby the fracture occurs after the dislocation as the humeral head impacts on the "anvil" of the posterior glenoid. This mechanism was proposed on the basis of a consistent pattern of injury, where all patients had an anatomic neck fracture, with the fracture line propagating from the reverse Hill-Sachs lesion.

DIAGNOSIS

Delays in diagnosis of posterior fracture-dislocations are common (36,41,42) due to many reasons, including late presentation by the patient, failure of the examiner to suspect the diagnosis, and inadequate radiographic evaluation (2,43) (Fig. 20-1). Elderly patients and those with other fractures are especially prone to be missed.

A posterior shoulder fracture-dislocation should be suspected when a patient complains of shoulder pain following a seizure. Keys to the diagnosis on physical examination include posterior glenohumeral fullness, flattening of the anterior aspect of the shoulder, and a prominent coracoid process. However, the most important finding on examination is an arm held in internal rotation with a mechanical block to passive external rotation. It may not even be possible to passively external rotate the patient's arm to neutral. This block occurs as a result of the engagement of the humeral head defect on the posterior glenoid (2,4,44) (Fig. 20-2A). The absence of pain on rotation of the shoulder during the examination is suggestive of a chronic condition (2). Rotator cuff tears and neurovascular injuries are uncommonly associated with posterior fracture-dislocations, but they must be ruled out (36,37,45).

It is also important to obtain a thorough past medical history of the patient including medical, neurologic, and psychological comorbidities, since these injuries are often associated with seizures, trauma, or alcohol withdrawal.

IMAGING

Common findings of posterior fracture-dislocations on standard anteroposterior (AP) plain radiographs of the shoulder include internal rotation of the proximal humerus (described as the "lightbulb sign"), overlap of the humeral head and glenoid, an indentation fracture line on the humeral head parallel to the glenoid and a small humeral head relative to the glenoid (2,35,46)

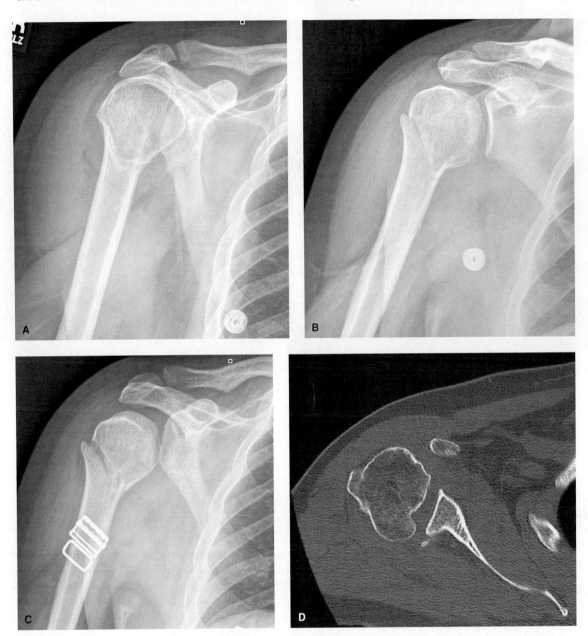

▲ **FIGURE 20-1:** **A:** Internal and **B:** External rotation anteroposterior (AP) plain radiographs of a posterior fracture-dislocation of the shoulder, with fracture line through the surgical neck of the proximal humerus. The extent of the injury was not fully appreciated on the initial postinjury images, although the typical, "lightbulb sign," can be seen on the internal rotation view **(A)**. **C:** Follow-up plain radiographs showed more obvious overlap of the humeral head and glenoid, an indentation fracture line on the humeral head parallel to the glenoid, and widening of the glenohumeral joint space, consistent with a posterior dislocation. **D:** Subsequent CT of the shoulder demonstrated a head-split component to the fracture, with the posterior fragment of the humeral head dislocated posteriorly.

(Fig. 20-1A–C). Widening of the joint space can occur in the rare case where there is interposition of the torn rotator cuff (47).

It is essential, however, to obtain an axillary radiograph to confirm or rule out the diagnosis. Although standard axial radiographs may be difficult to obtain since they require arm abduction, apical oblique (48), Velpeau (49), or modified axial radiographs (50) can be obtained without any manipulation of the arm.

Computed tomography (CT) scans are useful in confirming the diagnosis, when plain radiographs are inadequate, and to delineate the number of fracture fragments, the orientation of the fracture lines, as well as the size of the defect in the humeral head (Fig. 20-1D). CT can also detect occult anatomic neck fractures (51) and the presence of arthritic changes in the shoulder (2,52). The features of the fracture on the CT scan may determine whether the injury is acute or chronic (2).

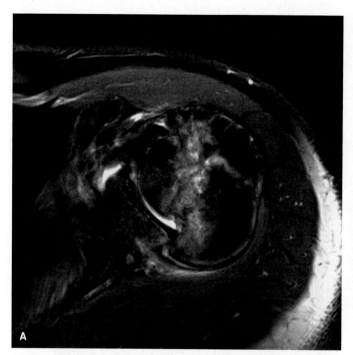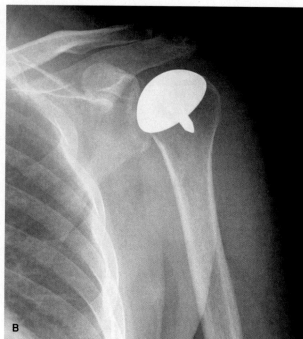

▲ **FIGURE 20-2: A:** Axial, T2-weighted MRI demonstrating a humeral head-splitting posterior fracture-dislocation of the shoulder, with the posterior fragment of the humeral head dislocated posteriorly. The injury went undetected in the acute period and the patient ultimately presented 5 months later with passive external rotation of the shoulder limited to negative 20 degrees. **B:** The patient was treated surgically with a humeral resurfacing.

If closed reduction of a fracture-dislocation is performed, it is also essential to carefully review postreduction imaging. Unrecognized fractures may become displaced upon reduction of the dislocation, which could jeopardize the vascularity of the humeral head and potentially lead to instability, avascular necrosis, and degenerative changes (22,53).

CLASSIFICATION

Robinson et al. (21) investigated 26 patients with 28 posterior fracture-dislocations of the shoulder and divided the cases into three subtypes based on the extent of the fracture and the involvement of the tuberosities.

- Type 1: Represents a Neer two-part anatomic neck fracture without associated tuberosity fractures. This was found in 6/28 cases (21%)
- Type 2: Represents a Neer three-part fracture involving the anatomic neck, as well as the lesser tuberosity. The lesser tuberosity fracture line propagates from the reverse Hill-Sachs lesion. This was found in 5/28 cases (18%)
- Type 3: Represents a Neer three-part fracture with a composite tuberosity "shield" fragment. This was found in 17/28 patients (61%). This fracture pattern consists of an anatomic neck fracture and a fracture involving both tuberosities. The tuberosities, however, form a composite "shield" fragment, as described by Edelson et al. (54) via an intact posterior periosteal

sleeve. The periosteal sleeve enabled the tuberosities to remain minimally displaced despite the presence of intertubercular comminution ("shattered shield" configuration) in some patients.

Chalidis et al. (53) added a fourth subtype, representing a Neer four-part fracture, in which the tuberosities are substantially displaced, in addition to the anatomic neck fracture. Isolated lesser tuberosity fractures, surgical neck fractures, and head-splitting fractures also occur with posterior fracture-dislocations of the shoulder, but were excluded from the Robinson et al. study (3,15,20,24,39).

TREATMENT AND OUTCOMES

Regardless of the type of fracture or the type of treatment, early recognition of posterior shoulder fracture-dislocations is crucial as late diagnosis results in poor outcomes (3). Reduction of a dislocated humeral head becomes difficult beyond 6 weeks, and late treatment is associated with painful and stiff shoulders (30). Treatment within 2 years of injury has been reported to result in better shoulder function in comparison with neglected or misdiagnosed cases (55).

There have been a number of described techniques for the treatment of posterior fracture-dislocations of the shoulder. These techniques differ based on patient age, the pattern and morphology of the fracture, the number

TABLE 20-1 Posterior Shoulder Fracture-Dislocation Classification and Treatment Algorithm Proposed by Checchia et al.

Group	Type of Fracture/Size of Reverse Hill-Sachs Lesion	Duration of Dislocation	Treatment
I	<20% lesion	Acute	Closed reduction and 6-wk immobilization in external rotation
II	Three-part fracture Anatomic neck fracture in young patient Tuberosity fracture	Acute	Open reduction and internal fixation
III	>20% but <50% lesion	Acute or chronic <6 mos	McLaughlin or modified McLaughlin procedure
IV A	>50% lesion 4-part fracture Anatomic neck fracture in older patient	Acute or chronic <12 mos	Hemiarthroplasty
B	Abnormal humeral head cartilage	Chronic 12 mos	
V	Glenoid arthritic changes	Chronic <2 yrs	Total shoulder arthroplasty
VI	Severe global arthritic changes	Chronic >2 yrs	Arthrodesis or resection arthroplasty

From: Checchia SL, Santos PD, Miyazaki AN. Surgical treatment of acute and chronic posterior fracture-dislocation of the shoulder. *J Shoulder Elbow Surg.* 1998;7(1):53–65.

of fracture fragments, the chronicity of the injury, the reducibility of the humeral head, the magnitude of the reverse Hill-Sachs lesion, and the presence or lack of soft tissue attachments to the fracture fragments (15,24). Treatment options include closed reduction alone, closed or open reduction followed by percutaneous pinning, open reduction and suture fixation, open reduction and internal fixation using locking plates and/or screws, and arthroplasty (hemiarthroplasty, standard or reverse total shoulder arthroplasty) (1,21,24,25,44,56–59). Checchia et al. (55) proposed a treatment algorithm and a classification based on the type of fracture, the size of the reverse Hill-Sachs lesion, and the duration of the dislocation. This algorithm included cases of posterior fracture-dislocations, as well as posterior dislocations with impression fractures alone. The algorithm is summarized in Table 20-1.

Treatment of isolated lesser tuberosity fractures associated with posterior shoulder fracture-dislocations has been described separately than other types of fractures. Therefore, management of this pattern of posterior fracture-dislocation will be discussed separately first, followed by an overview of treatment options for other fracture patterns.

Isolated Lesser Tuberosity Fracture Associated with Posterior Shoulder Fracture-Dislocation

Dislocations with nondisplaced lesser tuberosity fractures should be treated similarly to simple dislocations (60,61). Isolated, displaced tuberosity fractures can be

treated with closed reduction alone if the fracture reduces as a result of the joint reduction (35). However, even in these cases, some authors recommend open reduction and internal fixation to ensure a secure reduction of the lesser tuberosity and to allow a faster rehabilitation program (35). Displaced lesser tuberosity fractures that remain displaced after closed reduction require open reduction and internal fixation, generally with a tension band construct using heavy suture or wires (35,38,60). The lesser tuberosity can be either fixed anatomically or into the base of the reverse Hill-Sachs lesion if the shoulder is unstable (2). In the face of an irreducible posterior shoulder dislocation with an isolated lesser tuberosity fracture, an open reduction is also indicated. Internal fixation with a tension band construct using sutures or wires is recommended (35,44).

Regardless of the method of treatment, it is essential to obtain adequate reduction of the lesser tuberosity fragment for proper functioning of the subscapularis. The subscapularis is the only internal rotator that provides terminal internal rotation; therefore, patients suffering from subscapularis deficiency often complain of difficult with tucking in their shirts, reaching their back pockets, or fastening the bra strap behind their backs (35).

Other Fracture Patterns Associated with Posterior Fracture-Dislocations

Closed Reduction

When an anatomic neck fracture or head-split fracture exists, closed reduction of a posterior shoulder fracture-dislocation is more controversial. Some authors argue

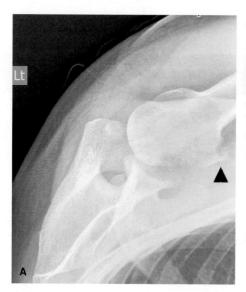 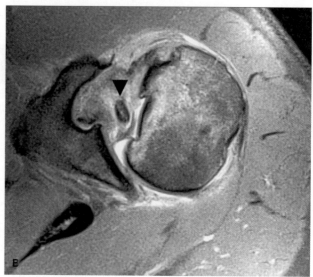

▲ **FIGURE 20-3:** **A:** Postreduction axillary plain radiograph showing persistent posterior subluxation of a lesser tuberosity posterior fracture-dislocation of the shoulder that occurred due to a seizure. The lesser tuberosity fracture is identified by the *arrowhead*. **B:** Subsequent MRI study demonstrated interposition of the long head of the biceps tendon in the fracture site (*arrowhead*) as the cause of the persistent subluxation (axial, T2-weighted image). This finding was confirmed intraoperatively, and the patient was treated with biceps tenodesis and open reduction and internal fixation of the lesser tuberosity fracture using a tension band technique with heavy suture. (Reprinted from: Ilaslan H, Bilenler A, Schils J, et al. Pseudoparalysis of shoulder caused by glenohumeral interposition of rotator cuff tendon stumps: A rare complication of posterior shoulder dislocation. *Skeletal Radiol.* 2013;42:135–139, with permission.)

that closed reduction may result in further displacement or avascular necrosis of the humeral head (27,28,32,62). Nevertheless, there are a number of reports of successful treatment with closed reduction (5,18,25,26,34,63). As a result, some authors (25) believe that if the fracture fragments have some contact then one attempt of gentle closed reduction under full-relaxant general anesthesia is acceptable. However, closed reduction is futile if the humeral head appears to be completely detached (25). Spontaneous reduction of displaced fracture fragments has been reported to occur with closed reduction of a dislocated humeral head (25,63). In these cases, nonoperative treatment (25) or limited percutaneous pinning (57) has been suggested.

Closed reduction is unlikely to be successful with chronic cases, especially 6 weeks after the injury. Acute dislocations may also be irreducible in a closed manner due to inadequate sedation or muscle relaxation, concomitant fractures around the shoulder, buttonholing of the humeral head through the posterior capsule and/or musculature, or interposition of soft tissue structures in the joint or between fracture fragments (46). Both the long head of the biceps tendon and the infraspinatus have been reported to be an interposing structure preventing closed reduction (29,46,63–66) (Fig. 20-3).

Traction in the "zero position" (155 degrees overhead and 45 degrees in front of the coronal plane) has been described as a technique to improve the success of closed reduction of posterior shoulder fracture-dislocations (46). In this position, all of the rotator cuff muscles as well as the biceps align along the scapular spine and humeral shaft. This allows the biceps to be reduced to its proper position. Moreover, traction in this position decreases the tension on the infraspinatus and permits the teres minor to move upward over the humeral head, pushing the head forward and reducing it into the joint (46).

Minimally Invasive Techniques

Other authors have recommended the use of arthroscopically assisted (67) or minimally invasive techniques (1,57), in addition to percutaneous fixation for posterior fracture-dislocations. Altay et al. (1) used a limited 5-cm incision centered over the glenoid to leverage the humeral head out of the dislocated position with a flat instrument, followed by percutaneous pin fixation. Shoulder motion was started at 3 weeks postoperatively. They reported their results on 10 patients with four-part posterior fracture-dislocations at mean 3.2-year follow-up. Nine patients had excellent results with mean Constant score of 95.7, no pain, no loss of fixation, and "minor" loss of range of motion. These patients did not demonstrate any signs of malunion, nonunion, avascular necrosis, or joint incongruity. The authors noted, however, that all patients with excellent results had at least 1 mm of the medial neck still attached to the humeral head. The one patient with a poor outcome developed avascular necrosis and did not have any neck portion attached to the humeral head. They concluded that patients who do not have any medial neck attached to the head should receive arthroplasty.

Ogawa et al. (25) studied 10 patients with posterior fracture-dislocations involving at least the anatomic neck, and found that in 9 patients, the fracture fragments reduced to within 10 mm of their anatomic position after reduction of the humeral head. Closed reduction was successful in two patients, whereas eight patients required an open reduction via a posterior approach using the interval between the teres minor and the infraspinatus. The authors argued that when the fracture fragments reduce by closed or open reduction, internal fixation is not essential since reduction indicates that a sleeve of tissue connecting and stabilizing all fragments is present. The last patient had a persistently displaced lesser tuberosity fragment following open reduction using a posterior approach. Eight of the ten patients had complete recovery of function at 2-year follow-up, one developed avascular necrosis and one had decreased range of motion due to the persistently displaced lesser tuberosity. On the basis of their findings, the authors recommended this technique when fracture fragments reduce with less than 10 mm of displacement, otherwise open reduction and internal fixation is required.

Open Reduction and Internal Fixation

Due to concerns of substantial risk of soft tissue injury and iatrogenic displacement of a humeral head fragment (27) with closed reduction, many authors prefer and advocate that reduction and fixation of posterior fracture-dislocations be performed in an open fashion under direct vision.

Two-, three-, and four-part fractures involving the anatomic neck or a head-split are treated either with open reduction and internal fixation or with arthroplasty. The decision between the two is often based on patient age, medical status, the degree of fragmentation, and the presumed devascularization of the humeral head and tuberosities (61). Although preoperative planning is imperative, often the final treatment choice is made intraoperatively after a thorough assessment of the fracture fragments and their vascularity. Therefore, even if the initial plan is to perform open reduction and internal fixation, it is important to be prepared for shoulder arthroplasty, either hemiarthoplasty or reverse total shoulder arthroplasty, as a back-up option and have all required components available. Patient age is a significant consideration in this decision-making process. Open reduction and internal fixation is almost always attempted in the acute setting in younger patients with good bone quality, regardless of the fracture pattern, due to the desire to maintain the patient's native bone, the high functional expectations, and the concerns about implant longevity in shoulder arthroplasty.

Previously, open reduction and internal fixation has been criticized for its high risk of avascular necrosis, nonunion of the humeral head, and poor outcomes (2,58,59,68). However, with newer surgical techniques and with the use of locking plates, recent studies have shown that the prevalence of these complications is lower than previously reported (21,69–71). Furthermore, recent studies demonstrate that the functional results of arthroplasty, particularly hemiarthroplasty, may be poorer than those achieved by successful open reduction and internal fixation (21).

A number of surgical approaches have been described for open reduction and internal fixation of posterior fracture-dislocations, including the deltopectoral (4,5,29,33,72), deltoid splitting (21), and superior subacromial approaches (73). The posterior approach (32,62,74–76) has been used for reduction of the dislocation, as it provides direct visualization of the dislocated humeral head and avoids any further injury to the anterior blood vessels. However, it cannot be used for internal fixation and it risks injury to the posterior vessels, which may be the sole blood supply after these injuries. The deltopectoral approach is the most commonly used and preferred approach, but has some limitations: Access to the dislocated humeral head at the posterior aspect of the glenoid may be difficult and the anterior soft tissues of the shoulder may be further injured (25). While posterior exposure is improved with the deltoid splitting and superior subacromial approaches, both of these approaches are limited by the course of the axillary nerve and thus fractures with more distal extension may not be accessible. In addition, they require dissection of the deltoid, which may lead to damage or dehiscence of this muscle (25).

Following the surgical approach, the first step is to reduce the dislocated humeral head using a combination of disengagement from the posterior glenoid, pressure from the posterior shoulder, and traction. Flat instruments, such as a Cobb elevator, may help with disengaging the humeral head and reduction. Temporary K-wire fixation may also be placed initially to prevent fracture displacement during open reduction of the dislocation (27). After reduction of the dislocated humeral head, the type of fixation used varies depending on the complexity of the fracture, as well as the bone quality. Two-part fractures involving the tuberosities or isolated head-splitting fractures may be treated with interfragmentary screws alone (77), while more complicated multipart fractures and anatomic or surgical neck fractures often require the use of locking plates and possible suture tension banding of the tuberosities (69,78,79). A tension band construct with heavy suture or wire may also be an appropriate fixation for isolated tuberosity fractures.

In Robinson et al.'s series (21), patients showed significant continued functional improvements within the first two postoperative years after open reduction and internal fixation, with median Constant score of 83.5 at 2 years. Loss of internal rotation was responsible for most of the functional loss on the score. Eighty-six percent (86%) of patients reported no pain, 9% had mild pain and 5% complained of moderate activity-related pain. Average shoulder forward flexion and abduction were 172 degrees and 169 degrees, respectively. All but two shoulders regained full external rotation; one lost 10 degrees and the other 24 degrees. Seventy-three percent (73%) of patients regained full internal rotation, while the others lost 5 to 45 degrees. No patients showed evidence of shoulder instability, rotator cuff weakness, or impingement. These results are superior to those reported for hemiarthroplasty (80–84).

It is important, as mentioned, to address these fracture-dislocations acutely as neglected or missed injuries become extremely difficult to reduce and extensive soft tissue and capsular dissection is required. Furthermore, malunion of the proximal humerus makes reconstructive procedures technically challenging (2). Even in the acute setting, however, open reduction and internal fixation carries potential postoperative risks, including the development of avascular necrosis, segmental fracture collapse, and hardware failure. Therefore, close surgical follow-up is essential.

Shoulder Arthroplasty

Traditionally, hemiarthroplasty was the most commonly advocated treatment for posterior fracture-dislocations of the shoulder, mainly due to the reported high risk of avascular necrosis or nonunion of the humeral head following open reduction and internal fixation (58,59). Neer in 1970 (59) recommended prosthetic replacement after his experience with 14 shoulders, reporting that the results of arthroplasty were better than open reduction and internal fixation, although still imperfect. Shaw (40) reported his results of bilateral hemiarthroplasties performed on a patient 3 to 4 weeks after suffering bilateral four-part posterior shoulder fracture-dislocations. Postoperatively, the patient achieved 90 degrees of forward elevation, 90 degrees of abduction, 20 degrees of external rotation, 45 degrees of extension, and 90 degrees of internal rotation, bilaterally. Hawkins et al. (24) suggested a treatment protocol for locked posterior fracture-dislocations, which included total shoulder arthroplasty if the duration of the dislocation is greater than 6 months or if there is significant damage to the glenoid and humeral head articular surfaces.

However, recent studies have suggested that the results of arthroplasty, specifically hemiarthroplasty, may be suboptimal (80–84). Outcomes, however, differ based on the chronicity of the dislocation and the specific fracture pattern. Chronic cases treated with hemiarthroplasty seem to perform better than acute cases,

and hemiarthroplasty may be the only treatment option for a chronic, missed fracture-dislocation in young or middle age patient when humeral head deformity prevents open reduction and internal fixation (55) (Fig. 20-2B). Functional results after hemiarthroplasty may also be better in fracture patterns that do not disrupt the tuberosities, such as head-splitting fractures. Since posterior fracture-dislocations mostly occur in middle age patients with higher functional demands, however, there has been concern about the long-term effects of arthroplasty and implant longevity.

Nevertheless, prosthetic replacement is still advocated by many authors for four-part fracture-dislocations, due to concerns with avascular necrosis, subchondral bone collapse, and subsequent bony incongruity (73,85,86). Arthroplasty is also recommended for multipart fractures in the elderly because of poor bone quality and fracture comminution that can make internal fixation not feasible, with reverse total shoulder arthroplasty becoming a more frequent option (55,56,61). When the glenoid articular surface is affected, total shoulder arthroplasty should be considered, again with reverse total shoulder arthroplasty as an option in the elderly. The series by Hawkins et al. (24) and Cheng et al. (56) demonstrated very good results for total shoulder arthroplasty with regard to pain relief and functional outcomes; however, patients still had difficulty with overhead activities and there was a 10% incidence of redislocation in both studies.

Arthroplasty after posterior fracture-dislocations may be technically difficult as it is challenging to judge the appropriate soft tissue tensioning and obtain stable fixation of the tuberosities (61). In chronic cases where a malunion has occurred, it is best to avoid performing osteotomy of the tuberosities as this can be associated with nonunion, secondary displacement, and a poor functional outcome (36,87,88). Furthermore, although the deltopectoral approach is the most common approach used for arthroplasty, extraction of the dislocated humeral head may be difficult from an anterior approach and some authors have recommended a second posterior incision if necessary to extract the humeral head (56).

More recently, reverse total shoulder arthroplasty has been suggested as a more reliable and more functional treatment option relative to hemiarthroplasty for posterior fracture-dislocations in the elderly (Fig. 20-4). Expert opinion indicates that this procedure seems to result in more favorable outcomes in older patients. However, to our knowledge, there are no published reports on the use of reverse total shoulder arthroplasty for posterior fracture-dislocations. Moreover, reverse total shoulder arthroplasty should be reserved for older patients and is not recommended for the typical middle-aged patients suffering a posterior shoulder

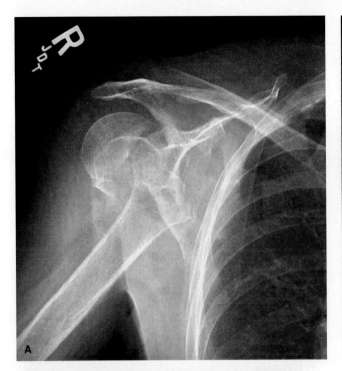

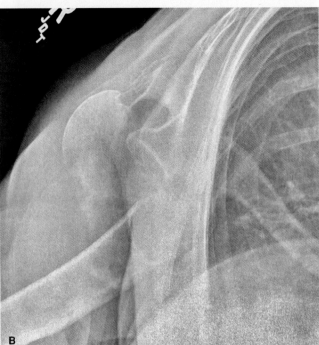

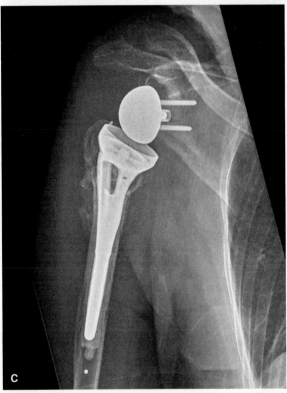

▲ **FIGURE 20-4:** **A:** Anteroposterior (AP) and **B:** axillary plain radiographs of a four-part posterior fracture-dislocation of the shoulder in an elderly patient, with fracture lines through the surgical neck, greater and lesser tuberosities. **C:** The patient presented more than a month after the injury and was treated surgically with reverse total shoulder arthroplasty.

fracture-dislocation, due to concerns about implant durability in this patient population.

Other Treatment Options

Other surgical treatment options have been reported for posterior fracture-dislocations of the shoulder,

including shoulder arthrodesis and resection arthroplasty (55,89). However, these procedures are typically not recommended as primary treatment options and are considered salvage procedures when extensive arthritis is present due to a very chronic fracture-dislocation in a young patient (55).

COMPLICATIONS

Avascular Necrosis

Although avascular necrosis may occur as a result of the initial fracture-dislocation, it is more common in patients who undergo open reduction and internal fixation for an anatomic neck fracture (27,90). The risk of avascular necrosis increases with the degree of fracture displacement, the extent of tuberosity involvement, as well as the chronicity of the injury prior to treatment (61). However, accurate reduction and stable internal fixation, even when performed late, has been reported to improve the likelihood of revascularization of the humeral head and decrease the risk of avascular necrosis (31,91). Reperfusion can occur via the intact posteromedial branches of the posterior humeral circumflex artery or, alternatively, by creeping substitution when all arterial flow and soft tissue attachment has been disrupted (2). Multiple long-term follow-up reports demonstrate that patients can show no evidence of avascular necrosis or head collapse after open reduction and internal fixation even when the humeral head fragments are found to be devoid of all soft tissue attachments intraoperatively (31,71,91).

Robinson et al. (21) found that all patients in their cohort had an intact posterior capsule and periosteal sleeve "hinge," possibly providing vascularity to the humeral head. This is likely to be the case if there is still a metaphyseal fragment attached to the inferomedial portion of the humeral head (25). Moreover, if the intertubercular grove is intact, the anterolateral ascending branch of the anterior humeral circumflex artery is likely to be preserved.

While avascular necrosis can lead to poor functional outcomes with the subsequent development of humeral head collapse, it may still be associated with satisfactory function if an anatomic reconstruction has been achieved (69,92).

Instability

In the study by Robinson et al. (21), 11 of 28 shoulders demonstrated posterior instability with neutral shoulder rotation after open reduction and internal fixation. This instability was a result of a reverse Hill-Sachs lesion, which caused the head to engage on the posterior glenoid leading to recurrent dislocation. Therefore, it is essential to assess for the presence and extent of this lesion at the time of surgery, including evaluation of the stability of the humeral head after open reduction and internal fixation to determine if adjunctive procedures are required. The reverse Hill-Sachs lesion can be addressed with several surgical options, based on defect size and chronicity. Elevation of the osteochondral defect with bone grafting may be possible in the acute setting, while transfer of the lesser tuberosity or structural allograft may be better options for bigger or more chronic defects (21). Hemiarthroplasty has been recommended when the reverse Hill-Sachs lesion is >50% of the articular surface (2,87).

Posttraumatic Arthritis

Radiographic signs of arthritic changes in the glenohumeral joint are common following posterior fracture-dislocations. Aparicio et al. (52) found that radiographic degenerative changes were present in the majority of cases they reviewed. Treatment is based on symptom severity, as patients' symptoms may not always correlate with the severity of radiographic changes. Symptomatic patients may benefit from initial nonoperative management, including activity modification, oral anti-inflammatories, and intra-articular cortisone injections. If symptoms worsen and fail to improve with nonoperative management, total shoulder arthroplasty may be indicated.

Stiffness

Shoulder stiffness is common in cases of posterior fracture-dislocation with a delay in treatment, posttraumatic degenerative changes, humeral head deformity, and avascular necrosis (2). Hemiarthroplasty has also been associated with decreased postoperative range of motion (56,80–82,93), especially in the elderly or in patients with malunion or nonunion of the tuberosities (81). Treatment of shoulder stiffness should address the underlying cause, once identified. In the absence of advanced degenerative changes or humeral head collapse, manipulation under anesthesia and/or arthroscopic capsular release followed by an intensive physical therapy regimen should be considered as a treatment option when range-of-motion fails to improve with nonoperative management (61). As noted above, advanced arthritic changes or humeral head collapse may be an indication for shoulder arthroplasty.

Other Complications

Other postoperative complications include infection, prominent hardware causing irritation, and subacromial impingement (21). Infections following open reduction and internal fixation may be treated with antibiotic therapy, irrigation and debridement, and hardware retention if fracture healing is not complete. Infections following arthroplasty are treated in a similar fashion to infections that occur after other shoulder arthroplasties, with implant removal and two-stage reimplantation usually required in a deep chronic infection. Prominent hardware may need to be removed after fracture healing is complete, but subacromial impingement is often resolved with a cortisone injection alone.

CONCLUSION

Posterior shoulder fracture-dislocations are uncommon injuries that are often caused by seizures, motor vehicle collisions, and falls. Since these injuries are frequently misdiagnosed, the clinician must have a high level of suspicion and perform a thorough physical examination with adequate radiographic evaluation. A block to passive external rotation beyond neutral is a key feature on examination that can aid in the diagnosis. There are many treatment options depending on the age of the patient, the chronicity of the injury, the pattern of the fracture, the quality of the bone, and the extent of comminution. Closed reduction may be attempted but is unlikely to be successful if the dislocation is older than 6 weeks. Open reduction and internal fixation is favored in young patients when possible, but in certain cases where the blood supply has been compromised, hemiarthroplasty may be the only solution. Reverse total shoulder arthroplasty has recently become a more common option in older patients.

References

1. Altay T, Ozturk H, Us RM, et al. Four-part posterior fracture–dislocations of the shoulder. Treatment by limited open reduction and percutaneous stabilization. *Arch Orthop Trauma Surg.* 1999;119(1–2):35–38.
2. Robinson CM, Aderinto J. Posterior shoulder dislocations and fracture-dislocations. *J Bone Joint Surg Am.* 2005;87(3):639–650.
3. Wilson JC, McKeever FM. Traumatic posterior dislocation of the humerus. *J Bone Joint Surg Am.* 1949;31A(1):160–172.
4. McLaughlin HL. Posterior dislocation of the shoulder. *J Bone Joint Surg Am.* 1952;24-A-3:584–590.
5. Dorgan JA. Posterior dislocation of the shoulder. *Am J Surg.* 1955;89(4):890–900.
6. Rowe CR. Prognosis in dislocations of the shoulder. *J Bone Joint Surg Am.* 1956;38-A(5):957–977.
7. May VR Jr. Posterior dislocation of the shoulder: Habitual, traumatic, and obstetrical. *Orthop Clin North Am.* 1980;11(2):271–285.
8. DePalma AF. Dislocations of the shoulder girdle. In: DePalma AF. ed. *Surgery of the Shoulder.* 3rd ed. Philadelphia, PA: Lippincott; 1983:428–511.
9. Ovesen J, Sojbjerg JO. Posterior shoulder dislocation. Muscle and capsular lesions in cadaver experiments. *Acta Orthop Scand.* 1986;57(6):535–536.
10. Warren R, Kornblatt I, Marchand R. Static factors affecting posterior shoulder stability. *Orthop Trans.* 1984;8:89.
11. Terry GC, Hammon D, France P, et al. The stabilizing function of passive shoulder restraints. *Am J Sports Med.* 1991;19(1):26–34.
12. O'Brien SJ, Schwartz RS, Warren RF, et al. Capsular restraints to anterior-posterior motion of the abducted shoulder: A biomechanical study. *J Shoulder Elbow Surg.* 1995;4(4):298–308.
13. Harryman DT 2nd, Sidles JA, Harris SL, Matsen FA 3rd. The role of the rotator interval capsule in passive motion and stability of the shoulder. *J Bone Joint Surg Am.* 1992;74(1):53–66.
14. Ovesen J, Nielsen S. Anterior and posterior shoulder instability. A cadaver study. *Acta Orthop Scand.* 1986;57(4):324–327.
15. Blasier RB, Soslowsky LJ, Malicky DM, et al. Posterior glenohumeral subluxation: Active and passive stabilization in a biomechanical model. *J Bone Joint Surg Am* 1997;79(3):433–440.
16. DeToledo JC, Lowe MR. Seizures, lateral decubitus, aspiration, and shoulder dislocation: Time to change the guidelines? *Neurology.* 2001;56(3):290–291.
17. DeToledo JC, Lowe MR, Ramsay RE. Restraining patients and shoulder dislocations during seizures. *J Shoulder Elbow Surg.* 1999;8(4):300–302.
18. Chattopadhyaya PK. Posterior fracture-dislocation of the shoulder. Report of a case. *J Bone Joint Surg Br.* 1970;52(3):521–523.
19. Neer CS, Brown TH Jr, McLaughlin HL. Fracture of the neck of the humerus with dislocation of the head fragment. *Am J Surg.* 1953;85(3):252–258.
20. Neer CS 2nd. Displaced proximal humeral fractures. Part I. Classification and evaluation. By Charles S. Neer, I, 1970. *Clin Orthop Relat Res.* 1987;(223):3–10.
21. Robinson CM, Akhtar A, Mitchell M, et al. Complex posterior fracture-dislocation of the shoulder. Epidemiology, injury patterns, and results of operative treatment. *J Bone Joint Surg Am.* 2007;89(7):1454–1466.
22. Bock P, Kluger R, Hintermann B. Anatomical reconstruction for reverse Hill-Sachs lesions after posterior locked shoulder dislocation fracture: A case series of six patients. *Arch Orthop Trauma Surg.* 2007;127(7):543–548.
23. Moseley HF. *Shoulder Lesions.* 3rd ed. Edinburgh and London: Churchill Livingstone; 1969.
24. Hawkins RJ, Neer CS 2nd, Pianta RM, et al. Locked posterior dislocation of the shoulder. *J Bone Joint Surg Am.* 1987;69(1):9–18.
25. Ogawa K, Yoshida A, Inokuchi W. Posterior shoulder dislocation associated with fracture of the humeral anatomic neck: Treatment guidelines and long-term outcome. *J Trauma.* 1999;46(2):318–323.
26. Bell HM. Posterior fracture-dislocation of the shoulder–a method of closed reduction; a case report. *J Bone Joint Surg Am.* 1965;47(8):1521–1524.
27. Hersche O, Gerber C. Iatrogenic displacement of fracture-dislocations of the shoulder. A report of seven cases. *J Bone Joint Surg Br.* 1994;76(1):30–33.
28. Neer CS 2nd. Prosthetic replacement of the humeral head: Indications and operative technique. *Surg Clin North Am.* 1963;43:1581–1597.
29. Richards RH, Clarke NM. Locked posterior fracture-dislocation of the shoulder. *Injury.* 1989;20(5):297–300.
30. Honner R. Bilateral posterior dislocation of the shoulders. *Aust N Z J Surg.* 1969;38(3):269–272.
31. Swamy G, Schemitsch EH. Humeral head fracture dislocation: Case report and review of the literature. *J Trauma.* 1998;44(2):377–380.

32. Fipp GJ. Simultaneous posterior dislocation of both shoulders. Report of a case. *Clin Orthop Relat Res.* 1966; 44:191–195.

33. Galanakis IA, Kontakis GM, Steriopoulos KA. Posterior dislocation of the shoulder associated with fracture of the humeral anatomic neck. *J Trauma.* 1997;42(6):1176–1178.

34. Taylor RG, Wright PR. Posterior dislocation of the shoulder. *J Bone Joint Surg Br.* 1952;34-B(4):624–629.

35. Hayes PR, Klepps S, Bishop J, et al. Posterior shoulder dislocation with lesser tuberosity and scapular spine fractures. *J Shoulder Elbow Surg.* 2003;12(5):524–527.

36. Gerber C. Chronic, locked anterior and posterior dislocations. In: Warner J, Iannotti J, Gerber C, eds. *Complex and Revision Problems in Shoulder Surgery.* Philadelphia, PA: Lippincott-Raven; 1997:99–116.

37. Roberts A, Wickstrom J. Prognosis of posterior dislocation of the shoulder. *Acta Orthop Scand.* 1971;42(4):328–337.

38. van Laarhoven HA, te Slaa RL, van Laarhoven EW. Isolated avulsion fracture of the lesser tuberosity of the humerus. *J Trauma.* 1995;39(5):997–999.

39. Neviaser JS. Posterior dislocations of the shoulder: Diagnosis and treatment. *Surg Clin North Am.* 1963;43:1623–1630.

40. Shaw JL. Bilateral posterior fracture-dislocation of the shoulder and other trauma caused by convulsive seizures. *J Bone Joint Surg Am.* 1971;53(7):1437–1440.

41. Heller KD, Forst J, Forst R. Differential therapy of traumatically-induced persistent posterior shoulder dislocation. Review of the literature. *Unfallchirurg.* 1995;98(1):6–12.

42. Hawkins RJ. Unrecognized dislocations of the shoulder. *Instr Course Lect.* 1985;34:258–263.

43. Jensen KL, Rockwood CA Jr. X-ray evaluation of shoulder problems. In: Rockwood CA Jr, Matsen FA 3rd, Wirth MA, Lippitt SB, eds. *The Shoulder.* Vol 1. 3rd ed. Philadelphia, PA: Saunders; 2004:187–222.

44. Tey IK, Tan AH. Posterior fracture-dislocation of the humeral head treated without the use of metallic implants. *Singapore Med J.* 2007;48(4):e114–e118.

45. Steinitz DK, Harvey EJ, Lenczner EM. Traumatic posterior dislocation of the shoulder associated with a massive rotator cuff tear: A case report. *Am J Sports Med.* 2003;31(6):1010–1012.

46. Ogawa K, Ogawa Y, Yoshida A. Posterior fracture-dislocation of the shoulder with infraspinatus interposition: The buttonhole phenomenon. *J Trauma.* 1997;43(4):688–691.

47. Tietjen R. Occult glenohumeral interposition of a torn rotator cuff. A case report. *J Bone Joint Surg Am.* 1982; 64(3):458–459.

48. Garth WP Jr, Slappey CE, Ochs CW. Roentgenographic demonstration of instability of the shoulder: The apical oblique projection. A technical note. *J Bone Joint Surg Am.* 1984;66(9):1450–1453.

49. Bloom MH, Obata WG. Diagnosis of posterior dislocation of the shoulder with use of Velpeau axillary and angle-up roentgenographic views. *J Bone Joint Surg Am.* 1967;49(5):943–949.

50. Wallace WA, Hellier M. Improving radiographs of the injured shoulder. *Radiography.* 1983;49(586):229–233.

51. Wadlington VR, Hendrix RW, Rogers LF. Computed tomography of posterior fracture-dislocations of the shoulder: Case reports. *J Trauma.* 1992;32(1):113–115.

52. Aparicio G, Calvo E, Bonilla L, et al. Neglected traumatic posterior dislocations of the shoulder: Controversies on indications for treatment and new CT scan findings. *J Orthop Sci.* 2000;5(1):37–42.

53. Chalidis BE, Papadopoulos PP, Dimitriou CG. Reconstruction of a missed posterior locked shoulder fracture-dislocation with bone graft and lesser tuberosity transfer: A case report. *J Med Case Rep.* 2008;2:260.

54. Edelson G, Kelly I, Vigder F, et al. A three-dimensional classification for fractures of the proximal humerus. *J Bone Joint Surg Br.* 2004;86(3):413–425.

55. Checchia SL, Santos PD, Miyazaki AN. Surgical treatment of acute and chronic posterior fracture-dislocation of the shoulder. *J Shoulder Elbow Surg.* 1998;7(1):53–65.

56. Cheng SL, Mackay MB, Richards RR. Treatment of locked posterior fracture-dislocations of the shoulder by total shoulder arthroplasty. *J Shoulder Elbow Surg.* 1997;6(1):11–17.

57. De Wall M, Lervick G, Marsh JL. Posterior fracture-dislocation of the proximal humerus: Treatment by closed reduction and limited fixation: A report of four cases. *J Orthop Trauma.* 2005;19(1):48–51.

58. Hawkins RJ, Switlyk P. Acute prosthetic replacement for severe fractures of the proximal humerus. *Clin Orthop Relat Res.* 1993;(289):156–160.

59. Neer CS 2nd. Displaced proximal humeral fractures. II. Treatment of three-part and four-part displacement. *J Bone Joint Surg Am.* 1970;52(6):1090–1103.

60. Ogawa K, Takahashi M. Long-term outcome of isolated lesser tuberosity fractures of the humerus. *J Trauma.* 1997;42(5):955–959.

61. Pereira DS, Zuckerman JD. Fracture-dislocations of the shoulder. In: Warren RF, Craig EV, Altchek DW, eds. *The Unstable Shoulder.* Philadelphia, PA: Lippincott-Raven; 1999:447–446.

62. Mills KL. Simultaneous bilateral posterior fracture-dislocation of the shoulder. *Injury.* 1974;6(1):39–41.

63. Samilson RL, Miller E. Posterior dislocations of the shoulder. *Clin Orthop Relat Res.* 1964;32:69–86.

64. Allard JC, Bancroft J. Irreducible posterior dislocation of the shoulder: MR and CT findings. *J Comput Assist Tomogr.* 1991;15(4):694–696.

65. Goldman A, Sherman O, Price A, et al. Posterior fracture dislocation of the shoulder with biceps tendon interposition. *J Trauma.* 1987;27(9):1083–1086.

66. Ilaslan H, Bilenler A, Schils J, et al. Pseudoparalysis of shoulder caused by glenohumeral interposition of rotator cuff tendon stumps: A rare complication of posterior shoulder dislocation. *Skeletal Radiol.* 2013;42(1):135–139.

67. Costa M, Sjolin S. Arthroscopically-assisted percutaneous fixation of a posterior fracture dislocation of the proximal humerus. *Ann R Coll Surg Engl.* 2006;88(1):78.

68. Des Marchais JE, Benazet JP. Evaluation of Neer's hemiarthroplasty in the treatment of humeral fractures. *Can J Surg.* 1983;26(5):469–471.

69. Wijgman AJ, Roolker W, Patt TW, et al. Open reduction and internal fixation of three and four-part fractures of the proximal part of the humerus. *J Bone Joint Surg Am.* 2002;84-A(11):1919–1925.

70. Robinson CM, Khan LA, Akhtar MA. Treatment of anterior fracture-dislocations of the proximal humerus by

open reduction and internal fixation. *J Bone Joint Surg Br.* 2006;88(4):502–508.

71. Kofoed H. Revascularization of the humeral head. A report of two cases of fracture-dislocation of the shoulder. *Clin Orthop Relat Res.* 1983;(179):175–178.

72. Din KM, Meggitt BF. Bilateral four-part fractures with posterior dislocation of the shoulder. A case report. *J Bone Joint Surg Br.* 1983;65(2):176–178.

73. Stableforth PG, Sarangi PP. Posterior fracture-dislocation of the shoulder. A superior subacromial approach for open reduction. *J Bone Joint Surg Br.* 1992;74(4):579–584.

74. Wirth MA, Butters KP, Rockwood CA Jr. The posterior deltoid-splitting approach to the shoulder. *Clin Orthop Relat Res.* 1993;(296):92–98.

75. Norwood LA, Matiko JA, Terry GC. Posterior shoulder approach. *Clin Orthop Relat Res.* 1985;(201):167–172.

76. Arden GP. Posterior dislocation of both shoulders; report of a case. *J Bone Joint Surg Br.* 1956;38-B(2):558–563.

77. Checchia SL. Treatment of locked anterior and posterior dislocations of the shoulder. In: Bigliani LU, Levine WN, Marra G, eds. *Fractures of the Shoulder Girdle.* New York, NY: Marcel Dekker; 2003:165–184.

78. Hawkins RJ, Bell RH, Gurr K. The three-part fracture of the proximal part of the humerus. Operative treatment. *J Bone Joint Surg Am.* 1986;68(9):1410–1414.

79. Iannotti JP, Ramsey ML, Williams GR Jr, et al. Nonprosthetic management of proximal humeral fractures. *Instr Course Lect.* 2004;53:403–416.

80. Robinson CM, Page RS, Hill RM, et al. Primary hemiarthroplasty for treatment of proximal humeral fractures. *J Bone Joint Surg Am.* 2003;85-A(7):1215–1223.

81. Boileau P, Krishnan SG, Tinsi L, et al. Tuberosity malposition and migration: Reasons for poor outcomes after hemiarthroplasty for displaced fractures of the proximal humerus. *J Shoulder Elbow Surg.* 2002;11(5):401–412.

82. Kralinger F, Schwaiger R, Wambacher M, et al. Outcome after primary hemiarthroplasty for fracture of the head of the humerus. A retrospective multicentre study of 167 patients. *J Bone Joint Surg Br.* 2004;86(2):217–219.

83. Wretenberg P, Ekelund A. Acute hemiarthroplasty after proximal humerus fracture in old patients. A retrospective evaluation of 18 patients followed for 2–7 years. *Acta Orthop Scand.* 1997;68(2):121–123.

84. Zyto K, Wallace WA, Frostick SP, et al. Outcome after hemiarthroplasty for three- and four-part fractures of the proximal humerus. *J Shoulder Elbow Surg.* 1998;7(2):85–89.

85. Tanner MW, Cofield RH. Prosthetic arthroplasty for fractures and fracture-dislocations of the proximal humerus. *Clin Orthop Relat Res.* 1983;(179):116–128.

86. Moeckel BH, Dines DM, Warren RF, et al. Modular hemiarthroplasty for fractures of the proximal part of the humerus. *J Bone Joint Surg Am.* 1992;74(6):884–889.

87. Cicak N. Posterior dislocation of the shoulder. *J Bone Joint Surg Br.* 2004;86(3):324–332.

88. Boileau P, Trojani C, Walch G, et al. Shoulder arthroplasty for the treatment of the sequelae of fractures of the proximal humerus. *J Shoulder Elbow Surg.* 2001;10(4):299–308.

89. Rowe CR, Zarins B. Chronic unreduced dislocations of the shoulder. *J Bone Joint Surg Am.* 1982;64(4):494–505.

90. Walch G, Boileau P, Martin B, et al. Unreduced posterior luxations and fractures-luxations of the shoulder. Apropos of 30 cases. *Rev Chir Orthop Reparatrice Appar Mot.* 1990;76(8):546–558.

91. Kaar TK, Wirth MA, Rockwood CA Jr. Missed posterior fracture-dislocation of the humeral head. A case report with a fifteen-year follow-up after delayed open reduction and internal fixation. *J Bone Joint Surg Am.* 1999;81(5):708–710.

92. Gerber C, Hersche O, Berberat C. The clinical relevance of posttraumatic avascular necrosis of the humeral head. *J Shoulder Elbow Surg.* 1998;7(6):586–590.

93. Mansat P, Guity MR, Bellumore Y, et al. Shoulder arthroplasty for late sequelae of proximal humeral fractures. *J Shoulder Elbow Surg.* 2004;13(3):305–312.

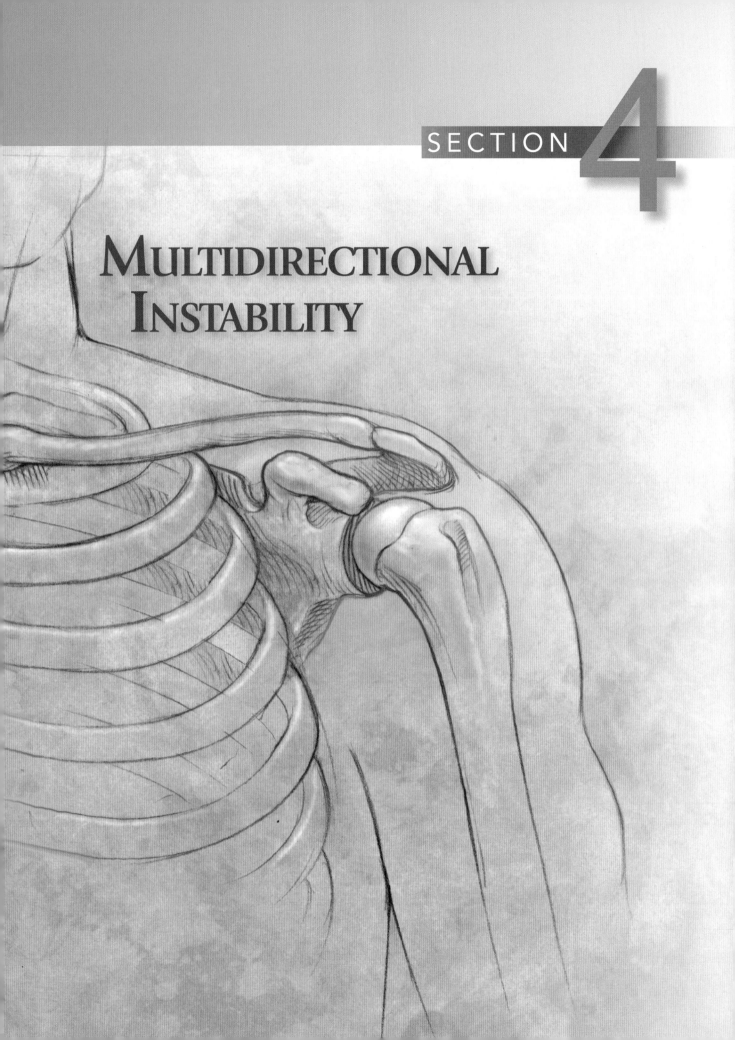

MULTIDIRECTIONAL INSTABILITY

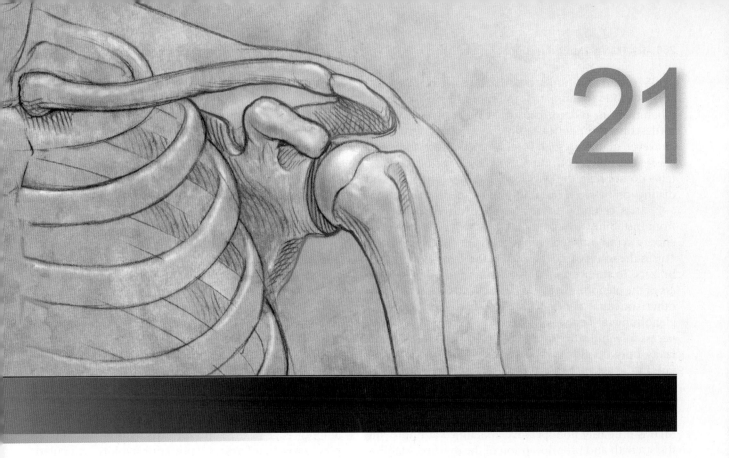

Why Rehabilitation Is the Most Effective Treatment Option for Multidirectional Shoulder Instability

Nicholas R. Slenker / Michael G. Ciccotti

INTRODUCTION

In 1980, Neer and Foster (1) first identified the complex shoulder condition known as multidirectional instability (MDI). They described it as "involuntary inferior and multidirectional subluxation and dislocation." This original article outlined the basis for much of our modern thinking about this condition. Today, MDI is generally considered to encompass symptomatic subluxation or dislocation of the glenohumeral joint in more than one direction, including the inferior, anterior, or posterior directions. The underlying pathoanatomy is multifactorial, including soft tissue laxity with subsequent capsular redundancy, or repetitive microtrauma as seen in overhead throwers and swimmers. Although basic science and clinical research have given us a better understanding of glenohumeral instability, the diagnosis and management of MDI remains a challenge.

Shoulder instability is best understood as a spectrum of disease. At one end of the spectrum is the most common type of instability, traumatic unidirectional instability, while atraumatic MDI lies at the other extreme. Historically, the acronyms

TUBS (traumatic, unilateral, Bankart lesion, surgery) and AMBRI (atraumatic, multidirectional, bilateral, rehabilitation, inferior capsular shift) have been used to describe shoulder instability in etiologic terms (2). However, many cases fall somewhere between these two classic examples. Unfortunately, these classification systems do not help the physician make the often difficult distinction between instability and hyperlaxity.

It is certainly most critical to distinguish laxity from instability. Instability is characterized by the presence of symptoms in conjunction with abnormal laxity. This is the result of a deficiency in the glenohumeral stabilizers. To some extent, the dynamic and static stabilizers of the glenohumeral joint are able to compensate for other structural deficiencies. So, objective measures of glenohumeral laxity, which may be abnormal, are not necessarily indicative of instability. Rather, symptomatic laxity only develops when compensatory mechanisms fail. In the absence of symptoms, the presence of a sulcus sign or the ability to subluxate the shoulder must not be inappropriately diagnosed as MDI.

Regardless of etiology, management of patients with MDI is primarily nonoperative and aimed at improving the strength and proprioception of the dynamic stabilizers of the glenohumeral joint and the periscapular muscles (1,3–6). In the recalcitrant case in which nonoperative treatment fails, surgical management is appropriate. There are several surgical techniques described to manage MDI, ranging from the classic open Neer inferior capsular shift to a multitude of arthroscopic procedures. Most of these procedures; however, have a much higher failure rate than operations designed for the treatment of unidirectional posttraumatic instability (3,7–10). This, along with a high success rate for nonoperative treatment in appropriately selected patients, makes rehabilitation the treatment of choice for MDI.

GLENOHUMERAL STABILITY

The glenohumeral joint is capable of a tremendous range of motion in multiple planes with a minimum of bony constraint. It requires both sufficient capsular pliability for normal function, as well as static and dynamic stabilizers to provide joint stability. Stabilizer deficiency yields instability, and therefore, treatment strategies focus on restoring or rehabilitating these structures.

Shoulder stability is imparted by a combination of static and dynamic stabilizers. Static stabilization of the joint is provided by its inherent bony and ligamentous structures. The soft tissue envelope of the joint capsule has discrete thickenings termed glenohumeral ligaments. The fibrocartilaginous labrum adds depth to the otherwise shallow glenoid fossa and serves as a site of attachment for the glenohumeral ligaments. Along with the labrum, the glenohumeral ligaments form the capsuloligamentous complex, which acts as the most important static stabilizer and is most effective at the extremes of glenohumeral joint motion.

The glenohumeral ligaments work through a pattern of reciprocal tension and relaxation throughout various shoulder positions. As a group, they render the shoulder stable through the full range of motion. The inferior glenohumeral ligament consists of discreet anterior and posterior bands that form a sling beneath the glenohumeral joint stabilizing the joint in positions of abduction and thereby preventing anterior, posterior, and inferior translations (11,12). The somewhat variable middle glenohumeral ligament provides anterior stability in the midrange of abduction, limiting external rotation, and inferior translation (13). The superior glenohumeral ligament (SGHL) and coracohumeral ligament stabilize the shoulder in the adducted position, primarily limiting inferior translation, and external rotation (14,15). Both the superior glenohumeral and coracohumeral ligaments also reinforce the rotator interval, which is a triangular portion of the capsule located between the superior edge of the subscapularis tendon and the anterior edge of the supraspinatus tendon. The interval plays a role in inferior and posterior stability, particularly when the arm is adducted and externally rotated (15).

The pathoanatomy of MDI is multifactorial, and involves both anatomic and neuromuscular abnormalities. The typical pathology observed in patients with MDI includes a large, patulous inferior pouch and a wide rotator interval. The pouch expands to varying degrees creating a global increase in capsular volume and thereby resulting in overall laxity (16). The type and quantity of collagen in the capsule has also been shown to be significantly altered in patients with MDI (17). Repetitive minor injuries to the joint capsule may eventually result in labral injury and global laxity over time. In contrast, not all patients with shoulder laxity develop symptoms of instability. Therefore, factors other than capsuloligamentous laxity must play a role in symptom development. These other factors include dysfunction of the dynamic stabilizers of the shoulder.

The most important dynamic stabilizing structures include the rotator cuff muscles and the scapular stabilizers (Fig. 21-1), which work optimally at midrange positions when the capsuloligamentous complex is most ineffective. The rotator cuff resists humeral head translation through the mechanism of concavity compression, in which the humeral head is centered into the glenoid by a balanced contact pressure imparted by the rotator cuff (18). Scapular stabilizers are also critical to dynamic joint stability, as these muscles are responsible for positioning the glenoid in space and altering glenoid version and inclination. Abnormal scapular kinematics have been reported in patients with MDI, manifesting as decreased scapular abduction and external rotation, or frank winging (19). This

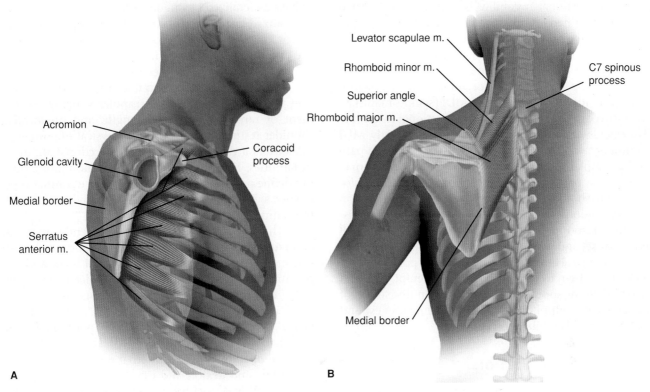

▲ **FIGURE 21-1:** Scapular stabilizing muscles.

dysfunction of the scapula may lead to an increase, and eventual overload, in the translational forces seen by the other stabilizing structures (18). The trapezius, serratus anterior, and rhomboid muscles all influence scapular movements.

Neuromuscular control is also an integral for the stability of the glenohumeral joint. Loss of strength or neuromotor coordination of the dynamic stabilizers can lead to an inability to properly center the humeral head within the glenoid. Electromyographic evidence has shown that patients with MDI have abnormal patterns of muscle activity when compared with controls. Specifically, changes in both the strength and timing of muscle firing were noted in the supraspinatus, infraspinatus, biceps, deltoid, and pectoralis major (20). Abnormal dynamic humeral head centering, as well as increased hand position errors with proprioceptive testing, has also been reported in these patients (21,22). These abnormal patterns of muscle recruitment and function result in increased glenohumeral translation.

CLINICAL PRESENTATION

Clinical suspicion is essential for the accurate diagnosis of MDI, given the myriad of presenting symptoms. Most patients present with insidious onset and nonspecific, activity-related pain in the second to third decade of life. Decreased strength and deteriorating athletic performance also may be reported. Presentation can range from vague generalized symptoms of pain to the complaints of frank instability. Between these extremes, patients typically report varying degrees of a painful "loose" shoulder, including the sensation of clicking, popping, and pain with overhead activities or sleeping.

Description of specific inciting activities can provide insight into the direction of instability. Anterior instability is classically provoked when the arm is in the throwing position of abduction and external rotation. Posterior instability can be elicited when the humerus is in the flexed and internally rotated position, as in pushing activities such as the bench press, push-ups, or blocking in football. Inferior instability is often associated with pain while carrying a heavy object. Frequently, patients learn to avoid these inciting activities.

Patients with generalized ligamentous laxity are especially prone to develop MDI (1). A history of symptomatic laxity in other joints, such as patellar instability or frequent ankle sprains should be elicited. Collagen disorders, such as Ehlers-Danlos syndrome, can also be a contributing factor and can be evaluated with genetic testing (23,24). The prevalence of MDI is higher in patients involved in repetitive overhead activities, particularly with volleyball, swimming, or gymnastics (18). These patients are likely predisposed to excel in these activities because of greater shoulder mobility; however, repetitive microtrauma may eventually lead to capsular damage over time.

Unidirectional instability is commonly associated with an identified lesion; therefore, MDI should be considered in the patient with unidirectional instability in the absence of an identifiable anatomic lesion. MDI should also be suspected in patients with a history of multiple failed instability procedures. The distinction must be made, however, between MDI (symptomatic laxity in two or more planes) and unidirectional instability associated with multidirectional hyperlaxity. Lastly, MDI should be considered in patients who present with pain and a complaint of instability but no history of trauma.

Some patients may be able to voluntarily dislocate their shoulders with selective muscle contraction and relaxation. In general, patients with willful dislocation respond poorly to surgical stabilization (4). Issues of secondary gain or psychiatric pathology must be considered. Patients who demonstrate positions that reproduce their instability but who attempt to avoid these positions should not be included in this subset of patients with willful dislocation, and generally respond well to surgical stabilization (25).

Physical Examination

A thorough physical examination is critical in order to not only confirm the diagnosis, but also to exclude other causes of shoulder pain, such as cervical radiculopathy, impingement lesions, and rotator cuff tears. A neurologic examination of the upper extremity and evaluation of the cervical spine should be performed to evaluate for referred pain.

Generalized hyperlaxity can be identified by elbow or knee hyperextension beyond 10 degrees, small finger metacarpophalangeal hyperextension more than 90 degrees, or the ability to abduct the thumb to the forearm with the wrist fully flexed (Fig. 21-2). If the patient has three out of four of these signs, they are believed to have generalized ligamentous laxity (26,27). If severe generalized ligamentous laxity is found, a genetic work-up for Ehlers-Danlos syndrome or other connective tissue disorders may be warranted, as surgical stabilization in these patients is less successful (23).

Examination of the shoulder begins with inspection for muscle atrophy and scapular winging. Assessment of range of motion, strength, and provocative shoulder testing follows. Various physical examination maneuvers are designed to detect directional shoulder instabilities. However, excessive translation alone does not define pathology. The key part of the examination is to elicit symptoms, such as pain and apprehension with translation testing (24).

The load-and-shift test is frequently used to evaluate glenohumeral translation. The humeral head is centered in the glenoid with an axial load, and the proximal humerus is then translated to determine laxity (28). Anterior and posterior drawer tests also evaluate laxity in these respective directions (29). More importantly, provocative testing must be performed. The apprehension test is performed with the shoulder in a position of abduction and external rotation for anterior instability, and flexion and internal rotation for posterior instability. A positive test produces a sense of pending subluxation or when the patient has involuntary guarding in the provocative position. The relocation test is then performed, which is positive when a stabilizing counterforce to the provocative position results in an improvement in symptoms (28).

One of the most important maneuvers in the MDI examination; however, is the sulcus test (Fig. 21-3), initially described by Neer and Foster (1). While a positive sulcus sign is not necessarily diagnostic of MDI, it does reflect inferior laxity (30,31). Inferior traction is placed on the affected arm adducted at the side in neutral rotation, looking for a sulcus below the lateral acromial

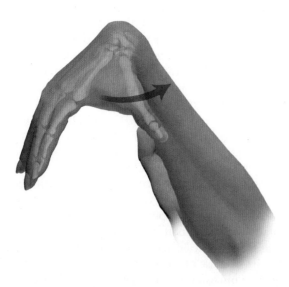

▲ **FIGURE 21-2:** Generalized hyperlaxity.

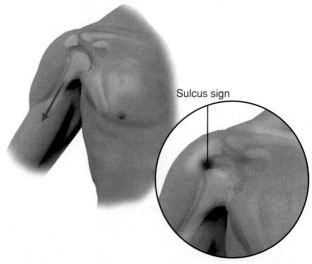

▲ **FIGURE 21-3:** Sulcus sign.

Sulcus sign

edge of the shoulder. The magnitude of translation reflects the integrity of the rotator interval, with greater than 2 cm of displacement of the humeral head from the acromion being indicative of a high degree of laxity (15). This maneuver is repeated with the arm in external rotation and in the abducted position. A persistent sulcus in external rotation suggests insufficiency of the rotator interval, whereas a persistent sulcus in abduction is indicative of inferior capsular laxity (1,12,32). These signs, however, are not considered abnormal unless the patient is symptomatic.

Imaging

Diagnosis of MDI is primarily clinical, but imaging is most important in ruling out other causes of shoulder pain and dysfunction. Plain radiographs are typically normal in MDI, but they should be evaluated for the presence of humeral head defects or glenoid bone defects. In cases of suspected bony deficiency, a CT scan should be obtained. Magnetic resonance arthrography may be more useful than MRI, improving definition of the glenoid labrum, rotator interval, and glenohumeral ligaments. Structural lesions such as labral tears may also be present as a result of either repetitive microtrauma or macrotrauma. Frequently, a patulous capsule, increased glenohumeral volume, and labral abnormalities are seen in MDI patients (33).

TREATMENT

Nonoperative Management

Numerous outcome studies of MDI have suggested that a rehabilitation program is the preferred initial treatment (1,3–6). The basic principles of every rehabilitation program are to improve the muscle strength and coordination of the rotator cuff and scapular stabilizers, in conjunction with patient education and avoidance of high-risk activities. There have been several rehabilitation protocols published; however, there is no clear evidence that any one is better than another.

Evaluation and treatment of scapulothoracic dyskinesia is typically the primary focus of therapy. Improving the dynamic positioning of the glenoid and instituting a proprioceptive exercise program can improve the efficiency of the dynamic glenohumeral stabilizers. Specifically, the muscles thought to be most important for scapular stability include the serratus anterior, rhomboids, and the trapezius. Preferential strengthening of the rotator cuff may also improve concavity compression, resulting in improved humeral head centering and a stronger opposition to shear forces. A minimum 6-month trial of therapy should be carried out in order to improve stability; however, many authors suggest that longer periods may be required (18,34).

Motivated patients typically respond well to these rehabilitation protocols, reporting diminished pain and improved stability. Recent reports by Nyiri et al. (35) and Kiss et al. (34) suggest that rehabilitation for MDI results in substantially increased strength in the muscles around the shoulder joint and increased neuromuscular control, which functionally reduces instability. Despite improved glenohumeral stability, they also noted that normal scapulothoracic rhythms and glenohumeral rhythms were not fully restored with rehabilitation alone. They did note; however, that a postoperative group undergoing therapy after a capsular shift was able to successfully restore normal muscle activation patterns.

The idea of strengthening the muscles around the shoulder to help with stability is not a new concept. In 1956, Rowe (36) reported that most patients with atraumatic shoulder instability responded favorably to an exercise program during short-term follow-up. Neer and Foster (1) recommended at least 1 year of physical therapy before considering surgery. Matsen et al. (6) described the differences between traumatic and atraumatic forms of instability and emphasized the importance of rehabilitation in atraumatic cases. However, none of these authors presented specific data detailing the results of nonoperative treatment in MDI.

In 1992, Burkhead and Rockwood (5) demonstrated the efficacy of nonsurgical management in atraumatic shoulder instability. Using a physician-directed home exercise program focused on strengthening the deltoid, rotator cuff, and scapular stabilizers, the authors reported good or excellent results in 88% (29 of 33) patients with atraumatic MDI. Their results also clearly demonstrated that patients with a traumatic subluxation had a much lower percentage of good or excellent results with an exercise program (12 of 74 shoulders; 16%) compared with the shoulders that had an atraumatic subluxation (53 of 66 shoulders; 80%). Because of the substantial difference in the number of successful outcomes in patients with traumatic versus atraumatic instability, the authors stressed that it is imperative to identify the etiology of shoulder instability if a successful result from conservative treatment is to be expected.

More recently, Misamore et al. (37) reported less encouraging long-term results after rehabilitation for MDI, but in a cohort of younger, athletic patients. They reported that at long-term follow-up, many patients had significant pain and instability or had elected to undergo surgical treatment. At 7 to 10 years follow-up, 40 of 57 patients (70%) had been treated surgically or had fair or poor ratings for their shoulders. Only 30% had a good or excellent result. The difference in the results between this study and that of Burkhead and Rockwood (5) likely have to do with this cohort being younger (mean age 19 years vs. 27 years), more involved in aggressive sporting activities, and all patients having significant laxity (grade II or greater). These reports indicate that athletic patients with MDI and those with instability associated with traumatic etiology may have a less favorable response to rehabilitation.

Surgical Management

Surgical intervention should be considered in patients who continue to experience debilitating symptoms despite completion of an appropriate rehabilitation regimen. The duration of therapy varies based on the presentation, symptom severity, activity level, and goals. Persistent instability with activities of daily living can be a compelling argument for surgery.

Several operative procedures have been developed for treating MDI, but most of these have a much higher rate of failure than operations designed for the treatment of unidirectional posttraumatic instability (3,7–10). One of the reasons for this may be that MDI represents a spectrum of possible pathology, making the diagnosis of the exact pathoanatomy more difficult. Therefore, it is imperative that surgical management should be individualized to address the specific anatomic cause of shoulder instability in a particular patient. Capsuloligamentous reconstructive techniques, which include open inferior capsular shift, thermal capsulorrhaphy, and arthroscopic plication, have been the most frequently performed procedures.

Neer and Foster (1) first described the open inferior capsular shift with a humeral-based T-capsular incision to address capsular redundancy in patients with MDI. Of the 36 patients (40 shoulders) reported in the original study, only one instance of recurrent subluxation postoperatively was reported. However, current criteria for successful outcomes in patients treated with surgical repair are much more stringent than those of Neer and Foster (1). Surgical success is now measured in terms of persistent apprehension, recurrent subluxation, validated condition-specific outcome measures, and the patient's ability to return to a previous level of sport rather than recurrent dislocation. Using these outcome parameters, more recently reported clinical outcome scores and stability rates were approximately 95% in two studies of inferior capsular shift for management of MDI. However, return-to-sport rates remain less than optimal. In a study of 40 patients with MDI treated with a modified open Bankart procedure, Altchek et al. (7) reported that 33 of 40 (83%) returned to full sport. They also noted that all throwing athletes had experienced decreased velocity at a mean of 3 years follow-up. More recently, Pollock et al. (38) reported that only 25 of 36 athletes (69%) were able to return to previous sporting activity following an inferior capsular shift.

Thermal capsulorrhaphy was introduced as an alternative to the open capsular shift procedure. While

it was attractive because it could be performed all arthroscopically, quickly, and easily, it has since been associated with chondrolysis, thermal nerve injury, and high failure rates (39,40). Hawkins et al. (40) reported failure rates as high as 60% with this procedure. Therefore, thermal capsulorrhaphy is no longer a recommended treatment option.

The advent of arthroscopic techniques permitted better recognition of the pathology associated with MDI, as well as a viable, less invasive treatment option for patients who require soft tissue repair. Numerous arthroscopic techniques have been developed for the treatment of MDI, which have produced clinical results equivalent or superior to open techniques and with less morbidity (41–45). Some studies specifically reported results in the athletic population. McIntyre et al. (43) reported on arthroscopic capsular shift in 19 shoulders and had good or excellent results in 95% with a 5% recurrence rate. Eighty-nine percent of athletes, including four swimmers, three football players, and two position baseball players, returned to their previous level of sport. Also using arthroscopic capsular shift, Treacy et al. (45) reported on 25 shoulders and found that 88% had a satisfactory result by the Neer system, with a 12% recurrence rate. Only 64% (7 of 11) of athletes were able to return to their previous sport. Gartsman et al. (42) also reported on a series of 47 shoulders with MDI treated with arthroscopic capsular plication. Postoperatively, 94% were rated good or excellent with a 2% recurrence rate. Eighty-five percent of mostly recreational athletes (22 of 26) were able to return to their desired level of sports participation.

Arthroscopic capsular plication is capable of restoring glenohumeral stability in patients with MDI. However, overly aggressive plications can result in glenohumeral motion loss, particularly in external rotation (46–48). Thus, the appropriate magnitude of plication is critical to the success of the procedure. It remains a subjective determination that must be individualized for each patient, making consistent results with surgery somewhat more problematic. This is especially true with the decision of whether or not the rotator interval should be closed. Clinically, satisfactory results have been obtained both with and without routine rotator interval closure (42). While there is no clear clinical evidence that rotator interval closure adds stability to a shoulder with MDI, biomechanical data does suggest that this may be indicated when laxity is not sufficiently reduced despite an adequate plication (46,49). However, the benefit must be weighed against its clinically and biomechanically described potential to significantly limit external rotation.

Another danger of surgical treatment is the close proximity of the axillary nerve to the inferior glenohumeral pouch. In anatomic studies, the nerve has been noted to be closest to the glenoid and joint capsule at the 6-o'clock position, at a mean of 12.4 mm from the glenoid, and a mean of 2.5 mm from the inferior glenohumeral ligament complex (50). Injury to this nerve has been reported after open, thermal, and arthroscopic procedures. An open approach facilitates direct identification and protection of the nerve, while the nerve is typically not visualized arthroscopically. Therefore, proper caution and understanding of this relationship are helpful in avoiding axillary nerve complications.

OUTCOME LITERATURE REVIEW

Table 21-1 summarizes the results of the available studies evaluating nonoperative treatment of MDI in specific patient populations. Despite widespread acceptance of nonoperative management as the initial treatment for MDI, a relatively small amount of data has been published looking at the outcomes of this strategy. There are four available studies in the literature specifically looking at nonoperative management. While three of the studies had a large number of patients (>55) for this fairly rare condition, one older study by Rowe et al. (4) only reported on 18 patients. Otherwise, all of these studies averaged extremely long follow-up periods, ranging from 44 to 96 months. All of the studies also utilized the Rowe score, or some modification of it, to evaluate patient outcomes, providing some degree of standardization across studies. Three out of four studies showed a majority of good to excellent results for nonoperative management of MDI (range, 76% to 83%), even at long-term follow-up. However, the fourth study, by Misamore et al. (37), only reported 30% good to excellent results after nonoperative treatment. The reason for this discrepancy is likely due to the fact that there was a significant difference between the patient population of this study and the other published reports. Misamore et al. (37) reported on a very active, young patient population, most of whom were involved in aggressive sporting activ-

ities and all of whom were graded as having significant laxity (grade II or higher). The mean age in this study was 19 years compared to 27 years in the Burkhead and Rockwood study (5), which showed a much higher success rate after rehabilitation for atraumatic MDI. Looking at these studies as a whole, it would indicate that nonoperative management will provide successful outcomes in the majority of patients with MDI. One group that may have a less favorable outcome with rehabilitation is the younger, very athletic patient with MDI.

Table 21-2 summarizes the results of the available studies evaluating operative treatment for MDI. Although all eight of these studies report an extremely high success rate after operative management for MDI, the majority of the studies have only small, nonhomogeneous patient groups with short follow-up. Three of the studies report on less than 25 patients, with the largest study not exceeding 50 patients. The average follow-up is significantly shorter than those published for nonoperative treatment, with two of the eight studies having less than 2 years of follow-up, while seven of the eight have a minimum follow-up of 26 months or less. There are a variety of scoring systems used across the different studies, making it difficult to confirm their consistency. The reported patient groups also represent a younger, more active population than those evaluated in the nonoperative studies, with the exception of the Misamore et al.'s study (37). It is important to note that the actual definition and diagnosis of MDI is highly variable across this literature, making comparisons between these different study groups problematic. Often times MDI reported in the literature may represent the clinical expression of a variety of anatomic lesions. Another difficulty in interpreting this data is that these reports reflect the evolving surgical treatment strategies for MDI. The initial three studies report on open techniques developed for capsular shift and plication, while the remaining five look at different

TABLE 21-1 **Summary of Studies Evaluating Nonoperative Treatment for Multidirectional Instability**

Authors	Number of Patients	Average Age (yrs)/Range (yrs)	Average F/U (mos)/Range (mos)	Scoring Instrument(s)	Good/Excellent Results with Nonoperative Treatment
Burkhead and Rockwood (5)	66 shoulders w/ atraumatic instability	25/NR	46/24–72	Rowe score	80% (53/66)
Rowe et al. (4)	18 patients w/ unilateral or bilateral voluntary shoulder dislocations	14/8–25	NR	Rowe score	83% (15/18)
Misamore et al. (37)	57 patients w/ MDI (younger, athletic patients)	19/13–34	96/84–120	Modified Rowe score	30% (17/57)
Kiss et al. (34)	62 shoulders w/ MDI	25/15–47	44/12–120	Constant score, Rowe score	76% (47/62)

F/U, follow up; NR, not reported.

TABLE 21-2   Summary of Studies Evaluating Operative Treatment for Multidirectional Instability

Authors	Operative Treatment	Number of Patients	Average Age (yrs)/ Range (yrs)	Average F/U (mos)/ Range (mos)	Scoring Instrument(s)	Good/ Excellent Results	Return to Preinjury Level
Neer and Foster (1)	Open inferior capsular shift	40 shoulders	24/15–55	22/6–60	Recurrent subluxation/ significant pain	Only one recurrent subluxation; 98% (39/40)	NR
Altchek et al. (7)	Open modified Bankart procedure	40 patients	22/15–32	36/24–84	Patient satisfaction	95% (38/40)	83% returned to full sport (33/40)
Pollock et al. (38)	Open inferior capsular shift	49 shoulders	23/16–42	61/24–132	Rating system (pain, ROM, activity)	94% (46/49)	69% returned to full sport (25/36)
Duncan and Savoie (41)	Arthroscopic inferior capsular shift	10 patients	29/16–49	24/12–36	Neer system	100% (10/10) satisfactory by Neer criteria	NR
McIntyre et al. (43)	Arthroscopic capsular shift	19 patients	23/15–52	34/25–52	Tibone and Bradley system	95% (18/19)	89% returned to full sport (17/19)
Treacy et al. (45)	Arthroscopic capsular shift	25 shoulders	26/15–39	60/36–80	Neer system	88% (22/25)	73% returned to full sport (8/11)
Gartsman et al. (42)	Arthroscopic capsular shift	47 shoulders	30/15–56	35/26–67	Rowe, Constant, ASES index	94% (44/47)	85% returned to full sport (22/26)
Baker et al. (51)	Arthroscopic capsular shift	40 patients	19/14–39	34/24–65	ASES score	Mean 91.4 of 100	86% returned to full sport (34/40)

F/U, follow-up; NR, not reported.

arthroscopic techniques. Again, this variability makes it difficult to compare the operative outcomes noted in these eight reports. Despite the inconsistencies found in these studies on operative treatment for MDI, one overwhelming principle in all eight studies was that their patients had all failed a significant trial of rehabilitation. With most of these studies having inclusion criteria of a failure of at least 6 months of rehabilitation, even these authors preferred initial nonoperative management of MDI. Due to the success of nonoperative management for the majority of patients with atraumatic instability, it appears that the only subset of these patients who may benefit from operative intervention are those who have already failed an exhaustive course of rehabilitation, and possibly the young, very active athlete.

CONCLUSION

Surprisingly little clinical evidence exists in the literature regarding the treatment of MDI. Of the few articles published, most are either review articles or outcomes of surgical techniques. The patient groups are small and nonhomogeneous; follow-up is short; and there is often great variability in even defining the patient population with MDI. That being said, there is a general consensus that the initial management of MDI should be rehabilitation.

Burkhead and Rockwood (5) reported a high degree of success treating a group of atraumatic MDI patients with rehabilitation. Their study demonstrated the importance of identifying the etiology of instability if a successful result from conservative treatment is to be expected. Specifically, it appears that patients with a traumatic subluxation of the shoulder do poorly with conservative management. Furthermore, the study by Misamore et al. (37) illustrates that rehabilitation may also not be effective for the younger, athletic patient population with MDI. Clearly, these studies indicate that proper patient selection is essential for the successful nonoperative treatment of a shoulder with MDI.

The natural history of MDI has not yet been clearly established. Most patients presenting with MDI are adolescents or young adults. In contrast, older adults are rarely diagnosed with MDI. This would imply that it may spontaneously improve with advancing age. This could be due to decreased laxity in the joint, decreased activity demands, or some other unknown factor. However, this does shed some light on the treatment outcomes reported for MDI. Nonoperative treatment is successful in the overwhelming majority of patients with atraumatic MDI, but the subsets of patients who appear to have less reliable outcomes tend to be younger and more athletic. These patients may just place too great a demand on their glenohumeral joint for rehabilitation and strengthening alone to improve stability. Also, if stability does increase with age, the very young patient may be too far away from any expected improvement.

Further studies are certainly needed to help aid in the proper diagnosis and treatment of this not uncommon shoulder pathology. Today, it remains a difficult condition to treat. Identifying the difference between instability and laxity is critical. Traumatic instability can be seen in the setting of hyperlaxity and must not be misdiagnosed as MDI. Nonoperative treatment appears successful in the vast majority of MDI patients who are motivated to participate in a program aimed at strengthening and improving proprioception of the dynamic stabilizers of the glenohumeral joint and the periscapular muscles. Many authors have urged that nonoperative treatment should be maintained up to 6 to 12 months before surgical intervention is even considered, as it is not without significant complications and also possible failure. Clearly, proper patient selection is essential for a successful outcome with rehabilitation. First, the patient with traumatic instability must be differentiated from atraumatic MDI, as they do much worse with nonoperative treatment. Also, a younger, more athletic patient with MDI may be more appropriate for earlier surgical intervention if they continue to be symptomatic despite a thorough effort at rehabilitation. Otherwise, a nonoperative program focused on improving and strengthening the dynamic stabilizers of the glenohumeral joint is considered the optimal treatment for the patient with MDI.

References

1. Neer CS 2nd, Foster CR. Inferior capsular shift for involuntary inferior and multidirectional instability of the shoulder: A preliminary report. *J Bone Joint Surg Am.* 1980;62(6):897–908.
2. Thomas SC, Matsen FA 3rd. An approach to the repair of avulsion of the glenohumeral ligaments in the management of traumatic anterior glenohumeral instability. *J Bone Joint Surg Am.* 1989;71(4):506–513.
3. Mallon WJ, Speer KP. Multidirectional instability: Current concepts. *J Shoulder Elbow Surg.* 1995;4:54–64.
4. Rowe CR, Pierce DS, Clark JG. Voluntary dislocation of the shoulder. A preliminary report on a clinical,

electromyographic, and psychiatric study of twenty-six patients. *J Bone Joint Surg Am.* 1973;55:445–460.
5. Burkhead WZ, Rockwood CA Jr. Treatment of instability of the shoulder with an exercise program. *J Bone Joint Surg Am.* 1992;74:890–896.
6. Matsen FA III, Thomas SC, Rockwood CA Jr. Glenohumeral instability. In: Rockwood CA Jr, Matsen FA III, eds. *The Shoulder. Vol 1.* Philadelphia, PA: Saunders;526–622.
7. Altchek DW, Warren RF, Skyhar MJ, et al. T-plasty modification of the Bankart procedure for multidirectional instability of the anterior and inferior types. *J Bone Joint Surg Am.* 1991;73:105–112.
8. Bigliani LU, Pollock RG, McIlveen SJ, et al. Shift of the posteroinferior aspect of the capsule for recurrent posterior glenohumeral instability. *J Bone Joint Surg Am.* 1995;77:1011–1020.
9. Cooper RA, Brems JJ. The inferior capsular-shift procedure for multidirectional instability of the shoulder. *J Bone Joint Surg Am.* 1992;74:1516–1521.
10. Hawkins RJ, Koppert G, Johnson G. Recurrent posterior instability (subluxation) of the shoulder. *J Bone Joint Surg Am.* 1984;66:169–174.
11. O'Brien SJ, Neves MC, Arnoczky SP, et al. The anatomy and histology of the inferior glenohumeral ligament complex of the shoulder. *Am J Sports Med.* 1990;18:449–457.
12. Warner JJ, Deng XH, Warren RF, et al. Static capsuloligamentous restraints to superior-inferior translation of the glenohumeral joint. *Am J Sports Med.* 1992;20:675–682.
13. Ferrari DA. Capsular ligaments of the shoulder. Anatomic and functional study of the anterior superior capsule. *Am J Sports Med.* 1990;18:20–29.
14. Turkel SJ, Panio MW, Marshall JL, et al. Stabilizing mechanisms preventing anterior dislocation of the glenohumeral joint. *J Bone Joint Surg Am.* 1981;63(8):1208–1217.
15. Harryman DT, Sidles JA, Harris SL, et al. The role of the rotator interval capsule in passive motion and stability of the shoulder. *J Bone Joint Surg Am.* 1992;20(6):53–66.
16. Schenk TJ, Brems JJ. Multidirectional instability of the shoulder: Pathophysiology, diagnosis, and management. *J Am Acad Orthop Surg.* 1998;6(1):65–72.
17. Rodeo SA, Suzuki K, Yamauchi M, et al. Analysis of collagen and elastic fibers in shoulder capsule in patients with shoulder instability. *Am J Sports Med.* 1998;26(5):634–643.
18. Ogston JB, Ludewig PM. Differences in 3-dimensional shoulder kinematics between persons with multidirectional instability and asymptomatic controls. *Am J Sports Med.* 2007;35(8)1361–1370.
19. Gaskill TR, Taylor DC, Millett PJ. Management of multidirectional instability of the shoulder. *J Am Acad Orthop Surg.* 2011;19(12):758–767.
20. Barden JM, Balyk R, Raso VJ, et al. Atypical shoulder muscle activation in multidirectional instability. *Clin Neurophysiol.* 2005;116(8):1846–1857.
21. Barden JM, Balyk R, Raso VJ, et al. Dynamic upper limb proprioception in multidirectional shoulder instability. *Clin Orthop Relat Res.* 2004;(420):181–189.
22. Inui H, Sugamoto K, Miyamoto T, et al. Three-dimensional relationship of the glenohumeral joint in the elevated position in shoulder with multidirectional instability. *J Shoulder Elbow Surg.* 2002;11(5):510–515.

23. Jerosch J, Castro WH. Shoulder instability in Ehlers-Danlos syndrome: An indication for surgical treatment? *Acta Orthop Belg.* 1990;56(2):451–453.

24. Bahu MJ, Trentacosta N, Vorys GC, et al. Multidirectional instability: Evaluation and treatment options. *Clin Sports Med.* 2008;27:671–689.

25. Fronek J, Warren RF, Bowen M. Posterior subluxation of the glenohumeral joint. *J Bone Joint Surg Am.* 1989; 71(2):205–216.

26. Beighton PH, Horan FT. Dominant inheritance in familial generalized articular hypermobility. *J Bone Joint Surg Br.* 1970;52:145–153.

27. Schwartz E, Warren RF, O'Brien SJ, et al. Posterior shoulder instability. *Orthop Clin North Am.* 1987;18:409–419.

28. Bahk M, Keyurapan E, Tasaki A, et al. Laxity testing of the shoulder: A review. *Am J Sports Med.* 2007;35(1): 131–144.

29. Gerber C, Ganz R. Clinical assessment of instability of the shoulder. With special reference to anterior and posterior drawer tests. *J Bone Joint Surg Br.* 1984;66(4): 551–556.

30. Emery RJ, Mullaji AB. Glenohumeral joint instability in normal adolescents. Incidence and significance. *J Bone Joint Surg Br.* 1991;73(3):406–408.

31. McFarland EG, Campbell G, McDowell J. Posterior shoulder laxity in asymptomatic athletes. *Am J Sports Med.* 1996;24(4):468–471.

32. Gagey OJ, Gagey N. The hyperabduction test. *J Bone Joint Surg Br.* 2001;83(1):69–74.

33. Dewing CB, McCormick F, Bell SJ, et al. An analysis of capsular area in patients with anterior, posterior, and multidirectional shoulder instability. *Am J Sports Med.* 2008;36(3):515–522.

34. Kiss J, Damrel D, Mackie A, et al. Non-operative treatment of multidirectional shoulder instability. *Intl Orthop.* 2001;24:354–357.

35. Nyiri P, Illyes A, Kiss R, et al. Intermediate biomechanical analysis of the effect of physiotherapy only compared with capsular shift and physiotherapy in multidirectional shoulder instability. *J Shoulder Elbow Surg.* 2010;19:802–813.

36. Rowe CR. Prognosis in dislocations of the shoulder. *J Bone Joint Surg Am.* 1956;38:957–977.

37. Misamore GW, Sallay PI, Didelot W. A longitudinal study of patients with multidirectional instability of the shoulder with seven- to ten-year follow-up. *J Shoulder Elbow Surg.* 2005;14(5):466–470.

38. Pollock RG, Owens JM, Flatow EL, et al. Operative results of the inferior capsular shift procedure for multidirectional instability of the shoulder. *J Bone Joint Surg Am.* 2000;82(7):919–928.

39. D'Alessandro DF, Bradley JP, Fleischli JE, et al. Prospective evaluation of thermal capsulorrhaphy for shoulder instability: Indications and results, two-to five-year follow-up. *Am J Sports Med.* 2004;32(1):21–33.

40. Hawkins RJ, Krishnan SG, Karas SG, et al. Electrothermal arthroscopic shoulder capsulorrhaphy: A minimum 2-year follow-up. *Am J Sports Med.* 2007;35(9):1484–1488.

41. Duncan R, Savoie FH 3rd. Arthroscopic inferior capsular shift for multidirectional instability of the shoulder: A preliminary report. *Arthroscopy.* 1993;9(1):24–27.

42. Gartsman GM, Roddey TS, Hammerman SM. Arthroscopic treatment of multidirectional glenohumeral instability: 2- to 5-year follow-up. *Arthroscopy.* 2001;17(3):236–243.

43. McIntyre LF, Caspari RB, Savoie FH 3rd. The arthroscopic treatment of multidirectional shoulder instability: Two-year results of a multiple suture technique. *Arthroscopy.* 1997;13(4):418–425.

44. Tauro JC. Arthroscopic inferior capsular split and advancement for anterior and inferior shoulder instability: Technique and results at 2- to 5-year follow-up. *Arthroscopy.* 2000;16(5):451–456.

45. Treacy SH, Savoie FH 3rd, Field LD. Arthroscopic treatment of multidirectional instability. *J Shoulder Elbow Surg.* 1999;8(4):345–350.

46. Provencher MT, Mologne TS, Hongo M, et al. Arthroscopic versus open rotator interval closure: Biomechanical evaluation of stability and motion. *Arthroscopy.* 2007;23(6):583–592.

47. Farber AJ, ElAttrache NS, Tibone JE, et al. Biomechanical analysis comparing a traditional superior-inferior arthroscopic rotator interval closure with a novel medial-lateral technique in a cadaveric multidirectional instability model. *Am J Sports Med.* 2009;37(6):1178–1185.

48. Plausinis D, Bravman JT, Heywood C, et al. Arthroscopic rotator interval closure: Effect of sutures on glenohumeral motion and anterior-posterior translation. *Am J Sports Med.* 2006;34(10):1656–1661.

49. Mologne TS, Zhao K, Hongo M, et al. The addition of rotator interval closure after arthroscopic repair of either anterior or posterior shoulder instability: Effect on glenohumeral translation and range of motion. *Am J Sports Med.* 2008;36(6):1123–1131.

50. Ball CM, Steger T, Galatz LM, et al. The posterior branch of the axillary nerve: An anatomic study. *J Bone Joint Surg Am.* 2003;85:1497–1501.

51. Baker CL 3rd, Mascarentas R, Kline AJ, et al. Arthroscopic treatment of multidirectional shoulder instability in athletes: A retrospective analysis of 2- to 5-year clinical outcomes. *Am J Sports Med.* 2009;37:1712–1716.

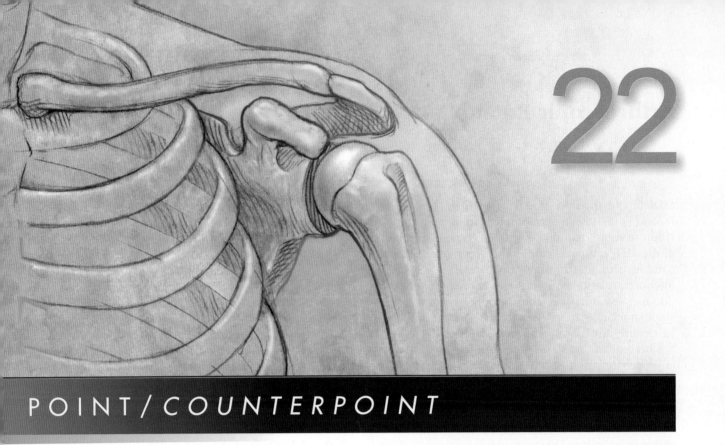

APPROPRIATE SURGICAL TREATMENT FOR MULTIDIRECTIONAL INSTABILITY

Capsular shift combined with rotator interval (RI) closure has become the preferred treatment for patients with multidirectional instability (MDI) and have failed conservative treatment. Recently, the need to perform an RI closure, as an additional measure to increase ultimate stability of the shoulder, has been scrutinized. Originally described as an open technique, advances in arthroscopy have led many to perform the surgery arthroscopically because it is less invasive and relatively easy to perform. However, there are still some who believe that an open RI closure is necessary. They point to the fact that many of the biomechanical studies that have been done on arthroscopic closure have failed to show any appreciable change in either posterior or inferior stability; therefore, open repair should still be the gold standard and should be applied in cases where RI closure is indicated. This section will review the indications for RI closure in the setting of MDI, the advantages of either arthroscopic or open techniques and whether RI closure remains a critical component of the treatment of patients with MDI.

Arthroscopic Rotator Interval Closure

Jeffrey Gagliano / Misty Suri /
Jeffrey S. Abrams

MDI of the shoulder was first described by Neer and Foster (1) in 1980 as "symptomatic humeral head translation in more than one direction." The anatomic basis of the MDI can result from a deficiency of the RI and a patulous shoulder capsule, which results in significant inferior translation. The emphasis has been made toward nonoperative management, including rotator cuff and scapular rehabilitation. The capsular shift combined with RI closure, initially described by Neer and Foster (1), has become the preferred treatment for those who have failed rehabilitation of the cuff and scapular stabilizers. Recently, the closure of the RI has been questioned as to whether it is a necessary part of the surgical procedure.

It is difficult to trace back to the original description of the RI as a discrete and defined anatomic entity within the shoulder. Due to its association with surrounding structures and pathologic conditions, this interval has been referred to in different contexts for decades. The illustrious career and life of Dr Charles Neer was decorated with extensive contributions to shoulder surgery. In 1970 Dr Neer (2) used the term "rotator interval" in a JBJS article about proximal humerus fractures. Ten years later, he further published on this anatomic space, as it related to shoulder instability and inferior capsular shift (1).

This triangular space that exists in the anterosuperior shoulder has a superior border composed of the anterior fibers of the supraspinatus (SSP) tendon, and an inferior border composed of the superior fibers of the subscapularis (SSC) tendon. The base of the triangle is delineated medially by the coracoid process and the apex of the triangle is defined laterally by the transverse humeral ligament. The superficial layer or roof of the space is composed of the coracohumeral ligament (CHL) and capsule most superficially, and the superior glenohumeral ligament (SGHL) exists on the deep surface of this tissue layer or "roof." The intra-articular portion of the long head of biceps tendon runs within the interval (3) (Fig. 22-1).

The RI has been implicated in shoulder pathology when it is either enlarged, such as instability, or when it is too tight, such as capsulitis. This chapter will focus on a lax or patulous RI and associated conditions. The role of the RI in shoulder instability is somewhat controversial and remains a topic of research and debate. Rowe and Zarins (4) provided some of the earliest evidence that the RI and associated structures contribute to glenohumeral instability. Harryman et al. (5) provided some of our most comprehensive and long-lasting understanding of the biomechanics of the shoulder, as it relates to the RI. In their cadaveric study, they analyzed glenohumeral motion and stability with the RI in its normal state, after RI sectioning and after imbrication. With sectioning of the interval, increased external rotation,

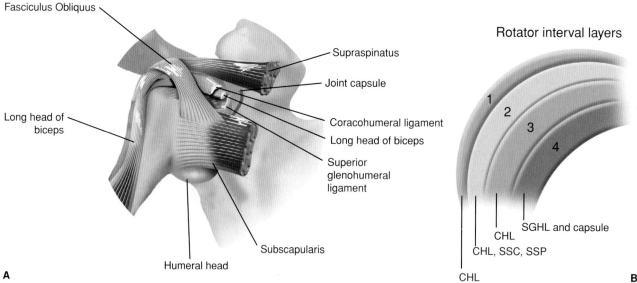

A

FIGURE 22-1: The rotator cuff interval. **A:** Diagrammatic representation of the boundaries. **B:** Rotator interval layers. SSP, supraspinatus; SSC, subscapularis; CHL, coracohumeral ligament; SGHL, superior glenohumeral ligament; LHB, long head of the biceps. (From Gaskill TR, Braun S, Millet PJ. Current concepts with video illustration. The rotator interval: Pathology and management. *Arthroscopy.* 2011;27(4):556–567.)

flexion, extension, and adduction occurred; and with imbrication of the interval, decreases occurred. Abduction and internal rotation were not significantly affected. This imbrication technique, or RI closure, was performed in a medial to lateral fashion via an open approach.

Harryman found that the humeral head underwent obligate translation on the glenoid, when testing glenohumeral range of motion (ROM). Most notably, there was increased translation in a superior and anterior direction when testing flexion, and in an inferior direction when testing adduction following RI closure. An increase in sulcus sign (inferior instability in adduction) was found with sectioning and a decrease with imbrication. Posterior drawer was increased with sectioning and decreased with imbrication.

Conclusions about RI function from Harryman study are as follows.

1. The RI contributes to limit glenohumeral flexion, extension, external rotation, and adduction.
2. The RI limits inferior instability/translation in adduction.
3. The RI limits posterior instability/translation in flexion and in abduction and external rotation (ABER).

RI imbrication or closure has been used during surgical stabilization procedures, sometimes in isolation, but most commonly as an additional measure to increase ultimate stability of the shoulder. Although this technique was originally described as an open procedure, the technique has been adapted for arthroscopic techniques, including arthroscopic stabilization. It is crucial to remember that open RI closure is a different procedure than that performed arthroscopically. These approaches result in a closure at nearly 90 degree orientations to one another. The open technique, as used by Harryman in their landmark biomechanical study, resulted in a medial-to-lateral closure, along the course of the RI fibers. The most commonly used arthroscopic procedures result in a superior–inferior closure across the interval's fibers. It is common to evaluate and close the RI in 30 degrees of external rotation and adduction in order to limit post-op external rotation losses (6–10).

RI closure will often be considered in cases of MDI, systemic hyperlaxity, or recurrent instability (11,12). Specific lesions of the RI can also be identified radiographically and incorporated into treatment plans, as shown by Vinson et al. (11). There is some evidence that MRI findings are predictable in cases of surgically proven RI pathology, including subcoracoid extravasation of contrast on MR arthrograms and CHL thickening. Therefore, surgical planning and decision making may be facilitated with thorough evaluation of preoperative MRI, in addition to history and physical examination.

Yamamoto et al. (12) evaluated two different superior–inferior RI closure techniques in cadaveric shoulders. Their closure techniques were either from the SGHL to the middle glenohumeral ligament (MGHL), or from the SGHL-SSC. Both techniques significantly decreased external rotation and horizontal abduction, and anterior translation in adduction only. Only the SGHL–MGHL technique showed a significant decrease in posterior translation in adduction, and anterior translation in ABER in the scapular plane. Neither technique reduced inferior translation. Therefore, the authors concluded that RI closure would enhance anterior–posterior stabilization during shoulder stabilization procedures.

Similar results were found by Plausinis et al. (13) when they compared one or two sutures used in an arthroscopic superior–inferior closure technique in a cadaveric model. No significant difference was found between one and two sutures, placed medially or laterally. RI closure did result in a decrease in anterior translation in the adducted shoulder, but no effect on posterior translation, and a slight decrease in flexion and external rotation ROM.

Isolated open versus arthroscopic closure was evaluated by Provencher et al. (14) in cadaver shoulders. Open closure was performed as per Harryman's published medial–lateral method with plication of the CHL. The arthroscopic technique was performed in a superior–inferior manner from the SGHL–MGHL to include the CHL. Notably, neither method improved posterior instability. Only the open method significantly improved anterior instability in adduction. Both techniques reduced the sulcus sign; however, the open method achieved greater stability in this direction. This finding is contrary to Yamamoto's findings in 2006. The arthroscopic method resulted in less loss of external rotation in adduction, but was still measureable with both techniques. The arthroscopic closure resulted in increased anterior stability in the ABER position over the open method.

Mologne et al. (15) further studied RI closure in a cadaveric model, attempting to evaluate it as a procedure being added to either anterior or posterior arthroscopic stabilization methods. They were able to show a significant improvement in anterior stabilization with the addition of RI closure. No difference in posterior or inferior instability was achieved with the addition of interval closure. In each case, a significant reduction of external rotation occurred in adducted and abducted positions, with a mean loss of 28 degrees. The authors concluded that RI closure can augment anterior stabilization procedures; however, it does not improve inferior or posterior instability. They cautioned that patient selection was important due to reduction of external rotation.

Orientation of interval closure was found to significantly alter stability in a cadaveric study by Farber et al. (16). This group compared superior–inferior closure to medial–lateral closure, via arthroscopic closure methods. Interestingly, they were able to show a significant improvement in posterior stabilization with glenohumeral ABER, when the closure was performed in a medial–lateral direction with a suture anchor placed in the humeral head. External rotation limitation was encountered with adduction using this technique, but normal ROM was maintained with abduction. Therefore, they concluded that a medial–lateral closure could be considered when addressing posterior instability.

A retrospective case-control study was performed by Chechik et al. (9) comparing recurrent instability after isolated arthroscopic Bankart repair (ABR) group and ABR with RI closure (ABR+ARIC) group. They found that patients with systemic joint hyperlaxity were more likely to have a poor functional outcome and recurrent instability, regardless of the procedures performed. Systemic joint hyperlaxity was more prevalent in the ABR+ARIC group (41%) versus the ABR group (28%). Recurrent dislocation was more common in the ABR group (13%) at a mean of 13 months post-op, compared to the ABR+ARIC group (8%) at a mean of 42 months post-op. They concluded that systemic joint hyperlaxity is a risk factor for recurrent dislocation after stabilization surgery, and that the addition of RI closure may improve shoulder stability.

PATIENT EVALUATION

Performing a detailed history and physical examination will elucidate the pathology in many cases. During the interview the patient should be questioned on the frequency, severity (ease of dislocation), duration, and prior nonoperative and operative treatments. The position(s) of the arm at the time of injury can also be helpful in determining the duration of the instability (17). In the setting of MDI, 30% of patients present with anterior traumatic dislocation (18,19). Patients often complain of pain, weakness, instability, and apprehension, and can report mechanical symptoms.

The sulcus sign has become a hallmark of evaluating inferior translation in patients with inferior and multidirectional instability. This sign is also useful to measure inferior laxity and is graded as grade 1 ≤1 cm, grade 2 1 to 2 cm, and grade 3 ≥2 to 3 cm. If the sulcus sign persists in ≥25 to 30 degrees external rotation, this suggests an incompetent RI (Fig. 22-2). The normal distance measured from the inferior aspect of the acromion to the superior aspect of the humeral head is 7 or 8 mm. The sulcus sign should also be compared to the contralateral side (19). It is not uncommon to have similar laxity in the contralateral shoulder, but is generally asymptomatic and nonpainful (20).

Muscle strength testing is an important part of the evaluation. Scaption and external rotation at 0 degrees should be tested to evaluate the rotator cuff for any weakness and possible concomitant tear. Supraspinatus and infraspinatus atrophy should be examined to evaluate for possible suprascapular neuropathy. A significant part of the shoulder examination should be focused on the exposed scapula and its supporting muscles. Weakness

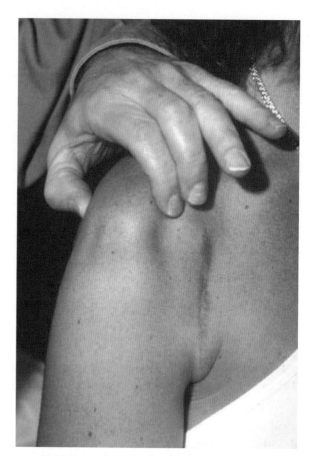

▲ **FIGURE 22-2:** The sulcus sign in a seated patient with multidirectional instability. A dimple is created below the acromion when inferior traction is applied.

or early fatigue can be a significant feature in patients with symptomatic MDI (20). Strength and motor testing should include the rotator cuff, scapula, and adjacent muscles. The evaluation should identify any isolated neurologic lesions (i.e., suprascapular or axillary nerves) or potentially, a more generalized situation (i.e., Parsonage-Turner or facioscapulohumeral (FSH) dystrophy).

Preoperative planning is essential for operative success. Preoperatively, the directions of laxity, degree of translation, presence of associated rotator cuff damage, and presence of associated labral damage should be performed. These factors are used together to assimilate the magnitude and balance of capsular tightening that is necessary intraoperatively.

PHYSICAL EXAMINATION

Anterior and posterior translation testing should be performed first in the relaxed supine position and graded 1, 2, or, 3. Grade 1: Up the face of the glenoid rim; grade 2: Perched on the glenoid rim; grade 3: Over the glenoid rim (Fig. 22-3). Testing for apprehension for pain or instability should also be performed. The relocation test may be done to confirm the diagnosis. The posterior Jahnke or "jerk" test is also useful (19).

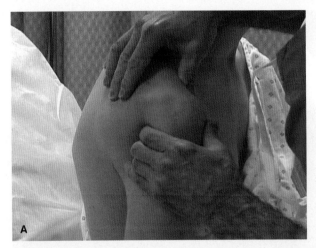 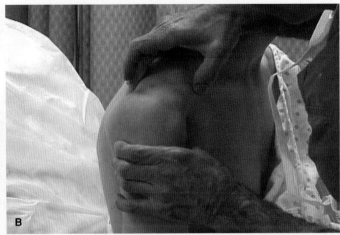

▲ **FIGURE 22-3:** The load-and-shift examination is applied to a patient to palpate and compare anterior and posterior translations. The opposite hand stabilizes the scapula. **A:** Anterior direction. **B:** Posterior direction.

MDI patients who are candidates for surgery should have failed 6 months of nonoperative management and treatment that includes physical therapy and anti-inflammatory medication. The physical therapy for scapular stabilization should start with scapular isometrics and closed chain exercises, then can progress to Blackburn exercises and higher level open chain therapeutic exercise (21). Avoidance of painful activities should be reduced or eliminated. Misamore et al. (22) reviewed patients who have chosen and failed nonoperative treatment in an 8-year study that attempted to identify improved patient selection and outcome in patients electing nonoperative treatment. In this study, failure or organized therapy for 3 months often determined a poor prognosis, and surgical intervention may become the preferred option.

Harryman (1992) demonstrated the significant reduction in the posterior–inferior laxity after a repair of the surgically created RI defect. As surgical treatment for shoulder instability shifted from open to arthroscopic, the view of this region changed from subdeltoid and bursal to articular. The types of interval closures changed with this perspective. Recent publications have made comparisons to Harryman's classic, but the arthroscopic superior–inferior closure is biomechanically distinct to the open medial–lateral closure that was originally described. Thereafter, the results of the open RI closure should not be extrapolated directly to the arthroscopic closure.

Appropriate patient selection for RI closure may be critical to the successful return to sports and demanding activities. The RI is an important adaptation of the shoulder to allow maximum rotation as in the overhead throwing athlete. Capsular plication and reduction of an enlarged inferior pouch has become an accepted and successful treatment for symptomatic hyperlaxity and MDI. However, the additional interval closure should be cautioned for patients who are overhead throwing athletes and cannot risk reduction of external rotation.

Anterior–superior capsular plicators can be added to augment or support the capsular reduction procedure with minimal risk. However, incorporating rotator cuff tendons or CHL should be reserved for individuals who will not be limited if terminal shoulder rotation is reduced by this procedure.

IMAGING

The diagnosis of MDI is primarily a clinical evaluation. Radiographs can show glenoid version abnormalities, hypoplasia, dysplasia, or bony defects; abnormalities in the humeral head can be revealed as well. Computed tomography can also be used to evaluate these structures (10). Magnetic resonance arthrography can show a distended patulous capsule in MDI, though this observation may not necessarily be pathologic (11). An increase in the dimensions of the RI in patients with MDI remains controversial (23–25).

SURGICAL TECHNIQUE

The operative treatment of patients with MDI begins with an examination under anesthesia. In a supine patient, the physician can make comparisons to both shoulders. The load-and-shift examination allows for an objective examination on the amount of humeral head translation relative to the stabilized glenoid in an anterior, inferior, and posterior direction. Placing one hand to secure the chest wall and scapula against the operative table, the other hand is free to compress the humeral head into the glenoid socket and gently translate with the arm in approximately 20 degrees abduction and neutral rotation. Additional testing is performed with ligament tensioning. To test anteriorly, the arm is abducted to 45 degrees and externally rotated to

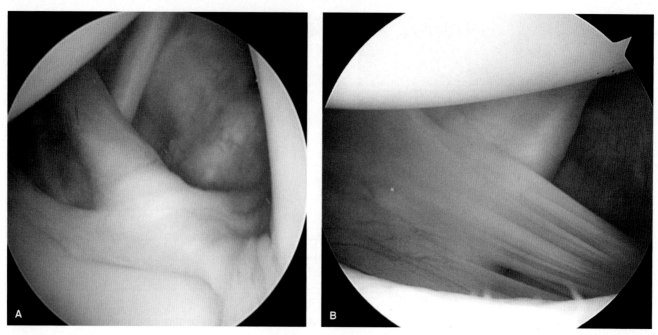

▲ **FIGURE 22-4:** Rotator interval in patients with multidirectional instability. **A:** Widened, stretched interval structures, including middle and superior glenohumeral ligaments. **B:** Thin deficient capsular tissue from repetitive strain.

45 degrees. To test inferiorly, the arm is externally rotated 45 to 60 degrees, and sulcus sign is reexamined. To test posteriorly, the arm is flexed to 60 degrees and internally rotated to 45 degrees. By positioning the humerus, the articular ligaments are pretensioned to test their ability to reduce translation. The examiner quantifies the translation in a grading system: Grade 1 is to the edge of the glenoid; grade 2 is over the edges of the glenoid; grade 3 is translated over the edge and reduces as the force is eliminated; and grade 4, the shoulder remains dislocated (26). The sulcus sign is often measured in centimeters as the interval between the acromion and the palpated humeral head (27).

The arthroscopic examination can be performed in the lateral decubitus or beach chair position. The lateral decubitus is preferred by some, since it allows global access to the articular capsule. Surgical capsule plication often requires access to multiple quadrants and is easily performed with the patients on their side and the shoulder supported in 30 degrees of abduction and 20 degrees forward flexion. The trunk and scapula are rotated posteriorly 20 degrees to position the glenoid parallel to the floor. Less traction via weights is required to minimize humeral head inferior translation. The surgical assistant can help distract the humeral head away from the glenoid, improving visualization and access to the inferior capsular structures.

The diagnostic scope begins with the RI, biceps, and superior exposed border of the SSC. The surgeon should observe size of the interval, quality of tissues, biceps stability with arm rotation, and rotator cuff integrity (Fig. 22-4). Articular-sided rotator cuff tears can be seen in this area and may be responsible for patients' painful findings. Gentle internal rotation of the humerus with a posterior drawer will allow improved visualization of the superior border of the SSC and capsular insertion to the humerus.

An anterior portal is created 1 cm inferior to the acromion and enters through the RI. Through this interval, the structures can be palpated, the biceps can be pushed into the visual field to see if tendon damage exists below the transverse ligament, and the coracoid can be palpated. Minor debridement of the central capsule overlying the interval will create a window allowing access to the bursal aspect of this region. The arthroscope can be advanced through this window, and a bursal perspective of the coracoid, CHL, and SSC can be assessed. The anterior, inferior, and posterior capsules, labrum, and articular cartilage structure are evaluated in sequential fashion. Labral tears, capsular pouches, and loss of definition of thickenings of the glenohumeral ligaments are documented. Additional attention is directed toward the superior labrum. A small series of patients with a superior labral anterior-to-posterior tear can present with similar physical findings. Although superior labral anterior and posterior tears (SLAP) repairs have recently been questioned due to complications, symptomatic MDI may be a reasonable indication for a suture anchor repair.

The instrumentation is then reversed, with the arthroscope being placed in the anterior portal. The articular structures are viewed with emphasis on the posterior–inferior capsule and labrum. Labral tissue

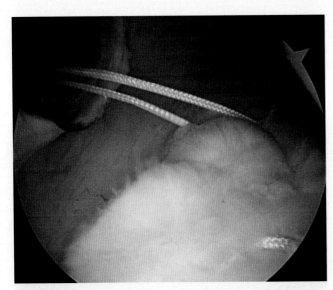

▲ **FIGURE 22-5:** Patients treated for MDI require inferior capsular plication to reduce the size of the pouch. Mattress sutures are placed to shorten the capsular ligaments, widen the labrum, and maintain a safe distance between the humeral head and the suture knots.

is carefully probed to see if it can support sutures, allowing for plication, or if additional anchors are required. As the scope is withdrawn, the capsular structures anterior and deep to the SSC tendon can be visualized.

Surgical repair begins with inferior plication (18,28). The capsular tissue is gently abraded with a rasp or shaving system with the suction turned off to minimize perforation. With the scope in the anterior portal, a curved suture hook allows placement of an absorbable monofilament suture at 6 o'clock position relative to the glenoid. A predetermined amount of capsule is selected using the 8-mm hook and secured to the glenoid (Fig. 22-5). The initial direction of repair is based on the categorization of anterior–inferior or posterior–inferior, based on patients' complaints, positions of greatest symptoms, and load-and-shift examination. When patients have greater posterior symptoms, the scope remains in the anterior portal and the plication proceeds posteriorly from inferior to superior. When anterior symptoms are most pronounced, the scope is placed in the posterior portal, and the anterior approach is used to plicate and shift the anterior–inferior capsule. Sutures are placed approximately 1 cm apart and can be placed as single sutures, mattress sutures, or figure-of-eight sutures, with knot placement lateral to the labral tissue. Softer braided sutures or monofilament sutures can be used to minimize articular cartilage irritation. Following the symptomatic side repair, the scope is switched to the opposite viewing portal, and the balancing capsular sutures are placed in the opposite capsule. The goal is to center the inferior glenohumeral ligament tension, reduce the size of the pouch, and advance the anterior and posterior bands of the inferior glenohumeral

ligaments superiorly, relative to their attachments on the glenoid.

The scope is placed in the posterior viewing portal to view and treat the RI. The bordering structures include the anterior glenoid rim medially, the SGHL and anterior edge of the SSP superiorly, and the MGHL and superior border of the SSC inferiorly, creating a triangular window. Anterior bursal structures that need to be appreciated are the coracoid and the CHL. A decision as to the location of the interval closure and which structures to include should be considered at this time.

The first concern is the location of the interval plication. The medial aspect of the interval can contact the coracoid base with internal rotation. Capsule plication medially will not produce the same effect, since it is an all-inside technique. If a surgeon elects to incorporate portions of the SSC or SSP tendons into the repair, this can produce a restriction of motion, since this normally occurring interval rotates above and below the coracoid process. A surgeon who chooses a laterally based plication may experience space restrictions and potential constriction of the pathway of the long head of the biceps and pulley system. To avoid these concerns, the central area of visualized interval minimizes risks of this dilemma.

The second concern is to choose the structures that should be included in the plication. The initial arthroscopic plications suggest the SGHL–MGHL interval. This is still the most commonly performed closure in an inferior-to-superior direction. Others believe that the superior border of the SSC can be incorporated, especially when the middle ligament is thin and provides minimal support. In patients with a large symptomatic sulcus, we could select the CHL in combination with the middle ligament. The humerus can be rotated during the placement of this suture to visualize potential impingement or restrictions before tying the suture. The superior interval contains the superior ligament running parallel to the biceps tendon. These sutures can be placed via an arthroscopic viewing portal and tied with a cannula, or the scope can be switched to a lateral bursal portal, and direct visualization of the bursal structures can be appreciated during knot placement.

The technique using a large clear anterior cannula begins with a curved suture hook (Fig. 22-6). Tissue selected at minimal is the middle capsular ligament, and can be further reinforced with corachumeral and/or SSC. A shuttle or monofilament suture is introduced into the joint capsule. Gently backing out the cannula, the capsular tissue covers the entrance of the cannula (Fig. 22-7). A perforating instrument is placed through the superior tissues, and the monofilament shuttling the suture is retrieved. One can elect to leave this type of suture or shuttle through a smooth-braided suture

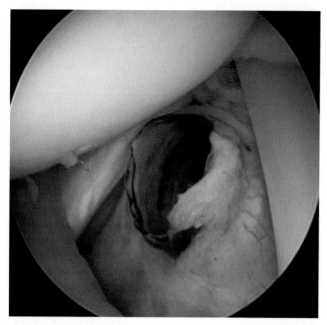

▲ **FIGURE 22-6:** A plastic cannula is placed within the rotator interval and is gently unscrewed to allow for the capsular tissue to close in front of the cannula opening.

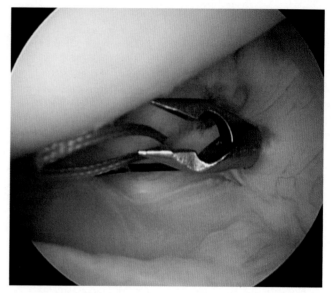

▲ **FIGURE 22-8:** A penetrating retrieving instrument is used to pierce the coracohumeral and superior glenohumeral ligament to create an oblique inferior-to-superior plication using braided sutures.

(Fig. 22-8). Generally, two parallel sutures are used to complete the closure along the lateral half of the interval (Fig. 22-9). This closure is inspected with ROM. The scope is switched to a lateral bursal portal and the plication is visualized from this perspective as well (Fig. 22-10). If additional fixation is performed, the bursal view allows further tensioning along the lateral aspect of the interval. Be aware of the long and short head of the biceps, since both can be accidently incorporated into an interval closure.

CONCLUSION

RI closure remains a topic of debate and continued research, as current literature does not provide the

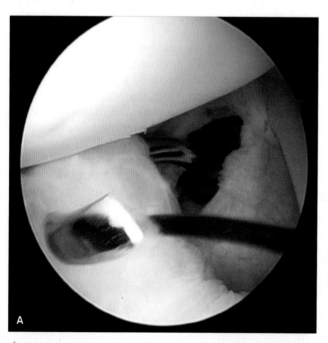

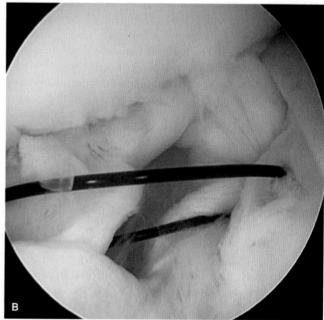

▲ **FIGURE 22-7:** A curved suture hook is introduced and penetrates coracohumeral ligament and middle capsular ligament. Additional fibers from the superior border of the subscapularis are added if tissue quality is deficient. **A:** Suture hook introduces monofilament suture. **B:** Suture is retrieved through superior glenohumeral ligament.

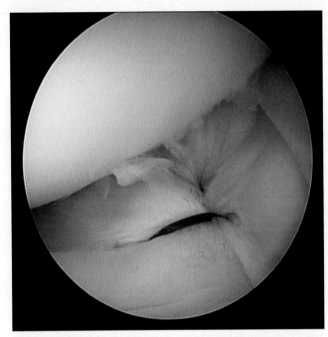

▲ **FIGURE 22-9:** Sutures can be tied within the cannula, completing the articular-viewed rotator interval closure.

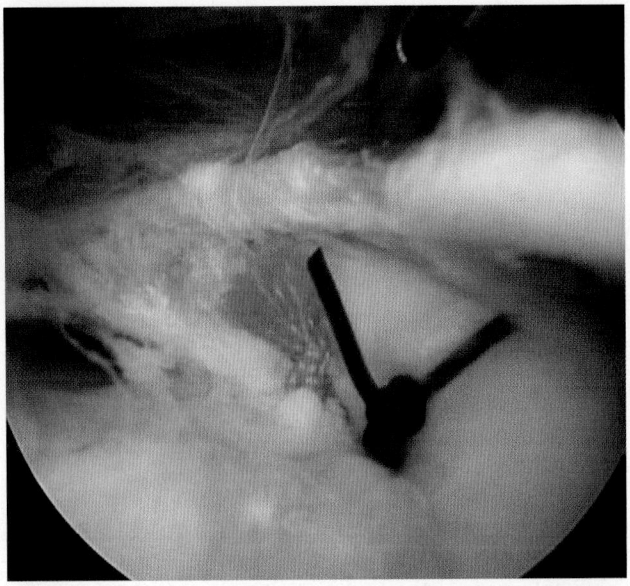

▲ **FIGURE 22-10:** A bursal view of the rotator interval closure. Adjacent structures including the coracoacromial ligament or short head of the biceps should be avoided.

surgeon with a clear-cut picture of when to use the technique and how it will affect glenohumeral kinematics. In addition, a variety of techniques have been developed with resulting differences in motion and stability. It appears that a certain degree of glenohumeral "stiffness" or loss of ROM can be expected in any case, most notably external rotation. However, subtle differences can be expected depending on how the ROM is tested and which technique is used to close the interval. Glenohumeral instability can be affected after RI closure; however, these changes will depend upon the surgical approach and technique used, and the position of the shoulder when the instability is assessed.

Open Rotator Interval Closure

M. Michael Khair / Sabrina Strickland

INTRODUCTION AND BACKGROUND

The RI is the space in the anterior–superior glenohumeral joint that is made by the superior border of the SSC tendon, the anterior border of the SSP tendon, and the coracoid process medially. It is triangular in shape and contains the MGHL, CHL, SGHL, tendon of the long head of the biceps, and a portion of the anterior capsule (3,8,29,30). While the structures themselves have been defined, the precise function of the RI, specifically with regards to shoulder instability, remains contested.

It has been shown that the RI plays a role in the stability of the glenohumeral joint (5,31–36). One of the first studies to examine the role of the RI in shoulder stability was published by Harryman et al. (5) In their report, the authors showed that when the capsule and the ligamentous structures within the RI are sectioned, passive glenohumeral extension, external rotation, flexion, and adduction, all increase. In the same study, the authors showed that a medial-to-lateral imbrication of the RI resulted in a decrease in magnitude of the same motions. The conclusion of the study, that the RI serves to limit excessive motion in the shoulder, specifically, posterior–inferior glenohumeral motion, has been used to justify the plication of RI tissues in some shoulder stabilization cases. As surgeons have moved to treating instability arthroscopically, many have continued to advocate for closure of the RI as an adjunct to other stabilization procedures (37–39). This is especially true in the patient diagnosed with MDI.

Patients who present with excessive shoulder laxity can either present with a history of acute trauma, or a series of repetitive overuse injuries that can eventually give rise to tissue insufficiency. Many patients will complain of shoulder instability or fatigue (10). On physical examination, there is often a sulcus sign if humeral translation is excessive. A persistent sulcus sign when the shoulder is externally rotated can be a sign of pathologic laxity (5,7,8). Radiographs can sometimes show inferior subluxation, though currently, MRI has become a popular imaging modality due to its soft tissue detail. Research has shown that findings on MRI, especially with regards to the dimensions of the RI, can be a significant clue in trying to diagnose patients with chronic instability (24).

While the RI is thought to be important to shoulder stability, when evaluating the patient with instability it is important to rule out all potential causes including anterior and posterior labral pathology, bony defects, humeral avulsion of the glenohumeral ligaments (HAGL), and genetic abnormalities such as Ehlers-Danlos syndrome.

Although isolated RI closure for instability has been reported to have excellent results (7), patient selection is critical and failure to recognize other causes of instability will yield poor results (40).

In cases where closure of the RI is indicated, surgery can be approached either through an open procedure or by arthroscopic techniques. The original paper by Harryman et al. (5) described open imbrication of the CHL with resultant decreases in both posterior and inferior translations of the glenohumeral joint. It is important to recognize that in their original paper, the authors describe a medial-to-lateral imbrication of the CHL. In addition to being used to justify open closure of the RI in certain situations, their findings have also been applied to arthroscopic RI closure despite fundamental differences in the method of interval closure. While techniques can differ, most authors have described arthroscopic interval closure as a shift of the MGHL in a cephalad direction, or a shift of the SSC tendon to the SGHL (37,38). Perhaps the most important difference is that arthroscopic plication of the RI is often done in a superior-to-inferior shift whereas open plications have been described as medial-to-lateral shifts. As a result, there is debate over whether the biomechanical data that has been generated by open RI closure studies can appropriately be used to justify arthroscopic RI closure.

Making the issue even more confusing is that recent attempts to replicate the findings of Harryman et al. have been largely unsuccessful. Provencher et al. (14) compared arthroscopic to open RI closure in 14 fresh-frozen cadaver shoulders. The open repair was modeled after the description given in Harryman et al. where the CHL is sectioned transversely and then sutured together in a "pants-over-vest" fashion. Their arthroscopic repair was modeled on the technique described by Gartsman et al. (37) and Taverna et al. (38), and involved plicating the tissue in the SGHL through the MGHL and including the CHL in the repair. Their results showed that posterior stability was not improved by either open or arthroscopic RI closure. Further, the shoulders undergoing open closure were the only specimens to have any improvement in sulcus stability. Neutral anterior stability was also only increased in the open group. Both open and arthroscopic closure increased anterior stability in 90 degrees of ABER. Loss of external rotation in neutral was found to be greater in the open repair specimens than in those that were arthroscopically repaired.

It is our stance that given the lack of convincing evidence in the literature supporting arthroscopic RI closure over open closure, and considering that many of the biomechanical studies that have been done on arthroscopic RI closure have failed to show any appreciable change in either posterior or inferior stability, that open repair is still the gold standard and should be applied in cases where RI closure is indicated.

SURGICAL TECHNIQUES AND PEARLS

We rarely indicate patients for an isolated RI closure. Often we perform RI closure in conjunction with a capsular shift. Thus, in this section, we will describe our most frequently performed operation for chronic shoulder instability which includes a description of open RI closure.

For our instability cases, we position the patient in the beach chair with the patient's head secured using a headrest and the shoulder prepped and the arm draped free. At our institution the vast majority of shoulder surgery is done with the patient under regional anesthesia, typically a supraclavicular block placed with the aid of ultrasound; however, we prefer general anesthesia for open cases to allow optimal relaxation and evaluation of both shoulders. An examination under anesthesia is then carried out paying special attention to the sulcus in both neutral and external rotation. A positive sulcus in external rotation or the history of a failed stabilization procedure leads us to highly consider an RI closure. The surgeon performing the operation is situated in the axilla. Depending on the number of assistants available, the forearm is sometimes placed in a McConnell ASIP (McConnell Orthopedic Manufacturing Co., Greenville, TX.) device to aide with arm positioning. Once the patient is positioned properly, the standard axillary incision extending from the coracoid process into the axilla following the anterior axillary fold is performed. The incision is extended toward the clavicle if more exposure is needed. The skin and subcutaneous tissue is incised with a No. 10 scalpel. Curved Metzenbaum scissors are used to undermine the subcutaneous tissue. The cephalic vein is identified and noted to demarcate the deltopectoral interval. The vein is freed and is taken laterally with the deltoid. Once the interval is identified and retracted using narrow Richardson retractors, the conjoined tendon is identified and the clavipectoral fascia just lateral to the tendon is incised and divided. It is released superiorly to the level of the CHL. The medial Richardson is repositioned so as to retract the conjoined tendon medially. The humerus is externally rotated and the long head of the biceps tendon and lesser tuberosity are identified. Working medially, the "soft spot" of the RI is identified as well as the superior and inferior borders of the SSC tendon. In patients with MDI, we find that the RI is often patent (Fig. 22-11). At this point, using the electrocautery device, the upper two-thirds of the SSC tendon is vertically transected approximately

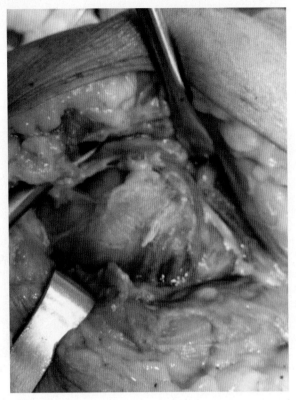

▲ **FIGURE 22-11:** The rotator interval bordered by the anterior supraspinatus tendon and the superior subscalpularis tendon.

1 cm medial to its insertion on the lesser tuberosity. Care is taken not to violate the underlying anterior capsule which can be quite adherent. After the vertical transection is completed, a small horizontal extension can be created in line with the SSC tendon fibers at the inferior portion of the vertical incision. This can help mobilize the SSC and free the capsule underneath. We tag the medial border of SSC in anticipation of repairing it. Using blunt dissection, or, if necessary, a periosteal elevator, the inferior SSC is elevated so as to have complete access to the anterior capsule from superior to inferior as well as from medial to lateral. The superior and inferior borders of the RI are tagged with two or three No. 2 Ethibond (Johnson and Johnson, New Brunswick, NJ) sutures (Fig. 22-12). The anterior capsule is "T'ed" by vertically releasing it at its insertion on the humeral head with a new No. 15 scalpel (Fig. 22-13). A horizontal incision is then made midway between the superior and inferior halves of the anterior capsule. Both the inferior and superior limbs are then tagged at their lateralmost border using more No. 2 Ethibond sutures. The inferior limb is then brought superiorly to be tightened and reattached at the point where the superior limb was released (Fig. 22-14). We prefer to use suture anchors for our capsular repair. If performing a capsular shift, three double-loaded suture anchors, typically Mitek G4 (DePuy Mitek, Raynham, MA), are placed at the lateral margin of the repair. The inferior limb is then shifted superiorly

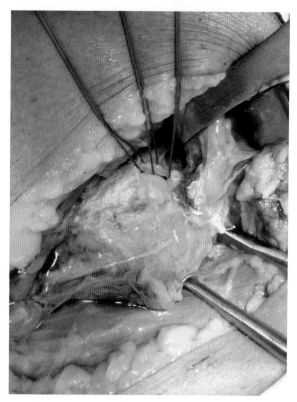

▲ FIGURE 22-12: Tagging of rotator interval.

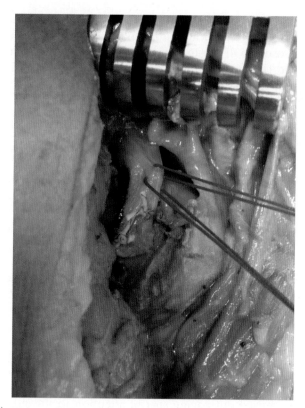

▲ FIGURE 22-14: Bringing the inferior limb superiorly to be tightened and reattached at the point where the superior limb was released.

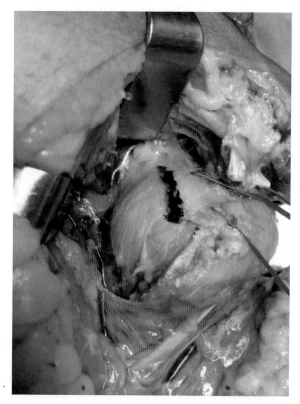

▲ FIGURE 22-13: Performing a "T-shaped" release of the anterior capsule by vertically releasing it at its insertion on the humeral head.

and one limb from each anchor is passed successively from inferior to superior through this limb achieving a reduction in both inferior and anterior capsular laxity. The superior limb is then sewn with the aid of the remaining suture to the superior two suture anchors in a "vest-over-pants" fashion. We tailor the tension of our repair to the individual demands of each shoulder, though in general, we repair the inferior capsular limb with the arm abducted 40 degrees and the shoulder in 40 degrees of external rotation. Once both of the capsular limbs are repaired, the previously tagged borders of the RI interval are sutured together in a medial-to-lateral fashion (Fig. 22-15). This completes both the capsular shift and the closure of the RI. The SSC tendon is repaired back to its lateral stump. We generally use two to three No. 2 Orthocord sutures (DePuy Mitek, Raynham, MA) tied in a figure-of-eight fashion being careful not to overtighten the musculotendinous unit. If we do not feel that the patient requires an anterior capsular shift we simply start the case by identifying the RI and place sutures at the superior and inferior borders both medially and laterally and tie the sutures down and check for stability as well as the degree of translation with the inferior translation. Once the shoulder feels stable we finish the interval closure carefully maintaining the degree of soft tissue tension that we have found to be optimal as far as stability and ROM. After we have thoroughly irrigated

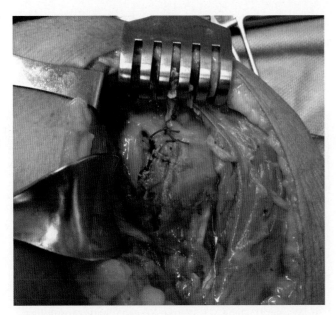

▲ **FIGURE 22-15:** The previously tagged borders of the RI interval are sutured together in a medial-to-lateral fashion.

the wound, we close and mark the deltopectoral interval loosely with nonabsorbable suture. The subcutaneous tissue is closed with buried No. 2 Vicryl sutures and the skin is closed with a running 4.0 monocryl subcuticular stitch. We do not routinely use a surgical drain but will do so if we feel it necessary at the time of closure.

CONCLUSION

Closure of the RI continues to be performed when treating patients with persistent shoulder instability. Much of the justification for closure of the RI comes from the original work of Harryman et al. (5) which showed that imbrication of the RI (in a medial-to-lateral fashion) decreased both inferior and posterior shoulder translations. Subsequently, as arthroscopy became the preferred method for treating the unstable shoulder, the same results were used to justify arthroscopic RI closure, despite the fact that the technique and the actual method of closure differed significantly. Current biomechanical research shows that arthroscopic closure and open closure are not equivalent in terms of decreasing shoulder translation (14). Open repair, it has been shown, can significantly decrease anterior translation and also significantly increase sulcus stability. Arthroscopic repair does neither. In addition, both open and arthroscopic RI closures failed to reduce posterior translation. As a result of this current research, and given the significant differences between those methods described by Harryman et al. and arthroscopic RI closure, it is our belief that if the surgeon is going to close the RI in hopes of achieving increased shoulder stability, the only reliable method for doing so is through an open incision.

References

1. Neer CS 2nd, Foster CR. Inferior capsular shift for involuntary inferior and multidirectional instability of the shoulder: A preliminary report. *J Bone Joint Surg Am.* 1980;62:897–908.
2. Neer CS 2nd. Displaced proximal humeral fractures. I. Classification and evaluation. *J Bone Joint Surg Am.* 1970;52(6):1077–1089.
3. Jost B, Coch PP, Gerber C. Anatomy and functional aspects of the rotator interval. *J Shoulder Elbow Surg.* 2000;9(4):336–341.
4. Rowe CR, Zarins B. Recurrent transient subluxation of the shoulder. *J Bone Joint Surg Am.* 1981;63:863–872.
5. Harryman DT 2nd, Sidles JA, Harris SL, et al. The role of the rotator interval capsule in passive motion and stability of the shoulder. *J Bone Joint Surg Am.* 1992;74(1):53–66.
6. Karas SG. Arthroscopic rotator interval repair and anterior portal closure: An alternative technique. *Arthroscopy.* 2002;18(4):436–439.
7. Field LD, Warren RF, O'Brien SJ, et al. Isolated closure of rotator interval defects for shoulder instability. *Am J Sports Med.* 1995;23:557–563.
8. Fitzpatrick MJ, Powell SE, Tibone JE, et al. The anatomy, pathology, and definitive treatment of rotator interval lesions: Current concepts. *Arthroscopy.* 2003;19(suppl 1): 70–79.
9. Chechik O, Maman E, Dolkart O, et al. Arthroscopic rotator interval closure in shoulder instability repair: A retrospective study. *J Shoulder Elbow Surg.* 2010;19(7):1056–1062.
10. Gaskill TR, Braun S, Millett PJ. Current concepts with video illustration. The rotator interval: Pathology and management. *Arthroscopy.* 2011;27(4):556–567.
11. Vinson EN, Major NM, Higgins LD. Magnetic resonance imaging findings associated with surgically-proven rotator interval lesions. *Skeletal Radiol.* 2007;36(5):405–410.
12. Yamamoto N, Itoi E, Tuoheti Y, et al. Effect of rotator interval closure on glenohumeral stability and motion: A cadaveric study. *J Shoulder Elbow Surg.* 2006;15(6):750–758.
13. Plausinis D, Bravman JT, Heywood C, et al. Arthroscopic rotator interval closure: Effect of sutures on glenohumeral motion and anterior-posterior translation. *Am J Sports Med.* 2006;34(10):1656–1661.
14. Provencher MT, Mologne TS, Hongo M, et al. Arthroscopic versus open rotator interval closure: Biomechanical evaluation of stability and motion. *Arthroscopy.* 2007;23(6): 583–592.
15. Mologne TS, Zhao K, Hongo M, et al. The addition of rotator interval closure after arthroscopic repair of either anterior or posterior shoulder instability: Effect on glenohumeral translation and range of motion. *Am J Sports Med.* 2008;36(6):1123–1131.
16. Farber AJ, ElAttrache NS, Tibone JE, et al. Biomechanical analysis comparing a traditional superior-inferior arthroscopic rotator interval closure with a novel medial-lateral technique in a cadaveric multidirectional instability model. *Am J Sports Med.* 2009;37(6):1178–1185.
17. Millet PJ, Clavert P, Warner JJ. Arthroscopic management of anterior, posterior, and multidirectional shoulder instability: Pearls and pitfalls. *Arthroscopy.* 2003;19(suppl 1):86–93.

18. Stokes DA, Savoie FH, Field LD, et al. Arthroscopic repair of anterior glenohumeral instability and rotator interval lesions. *Orthop Clin N Am.* 2003;34:529–538.

19. Ramappa AJ, Hawkins RJ, Suri M. Shoulder disorders in the overhead athlete. *Instr Course Lect.* 2007;56:35–43.

20. Abrams JS. Special shoulder problems in the throwing athlete: Pathology, diagnosis, and nonoperative management. *Clin Sports Med.* 1991;10:839–870.

21. Burkhart SS, Morgan CD, Kibler WB. The disabled throwing shoulder: Spectrum of pathology Part III: The SICK scapula, scapular dyskinesis, the kinetic chain, and rehabilitation. *Arthroscopy.* 2003;19(6):641–661.

22. Misamore GW, Sallay PI, Didelot W. A longitudinal study of patients with multidirectional instability of the shoulder with seven- to ten-year follow-up. *J Shoulder Elbow Surg.* 2005;14(5):466–470.

23. Dewing CB, McCormick F, Bell SJ, et al. An analysis of capsular area in patients with anterior, posterior, and multidirectional shoulder instability. *Am J Sports Med.* 2008;36(3):515–522.

24. Kim KC, Rhee KJ, Shin HD, et al. Estimating the dimensions of the rotator interval with use of magnetic resonance arthrography. *J Bone Joint Surg Am.* 2007;89(11):2450–2455.

25. Provencher MT, Dewing CB, Bell SJ, et al. An analysis of the rotator interval in patients with anterior, posterior, and multidirectional shoulder instability. *Arthroscopy.* 2008;24(8):921–929.

26. Hawkins RJ, Abrams JS, Schutte JP. Multidirectional instability of the shoulder: An approach to diagnosis. *Ortho Trans.* 1987;11:246.

27. Nobuhara K, Ikeda H. Rotator interval lesion. *Clin Orthop Related Res.* 1987;223:44–50.

28. Gaskill TR, Taylor DC, Millet PJ. Management of multidirectional instability of the shoulder. *J Am Acad Orthop Surg.* 2011;19(12):758–767.

29. Cole BJ, Rodeo SA, O'Brien SJ, et al. The anatomy and histology of the rotator interval capsule of the shoulder. *Clin Orthop Relat Res.* 2001;(390):129–137.

30. Plancher KD, Johnston JC, Peterson RK, et al. The dimensions of the rotator interval. *J Shoulder Elbow Surg.* 2005;14(6):620–625.

31. Blasier RB, Guldberg RE, Rothman ED. Anterior shoulder stability: Contributions of rotator cuff forces and the capsular ligaments in a cadaver model. *J Shoulder Elbow Surg.* 1992;1(3):140–150.

32. Itoi E, Berglund LJ, Grabowski JJ, et al. Superior-inferior stability of the shoulder: role of the coracohumeral ligament and the rotator interval capsule. *Mayo Clin Proc.* 1998;73(6):508–515.

33. Ovesen J, Nielsen S. Posterior instability of the shoulder. A cadaver study. *Acta Orthop Scand.* 1986;57(5):436–439.

34. Ovesen J, Nielsen S. Stability of the shoulder joint. Cadaver study of stabilizing structures. *Acta Orthop Scand.* 1985;56(2):149–151.

35. Selecky MT, Tibone JE, Yang BY, et al. Glenohumeral joint translation after arthroscopic thermal capsuloplasty of the rotator interval. *J Shoulder Elbow Surg.* 2003;12(2):139–143.

36. Warner JJ, Deng XH, Warren RF, et al. Static capsuloligamentous restraints to superior-inferior translation of the glenohumeral joint. *Am J Sports Med.* 1992;20(6):675–685.

37. Gartsman GM, Taverna E, Hammerman SM. Arthroscopic rotator interval repair in glenohumeral instability: Description of an operative technique. *Arthroscopy.* 1999;15(3):330–332.

38. Taverna E, Sansone V, Battistella F. Arthroscopic treatment for greater tuberosity fractures: Rationale and surgical technique. *Arthroscopy.* 2004;20(6):e53–e57.

39. Wolf RS, Zheng N, Iero J, et al. The effects of thermal capsulorrhaphy and rotator interval closure on multidirectional laxity in the glenohumeral joint: A cadaveric biomechanical study. *Arthroscopy.* 2004;20(10):1044–1049.

40. Levine WN, Arroyo JS, Pollock RG, et al. Open revision stabilization surgery for recurrent anterior glenohumeral instability. *Am J Sports Med.* 2000;28(2):156–160.

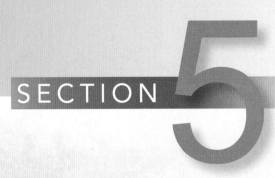

SECTION 5

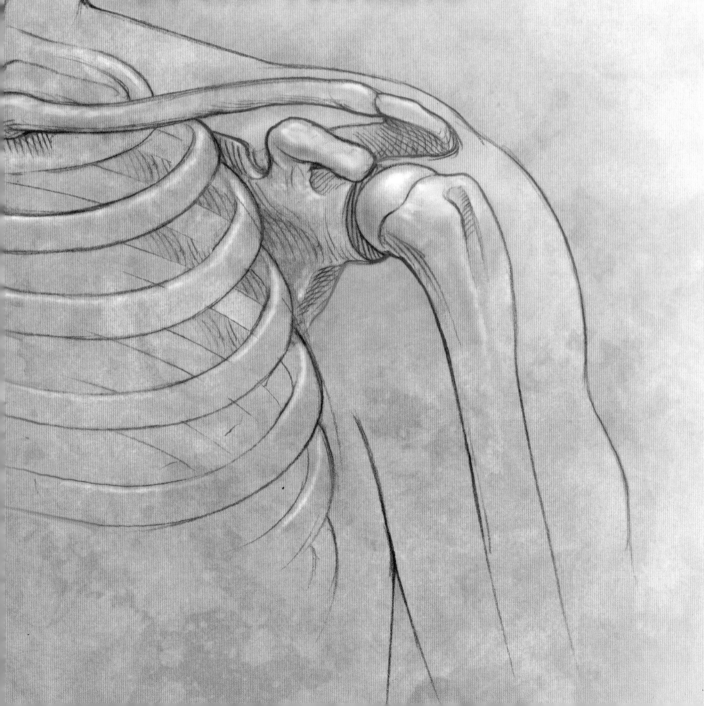

SHOULDER INSTABILITY IN THE ATHLETE

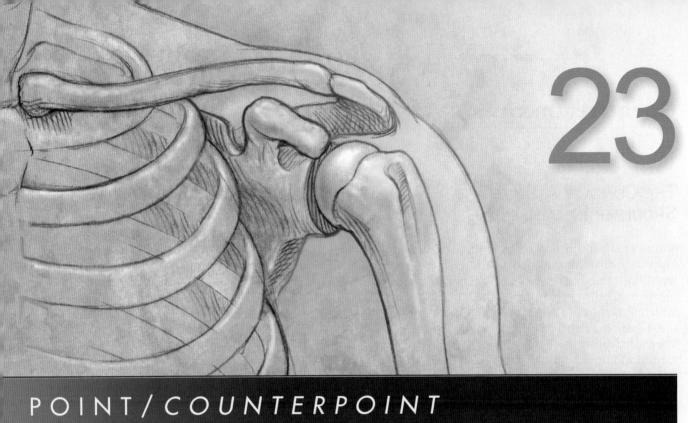

POINT / COUNTERPOINT

STABILIZING THE CONTACT ATHLETE

*T*he contact athlete with recurrent instability is perhaps the most challenging patient to treat. The relatively high recurrence rate after arthroscopic stabilization has led many surgeons to rethink the manner in which stabilization for the contact athlete with shoulder instability is performed. The literature generally favors open stabilization techniques over arthroscopic techniques with regard to contact athletes. However, open stabilization is not without complications and many surgeons still point to good published and anecdotal results as a way of justifying arthroscopic stabilization. The following chapters will address this fascinating topic including indications, surgical technique, and results.

Open Treatment

Demetris Delos / Scott A. Rodeo

THE CONTACT ATHLETE AND SHOULDER INSTABILITY

Shoulder instability is a common problem in athletes, especially those in collision sports such as football, wrestling, and hockey, where the rate of glenohumeral instability events can approach 0.4 per 1,000 athlete exposures (1). In a military cadet population, the 1-year incidence was reported to be 2.8% (2). These instability events are associated with significant morbidity and often lead to significant time lost from sport (1). Furthermore, the risk of future instability events is high, with a rate of recurrence reported to be 72% in one series (3) of patients younger than 23 years and 87% in another series of patients aged 15 to 20 years (4).

THE ROLE OF SURGICAL STABILIZATION IN REDUCING THE RISK OF RECURRENT INSTABILITY

In order to limit the risk of recurrence in athletes and the associated sequelae, early stabilization is often recommended as conservative treatment has had limited success. In a prospective cohort study by Robinson et al. (4), the authors reported that individuals aged 15 to 35 years who had sustained their first glenohumeral dislocation and were treated conservatively with a sling and physical therapy had over a 55% chance of recurrent instability (subluxation or dislocation event) within 2 years. The risk was shown to increase with decreasing age and with male gender. Similar high rates of recurrent instability in young athletes after conservative treatment for first-time dislocations has been shown by numerous other groups (3,5,6). In a follow-up prospective, randomized, double-blind trial by Robinson et al. (7) comparing primary arthroscopic stabilization to arthroscopic examination and lavage alone, the authors reported a significant reduction in the risk of further dislocation (76%) and recurrent instability episode (82%) in the group that underwent Bankart repair. Patients that underwent stabilization were also more likely to return to sport compared to the group that did not undergo stabilization. Other groups have also reported on their series of patients that underwent acute surgical stabilization for first-time traumatic dislocation with positive results (8).

The high rate of recurrence in young patients, especially athletes, has prompted many surgeons to recommend operative management for first-time dislocators. Several key factors we take into consideration before recommending surgery for first-time dislocators include the following.

1. Age and activity level: Younger patients tend to be more active and are particularly prone to recurrent instability as described above.
2. Expectations/desired goals: Those individuals who wish to return to contact sports, especially of the collision-type, may be at higher risk for repeat instability episodes and therefore, we typically are more aggressive at treating these individuals surgically.
3. Generalized ligamentous laxity: A careful history should be obtained to determine the mechanism of injury (i.e., traumatic vs. atraumatic cause). For patients with generalized ligamentous laxity that sustained an initial *atraumatic* instability episode we recommend first treating with conservative measures such as physical therapy and activity modification rather than surgery.
4. Prior contralateral glenohumeral dislocation: Patients that sustained a previous contralateral dislocation treated either with or without surgery should first be investigated for generalized ligamentous laxity in order to rule out underlying collagen disorders and if that portion of the history/physical examination is positive they should be treated accordingly. In general, we favor treating the more symptomatic/problematic side with a stabilization procedure if they have not yet undergone surgery and are more aggressive with treating a first-time dislocation if the contralateral shoulder has had instability.
5. Bone loss (Hill–Sachs lesion, bony Bankart): We prefer to operate on first-time dislocators who present with large bone defects on the humerus (Hill–Sachs lesions) and/or with glenoid avulsion fractures associated with the instability event (bony Bankart) due to the higher risk of recurrent instability (9–12).

OPEN SHOULDER STABILIZATION VERSUS ARTHROSCOPIC STABILIZATION

Though the literature supports surgical stabilization of the contact athlete who presents with primary or recurrent glenohumeral instability, the risk of recurrent instability episodes after primary arthroscopic stabilization is substantial. In the series by Robinson et al. (7), there was a 7% rate of redislocation in the group that underwent Bankart repair. Owens et al. (8) reported a redislocation rate of 14.3% in their military population that underwent acute arthroscopic stabilization after a primary dislocation at a mean follow-up of 11.7 years. A recent report from our institution (13) found that patients younger than age 20 with anterior glenohumeral instability that underwent arthroscopic Bankart repair had a recurrence rate as high as 37.5% at an average follow-up of 33 months.

The relatively high recurrence rate after arthroscopic stabilization in some series has led surgeons to rethink the manner in which stabilization for the contact athlete with shoulder instability is performed. The literature generally favors open stabilization techniques over arthroscopic techniques with regards to contact athletes. In the retrospective review by Rhee et al. (14) evaluating 48 shoulders in collision athletes (16 arthroscopically repaired, 32 open), the rate of instability was doubled in patients undergoing arthroscopic stabilization compared to open (25% vs. 12.5%, respectively).

Pagnani and Dome (15) reviewed their series of 58 patients who participated in American football that underwent open treatment for recurrent anterior instability. The mean age was 18.2 years and the mean follow-up was 37 months. In this series, none of the patients sustained postoperative dislocations, and only two experienced recurrent subluxation. Fifty-two of the fifty-eight subjects returned to competitive football for at least 1 year and only one had to quit playing due to recurrent instability.

In a randomized controlled trial comparing arthroscopic to open Bankart repair, Bottoni et al. (16) found no significant clinical difference between the two groups and no statistically significant difference in the rate of recurrent instability. Fabbriciani et al. (17) also reported no significant clinical differences between patients treated with open or arthroscopic methods in their randomized controlled trial. Nevertheless, in a recent systematic review and meta-analysis comparing arthroscopic to open repairs for recurrent shoulder instability (18), the authors reported that after pooling the data from 18 studies (including four randomized clinical trials) arthroscopic stabilization procedures were associated with higher rates of recurrent instability (18% vs. 8%) and reoperation (relative risk = 2.32). Open stabilization approaches were also more effective at allowing patients to return to sport and previous work (relative risk = 0.87) (18).

THE ADVANTAGES OF OPEN GLENOHUMERAL STABILIZATION

We believe there are several specific advantages to performing an open glenohumeral stabilization, especially in the context of the contact athlete with primary or recurrent anterior instability. These patients represent the most challenging instability group, considering the nature of their activities, the high loads often experienced across the joint, and their (typically) young age. Therefore, they require the most robust and effective repair possible in order to minimize the risk of recurrence. The most important advantages of open treatment for shoulder instability are outlined below.

1. **Better selective tensioning of the glenohumeral capsule by a capsular shift performed with the arm set at the desired position. This cannot typically be done with arthroscopic techniques as visualization becomes limited with the shoulder placed in abduction and external rotation.**

In Neer and Foster's (19) landmark paper from 1980, the authors described the open inferior capsular shift for instability of the shoulder, which is still practiced in various forms today. In the original manuscript, Neer and Foster (19) stressed the importance of tensioning the capsule with the shoulder in slight flexion and 10 degrees of external rotation. In their glenoid-based modification to the open capsular shift, Altchek et al. (20) described performing the repair with the shoulder in 40 degrees of external rotation and 45 degrees of abduction. Bak et al. (21) described a subscapularis sparing open capsular shift which was performed with the shoulder in 45 degrees of abduction and neutral rotation. We currently prefer to perform the capsular shift with the shoulder positioned in approximately 30-degree forward flexion, 30 to 40 degrees of external rotation, and 30 to 40 degrees of abduction. However, this can also vary depending on the type of activities and position that the contact athlete plays. Thus, for instance, an American football lineman who typically plays with his arms in front of him can tolerate a more substantial capsular shift than a throwing athlete whose throwing motion requires a significant amount of abduction and external rotation in order to be effective.

Open shoulder stabilization allows this selective arm positioning which is otherwise difficult to reproduce arthroscopically. Abduction and external rotation of the shoulder can severely limit visualization of the structures of interest and make both the reduction portion and the repair portion difficult to perform arthroscopically.

2. **Open treatment allows for overlapping of the capsule which can strengthen the capsule and improve resistance to subluxation and dislocation (pants over vest)**

Open repairs allow the surgeon to incise the capsule longitudinally producing two leaflets (superior and inferior) (19–21). These leaflets can then be advanced (shifted) in opposite directions and sutured in place. In this manner, tensioning of the capsule by overlapping the superior and inferior leaflets can be performed to the appropriate degree. In vitro studies have shown that the degree of capsular volume reduction is proportional to the magnitude of the capsular shift (22). This is technically difficult to do arthroscopically, as arthroscopic stabilization relies on capsular plication rather than a formal capsular shift with advancement of the leaflets.

3. **Open treatment allows for better identification of the rotator interval lesion and for closure of the defect**

The importance of the rotator interval in glenohumeral instability has been recognized for several decades now, though its exact role and significance is still debated. Harryman et al. (23) published an oft-quoted article in 1992 describing their method for open closure of the rotator interval. In brief, after the authors sectioned the coracohumeral ligament, they then imbricated the two ends together in a pants-over-vest fashion in the medial–lateral direction (23). This resulted in decreased inferior translation in the adducted shoulder and decreased posterior translation in flexion. Provencher et al. (24) noted the difficulty in extrapolating these results to the arthroscopic setting where the interval is typically closed in a superior–inferior fashion rather medial–lateral. In addition, with the arthroscopic method it is the middle and superior glenohumeral ligaments that are typically approximated in order to close the interval, whereas with the open method the structure involved is the coracohumeral ligament. These important distinctions (namely the vector of repair and the tissues utilized for the closure) have led to distinct differences in terms of biomechanical results. In the cadaveric study by Provencher et al. (24) comparing arthroscopic to open rotator interval closure, the authors reported that both sulcus stability and anterior stability with the shoulder in the neutral position were improved with the open closure but not with the arthroscopic technique.

We believe that an open Bankart/stabilization procedure allows for better identification of the interval lesion and the coracohumeral ligament. Likewise, for the reasons stated above it is easier to close the defect. In addition, there are yet no reliable methods of identifying rotator interval pathology from the intra-articular examination (25,26).

4. **Open stabilization allows for treatment of glenoid bone defects**

Burkhart and De Beer (9) reported on the poor outcomes of arthroscopic stabilization procedures in the context of glenoid bone deficiency. The authors found that patients treated arthroscopically for recurrent instability with significant bone defects had a 67% recurrence rate, whereas those without significant bone defects had a 4% recurrence rate. The numbers are even more striking in contact athletes: This subset of patients had an 89% recurrence rate if they had significant bone defects, whereas those without significant bone defects had a 6.5% recurrence rate (9). For anterior glenoid bone defects greater than 25% to 30% of the width of the glenoid (i.e., less than 4 mm of bone remaining anterior to the bare spot as determined arthroscopically), it is usually recommended that surgical reconstruction of the defect be performed due to the inherent lack of stability and poor clinical outcomes associated with this degree of bone loss (9–11,27). In order to assess the degree of glenoid bone loss, we typically perform preoperative CT and use the best-fit circle method to quantify the degree of bone loss (28,29).

The most popular methods for glenoid augmentation are the Bristow and Latarjet procedures—both involve transfer of the coracoid process to the region of the glenoid defect; the Bristow procedure involves fixing the graft along its long axis, whereas the Latarjet places the graft perpendicular to its long axis (parallel to the glenoid arc). Though several authors have described arthroscopic methods of performing the Latarjet (30,31), this is a technically difficult procedure that has yet to gain widespread acceptance. Proper positioning of the graft is critical—if it is placed too medial then it will not function as intended and will risk recurrent instability, whereas if it is too lateral it may harm the articular surfaces and possibly lead to osteoarthritis (32,33). In our experience, by performing the Latarjet procedure open, one can harvest the coracoid graft safely and place it along the anterior glenoid in the appropriate manner with less risk of malalignment and hardware malposition.

5. **Humeral avulsion of glenohumeral ligament (HAGL) lesions can often only be repaired through an open approach**

HAGL lesions are relatively rare injuries reported in 1% to 9% of shoulder instability patients that have recently garnered greater attention and recognition. These lesions can occur with the arm in hyperabduction and external rotation and involve avulsion of the inferior glenohumeral ligament (IGHL) from its humeral attachment. Though these lesions can sometimes be addressed arthroscopically, they are typically difficult to access without an open approach. In addition, concomitant injuries (34), subscapularis avulsions (35), and glenoid bony defects (36) have been reported which may be difficult to address arthroscopically. The literature on this subject is limited, and to date the largest series reported included patients treated with an open approach using suture anchors (37).

Authors' Preferred Surgical Technique

The patient is placed in the beach chair position with all bony prominences well padded. We prefer to use interscalene regional anesthetic blocks; however, we will consider general anesthesia and paralysis in larger patients in order to make the exposure less difficult. The incision is made in anterior axillary fold. The deltopectoral interval is developed and the cephalic vein is carefully retracted medially. We perform a subscapularis tenotomy, incising the tendon approximately 1 cm medial from the bicipital groove to ensure sufficient tendon stump for later repair. A vertical capsulotomy is performed on the lateral side off the humerus and a transverse incision is made between the middle glenohumeral ligament (MGHL) and the IGHL. If a Bankart lesion is present, we will repair it with suture anchors placed along the anteroinferior glenoid (usually at least three anchors, single-loaded). These sutures are then passed through the capsulolabral complex in mattress fashion and tied outside the capsule. We then set the arm position for the capsular shift and perform it accordingly. In general we prefer to use suture anchors laterally on the humerus to complete the repair; however, one may also leave a capsular flap to suture to when performing the lateral capsular shift. We then close the rotator interval in adduction and approximately 30 to 40 degrees of external rotation. The subscapularis tenotomy is then repaired and the wound is closed in layers as per routine.

Our postoperative rehabilitation protocol includes early motion in a protected range. Elevation in the plane of the scapula is allowed, with avoidance of excessive external rotation in order to protect the subscapularis tendon and capsular repairs. Codman and pendulum exercises are permitted in the immediate postoperative period. Motion is gradually progressed after 3 to 4 weeks, with specific limits determined based on the degree of capsular tensioning that was performed. Gentle strengthening exercises are introduced at 6 weeks, with a gradual progression over time. Return to contact sports typically requires 5 to 6 months, with an individualized program based on return of shoulder motion, strength, proprioception, and overall function. The surgeon should work closely with the physical therapist throughout the rehabilitation process.

Despite the effectiveness of the procedure, there are complications specific to open stabilization that must be recognized. The subscapularis repair may fail and the tendon may rupture. Greis et al. (38) noted an incidence of subscapularis tendon disruption after open stabilization of 4.5%. Stiffness is also a concern (39–41), which is why we prefer to mobilize the joint in the early postoperative period within limits. There is also a risk of neurovascular injury; in one series of 282 patients (42) that underwent anterior reconstruction for recurrent glenohumeral instability, 23 patients (8.2%) had a neurologic deficit after surgery, with complete resolution in 18 of the 23. The axillary nerve can be injured when handling the inferior capsule and during the subscapularis tenotomy and the musculocutaneous nerve may be injured with retraction of the conjoint tendon. In addition, there is a risk of infection, particularly *Propionibacterium acnes*, with a reported incidence of 0% to 6% (43,44).

Conclusions

Glenohumeral instability in the contact athlete is a challenging clinical problem. Shoulder stabilization procedures have proven effective compared to nonoperative treatments; however, the rate of recurrent instability after arthroscopic stabilization is still relatively high in the young athlete participating in collision sports. In order to minimize the risk of repeat subluxation or dislocation events we recommend consideration for open stabilization methods rather than arthroscopic in contact/collision athletes. Open treatment allows for better tensioning of the capsule, better visualization and ability to close the rotator interval when needed, and the ability to address concomitant pathoanatomy such as glenoid bone defects. The literature has generally favored open stabilization over arthroscopic in contact athletes, and we believe open shoulder stabilization procedures should still be considered the gold standard, especially in the context of contact and collision athletes.

Arthroscopic Treatment

Evan Argintar / James E. Tibone

Shoulder instability is commonly occurring in contact athletes. Between 1989 and 2004, the National Collegiate Athletic Association (NCAA) injury database was queried for all glenohumeral instability events. An incidence rate of 0.12 injuries per 1,000 athlete exposures was demonstrated. Men's football was the sport with the greatest injury rate, with 0.40 injuries per 1,000 athlete exposures. Athletes sustained more glenohumeral instability events during games than practices (incidence rate ratio [IRR], 3.50; 95% confidence interval [CI], 3.29 to 3.73), and male athletes sustained more injuries than did female athletes (IRR, 2.67; 95% CI, 2.43 to 2.93). Time lost to sport greater than 10 days occurred in 45% of glenohumeral instability events (1).

The operative treatment of anterior shoulder stability is commonly indicated and is clinically successful in a high percentage of cases. Arthroscopic technique allows for accurate detection of shoulder pathology, the re-establishment of normal glenolabral anatomy with minimal soft tissue disruption, optimized cosmesis, and minimized capsular and musculotendinous scarring inherent with open stabilization procedures.

Contact athletes make up a unique subset of a standard patient population. The anticipated recurring force to a contact athlete's shoulder places joint stability at heightened postoperative risk for recurrence. One review of 29 athletes showed that compared with noncollision athletes, the collision athlete group yielded a higher failure rate (28.6% vs. 6.7%) (45). For these reasons, shoulder stability may be more important than full range of motion. Historical clinical evidence has demonstrated

the superiority of open treatment (15,45). Using proper patient selection coupled with rigid adherence to current surgical technique, we argue the same clinical results can be achieved with arthroscopic surgical management.

Although in-season management has been shown to have short-term success (46), contact athletes, who require a full return to a high-impact high level of fitness to perform their sport and/or job should have operative management after primary instability events. Arthroscopic management should be utilized, and clinical success is dependent on several technical aspects that must be routinely implemented during all surgical interventions.

We routinely utilize the lateral decubitus position. This position allows the surgeon free movement around the head of the patient, allowing for greater ease for anterior, and especially, posterior instrumentation. In addition, the shoulder is positioned in a 30- to 40-degree abduction and forward flexion with 6.80 kg (15 lb) of traction.

We use three standard portals (Fig. 23-1). An initially posterior-lateral portal is placed in the humeral soft spot which is typically located 2 cm inferior and 1 cm medial to the posterior-lateral corner of the acromion. Using a spinal needle to assist, under arthroscopic visualization, an anterior portal is made off the anterior edge of the acromion. Intra-articularly, after introduction, the cannula is placed superior to the long bicep tendon. A second anterior portal is placed directly off the lateral edge of the coracoid process. Intra-articular placement of this cannula is directly off the superior edge of the subscapularis tendon. This cannula is placed on the inferior side of the biceps tendon, which anatomically keeps the two anterior cannulas separated (Fig. 23-2).

Routine diagnostic shoulder arthroscopy should initially be performed. Contact athletes often have concomitant pathology, including posterior and/or superior labral tears. If present, these lesions must additionally be treated and repaired.

After diagnostic arthroscopy is complete, Bankart lesion mobilization is the first, and perhaps, most important technical component for successful arthroscopic management of anterior shoulder instability. Often, the torn labrum is scarred to the glenoid in a more medial position, such that the normal anatomic labral bumper is well medial of the joint surface. Using a freer, the anterior–inferior glenohumeral ligament (AIGHL) is separated from the glenoid bluntly. Often, once an edge is created, the separation between the labrum and glenoid is propagated distally with a basket cutter. Care must be taken to protect the axillary nerve with the inferior

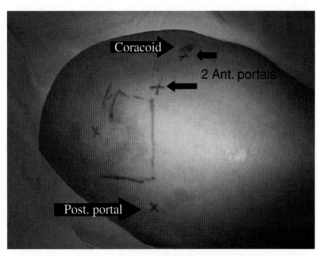

▲ FIGURE 23-1: Arthroscopic portals.

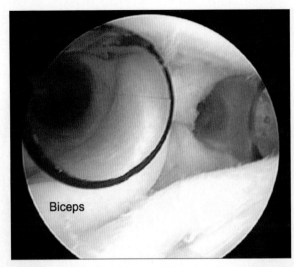

▲ **FIGURE 23-2:** Anterior portals separated by long head of bicep tendon.

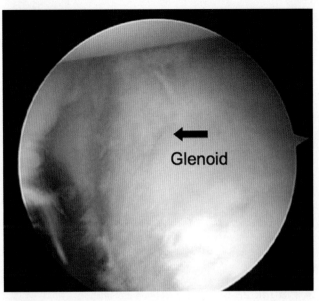

▲ **FIGURE 23-4:** Arthroscope in anterior superior cannula—perspective of Bankart lesion.

glenolabral release. Upon completion, the subscapularis muscle should be visible between the separated labrum and the anterior glenoid edge (Fig. 23-3).

The arthroscope should then be placed in the anterior-superior portal, and a cannula should be inserted in the posterolateral incision. We find moving the camera anteriorly helps to confirm satisfactory soft tissue dissection. In addition, from this perspective, improved visualization of the glenoid is obtained (Fig. 23-4). Here, using a burr, curette, or a high-speed shaver, the glenoid can be prepared with a goal of creating a bleeding boney bed for the ensuing labral repair. Care must be taken to conserve bone while creating a rough bleeding surface for Bankart repair.

Proper anchor insertion should begin inferiorly, and at the 5:30 clock position. For improved visualiza-

tion and inferior joint access, a towel roll can be placed under the axilla. Anchor insertion should be placed up on the rim of the glenoid (Fig. 23-5). Medial anchor placement, below the glenoid rim, leads to ineffective ligament tensioning, creating an anterior labral periosteal sleeve avulsion (ALPSA) lesion. Anchors placed excessively high on the glenoid surface places ligaments against cartilage, which has poorer healing characteristics.

Once the anchor is placed, the inferior suture should be identified and retrieved from the posterior portal. From the anterior–inferior portal, a shuttling suture should be passed through the capsule and under the Bankart lesion, inferior to the placement of the anchor, and retrieved from the posterior portal. This

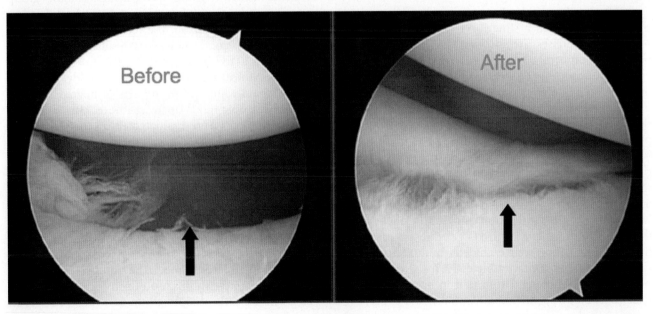

▲ **FIGURE 23-3:** Bankart mobilization.

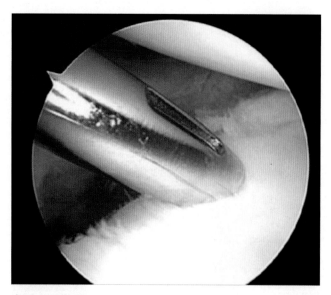

▲ **FIGURE 23-5:** Correct placement of anchors.

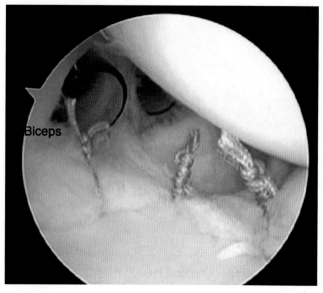

▲ **FIGURE 23-6:** Final arthroscopic Bankart repair.

creates an inferior to superior capsular shift in addition to the labral repair. Once the original suture has been threaded through the shuttling suture, it should be brought anteriorly. This suture end should serve as the post. We typically tie a sliding knot backed up with three alternating half-hitch knots. Attention should be made to direct the sutures medially, in an effort the remove the suture knot from close proximity to the articular surface (Fig. 23-6). These steps should be repeated incrementally, as the labrum is restored from an inferior to superior direction. We routinely place a minimum of four anchors in the glenoid (47), and we routinely incorporate the MGHL, if robust, in the more superior labral repairs. Unless additional labral pathology is present, sutures do not need to be placed in posterior or superior locations.

After arthroscopic Bankart repair, the patient should be placed in a sling for 1 week. Active ranges of motion exercises are incorporated into organized physical therapy from 1 to 6 weeks. Light weights can be employed from 6 to 12 weeks, and heavy weights may be included in therapy from 12 weeks to 6 months. During this period, no weight training should occur posterior to the coronal plane of the body, including military press. Contact sports may be resumed at 6 months.

The success of arthroscopic treatment for anterior shoulder instability is documented in the current orthopedic literature. In 2004, Ide et al. reviewed 55 young athletes (contact and noncontact) that underwent arthroscopic stabilization using suture anchors. In this population, athletes with a large bone loss of glenohumeral articulation were excluded from the study. The recurrence rate in contact athletes (9.5%, 2 of 21) was not statistically different from that in noncontact athletes (6%, 2 of 34) (48). In 2005, Mazzocca et al. (49) retrospectively evaluated 18 contact athletes and found

that 100% of all collision and contact athletes returned to organized high school or college sports.

In 2006, Larrain et al. reviewed the clinical outcomes at 4 to 9 years for 39 rugby players with acute anterior shoulder instability. Twenty percent of patients had acute instability, and of the remaining group, only 5% had surgery after their second episode of instability. Players with bone humeral deficiencies greater than one-fourth of the articular humeral head, bone glenoid deficiencies greater than 25% of the glenoid surface area, capsular laxity with poor tissue quality, and/or HAGL were excluded from the study. The results of the arthroscopic reconstructions were evaluated by use of the Rowe scale and analyzed according to stability and range of motion. Good or excellent results were found in 94.9% of cases in the acute instability group. In the acute instability group there were two cases of recurrence (5.1%) while playing rugby. In comparison, the recurrent stability group (158 patients), good-to-excellent results were found in 91.8%, with 10 recurrence (8.3%) (50).

The clinical results of anterior shoulder stabilization in contact athletes have been compared between the arthroscopic and open methods. In 2006, 48 collision athletes were evaluated using the visual analog scale, Rowe, and Constant scores. These authors found improvements after both open and arthroscopic surgeries; however, no statistically significant difference was found between the arthroscopic and open repair groups in these three outcome measures. Thirty-seven athletes (83%) returned to near preinjury sports activity levels (≥90% recovery) after operation. There were eight (16.5%) instances of postoperative instability among the collision athletes studied. The number of shoulders with postoperative subluxation or dislocation was four (25%) in the arthroscopic group and four (12.5%) in the open group ($p = 0.041$) (14).

Certain situations do exist that may require open surgical management for treatment of anterior shoulder instability in contact athletes. Specifically, patients with prior failed arthroscopic treatment (51), excessive capsular scarring, and/or patients with glenoid bone deficiency and/or large Hill–Sachs lesions (9) may be candidates for open surgery. Coracoid, iliac crest and/ or allograft transfer procedures in addition to, or instead of standard arthroscopic Bankart repair should be performed.

Efforts to stratify the risk of arthroscopic shoulder instability recurrence has been attempted using the instability severity index score (52). Using risk factors including patient age under 20 years at the time of surgery, involvement in competitive or contact sports or those involving forced overhead activity, shoulder hyperlaxity, a Hill–Sachs lesion present on an anteroposterior radiograph of the shoulder in external rotation and/or loss of the sclerotic inferior glenoid contour, patients with preoperative scores greater than six were identified as having unacceptable levels of risk for recurrence (70%) to warrant arthroscopic surgery. For these patients, instead Bristow–Laterjet procedures were recommended (52).

Although the mentioned studies demonstrate a large range of postarthroscopic repair shoulder instability clinical success, those studies excluding contact athletes with glenoid bone loss demonstrated recurrence rates similar to open Bankart repair (53).

Contact athletes are at a high risk for redislocation after stabilization for anterior shoulder instability. Traditional surgical management has demanded open treatment. With the proper patient exclusion of contact athletes needing open procedures, successful clinical outcomes can be achieved with arthroscopic technique in the remaining athletes. Operating on this group after the primary dislocation event will allow arthroscopic treatment to be used in almost all operative cases.

References

1. Owens BD, Agel J, Mountcastle SB, et al. Incidence of glenohumeral instability in collegiate athletics. Am J Sports Med. 2009;37(9):1750–1754.
2. Owens BD, Duffey ML, Nelson BJ, et al. The incidence and characteristics of shoulder instability at the United States Military Academy. Am J Sports Med. 2007;35(7):1168–1173.
3. Hovelius L, Olofsson A, Sandström B, et al. Nonoperative treatment of primary anterior shoulder dislocation in patients forty years of age and younger. a prospective twenty-five-year follow-up. J Bone Joint Surg Am. 2008;90(5):945–952.
4. Robinson CM, Howes J, Murdoch H, et al. Functional outcome and risk of recurrent instability after primary traumatic anterior shoulder dislocation in young patients. J Bone Joint Surg Am. 2006;88(11):2326–2236.
5. Arciero RA, Wheeler JH, Ryan JB, et al. Arthroscopic Bankart repair versus nonoperative treatment for acute, initial anterior shoulder dislocations. Am J Sports Med. 1994;22(5):589–594.
6. Bottoni CR, Wilckens JH, DeBerardino TM, et al. A prospective, randomized evaluation of arthroscopic stabilization versus nonoperative treatment in patients with acute, traumatic, first-time shoulder dislocations. Am J Sports Med. 2002;30(4):576–580.
7. Robinson CM, Jenkins PJ, White TO, et al. Primary arthroscopic stabilization for a first-time anterior dislocation of the shoulder. A randomized, double-blind trial. J Bone Joint Surg Am. 2008;90(4):708–721.
8. Owens BD, DeBerardino TM, Nelson BJ, et al. Long-term follow-up of acute arthroscopic Bankart repair for initial anterior shoulder dislocations in young athletes. Am J Sports Med. 2009;37(4):669–673.
9. Burkhart SS, De Beer JF. Traumatic glenohumeral bone defects and their relationship to failure of arthroscopic Bankart repairs: Significance of the inverted-pear glenoid and the humeral engaging Hill-Sachs lesion. Arthroscopy. 2000;16(7):677–694.
10. Itoi E, Lee SB, Berglund LJ, et al. The effect of a glenoid defect on anteroinferior stability of the shoulder after Bankart repair: A cadaveric study. J Bone Joint Surg Am. 2000;82(1):35–46.
11. Montgomery WH, Wahl M, Hettrich C, et al. Anteroinferior bone-grafting can restore stability in osseous glenoid defects. J Bone Joint Surg Am. 2005;87(9):1972–1977.
12. Bigliani LU, Newton PM, Steinmann SP, et al. Glenoid rim lesions associated with recurrent anterior dislocation of the shoulder. Am J Sports Med. 1998;26(1):41–45.
13. Voos JE, Livermore RW, Feeley BT, et al. Prospective evaluation of arthroscopic bankart repairs for anterior instability. Am J Sports Med. 2010;38(2):302–307.
14. Rhee YG, Ha JH, Cho NS. Anterior shoulder stabilization in collision athletes: Arthroscopic versus open Bankart repair. Am J Sports Med. 2006;34(6):979–985.
15. Pagnani MJ, Dome DC. Surgical treatment of traumatic anterior shoulder instability in american football players. J Bone Joint Surg Am. 2002;84-A(5):711–715.
16. Bottoni CR, Smith EL, Berkowitz MJ, et al. Arthroscopic versus open shoulder stabilization for recurrent anterior instability: A prospective randomized clinical trial. Am J Sports Med. 2006;34(11):1730–1737.
17. Fabbriciani C, Milano G, Demontis A, et al. Arthroscopic versus open treatment of Bankart lesion of the shoulder: A prospective randomized study. Arthroscopy. 2004;20(5):456–462.
18. Lenters TR, Franta AK, Wolf FM, et al. Arthroscopic compared with open repairs for recurrent anterior shoulder instability. A systematic review and meta-analysis of the literature. J Bone Joint Surg Am. 2007;89(2):244–254.
19. Neer CS, Foster CR. Inferior capsular shift for involuntary inferior and multidirectional instability of the shoulder. A preliminary report. J Bone Joint Surg Am. 1980;62(6):897–908.
20. Altchek DW, Warren RF, Skyhar MJ, et al. T-plasty modification of the Bankart procedure for multidirectional instability of the anterior and inferior types. J Bone Joint Surg Am. 1991;73(1):105–112.

21. Bak K, Spring BJ, Henderson JP. Inferior capsular shift procedure in athletes with multidirectional instability based on isolated capsular and ligamentous redundancy. *Am J Sports Med.* 2000;28(4):466–471.
22. Wiater JM, Vibert BT. Glenohumeral joint volume reduction with progressive release and shifting of the inferior shoulder capsule. *J Shoulder Elbow Surg.* 2007;16(6):810–814.
23. Harryman DT, Sidles JA, Harris SL, et al. The role of the rotator interval capsule in passive motion and stability of the shoulder. *J Bone Joint Surg Am.* 1992;74(1):53–66.
24. Provencher MT, Mologne TS, Hongo M, et al. Arthroscopic versus open rotator interval closure: Biomechanical evaluation of stability and motion. *Arthroscopy.* 2007;23(6):583–592.
25. Provencher MT, Dewing CB, Bell SJ, et al. An analysis of the rotator interval in patients with anterior, posterior, and multidirectional shoulder instability. *Arthroscopy.* 2008;24(8):921–929.
26. Provencher MT, Mologne TS, Romeo AA, et al. The use of rotator interval closure in the arthroscopic treatment of posterior shoulder instability. *Arthroscopy.* 2009;25(1):109–110.
27. Lo IKY, Parten PM, Burkhart SS. The inverted pear glenoid: An indicator of significant glenoid bone loss. *Arthroscopy.* 2004;20(2):169–174.
28. Sugaya H, Moriishi J, Dohi M, et al. Glenoid rim morphology in recurrent anterior glenohumeral instability. *J Bone Joint Surg Am.* 2003;85-A(5):878–884.
29. Saito H, Itoi E, Sugaya H, et al. Location of the glenoid defect in shoulders with recurrent anterior dislocation. *Am J Sports Med.* 2005;33(6):889–893.
30. Boileau P, Mercier N, Roussanne Y, et al. Arthroscopic Bankart-Bristow-Latarjet procedure: The development and early results of a safe and reproducible technique. *Arthroscopy.* 2010;26(11):1434–1450.
31. Lafosse L, Boyle S. Arthroscopic Latarjet procedure. *J Shoulder Elbow Surg.* 2010;19(2 suppl):2–12.
32. Hovelius LK, Sandström BC, Rösmark DL, et al. Long-term results with the Bankart and Bristow-Latarjet procedures: Recurrent shoulder instability and arthropathy. *J Shoulder Elbow Surg.* 2001;10(5):445–452.
33. Hovelius L, Sandström B, Sundgren K, et al. One hundred eighteen Bristow-Latarjet repairs for recurrent anterior dislocation of the shoulder prospectively followed for fifteen years: Study I–clinical results. *J Shoulder Elbow Surg.* 2004;13(5):509–516.
34. Shah AA, Selesnick FH. Traumatic shoulder dislocation with combined bankart lesion and humeral avulsion of the glenohumeral ligament in a professional basketball player: Three-year follow-up of surgical stabilization. *Arthroscopy.* 2010;26(10):1404–1408.
35. Coates MH, Breidahl W. Humeral avulsion of the anterior band of the inferior glenohumeral ligament with associated subscapularis bony avulsion in skeletally immature patients. *Skeletal Radiol.* 2001;30(12):661–666.
36. Bhatia DN, DasGupta B. Surgical treatment of significant glenoid bone defects and associated humeral avulsions of glenohumeral ligament (HAGL) lesions in anterior shoulder instability. *Knee Surg Sports Traumatol Arthrosc.* 2013;21(7):1603–1609.
37. Bokor DJ, Conboy VB, Olson C. Anterior instability of the glenohumeral joint with humeral avulsion of the glenohumeral ligament. A review of 41 cases. *J Bone Joint Surg Br.* 1999;81(1):93–96.
38. Greis PE, Dean M, Hawkins RJ. Subscapularis tendon disruption after Bankart reconstruction for anterior instability. *J Shoulder Elbow Surg.* 1996;5(3):219–222.
39. Karlsson J, Magnusson L, Ejerhed L, et al. Comparison of open and arthroscopic stabilization for recurrent shoulder dislocation in patients with a Bankart lesion. *Am J Sports Med.* 2001;29(5):538–542.
40. Regan WD, Webster-Bogaert S, Hawkins RJ, et al. Comparative functional analysis of the Bristow, Magnuson-Stack, and Putti-Platt procedures for recurrent dislocation of the shoulder. *Am J Sports Med.* 1989;17(1):42–48.
41. Rosenberg BN, Richmond JC, Levine WN. Long-term followup of Bankart reconstruction. Incidence of late degenerative glenohumeral arthrosis. *Am J Sports Med.* 1995;23(5):538–544.
42. Ho E, Cofield RH, Balm MR, et al. Neurologic complications of surgery for anterior shoulder instability. *J Shoulder Elbow Surg.* 1999;8(3):266–270.
43. McFarland EG, O'Neill OR, Hsu CY. Complications of shoulder arthroscopy. *J South Orthop Assoc.* 1997;6(3):190–196.
44. Mair SD, Hawkins RJ. Open shoulder instability surgery. Complications. *Clin Sports Med.* 1999;18(4):719–736.
45. Cho NS, Hwang JC, Rhee YG. Arthroscopic stabilization in anterior shoulder instability: Collision athletes versus noncollision athletes. *Arthroscopy.* 2006;22(9):947–953.
46. Buss DD, Lynch GP, Meyer CP, et al. Nonoperative management for in-season athletes with anterior shoulder instability. *Am J Sports Med.* 2004;32(6):1430–1433. Erratum in: *Am J Sports Med.* 2004;32(7):1780.
47. Boileau P, Villalba M, Héry JY, et al. Risk factors for recurrence of shoulder instability after arthroscopic Bankart repair. *J Bone Joint Surg Am.* 2006;88(8):1755–1763.
48. Ide J, Maeda S, Takagi K. Arthroscopic Bankart repair using suture anchors in athletes: Patient selection and postoperative sports activity. *Am J Sports Med.* 2004;32(8):1899–1905.
49. Mazzocca AD, Brown FM Jr, Carreira DS, et al. Arthroscopic anterior shoulder stabilization of collision and contact athletes. *Am J Sports Med.* 2005;33(1):52–60.
50. Larrain MV, Montenegro HJ, Mauas DM, et al. Arthroscopic management of traumatic anterior shoulder instability in collision athletes: Analysis of 204 cases with a 4- to 9-year follow-up and results with the suture anchor technique. *Arthroscopy.* 2006;22(12):1283–1289.
51. Kim SH, Ha KI, Kim YM. Arthroscopic revision Bankart repair: A prospective outcome study. *Arthroscopy.* 2002;18(5):469–482.
52. Balg F, Boileau P. The instability severity index score. A simple pre-operative score to select patients for arthroscopic or open shoulder stabilisation. *J Bone Joint Surg Br.* 2007;89(11):1470–1477.
53. Uhorchak JM, Arciero RA, Huggard D, et al. Recurrent shoulder instability after open reconstruction in athletes involved in collision and contact sports. *Am J Sports Med.* 2000;28(6):794–799.

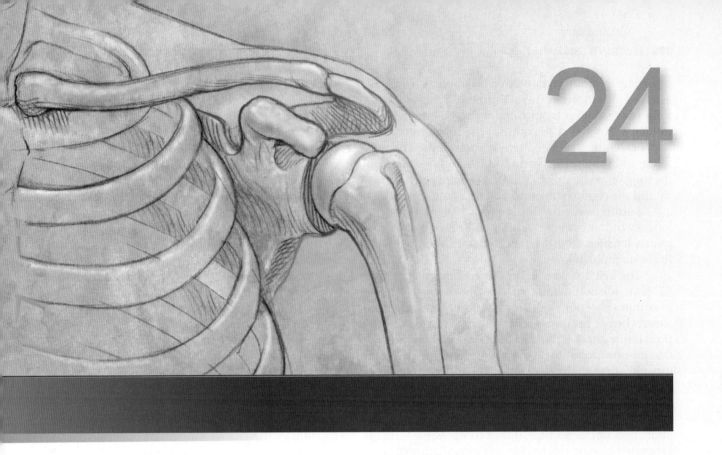

TREATMENT OF ANTERIOR INSTABILITY IN THE THROWING ATHLETE: DOS AND DON'TS

Michael E. Angeline / David W. Altchek

INTRODUCTION

For the overhead athlete, the specific act of throwing places an extreme demand on the shoulder. In response to these repetitive throwing activities, several adaptive changes have been described including increased glenohumeral external rotation, increased humeral head and glenoid retroversion, and anterior capsular laxity (1–4). These compensatory changes play an integral role in the delicate balance between the static and dynamic stabilization systems of the shoulder, which allow an asymptomatic throwing athlete to function normally.

The overhead throwing motion has six sequential phases: Wind-up, early/late cocking, acceleration, deceleration, and follow-through. Within this throwing cycle, potential energy is generated and efficiently converted into kinetic energy that is transferred to the baseball (5). When the throwing shoulder is subject to applied stresses at a rate that exceeds the tissue's maximum load to failure, acute or chronic/progressive damage to the shoulder's stabilizing structures can occur (6). This is especially true for the rotator cuff and capsulolabral complex, which are at risk for injury due to the large forces generated and rapid changes encountered during the throwing motion. Recent work by Shimizu et al. (7) assessed alterations in stress distribution across the glenoid cavity caused by pitching using CT osteoabsorptiometry. Compared to controls, the throwing athletes had a bicentric density pattern greatest in the anteroinferior and posterior segments. These findings highlight the long-term stress distributions across the glenoid cavity and the regions subject to potential injury.

Further work by Fleisig et al. (8) examined the kinetics of the pitching motion and noted two critical points at which these dynamic and static shoulder stabilizers are prone to injury.

The first instant is in the late cocking phase where 67 Nm of shoulder internal rotation torque and a maximum anterior shear force of 380 N are generated shortly before the arm reaches maximum external rotation. If this internal rotation torque is increased and the maximum anterior shear force is exceeded, the anterior capsulolabral complex can tear on either the glenoid side, in the midportion, or on the humeral side (9). The second critical instant during the throwing motion is just after ball release where 97 Nm of horizontal abduction torque and 1,090 N of compressive force are generated placing the rotator cuff musculature at risk.

The significant shear force across the anterior shoulder seen during the late cocking and early acceleration phases of throwing results in an increased load at the anterior capsule. In the case of anterior instability, there is a subsequent increase in this load resulting in failure of the capsuloligamentous system. This injury and subsequent laxity can be microtraumatic in nature resulting in a plastic deformation of the capsular ligaments or acute in nature (10). In this chapter, we will examine micro and acute anterior instability as it relates to anterior shoulder laxity and increased anterior translation during throwing. The pathomechanics/anatomy, presenting history and physical examination findings along with our preferred treatment interventions and postoperative rehabilitation will be reviewed.

PATHOMECHANICS OF ANTERIOR INSTABILITY

Anterior instability in the throwing athlete can be due to occult microinstability resulting from acquired capsular laxity, which allows increased humeral head translation with arm motion or it can be due to a single dislocation/subluxation episode.

While some anterior glenohumeral laxity may be a protective adaptation, microinstability is assumed to be a true pathologic laxity and the result of repetitive tensile loading due to scapular protraction or repetitive external loading (11). It may also be secondary to posterosuperior translation of the humeral head in the

abducted and externally rotated position due to posterior shoulder tightness/glenohumeral internal rotation deficit (GIRD). This posterior tightness subsequently results in redundancy of the anterior capsule because it is not stretched over the cam of the anterior edge of the humerus (11,12). Using a cadaveric model, Grossman et al. (13) found that posterior shoulder tightness resulted in a posterosuperior displacement of the humeral head with respect to the glenoid and increased anterior translation as compared to those shoulders without tightness. In the setting of microinstability, the challenge for the clinician is to distinguish adaptive capsular laxity and increased functional translation, which is advantageous for achieving maximal ball velocity and pathologic laxity that results in anterior instability.

An acute traumatic instability episode is uncommon in the throwing athlete. However, a subluxation event can occur when the athlete attempts to acutely increase their velocity. The maximal internal rotational velocity of a baseball pitcher has been shown to reach 6,100 to 7,510 degrees/sec (8). By increasing external rotation in the late cocking phase of throwing, the arc of rotation is expanded and subsequently the velocity can be optimized. If the internal rotation torque is increased however to the point where the maximum anterior shear force of the shoulder is exceeded, the anterior capsulolabral complex can tear acutely. This disruption can occur on either the glenoid side (Bankart lesion), in the midportion of the capsule, or as a humeral avulsion of the glenohumeral ligament (HAGL) lesion (1,9).

Two recent retrospective reviews of patients treated surgically for recurrent anterior shoulder instability found the incidence of isolated midsubstance capsular tears to be between 2% and 4% (14,15). While not as common as a Bankart lesion, an isolated capsular tear should be considered in the throwing athlete presenting with anterior instability.

PATHOANATOMY OF ANTERIOR INSTABILITY

The capsuloligamentous complex of the glenohumeral joint is composed of the superior, middle, and inferior glenohumeral ligaments along with the coracohumeral ligament.

It is important to note that these ligaments are actually thickenings of the shoulder capsule that assume their structural properties based on the position of the arm in space and their collagen orientation at the attachment site on the glenoid and humerus (16). On the basis of anatomic studies, the inferior glenohumeral ligament (IGHL) complex is a hammock-like structure with anchor points on the anterior and posterior sides of the glenoid (17). At 90 degrees of abduction and external rotation, the anterior band of the IGHL spans the midportion of the anterior glenohumeral joint and functions as the main restraint to anterior and inferior translations of the humerus (16,17).

For the throwing athlete with anterior instability, the capsular structure at risk is the anterior band of the IGHL. It originates from the anterior labrum and attaches to the glenoid through two separate mechanisms. The first is a direct attachment of collagen fibers to the glenoid labrum and the second is an indirect attachment with the collagen fibers blending together with the periosteum. The humeral insertion is located on the inferior margin of the articular surface around the anatomic neck and below the lesser tuberosity (17).

In terms of its vascular anatomy, the glenohumeral capsule has consistent contributions from the anterior/posterior circumflex, circumflex scapular and suprascapular arteries. These dominant vessels enter the capsule superficially and from the periphery. In addition, they run horizontally toward the midcapsule and deeper layers in a centripetal fashion (18). This has clinical significance when thinking about the surgical approach, as a horizontal capsular incision will run parallel to the dominant capsular vessels, while vertical incisions may cross them.

Looking at the ultimate load to failure of the anterior band of the IGHL, two separate studies by McMahon et al. (19,20) found no significant difference when failure occurred either at the glenoid insertion, in the midsubstance of the ligament, or at the humeral insertion. In addition, recent work by Moore et al. (21) using continuous and discrete finite element models suggested that the glenohumeral capsule should be evaluated as a continuous sheet rather than several discrete structures. These findings suggest that the clinician should consider the complex interactions between each capsular region when evaluating a throwing athlete that has sustained an acute instability episode.

HISTORY AND PHYSICAL EXAMINATION

During the throwing motion, the anterior capsuloligamentous system is subject to repetitive load by the anterior forces of the humeral head on the glenoid as the arm is repeatedly cocked in abduction, external rotation, and extension. Poor throwing mechanics and failure of the dynamic stabilizers will contribute to this overload. Baseball pitchers with occult anterior instability will complain of pain in the late cocking phase when the anterior static restraints are stressed or during follow-through if the glenohumeral decelerators do not appropriately stabilize the joint (22).

In the case of an acute instability episode where the athlete has sustained a disruption along any point of the capsuloligamentous system, they will note a sense of the humeral head subluxating over the glenoid rim during the late cocking phase of the throwing cycle. The athlete may also note decreased velocity or "dead arm" symptoms. It is crucial for the clinician to determine which phase of the throwing motion or arm position reproduces the athlete's symptoms. If the symptoms occur just after ball release, the pathology may be related to the rotator cuff more so than the anterior stabilizing structures of the shoulder (8).

The goal of the physical examination is to isolate the portions of the restraint system that are responsible for producing the athlete's symptoms. Our examination starts first with a visual assessment of the athlete's gross musculature. Poor global muscle bulk may signify a nutritional abnormality while atrophy within the infraspinatus fossa can represent chronic rotator cuff dysfunction or suprascapular nerve injury. Next, a postural assessment is performed, which is critical in the younger athlete. We look for any evidence of shoulder depression, increased or decreased lumbar lordosis, a change in pelvic tilt (anterior tilt), and any presence of a reduced thoracic kyphotic curvature. Presence of any of these abnormalities may contribute to poor throwing mechanics and should be addressed.

Scapular observation is performed next. Any evidence of altered scapular position can potentially produce a dynamic scapular dyskinesis in the throwing cycle, which can affect glenohumeral kinematics and lead to injury (23). Range of motion is assessed in various degrees of shoulder adduction and 90 degrees of abduction. An individual's total arc of motion (TAM), the sum of the internal and external ranges of motion, should be considered during the examination as a measure of capsular laxity (12,24). In throwers, there is a decrease in internal rotation and an increase in external rotation as compared to the nondominant arm.

The TAM however is the same on both shoulders (25). When the internal rotation and TAM are decreased in the dominant arm alone, glenohumeral kinematics are altered and a resultant increase in throwing related injuries can occur (10). In a cohort study performed by Shanley et al. (26), it was found that a passive shoulder internal rotation loss of greater the 25 degrees as compared bilaterally was a predictor of arm injury for high school softball and baseball players.

Looking specifically at external rotation in the throwing athlete, an increase in external rotation of the dominant shoulder compared with the nondominant shoulder can be an expected manifestation of normal laxity as previously discussed. In the setting of an acute capsular tear; however, the athlete will present with increased external rotation at 90 degrees of abduction with no endpoint. This finding is crucial to diagnose an acute capsular injury in the throwing athlete presenting with symptoms of anterior instability.

The rotator cuff and internal rotators of the shoulder are next assessed by attempting to elicit symptoms or weakness on resistance maneuvers. Electromyography (EMG) evaluation of the muscular firing patterns about the shoulder during the throwing motion demonstrated that the pectoralis major, serratus anterior, latissimus dorsi, and subscapularis had the highest activity during the acceleration phase of the throw. These muscles eccentrically contract to protect the anterior part of the shoulder joint. In contrast, the rotator cuff musculature and larger core musculature had the highest forces during the deceleration phase (23). Work using dynamic intramuscular EMG, demonstrated that throwing athletes with chronic anterior instability had a marked decreased activity in the internal rotators of the shoulder during all phases of the pitching sequence (27).

A mild increase in activity was noted in the biceps and the supraspinatus suggesting a compensatory mechanism. This muscular imbalance is thought to contribute to the problem of anterior instability in the throwing athlete, especially in the occult setting.

Ligamentous stability is tested on both shoulders in the anterior, posterior, and inferior directions. The goal of the examination is to differentiate adaptive laxity from pathologic laxity and determine whether the different maneuvers reproduce the patient's symptoms. We approach the examination in the same manner no matter what the patient's presenting complaints include.

The first assessment is to elicit a sulcus sign with the patient in the seated position. Typically, the throwing athlete will exhibit a 1 to 2 plus sulcus, which correlates with 1 to 3 cm of inferior displacement (10). The presence of 3 cm or more of inferior displacement (3 plus sulcus) is usually associated with pathologic inferior instability.

Anterior and posterior instability is examined with the patient in the supine position. After applying an axial load at the elbow to center the humeral head on the glenoid, the examiner translates the humeral head on the glenoid. It is important to note that the force vector for evaluating anterior instability is in an anteroinferior direction and not a straight anterior direction due to the associated pathology with the anterior IGHL complex. Our grading system has been previously described and is as follows: 1+, increased translation compared with the opposite shoulder without distinct subluxation of the humeral head over the glenoid; 2+, noted subluxation over the glenoid rim can be produced; 3+, the humeral head can be displaced and locked over the glenoid rim (10). It is not uncommon for the throwing athlete to have 1+ anterior laxity and 2+ posterior laxity. However, the presence of 2+ or greater anterior laxity signifies the presence of a pathologic condition (28).

It has been our experience that athletes presenting with an acute Bankart lesion will have at least 2+ anterior laxity whereas those athletes with a purely capsular injury may only display 1+ anterior laxity. The Jobe relocation test is also performed to further evaluate for the presence of subtle instability (1).

The findings obtained from the history and physical examination are combined with diagnostic radiographic imaging and magnetic resonance imaging (MRI). Radiographs obtained include a true anteroposterior (AP) view of the shoulder, AP of the shoulder in internal rotation, an outlet view, a West Point axillary view, and a Stryker notch view. In most cases, the plain radiographic views will rarely yield any diagnostic information within this patient population. As a result, we have frequently used MRI to provide further information regarding the anterior shoulder pathology and refine the diagnosis.

It has become our standard to not inject any contrast agents into the shoulder when performing an MRI. The contrast can subtly change the capsular morphology and make it difficult to identify any acute capsular injury. Using a three-channel shoulder coil, our typical MRI series evaluating anterior instability in the throwing athlete utilizes axial, oblique coronal, and oblique sagital fast spin echo techniques. With these images, the capsulolabral complex is evaluated for compromise.

In the setting of an acute Bankart tear in the throwing athlete, there will be a detachment of the labroligamentous complex from the glenoid with a disrupted periosteum (29). It is important to note that the cardinal event, which caused the disruption, is the result of a subluxation of the humeral head and not a frank dislocation. As a result, no Hill-Sachs impaction fracture will be typically noted. Unlike a Bankart tear, imaging evaluation of pure capsular injuries is usually difficult.

In the acute setting, MRI findings will depict prominent extracapsular soft tissue edema seen adjacent to the humeral attachment of the IGHL without frank avulsion at the humerus (Fig. 24-1). Capsular thickening may be the only imaging finding in the chronic setting. The diagnosis of a HAGL lesion is made by identifying the extracapsular soft tissue edema along with changes in the configuration of the axillary pouch, which assumes a J-shaped configuration (29).

TREATMENT OF ANTERIOR INSTABILITY

The primary goal in treating the throwing athlete with anterior instability is to regain glenohumeral stability while preserving an adequate range of motion to resume function. This can be accomplished with either nonsurgical or surgical interventions. In the case of microinstability where there is no evidence of any specific pathology within the labroligamentous complex, it has been our approach to treat the athlete with an extensive rehabilitation program first.

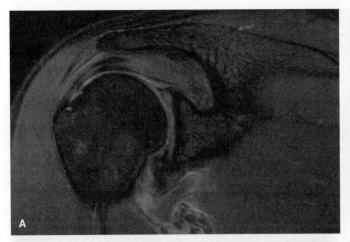

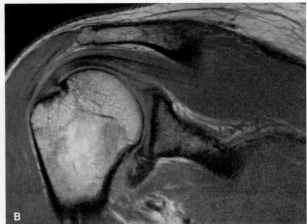

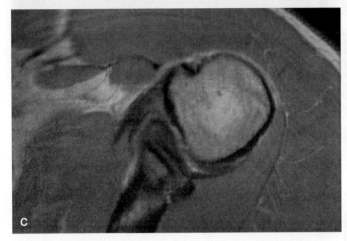

▲ **FIGURE 24-1:** MRI of the left shoulder utilizing oblique coronal **(A,B)** and axial **(C)** fast spin echo techniques. These images demonstrate extracapsular soft tissue edema and an anterior capsular tear with injury at both the humerus and the scapula. Inferiorly, the greatest injury is at the humeral margin.

This program is divided into three overall phases. The goal of the first phase is to restore full shoulder range of motion, normal flexibility, strength, and scapulohumeral rhythm. It is within this phase that upper extremity endurance is emphasized with the minimum criteria for advancement to the next phase being isokinetic internal rotation strength of at least 85% as compared to the unaffected side. The main focus of the second phase is to restore normal neuromuscular function and maintain strength and flexibility of the affected shoulder. In order to progress to the next phase, the goal is for the athlete to have isokinetic internal rotation/external rotation strength at least equal to the unaffected side as well as greater than 66% isokinetic external rotation/internal rotation strength ratio.

The third phase focuses on an independent sport specific program, which in the case of the throwing athlete would include a throwing program. Within the throwing program, the focus is on more volume of throws at a shorter distance. If the athlete continues to have significant pain and feeling of instability after completing this program then surgical intervention is warranted and an arthroscopic capsular plication is performed. With this technique, the senior author has recently demonstrated a 90% return to overhead sport (30).

In the setting of an acute Bankart lesion resulting in anterior instability, it has been our experience that nonoperative treatment is rarely successful for the throwing athlete.

Our approach has been to intervene early when this pathology is present in order to prevent further damage to the shoulder and to help increase the athlete's chances of returning to competitive play. We have found that by intervening early most of these stabilizations can be performed arthroscopically.

The basic premise of our surgical approach is to restore the labroligamentous complex back to its anatomic position. We do not over constrain the shoulder as this can alter the glenohumeral kinematics during the throwing cycle. Regional supraclavicular block anesthesia is used for all shoulder stabilization procedures along with a general anesthetic. This ensures complete relaxation of the operative extremity. The patient is positioned in a modified beach chair position with the use of a beanbag and a commercial arm holder. A careful examination of the shoulder under anesthesia is then performed as described previously. Following this examination, a diagnostic arthroscopy is performed through a standard posterior portal only with the use of a 30-degree arthroscope. Before making any other portals,

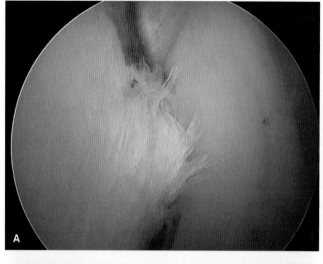

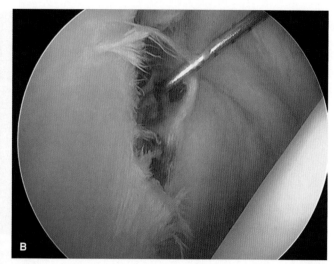

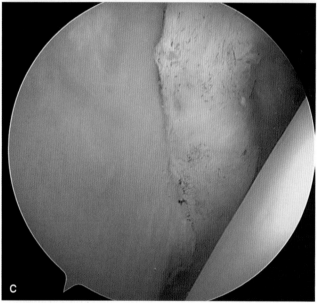

▲ **FIGURE 24-2:** Arthroscopic images of the right shoulder in a professional major league pitcher demonstrating an acute Bankart injury sustained after a subluxation event in which the athlete attempted to increase his velocity during a pitch **(A,B)**. A horizontal mattress suture configuration was utilized with knotless anchors to anatomically reduce and fix the anterior inferior labroligamentous complex **(C)**.

the presence of tissue injury should be demonstrated and consistent with the clinical and imaging findings.

The anterior inferior labrum has little anatomic variability and a tear or detachment in this region is significant (Fig. 24-2A,B). After arthroscopic confirmation of the anterior inferior labral tear, the definitive surgical procedure is carried out. Occasionally, we will use a 70-degree arthroscope during the repair process in order to achieve optimal visualization of the pathology.

For our stabilization procedures, we prefer to make a rotator interval portal with the use of a 5-mm cannula for suture management and a low anterior inferior portal with an 8.5-mm cannula for anchor placement and suture passage. Our current technique utilizes knotless anchor fixation with the sutures shuttled in a horizontal mattress configuration. The arm is positioned at 60 degrees of abduction, neutral forward flexion and between 60 and 80 degrees of external rotation

when tensioning each anchor during the repair. Again, our goal is to restore the anatomy of the labroligamentous complex and not to overconstrain the shoulder (Fig. 24-2C).

For the athlete with an acute capsular tear not involving the labrum, our approach of an early surgical intervention seeking to restore the anatomy without overconstraining the shoulder remains the same. The set-up is similar to that previously described for those patients presenting with a Bankart lesion. We perform a diagnostic arthroscopy in the modified beach chair position in order to fully define the pathology and tear configuration. Figure 24-3 demonstrates an acute capsular tear, while Figure 24-4 demonstrates an acute-on-chronic tear. It has been our experience that these capsular tears cannot be treated arthroscopically but instead should be repaired in an open fashion. After completion of the diagnostic arthroscopy, the head of the bed is

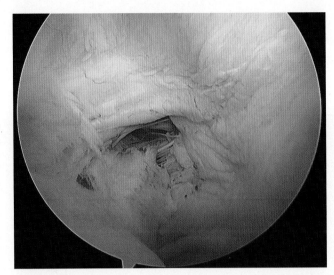

▲ **FIGURE 24-3:** Arthroscopic image of a professional major league pitcher's left shoulder demonstrating an acute capsular tear. This tear correlates with the MRI seen in Figure 24-1.

positioned at an approximate 45-degree angle. The skin incision extends from the axillary fold toward the lateral aspect of the coracoid. The deltopectoral interval is then identified and the cephalic vein is exposed and retracted laterally. Next, the coracoid and clavipectoral fascia are incised and a blunt retractor is placed under the conjoint tendon to expose the subscapularis tendon.

Depending on the location of the capsular tear, the subscapularis can be split at the junction of the upper two-thirds and lower one-third or divided laterally in an oblique fashion. If a HAGL lesion is present or the capsular tear is along the lateral aspect of the capsule, visualization and correct tensioning can be difficult through a split in the subscapularis. In this situation, the subscapularis tendon is divided laterally.

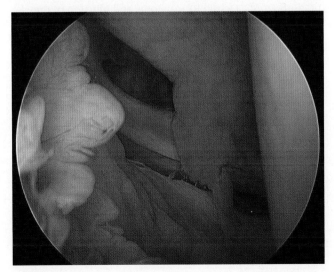

▲ **FIGURE 24-4:** Arthroscopic image of a professional major league pitcher's right shoulder demonstrating an acute-on-chronic capsular tear.

After the anterior capsule has been exposed, the repairs are performed with either direct suturing in the case of a midsubstance tear or with suture anchor fixation along the humeral insertion in the case of HAGL lesions, far lateral tears or tears in which the tissue quality is poor. A modified Mason-Allen stitch is utilized when suture anchors are placed otherwise a horizontal mattress suture configuration is utilized. Final capsular repair is again performed with the arm in 60 degrees of abduction, neutral forward flexion and between 60 and 80 degrees of external rotation. The shoulder is then re-examined and an endpoint to external rotation in the abducted position should be restored. The subscapularis is then repaired anatomically to ensure that no shortening occurs and a standard subcutaneous and subcuticular skin closure is performed.

POSTOPERATIVE REHABILITATION

Our rehabilitation program is similar for all stabilization procedures including capsular repairs. It follows along the guidelines of criteria-based and patient-specific progression emphasizing early, controlled motion with external rotation and extension advanced slowly in order to protect the repair and avoid excessive stretching of the anterior capsule. Overhead activities are progressed last.

The overall program is divided into five total phases with the three final phases being similar to those previously described for treating microinstability with no evidence of any specific pathology. In the first phase of the rehabilitation program, the goal is to promote healing while reducing inflammation, pain, and swelling. Active assisted elevation in the plane of the scapula to 90 degrees is emphasized along with scapular mobility, submaximal deltoid isometrics in neutral rotation and external rotation to neutral or 30 degrees in the case of an open procedure. A shoulder immobilizer is worn at all times when the athlete is not exercising. For those athletes who have undergone a capsular repair, this first phase is critical in order to prevent excessive stretching of the anterior capsule. As a result, this initial phase is typically extended over a longer period of time.

Once elevation in the scapular plane and external rotation to neutral or 30 degrees have been achieved, the athlete can be advanced to the second phase, which focuses on restoring scapular and rotator cuff strength along with increasing the active assisted external rotation motion. In the case of arthroscopic stabilizations, the limit of external rotation is 45 degrees and for open procedures the limit is 60 degrees. The shoulder immobilizer is gradually weaned off during this phase and again athletes who have undergone a capsular repair typically are slowly advanced within this phase as well in order to protect the anterior capsule. The remaining three phases have again been previously discussed. It has been our practice that the interval throwing programs are not started until after 6 to 8 months from the date of surgery. Athletes who have undergone a capsular repair may take over a year in order to get back to competitive play given the slow progression through the rehabilitation program.

S U M M A R Y

Treating the throwing athlete for anterior instability can be a challenging undertaking for the clinician. By combining the history and physical examination findings with diagnostic imaging, the clinician should be able to identify the distinct cause of anterior instability in the throwing athlete. The overall goal is to address the pathology encountered, restore joint stability, and return the athlete to their sport. This can be accomplished with either nonoperative rehabilitation or operative intervention. In the case of operative stabilization, over tensioning the labroligamentous complex should be avoided in order to prevent loss of motion or altered glenohumeral kinematics. The position of the arm during surgery is critical in determining the appropriate tension necessary to restore stability (22). Along with the importance of the operative intervention in addressing the anterior instability, we consider the postoperative rehabilitation protocol as crucial in returning the athlete to competitive play. Through the use of criteria-based and patient-specific progression, the athlete can have a safe timeline for a return to throwing.

References

1. Drakos MC, Rudzki JR, Allen AA, et al. Internal impingement of the shoulder in the overhead athlete. *J Bone Joint Surg Am.* 2009;91(11):2719–2728.
2. Crockett HC, Gross LB, Wilk KE, et al. Osseous adaptation and range of motion at the glenohumeral joint in professional baseball pitchers. *Am J Sports Med.* 2002;30(1):20–26.
3. Osbahr DC, Cannon DL, Speer KP. Retroversion of the humerus in the throwing shoulder of college baseball pitchers. *Am J Sports Med.* 2002;30(3):347–353.
4. Bigliani LU, Codd TP, Connor PM, et al. Shoulder motion and laxity in the professional baseball player. *Am J Sports Med.* 1997;25(5):609–613.
5. Ouellette H, Labis J, Bredella M, et al. Spectrum of shoulder injuries in the baseball pitcher. *Skeletal Radiol.* 2008;37(6):491–498.
6. Kvitne RS, Jobe FW. The diagnosis and treatment of anterior instability in the throwing athlete. *Clin Orthop Relat Res.* 1993;291:107–123.
7. Shimizu T, Iwasaki N, Nishida K, et al. Glenoid stress distribution in baseball players using computed tomography osteoabsorptiometry: A pilot study. *Clin Orthop Relat Res.* 2012;470(6):1534–1539.
8. Fleisig GS, Andrews JR, Dillman CJ, et al. Kinetics of baseball pitching with implications about injury mechanisms. *Am J Sports Med.* 1995;23(2):233–239.
9. Bigliani LU, Pollock RG, Soslowsky LJ, et al. Tensile properties of the inferior glenohumeral ligament. *J Orthop Res.* 1992;10(2):187–197.
10. Altchek DW, Dines DM. Shoulder injuries in the throwing athlete. *J Am Acad Orthop Surg.* 1995;3(3):159–165.
11. Kibler WB, Thomas SJ. Pathomechanics of the throwing shoulder. *Sports Med Arthrosc.* 2012;20(1):22–29.
12. Whiteley R, Oceguera MV, Valencia EB, et al. Adaptations at the shoulder of the throwing athlete and implications for the clinician. *Tech Should Surg.* 2012;13:36–44.
13. Grossman MG, Tibone JE, McGarry MH, et al. A cadaveric model of the throwing shoulder: A possible etiology of superior labrum anterior-to-posterior lesions. *J Bone Joint Surg Am.* 2005;87(4):824–831.
14. Mizuno N, Yoneda M, Hayashida K, et al. Recurrent anterior shoulder dislocation caused by a midsubstance complete capsular tear. *J Bone Joint Surg Am.* 2005;87(12):2717–2723.
15. Rhee YG, Ha JH, Park KJ. Clinical outcome of anterior shoulder instability with capsular midsubstance tear: A comparison of isolated midsubstance tear and midsubstance tear with Bankart lesion. *J Shoulder Elbow Surg.* 2006;15(5):586–590.
16. O'Brien SJ, Schwartz RS, Warren RF, et al. Capsular restraints to anterior-posterior motion of the abducted shoulder: A biomechanical study. *J Shoulder Elbow Surg.* 1995;4(4):298–308.
17. Burkart AC, Debski RE. Anatomy and function of the glenohumeral ligaments in anterior shoulder instability. *Clin Orthop Relat Res.* 2002;400:32–39.
18. Andary JL, Petersen SA. The vascular anatomy of the glenohumeral capsule and ligaments: An anatomic study. *J Bone Joint Surg Am.* 2002;84-A(12):2258–2265.
19. McMahon PJ, Tibone JE, Cawley PW, et al. The anterior band of the inferior glenohumeral ligament: Biomechanical properties from tensile testing in the position of apprehension. *J Shoulder Elbow Surg.* 1998;7(5):467–471.
20. McMahon PJ, Dettling J, Sandusky MD, et al. The anterior band of the inferior glenohumeral ligament. Assessment of its permanent deformation and the anatomy of its glenoid attachment. *J Bone Joint Surg Br.* 1999;81(3):406–413.
21. Moore SM, Ellis B, Weiss JA, et al. The glenohumeral capsule should be evaluated as a sheet of fibrous tissue: A validated finite element model. *Ann Biomed Eng.* 2010;38(1):66–76.
22. Payne LZ, Altchek DW. The surgical treatment of anterior shoulder instability. *Clin Sports Med.* 1995;14(4):863–883.

23. Eckenrode BJ, Kelley MJ, Kelly JD 4th. Anatomic and biomechanical fundamentals of the thrower shoulder. *Sports Med Arthrosc.* 2012;20(1):2–10.

24. Laudner K, Meister K, Noel B, et al. Anterior glenohumeral laxity is associated with posterior shoulder tightness among professional baseball pitchers. *Am J Sports Med.* 2012;40(5):1133–1137.

25. Kibler WB, Sciascia A, Moore S. An acute throwing episode decreases shoulder internal rotation. *Clin Orthop Relat Res.* 2012;470(6):1545–1551.

26. Shanley E, Rauh MJ, Michener LA, et al. Shoulder range of motion measures as risk factors for shoulder and elbow injuries in high school softball and baseball players. *Am J Sports Med.* 2011;39(9):1997–2006.

27. Glousman R, Jobe F, Tibone J, et al. Dynamic electromyographic analysis of the throwing shoulder with glenohumeral instability. *J Bone Joint Surg Am.* 1988;70(2): 220–226.

28. Altchek DW, Warren RF, Wickiewicz TL, et al. Arthroscopic labral debridement. A three-year follow-up study. *Am J Sports Med.* 1992;20(6):702–706.

29. Omoumi P, Teixeira P, Lecouvet F, et al. Glenohumeral joint instability. *J Magn Reson Imaging.* 2011;33(1): 2–16.

30. Jones KJ, Kahlenberg CA, Dodson CC, et al. Arthroscopic capsular plication for microtraumatic anterior shoulder instability in overhead athletes. *Am J Sports Med.* 2012; 40(9):2009–2014. Epub 8/6/2012.

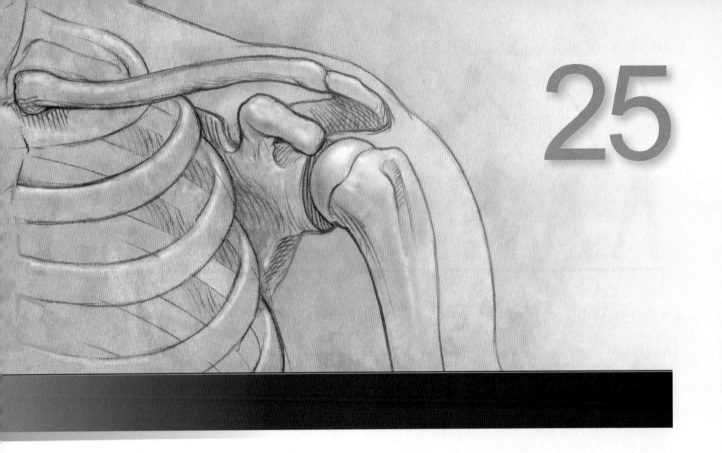

25

POSTERIOR INSTABILITY CAUSED BY "BATTER'S SHOULDER"

Richard W. Kang / Phillip N. Williams /
Ekaterina Urch / Thomas C. Harris /
Joshua S. Dines

INTRODUCTION

Although the throwing motion of baseball players has been thoroughly investigated, the baseball batting swing has received less attention despite obvious interest by players and fans alike in powerful hits and home runs. The baseball batting swing accounts for injuries to the shoulder, back, and knee. The forces imparted on the shoulder during the swing, however, can have potential deleterious effects. Specifically, the lead shoulder of a swing can undergo tremendous forces, especially when a pitch is missed. Repetitive loads on the lead shoulder can cause posterior instability, which we refer to as "Batter's Shoulder."

This chapter will review the pathomechanics, clinical presentation, imaging, treatment options, and initial clinical results of batter's shoulder.

MECHANICS OF BATTING

Electromyographic analyses of targeted muscle groups have provided important information on muscle activation during the batting swing (1–4). Results from these studies

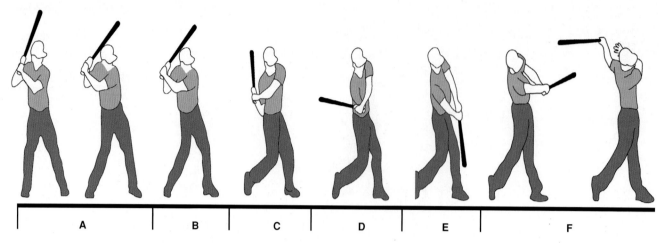

▲ FIGURE 25-1: Phases of the batting swing.

have helped improve our understanding of the mechanics that can lead to injury, optimize batting performance, and design specific training and rehabilitation regimens. Shaffer et al. (4) have divided the batting swing into four distinct phases: (1) Wind up—begins as the lead heel leaves the ground and ends as the lead toe re-establishes ground contact; (2) Preswing—begins as the lead forefoot strikes the ground and ends as the swing begins; (3) Swing has three subdivisions: (a) Early—begins as the bat moves forward until perpendicular with the ground, (b) Middle—continues until the bat is parallel with the ground, (c) Late—continues until ball contact; and (4) Follow through—begins with ball contact and ends as the lead shoulder reaches maximum abduction and external rotation (Fig. 25-1). The authors found that posterior deltoid activity was highest in preswing, but seemed to be more important in positioning than power generation. Similar to a golfer, a baseball batter generates bat speed using a kinetic link to transfer momentum to smaller adjacent segments (5,6). A majority of the force and speed is generated in the core and lower extremity and translated into rotational velocities of 937 degrees/sec at the shoulder and 1,160 degrees/sec at the arms immediately prior to ball contact. These forces allow the bat to rotate at 1,588 degrees/sec with a resultant linear bat velocity of 31 m/sec (5).

PATHOPHYSIOLOGY

During the batting swing, high rotational velocities coupled with the weight of the bat lead to a tremendous amount of force at the shoulders. For this reason, baseball players are susceptible to an uncommon but often disabling type of posterior instability known as batter's shoulder. In this entity posterior instability leads to episodic subluxation of the lead shoulder during the baseball swing (1).

A missed outside pitch is considered to be the predominant proposed mechanism of injury that leads to batter's shoulder (7). When the bat fails to make contact with the pitched ball, there is no counterforce to offset the dynamic posterior pulling force of 500 N during a swing.

In addition, reaching for an outside pitch increases the abduction angle of the shoulder during the swing. This increase in abduction angle can subsequently result in increased glenohumeral shear forces. In a preliminary study, Andrews found an average shoulder abduction angle of 105 degrees for outside pitches versus 90 degrees for inside pitches (7). The American Sports Medicine Institute group hypothesized that the increased shoulder abduction angle may increase shear forces across the joint. Given these angles, the torque generated for an outside pitch can be approximately 13.5% greater than that of an inside pitch. Therefore, during a missed pitch, it is believed that there is no counterforce to the baseball swing, leading to over loading of shoulder dynamics and an excessive pulling force in the lead shoulder.

Furthermore, the stabilizing muscles around the shoulder are recruited when the bat makes contact with the ball. A missed ball can fail to recruit these surrounding muscles, and prevent their important shoulder stabilization function.

CLINICAL PRESENTATION

Patients typically recall a specific event, where they feel a sensation of instability after reaching for an outside pitch or missing a pitch. After this event, patients may feel discomfort or pain with certain provocative positions, especially with forward flexion, adduction, and internal rotation (8).

The physical examination may be positive for a positive load and shift test, jerk test, or Kim test. The combination of the jerk and Kim tests has been shown to be about 97% sensitive for a posteroinferior labral lesion (3).

IMAGING

Plain radiographs should include an axillary view in addition to the other standard views of the shoulder. The radiographs should rule out any fractures or dislocations. In addition, the radiographs should be evaluated for reverse Hill–Sachs lesions, glenoid hypoplasia or retroversion, as well as any bony avulsions of the glenohumeral ligaments.

Magnetic resonance imaging (MRI) is used to evaluate the labrum and the capsule, and any associated chondral lesions. The presence of a Kim lesion should also be ruled out on the MRI (2).

A computed tomography (CT) scan, although less frequently used in the setting of "Batter's Shoulder," can be used to evaluate for glenoid version, humeral version, and reverse Hill–Sachs lesions.

TREATMENT

Nonoperative management is the initial course of treatment for athletes with batter's shoulder. This treatment course includes physical therapy directed toward rotator cuff strengthening, scapular stabilizing exercises, and improving range of motion. Surgical management is indicated if the patient fails at least 12 weeks of concerted nonoperative management.

Surgical treatment will likely involve an arthroscopic posterior labral repair. Although the operation can be performed in a beach chair position, our preference is the lateral decubitus position. Before prepping and draping, an examination under anesthesia is performed to determine the degree of instability. The posterior portal is made slightly more lateral than usual to facilitate anchor placement for the posterior labral repair. A complete diagnostic arthroscopy is performed initially. Then, the arthroscope is switched to the anterior portal to visualize the torn posterior labrum (Fig. 25-1). The labrum is mobilized using an elevator through the posterior portal. The bony surface is then prepared with the mechanical shaver (Fig. 25-2). Anchors are then placed starting at about the 5:30 position relative to the face of the glenoid in a left shoulder (Fig. 25-3). Using an accessory posterior portal, a tissue-piercing device is used to capture the appropriate amount of capsulolabral tissue to incorporate into the repair (Fig. 25-4). Arthroscopic knots are used to secure the labrum to the glenoid (Fig. 25-5). This sequence is repeated moving superiorly along the face of the glenoid with sequential anchors being placed at 4:30 and 3:30 positions. Occasionally more anchors will be needed if the tear extends into the biceps anchor.

The postoperative rehabilitation protocol involves a sling for 2 weeks. This is followed by physical therapy with a focus on passive range of motion for 6 weeks. After 6 weeks, active range of motion can begin. Then, after the 12-week mark, strength training and hitting

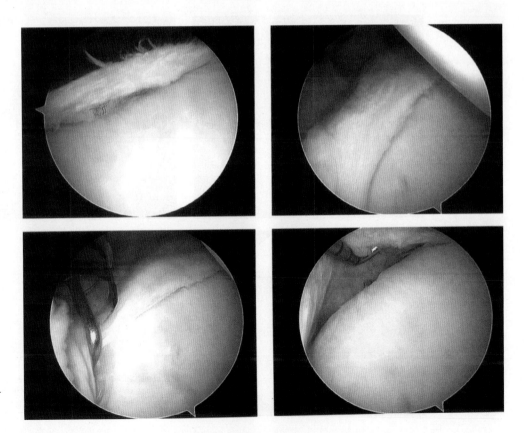

▶ **FIGURE 25-2:** Torn posterior labrum viewed from the anterior portal.

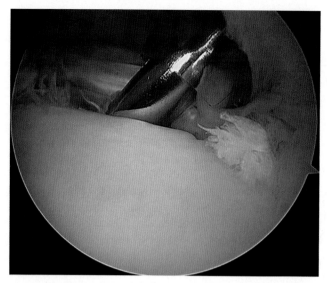

▲ FIGURE 25-3: Preparation of bony glenoid surface and debridement of frayed labral tissue using mechanical shaver.

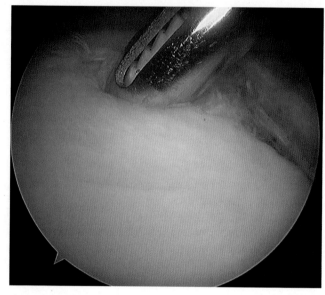

▲ FIGURE 25-4: Implantation of suture anchor onto glenoid rim.

off a tee can be started. They can progress to taking live pitches at 6 months postoperatively.

CLINICAL RESULTS

Wanich et al. have conducted the only published study on "Batter's Shoulder" (9). Their retrospective review had 14 participants with an average age of 20 years old (range 17 to 33 years old). The study consisted of four professional, six college, and four high school athletes. The inclusion criteria consisted of a history of batting-induced shoulder instability. Participants were excluded if they had a history of traumatic injury to the shoulder or prior shoulder pathology. The average follow-up was 1.2 years (range, 7 to 35 months).

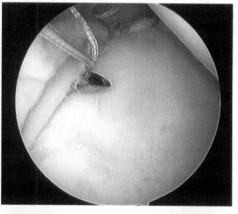

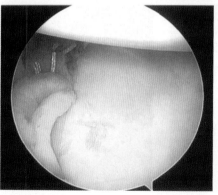

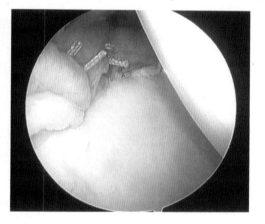

▲ FIGURE 25-5: Tissue-piercing device used to shuttle suture through the capsulolabral complex and arthroscopic knot to bring the capsulolabral complex to the glenoid rim.

Posterior laxity was demonstrated on all 14 patients and 12 had a positive O'Brien's sign. Twelve out of fourteen patients also demonstrated evidence of posterior labral tearing on MRI. Twelve out of fourteen failed conservative management and went onto surgical treatment. Ten players underwent arthroscopic posterior labral repair and two underwent labral debridement without repair. The average return to sport was 6.5 months. Both players managed conservatively had

excellent outcomes, while 11 out of 12 (92%) surgically treated players had excellent outcomes. The single player with a poor outcome also had a concomitant glenoid osteochondral lesion, which may have contributed to the lack of improvement despite operative intervention. The authors acknowledged several limitations to their study including the retrospective study design, limited numbers of participants, and lack of long-term follow-up.

SUMMARY

Batter's shoulder is a rare and only recently recognized entity. This condition consists of posterior shoulder instability caused by a missed attempt at hitting a pitch, especially with an outside pitch. The lack of counterforce from hitting a ball transmits increased forces on the posterior capsulolabral complex of the lead shoulder during batting.

Nonoperative management is first-line treatment. If a player fails this initial management, an arthroscopic posterior labral repair versus debridement is performed. After operative treatment, the player can expect to return to play after approximately 6 to 7 months. Initial results from a small, retrospective series demonstrate greater than 90% excellent results (9). These findings are similar to current literature for arthroscopic treatment of posterior instability. Williams et al. (10) performed arthroscopic posterior stabilization on 27 patients and were able to eliminate pain and instability in 92% of their patients with a 5.1-year mean follow-up. Lenart et al. (11) also performed arthroscopic

posterior stabilization on 34 patients with a success rate of 92%, and there was significant improvement in validated shoulder outcome measurements from preoperative measurements. In a series of 100 athletes by Bradley et al. (12), 89% returned to full sport without recurrence of instability. In a study of 33 patients, Provencher et al. (13) achieved stabilization in 88% at a mean follow-up of 39 months. In a series of 27 patients, Kim et al. (14) were able to successfully treat 26 out of 27 patients with arthroscopic posterior labral repair and capsular shift techniques. Savoie et al. (15) had a 97% success rate in 92 patients at a mean of 28 months postoperatively . Despite these successful outcomes, the natural history and true prognosis for batter's shoulder must be further elucidated by longer-term follow-up studies.

Based on initial results, we predict good-to-excellent results for most players with batter's shoulder who undergo proper treatment. In addition, since the nonthrowing arm is affected in most cases, there is a high likelihood of return to play.

References

1. Fleisig GS, Dun S, Kingsley D. Biomechanics of the shoulder during sports. In: Wilk KE, Reinold MM, Andrews JR, eds. *The Athlete's Shoulder.* 2nd ed. Philadelphia, PA: Churchill Livingstone; 2009:365–384.
2. Kim SH, Ha KI, Yoo JC, et al. Kim's lesion: An incomplete and concealed avulsion of the posteroinferior labrum in posterior or multidirectional posteroinferior instability of the shoulder. *Arthroscopy.* 2004;20(7): 712–720.
3. Kim SH, Park JS, Jeong WK, et al. The Kim test: A novel test for posteroinferior labral lesion of the shoulder–a comparison to the jerk test. *Am J Sports Med.* 2005; 33(8):1188–1192.
4. Shaffer B, Jobe FW, Pink M, et al. Baseball batting. An electromyographic study. *Clin Orthop Relat Res.* 1993; (292):285–293.
5. Welch CM, Banks SA, Cook FF, et al. Hitting a baseball: A biomechanical description. *J Orthop Sports Phys Ther.* 1995;22(5):193–201.
6. Wolf EM, Eakin CL. Arthroscopic capsular plication for posterior shoulder instability. *Arthroscopy.* 1998; 14(2):153–163.
7. Philips BB, Andrews JR, Fleisig GS. Batter's shoulder: posterior instability of the lead shoulder, A biomechanical evaluation. Paper presented at: Alabama Sports Medicine and Orthopaedic Center, 2000; Birmingham, Alabama.
8. Hawkins RJ, Koppert G, Johnston G. Recurrent posterior instability (subluxation) of the shoulder. *J Bone Joint Surg Am.* 1984;66(2):169–174.
9. Wanich T, Dines J, Dines D, et al. "Batter's Shoulder:" Can athletes return to play at the same level after operative treatment? *Clin Orthop Relat Res.* 2012;470(6): 1565–1570.
10. Williams RJ 3rd, Strickland S, Cohen M, et al. Arthroscopic repair for traumatic posterior shoulder instability. *Am J Sports Med.* 2003;31(2): 203–209.
11. Lenart BA, Sherman S, Mall NA, et al. Arthroscopic repair for posterior shoulder instability. *Arthroscopy.* 2012;28(10):1337–1343.

12. Bradley JP, Baker CL, Kline AJ, et al. Arthroscopic capsulolabral reconstruction for posterior instability of the shoulder. *Am J Sports Med.* 2006;34(7): 1061–1071.

13. Provencher MT, Bell SJ, Menzel KA, et al. Arthroscopic treatment of posterior shoulder instability: Results in 33 patients. *Am J Sports Med.* 2005;33(10):1463–1471.

14. Kim SH, Ha KI, Park JH, et al. Arthroscopic posterior labral repair and capsular shift for traumatic unidirectional recurrent posterior subluxation of the shoulder. *J Bone Joint Surg Am.* 2003;85-A(8):1479–1487.

15. Savoie FH 3rd, Holt MS, Field L, et al. Arthroscopic management of posterior instability: Evolution of techniques and results. *Arthroscopy.* 2008;24(4):389–396.

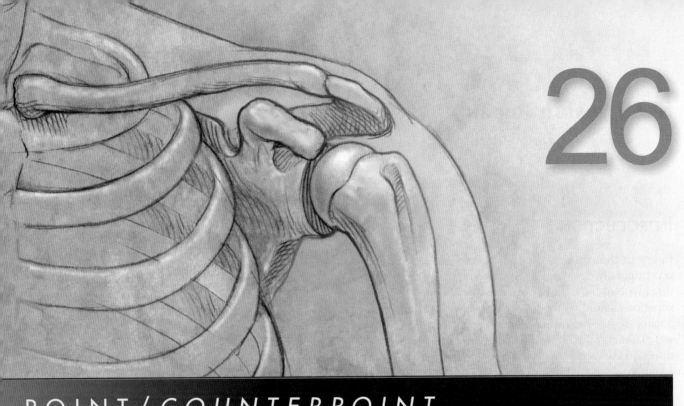

26

POINT/COUNTERPOINT

SLAP Tears

*T*he role of the long head of the biceps tendon is a subject of much debate. Those who believe that it plays an important role with regard to shoulder mechanics advocate for superior labral anterior to posterior (SLAP) repair in the presence of a type II SLAP lesion. Others argue that the LHB tendon is a vestigial structure that athletes and other patients can do without. In these situations, tenodesis or even biceps transfer to the conjoint tendon has been described. In the following chapters, the role of the long head biceps will be debated. Based on the presumed role, each author will highlight their preferred technique for superior labral–biceps anchor pathology.

SLAP Lesion Repair

Neal S. ElAttrache / Kaitlin M. Carroll / Michael B. Banffy

INTRODUCTION

Injury to the superior glenoid labrum–biceps complex was originally described by Andrews et al. (1) as a lesion that involved the labrum from the anterior portion of the superior glenoid to the posterior glenoid including the anchor of the long head of the biceps tendon. SLAP tears were later classified by Snyder into types I to IV classification (2,3). In recent years, arthroscopic procedures have advanced and there is a better understanding of labral pathologies and its pathomechanics.

The biceps and labral complex, consisting of the labrum and its attachments to the long head of the biceps, must be looked at synergistically to fully understand the function and anatomical position of these two structures. The biceps and superior labrum act in concert with one another, but they also have independent functions. Together, the biceps and the labrum play a crucial role in the stability and function of the glenohumeral joint. Microtrauma from repetitive overhead activities, or trauma from a fall on an outstretched arm or sudden traction on the shoulder are common etiologies of the labrum–biceps complex injuries (3,4). SLAP lesions can be the cause of shoulder pain and weakness and occasionally instability, especially in overhead athletes.

Diagnosing SLAP lesions on physical examination remains challenging due to the lack of specific testing and often-concomitant pathologies. Pathologies such as AC joint sprains and arthritis or rotator cuff tears can cause similar symptoms (5). Athletes complain of shoulder pain and weakness, especially with throwing, and often a decrease in velocity. Batters in baseball may complain of pain in their lead shoulder. There are many physical examination tests that have been described to diagnose a SLAP tear; however, there is no single specific test that can diagnose a SLAP tear (6–10). The treatment is determined based on clinical examination as well as an MR arthrogram and the treatment varies based on the type of tear and clinical findings (6,8,11,12). Treatment options include nonsurgical options (formal physical therapy and strengthening) or surgical treatments (SLAP repair, biceps tenodesis).

The relationship of the biceps to the superior labrum is critical to the overhead athlete for shoulder stability particularly in the extremes of motion. A biceps tenodesis creates a nonanatomic construct that clearly does not restore shoulder stability. To date, there is no data in the literature about the return of elite overhead athletes after biceps tenodesis. A tenodesis should not be performed in a structurally normal biceps unless the biceps is viewed as a vestigial structure, and biomechanical data is completely disregarded.

ANATOMY

Superior Labrum

Understanding the superior labrum is essential in the diagnosis and treatment of SLAP tears. In the superior hemisphere of the shoulder, the labrum is a fibrocartilaginous tissue and often meniscoid. The anterior superior labrum provides the attachment for the superior glenohumeral ligament (SGHL), middle glenohumeral ligament (MGHL), and occasionally a vertical inferior glenohumeral ligament (IGHL). There are very few biceps fibers in the anterior superior labrum (Fig. 26-1). The biceps tendon has a shared origin with the posterosuperior labrum and the supraglenoid tubercle of the glenoid (Fig. 26-2).

Shoulder stability will be disrupted if the attachments of the glenohumeral ligaments are disrupted. Superior labral avulsions that extend 1 cm anterior and 1 cm posterior to the biceps will cause a significant increase in anterior–posterior translations, superior–inferior translations, as well as external rotation (13). Marked instability increases as the tear involves more of the posterior and superior quadrant (13). These abnormal translations then allow "edge loading" of the humeral head on the glenoid that causes pain at extremes of motion and symptoms of instability.

Long Head of the Biceps

The biceps functions independently from the labrum, but its pathology and pathomechanics work in conjunction with the labrum. The long head of the biceps rotates with the humeral head from anterior superior in an oblique position during internal rotation to a posterior superior oblique position in external rotation at 120 degrees. Intra-articular length of biceps is the shortest and the tension is highest during extreme rotation and abduction such as during the throwing motion. The increased tension in the biceps tendon depresses the humeral head acting as a dynamic stabilizer increases concavity compression assuming an

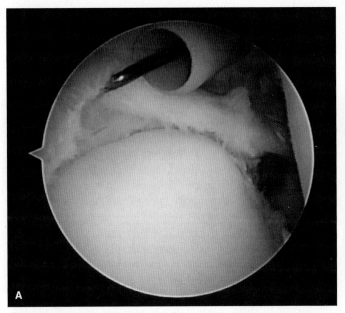
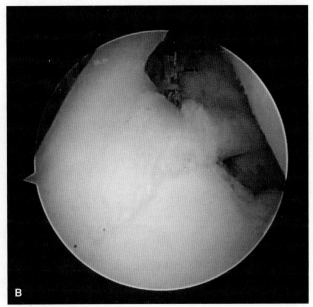

▲ **FIGURE 26-1:** Anterosuperior labral injury **(A)** pre- and **(B)** postrepair.

intact labrum. Dynamic loading of the biceps shifts the humeral head's center of rotation more toward the center of the glenoid. For the biceps to act as a dynamized ligament at the extremes of motion, the superior labrum must be stable (13). If the superior labrum is avulsed or loose, not only will the attachment of the SGHL and MGHL be disrupted, but the secondary stabilizing role of the biceps will also be deficient (13). In the overhead athlete the biceps plays a critical role in the extremes of motion and should not be considered a structure that can be released or repositioned without consequence.

DIAGNOSIS

Diagnosing a SLAP tear in an athlete can be difficult based on false positive effects of other injuries in the shoulder. SLAP tears often present with similar findings as a rotator cuff tear and can be associated with concomitant pathologies (6,14). Athletes complain of pain, clicking, weakness, and instability. Their symptoms are more pronounced with overhead activities or at the extremes of motion or exertion. On physical examination, there are a variety of tests that can be done to diagnose a SLAP tear (Speed, Yergason, O'Brien, Jobes relocation test) but

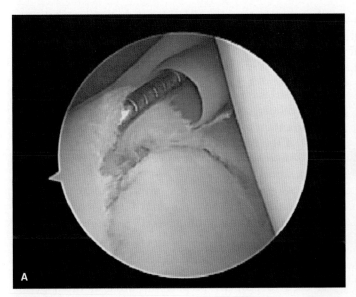
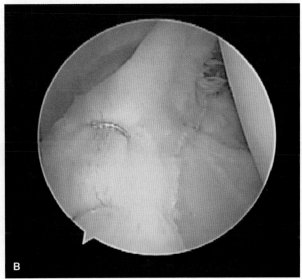

▲ **FIGURE 26-2:** Posterosuperior labral injury **(A)** pre- and **(B)** postrepair.

there is no single test that can accurately determine a SLAP tear with a high specificity and/or sensitivity. Physical examination findings include shoulder pain both posterior and anterior at extremes of motion. There is minimal to no pain at rest or with functional range of motion (ROM). At full-end ROM there may be pain with edge loading. On clinical examination, one must determine all potential sources of pain and determine if the labral tear causes disruption of stability independent of biceps signs and symptoms.

TREATMENT OPTIONS

Nonsurgical Option

Initially, SLAP tears should be treated nonoperatively with rest for 4 to 6 weeks. Patients should undergo a formal physical therapy protocol including the use of nonsteroidal anti-inflammatories. Overhead throwing athletes will undergo a throwing mechanics program focusing on full-body kinematics. The goal is to restore the ROM in the overhead athlete to "normal" and avoid excess stress on the anterior capsule. Physical therapy will help optimize lower extremity and trunk strength. In addition, the program will help strengthen scapular rotators and stabilizers, rotator cuff, and power muscles of the shoulder. Beyond strengthening, the protocol will help increase endurance and stress the need for proper mechanics. Rehabilitation may involve extensive stretching, and attention to scapulothoracic mechanics. Anatomic surgical repair should be considered if nonoperative treatment fails.

Surgical

For those that fail nonoperative treatment, surgical treatment should be considered to address labral pathology. During the arthroscopy, a dynamic diagnostic arthroscopy should be done to consider the type of SLAP tear present, identify any biceps pathology, and test labral stability (Table 26-1). Once the pathology is identified,

TABLE 26-1 Surgical Decision Making Based on Tear Classification

Classification Type	Surgical Treatment
Type I (and unstable flaps)	Debridement
Type II	Stabilize biceps anchor
Type III	Excise vs. repair bucket-handle tear
Type IV	III + stabilize biceps anchor vs. tenodesis

it is necessary to identify the relationship to ligament morphology to determine the location of fixation. There should be no fixation at the base of the biceps; instead it should be anterior and posterior to the biceps itself.

Surgical Decision Making

Before repairing a SLAP lesion, one must determine the patient's activity level, type of sport, and age. The ideal surgical candidate patient is the active patient less than 40 years of age that participates in overhead or contact sports, heavy lifting, pushing, or pulling. Patients that have a traumatic etiology of their SLAP lesions also have better outcomes (14).

Avoid repair in significant glenohumeral chondromalacia especially with subchondral bone deformity on post margin as the increased constraint from the SLAP repair may lead to increased pain. A repair should not be done in the setting of adhesive capsulitis and with caution in those with concomitant rotator cuff repairs. If there is any biceps subluxation, a tenodesis should be performed. Similarly, if the biceps is severely damaged consider a tenotomy or tenodesis and treat the labrum depending on stability and ligament morphology.

In the physiologically young patient, and particularly in the overhead athletes, it is important to stabilize the labrum anterior and posterior to the biceps without constraining biceps excursion. Type II and complex SLAP lesions should be anatomically restored. If there is a type IV tear, and a large bucket-handle fragment contains the attachment for the glenohumeral ligaments, an attempt should be made to repair the labrum and biceps delamination if possible.

SURGICAL PEARLS

We prefer to repair SLAP lesions and other intra-articular pathology in the lateral decubitus position. This position allows increased mobility within the glenohumeral joint to adequately assess and treat all pathologies.

It is very necessary to determine the relationship of the SLAP lesion to the glenohumeral ligament pathology; this will determine the location of our anchor points. It is important to avoid placing anchors and sutures at the base of the biceps as this will over constrain the biceps and lead to a higher failure rate, recurrent pain, and loss of motion.

After determining the proper fixation points, we utilize the portal of Wilmington for anchor placement and suture shuttling along with our normal anterior superior portal. When using the transrotator cuff portal, it is critical to remain medial to the rotator cuff cable. Prior to anchor placement, a rasp or mechanical shaver is used to properly prepare the bone at the superior aspect of the glenoid to enhance labral healing. We have

TABLE 26-2 Postoperative Rehabilitation Table

Time (Weeks)	Goal
0–1 week	• Sling for comfort • Active elbow motion • Active assisted elevation to salute position.
1–3	• Codman circumduction • Scapular retraction • Scapular isometrics
3–6	• Progressive AROM/AAROM overhead • Limit ER to 90 degrees
6–16	• Full AROM • Scapular stab program • Rotator cuff program • Posterior capsule stretching
16–28	• Interval throwing
28+	• Progress to full competitive throwing

found that a vertical mattress stitch appropriately recreates the anatomic meniscoid position of the superior labrum. Our preference is to utilize 2.4- or 2.9-mm knotless anchors to eliminate suture abrasion on chondral surfaces, synovium, and the rotator cuff tendons. These anchors are also cannulated to provide an extra channel for marrow elements to be released to enhance the biologic healing response between the bone and labrum.

Postoperative rehabilitation is critical to the success of SLAP repair. Active assisted ROM is initiated immediately with active elbow and wrist ROM. Starting week 3, we begin progressive active ROM, limiting external rotation to 90 degrees. Starting week 6, we begin full active ROM with posterior capsule stretching. Interval throwing begins at week 16 with progression to full return to play at 6 to 9 months (Table 26-2).

RESULTS

Injuries to the superior labrum are commonly seen in overhead athletes, and returning to high level of activities in athletes is challenging after repair. Patients with a history of acute SLAP tears are more frequently nonresponders to nonsurgical treatment, and patients with an acute traumatic injury have a higher success rate with surgery (14). Edwards et al. (15) found that 50% of athletes are successful to return to sports with nonoperative treatment, but a high level of activity and return to overhead sports at same level was difficult to achieve (66%). Therefore, nonoperative treatment should be considered for isolated SLAP tears, but if symptoms persist or the patient is a high-level athlete, surgical treatment should be considered.

Returning to activity after a SLAP repair varies, particularly if the patient is an overhead athlete (14–20). Morgan et al. reported on type II SLAP tears in overhead athletes and nonthrowers with an acute injury. Their results were 97% "good to excellent" in nonthrowers, and 83% of throwers subjectively felt that they returned to their same level of play after surgery. Rhee et al. (20) had 86% "good to excellent" results with 50% of throwers returning to their previous level of play. In this study, Rhee et al. found that throwing athletes had more satisfactory results than nonthrowing athletes. Based on the literature, throwing athletes can return to high level of activities with surgical intervention and a proper rehabilitation protocol.

Elite overhead throwing athletes are more of a treatment challenge, particularly with regard to getting them to return to their previous levels of play. In a study of 23 collegiate/professional throwers that underwent a SLAP repair, 57% returned to their prior level of play (18). A more critical look at the data showed that 80% of players treated for an isolated SLAP lesion returned to play, whereas only 12.5% of players with combined labral repair and partial-thickness rotator cuff tear returned to play. Return to play in players with labral and rotator cuff pathology is far lower than return to play in throwers with isolated SLAP repair, indicating that rotator cuff pathology is a major contributing factor to failure of SLAP treatment. According to Neuman et al. (17), players perceived that they returned to 84.1% of their preinjury level and had a KJOC score of 73.6. SLAP repairs have a high rate of overall satisfaction, but the outcome is less predictable in overhead athletes (16,17).

Failure after SLAP repair can result from any or all of the following: Poor patient selection, technical errors such as over constraining the biceps and or capsular ligaments, or unnecessary additional capsular plication. Prominent implants and suture abrasion can cause irritation that results in persistent pain after surgery. In addition, a failure to treat coexisting pathology or to correct predisposing mechanics can result in a failed repair.

CONCLUSION

While several treatment options for SLAP tears have been posited, only anatomic SLAP repair has been clinically shown to return high-level overhead athletes back to their prior level of play. Some authors have argued for tenodesis in place of anatomic SLAP repair. However, in addition to this procedure not restoring shoulder stability, there are no published clinical outcomes of tenodesis in high-level athletes that would support its use. Given our surgical technique and treatment, you can expect 80% of athletes will return to same level of competition after a SLAP repair. It is for this reason that we advocate for anatomic SLAP repair in the setting of SLAP tears.

Biceps Tenodesis

Kirk A. Campbell / Eric J. Strauss / Nikhil N. Verma / Anthony Romeo

INTRODUCTION

Tears of the superior glenoid labrum are a cause of shoulder pain and disability, especially in overhead athletes such as pitchers, swimmers, and volleyball players. First described by Andrews et al. (21) in 1985 in their report of findings at the time of shoulder arthroscopy in a group of 73 high-level overhead athletes, superior labral tears were further characterized in 1990 by Snyder et al. (2) who coined the term "SLAP lesion". Snyder devised a four-part arthroscopic classification system to describe the fraying or detachment of the superior labrum anterior and posterior to the biceps anchor, with type II lesions in which both the superior labrum and biceps anchor are detached from the superior glenoid rim being the most common variant.

Although SLAP tears have become a very important clinical entity, especially in overhead throwers, the prevalence of SLAP tears is thought to be very low (22). SLAP tears have a reported prevalence between 1.2% and 26%, but in their original description and classification of these lesions Snyder et al. (2) found a 4% incidence of SLAP tears in 700 consecutive shoulder arthroscopies (4,6,22). In another study involving a series of 2,375 consecutive shoulder arthroscopies Snyder et al. (23) found an incidence of SLAP tears of 5.9% (140 SLAP tears) and, of these, only 28% were isolated SLAP lesions. Interestingly, they found that 72% of the cases of SLAP tears were associated with other shoulder pathology such as rotator cuff tears (40% incidence of partial or full-thickness tear), Bankart lesions or humeral head lesions, which highlights the fact that the clinician should be cognizant to look for concomitant pathologies when treating SLAP pathology. In addition, anatomic variations and age-related changes in the superior labrum have made it more difficult to clearly determine the true incidence of SLAP tears. A recent prospective study of 3,395 shoulder arthroscopies also showed that prevalence of SLAP lesions was low and isolated SLAP lesions were found in only 5.4% (182 cases) of their cases (24). Based on these reports from high volume, experienced shoulder surgeons, clinicians can evaluate their own practice to avoid overtreatment of degenerative SLAP pathology or anatomic variants which can lead to increased risk of complications.

The SLAP type II lesion has been the most clinically important superior labral pathology and the management of these lesions has been a controversial topic in sports medicine and shoulder surgery literature. The management of this lesion has generally been dependent on patient characteristics with considerations made to age and activity level. At the present time, there are several schools of thought on how to appropriately manage superior labral tears with most surgeons recommending arthroscopic repair with suture anchors to relieve pain and prevent glenohumeral instability. While current data demonstrates good to excellent outcomes following repair of type II SLAP lesions, the majority of studies in the literature are of level 3 and level 4 evidence and mixes patients of variable age, various injury mechanism, and activity level. A recent systematic review reported good to excellent satisfaction in 83% of treated patients and an overall 73% return to preinjury level of athletic participation (16). However, a closer look demonstrates that the results of arthroscopic SLAP repair in overhead, throwing athletes are less consistent, with clinical studies demonstrating a return to preinjury level of sports participation ranging from 22% to 84% (6,19,25) (Table 26-3). Of 19 baseball players treated with arthroscopic suture anchor fixation of type II SLAP tears, Ide et al. (25) reported that 12 players (63%) had a complete return to play without pain or functional limitation at a mean follow-up of 3.5 years. It is believed that persistent pain and limitation of ROM following SLAP repair is the reason behind these low rates of return to overhead athletics (26,30). Some authors attribute the incidence of post-SLAP repair shoulder pain to the rigidity of the suture anchor fixation construct with a consequent loss of physiologic motion at the labral–biceps anchor junction, while others theorize that the highly innervated proximal portion of the biceps tendon acts as the primary pain generator following injury or surgery. Concomitant injuries such as rotator cuff tear has also been correlated with inability to return to sport (18). In addition, articular injury from hardware or suture, stiffness, and failure of healing may all contribute to persistent symptoms following repair. The low rate of return to play and the potential for continued symptoms postoperatively have led some authors to look for alternative treatment methods for managing isolated type II SLAP lesions.

Recently, some authors have proposed long head biceps tenodesis, which maintains the length–tension relationship of the long head of biceps, as a surgical

(text continues on page 319)

TABLE 26-3   Recent Results of Type II SLAP Repair with Suture Anchor in Overhead Athletes

Author	Year	Study Type	Follow-up	Avg. Age	Total No. of Patients	Amount Overhead Athletes	Overall% Good to Excellent Satisfaction	Overall% Return to Preinjury Level of Play (Overhead Athlete)	Baseball/ Softball Overhead Throwing Athlete% Return to Preinjury Level of Play	Notes
Morgan et al. (19)	1998	Retrospective case series	1 yr	33 yrs (range, 15 to 72 yrs)	102	53	97	NA	84	31% rate of RTC tears
Kim et al. (26)	2002	Retrospective case series	2.75 yrs	26 yrs (16 to 35 yrs)	34	18	94	22	NA	
Ide et al. (25)	2005	Retrospective case series	3.4 yrs	24 yrs (15 to 38 yrs)	40	40	90	75	63	30 patients with partial thickness RTC tears. Mean modified Rowe scores 92.1
Enad et al. (27)	2007	Retrospective case series	2.5 yrs	31.6 yrs (22 to 41 yrs)	27	NA	89	NA	NA	77% overall return to pre-injury level of play. Overall mean ASES score 86.9. Mean UCLA score 30.4.
Enad and Kurtz (28)	2007	Retrospective case series	2.4 yrs	31.6 yrs (22 to 41 yrs)	36	NA	92	NA	NA	94% return to duty rate in active duty military personnel
Yung et al. (29)	2008	Prospective cohort	2.3 yrs	24.2 yrs (15 to 38 yrs)	16	13	92	NA	NA	94% return to preinjury level of play
Boileau et al. (30)	2009	Prospective cohort	2.9 yrs	ª37 yrs (19 to 57 yrs)	25 (10 suture anchor repair and 15 biceps tenodesis)	15 (7 in SLAP repair group)	40	NA	NA	Overall 20% of suture anchor repair patients return to preinjury sports, while 87% of the biceps tenodesis patients returned to preinjury sports

(continued on page 318)

TABLE 26-3 Recent Results of Type II SLAP Repair with Suture Anchor in Overhead Athletes (continued)

Author	Year	Study Type	Follow-up	Avg. Age	Total No. of Patients	Amount Overhead Athletes	Overall% Good to Excellent Satisfaction	Overall% Return to Preinjury Level of Play (Overhead Athlete)	Baseball/ Softball Overhead Throwing Athlete% Return to Preinjury Level of Play	Notes
Brock-meier et al. (14)	2009	Retrospective case series	2.7 yrs	36 yrs (14 to 49 yrs)	47	28	87	74	64	Median ASES scores 97 and L'Instalata scores 93
Neuman et al. (31)	2011	Retrospective case series	3.5 yrs	24 yrs (16 to 48 yrs)	30	30	93.3	84.1	79.5	Mean time to return to play 11.7 mos. Avg ASES scores 87.9 and KJOC score 73.6
Neri et al. (18)	2011	Retrospective case series	3.2 yrs	25 yrs (18 to 45 yrs)	23	23	96	57	NA	Presence of a partial-thickness RTC correlated with inability to return to preinjury level status (12.5% vs. 80%) after SLAP repairs.
[b]Sayde et al. (16)	2012	Systematic review	NA	NA	506	198	83	63	76	327 type II SLAP tears were repaired with suture anchors. 169 with tacks and 10 with staples

NA, not available; RTC, rotator cuff tear; ASES, American Shoulder and Elbow Society; KJOC, Kerlan-Jobe Orthopaedic Clinic Shoulder and Elbow; Avg, average; #, number.

[a]Age of suture anchor repair group.

[b]Systematic review of SLAP repair in throwing athletes.

alternative to repair for patients with isolated type II SLAP lesions. Biceps tenodesis is a straightforward procedure with reliable outcomes, a shorter recovery period, and a low complication rate. In this chapter we will present a discussion of the evidence to support repair versus biceps tenodesis in the management of type II SLAP tear.

ANATOMY AND BIOMECHANICS

The glenoid labrum is a rounded or triangular fibrocartilaginous tissue that lines the edge of the glenoid and contributes to shoulder stability by increasing the depth of the glenoid cavity and facilitating concavity compression (32,33). The labrum receives its vascular supply from the suprascapular, circumflex scapular, and posterior humeral circumflex arteries, which all penetrate the labrum from the periphery in a circumferential and radial pattern (32). As a result of this pattern of blood flow, the inner portion of the labrum is avascular and the superior and anterosuperior labrum have the poorest vascularity which places SLAP tears at risk for impaired healing (32,34,35). The superior glenoid labrum serves as the anchor site for the insertion of long head of the biceps and the SGHL, MGHL, and IGHL. The anterosuperior labrum has several recognized normal variants; in a study by Rao et al. (36), it was found that the three most common variants occurred in 13.4% of the 546 patients undergoing shoulder arthroscopy. These variants included the sublabral foramen with a cord-like MGHL occurring in 8.6% of the patients, sublabral foramen in 3.3% of patients, and 1.5% of patients having an absent anterosuperior labrum with a cord-like MGHL (Buford complex) (Fig. 26-3) (35,36) Similarly, there

are clinically relevant anatomic variations in the site of the long head of biceps origin from the glenoid labrum with roughly 60% of its fibers arising from the supraglenoid tubercle and the other 40% arising from the superior labrum (34,37). It is important to be aware of these anatomic variations, which if misdiagnosed as a SLAP lesion and "repaired" can lead to pain, significant loss of external rotation, and stiffness.

The exact function of the superior labrum and biceps complex are not fully understood. The intact labrum improves joint stability while enhancing concavity compression and as previously mentioned, increases the effective diameter of the glenoid (35). Biomechanics studies on human cadavers have attempted to further elucidate superior labral function suggesting a role in glenohumeral stability; biomechanical study has demonstrated that creation of a type II SLAP lesion results in significantly decreased torsional rigidity and significantly increased strain on the anterior band of IGHL when the shoulder was in the vulnerable abducted and externally rotated position, which is common in overhead athletes (38). Further it was also shown that the long head of the biceps contributed to anterior glenohumeral joint stability by increasing the shoulder's resistance to torsional forces in the abducted and externally rotated position (35,37–39). Cadaveric studies have shown that the long head of the biceps functions as a head depressor and restricts glenohumeral translation in all directions, but more so in the anterior and inferior directions. Accordingly any destabilization of the long head of the biceps led to increased glenohumeral translation (40). Burkart et al. (41) also found increased glenohumeral translation with shoulder abduction after a simulated type II SLAP lesion and repair of the SLAP lesion reduced the inferior translation and restored glenohumeral stability. Recently Patzer et al. (42) showed that the repair of SLAP tears without associated long head of the biceps tenotomy was able to nearly restore baseline glenohumeral stability and also reduce the increased load on the long head of the biceps, which was present after the SLAP tear. Interestingly they also noted that, after a biceps tenotomy the repair of the SLAP tear no longer affected glenohumeral stability.

Although these cadaveric studies have increased our understanding of the role of the superior labrum and biceps complex, the results are an oversimplification of the clinical scenario because these biomechanical studies are not able to account for all of the complex interactions that occur between the rotator cuff muscles, glenohumeral ligaments, and other structures during shoulder motion. In addition, these studies use normal shoulder with artificially created SLAP lesions which fail to account for the complex mechanism by which SLAP tears occur in the overhead athlete. Electromyography (EMG) data highlight some of the shortcomings of

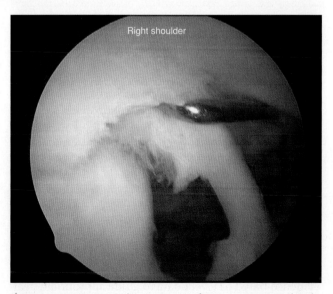

▲ **FIGURE 26-3:** Arthroscopic view from posterior portal, right shoulder, demonstrating a Buford Complex. This normal anatomic variant is notable for an absence of the anterior superior labrum with cord-like middle glenohumeral ligament complex.

biomechanics studies and have cast doubt on the exact role of the long head biceps in shoulder function. Multiple authors have demonstrated that following immobilization of the elbow, no significant shoulder-related biceps activity on EMG is noted during active shoulder motion (43,44). However, Glousman et al. (44) showed that there was increased biceps activity during pitching in athletes with anterior shoulder instability, which suggests a secondary role for the biceps in anterior glenohumeral stability. It has also been suggested that biceps activity at the elbow and not the shoulder may account for the stabilizing effect of the biceps on the glenohumeral joint (37). As suggested by these apparently conflicting findings, further research is needed in this area to clearly understand the role of the superior labrum in normal shoulder function, the effect of removing the LHB from the shoulder, and to determine if there is a need to repair the superior labrum following biceps tenotomy or tenodesis.

CLINICAL PRESENTATION AND DIAGNOSIS

The clinical diagnosis of a SLAP tear can be a diagnostic challenge and a careful history and physical examination are a key part of the workup. Typically an overhead throwing athlete will present with complaints of anterior shoulder pain, which can be associated with difficulties performing overhead activities and/or a decreased throwing velocity (4,33). Presentation may also include complaints of popping, clicking, catching, weakness, or stiffness. The fact that SLAP tears are commonly associated with other shoulder pathology such as rotator cuff tears or instability adds to the diagnostic challenge. A variety of provocative tests have been used to try and identify SLAP lesions. These tests include O'Brien active compression test, biceps load II test, dynamic labral shear test, crank test, Speed test, pain provocation test, SLAP apprehension test, resisted supination-external rotation test, Jobe test, and anterior slide test. Unfortunately none of these clinical tests have a high sensitivity or specificity for diagnosing SLAP tears. In a prospective study of the biceps load test II with arthroscopic confirmation, Kim et al. (45) found that the test had close to a 90% sensitivity and 97% specificity for diagnosing type II SLAP lesions. However, Cook et al. (7) examined the diagnostic accuracy of five clinical tests, including the biceps load II test, for diagnosis of SLAP lesions and found that none of the test demonstrated any clinical utility in diagnosing SLAP lesions, which highlights the diagnostic challenge that SLAP lesions present. Proper diagnosis required correlation of clinical history, complete physical examination, imaging studies and finally, arthroscopic confirmation.

IMAGING

In the patient with a suspected labral tear, imaging studies should start with plain radiographs, which will allow one to assess for any concomitant pathology such as glenohumeral or acromioclavicular joint arthritis. MRI is the gold standard for imaging biceps–labral pathology and MR arthrogram provides added accuracy in diagnosing SLAP tears. Connell et al. (46) found that MRI had 98% sensitivity and 89.5% specificity for identifying superior labral lesions, while the literature on MR arthrography has found it to have sensitivity that ranges from 82% to 100% and specificity that ranges from 71% to 98% (47–49). SLAP tears are generally best appreciated on the coronal oblique imaging.

DIAGNOSTIC ARTHROSCOPY

Although the history, physical examination, and imaging play a large role in the diagnosis of SLAP tears, diagnostic shoulder arthroscopy remains the definitive way of diagnosing labral pathology (4,49). Some labral tears may be easily identified by visual inspection combined with gentle probing of the superior labrum and biceps complex. However, it may be necessary to perform a dynamic arthroscopic evaluation, in which the arm is placed in the cocking position of abduction and external rotation and an occult SLAP tear with labral peel back may be identified (50). It is imperative that a complete diagnostic arthroscopy is performed, including both the glenohumeral joint and subacromial space, because SLAP lesions are highly associated with other shoulder pathology.

SURGICAL TREATMENT OF SLAP LESIONS

The indications for surgery remain controversial and are dependent on a variety of patient-specific factors. If the patient remains symptomatic after 3 months of nonoperative management including nonsteroidal anti-inflammatories, intra-articular corticosteroid injections, and physical therapy, surgical intervention should be considered. Once the SLAP tear is confirmed at arthroscopy treatment options may include arthroscopic debridement, arthroscopic SLAP repair, arthroscopic or open biceps tenodesis, or biceps tenotomy (4,22,35).

The greatest controversy exists in the treatment of type II SLAP tears and there is currently limited evidence-based or level I data to guide appropriate treatment. Despite the lack of clear guidelines Zhang et al. (51) have recently shown that surgeons are performing significantly more arthroscopic SLAP repairs each year.

In the patient with an isolated type II SLAP tear the current literature has favored arthroscopic repair with suture anchors. Although there are numerous studies on the short-term outcomes of patients after arthroscopic type II SLAP repair, these studies have been mainly retrospective in nature and include patients of varying age and activity level.

Overall, the percentage of good and excellent results after type II SLAP repair have been found to be between 40% and 94% (16,52). However, the results in overhead athletes have been inferior in comparison (Table 29b-1). In a recent systematic review of type II SLAP repair in athletes, Sayde et al. (16) found that following arthroscopic SLAP repair, overhead athletes had a 63% return to play at their preinjury level compared to a 73% return to play rate for the overall study cohort (16). Gorantla et al. (52) retrospectively reviewed the outcomes of arthroscopic repair of type II SLAP lesions in a group of athletes and found that while the procedure had a high satisfaction rate (93.3%), only 84.1% were able to return to their preinjury level of function. Despite these apparently good results, throwing athletes have a lower return to preinjury activity level compared to other overhead athletes. Neuman et al. (31) found that only 79.5% of the treated baseball and softball players were able to return to preinjury activity level compared to 93.9% of the other overhead athletes. Cohen et al. (53) found that only 32% of the professional baseball players who underwent arthroscopic SLAP repair were able to return to the same level of professional baseball. While arthroscopic repair of type II SLAP lesions leads to improvements in routine daily activities, the results have been inconsistent in returning overhead throwing athletes back to their preinjury level of participation.

REASONS FOR PERSISTENT SYMPTOMS FOLLOWING SLAP REPAIR

Though a variety of techniques and instrumentation are available, arthroscopic SLAP repair focuses on the central premise of reestablishing normal anatomic fixation of the superior labrum and long head of the biceps origin to the superior surface of the glenoid. Persistent symptoms following SLAP repair can be attributed to a variety of potential etiologies. Continued postoperative pain can occur secondary to the superior labrum failing to heal to the superior glenoid due to the poor vascularity present in this region, postoperative scar tissue formation, the rigidity of the suture anchor fixation construct with a consequent loss of physiologic motion at the labral–biceps anchor junction, and restriction of excursion of the highly innervated proximal portion of the long head of the biceps tendon (Fig. 26-4). In addition, chondrolysis or chondral injury from prominent hardware or suture knots has been described and meticulous technique is required to minimize the risk of articular damage or injury (Fig. 26-5). In addition, over-constraint of the anterior capsule and ligamentous structures including the SGHL, MGHL, and the anterior band of the IGHL may contribute to limitation of postoperative ROM, specifically external rotation, which may be another complicating factor with respect to return to overhead athletic activity. Even small losses of external rotation may significantly impact the ability to generate velocity during pitching and limit an athlete's ability to return to sport. Based on the finding of persistent pain and functional disability following type II SLAP repair, biceps tenodesis has been proposed as an alternative to repair in the primary or revision management of SLAP

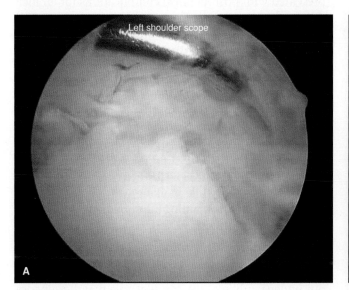

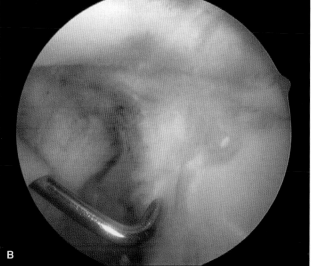

▲ **FIGURE 26-4:** Repeat arthroscopy of a 54-year-old male with persistent shoulder pain 8 months following SLAP repair. Findings include failure of healing of the superior labrum **(A)** with chondral damage of the superior glenoid and synovitis of the superior recess **(B)**.

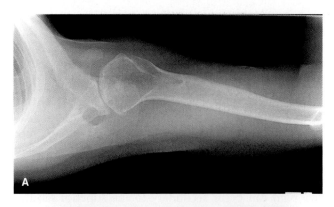

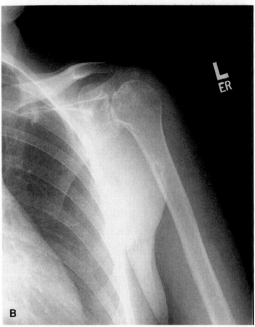

▲ **FIGURE 26-5:** Radiographs (AP and Axillary, left shoulder) of a 19-year-old male who presented with worsening pain and motion loss 18 months following labral repair. Radiographs demonstrate joint space destruction and osteophyte formation consistent with rapid chondrolysis following the repair.

lesions. Biceps tenodesis as the primary surgical treatment method alleviates a number of these potential sources of postoperative failure following SLAP repair by changing the biomechanical environment at the superior labrum–biceps origin.

BICEPS TENODESIS AS THE PROCEDURE OF CHOICE

In a recent study by Boileau et al. (30), the authors demonstrated that arthroscopic biceps tenodesis using an interference screw fixation was an effective treatment method for isolated type II SLAP lesions. After the biceps tenodesis, 93% of patients were satisfied or very satisfied and 87% of them were able to return to their preinjury level of athletic participation, compared to patients treated

with arthroscopic SLAP repair who had only a 40% satisfaction rate and a 20% return to their preinjury level of athletic participation (30). In addition, a high percentage of patients in the repair group required revision or secondary procedures compared to none in the tenodesis group. A further analysis of the data, however, reveals that the study group did not contain any overhead throwing athletes, and that the average age of each group was significantly higher than the typical age range of collegiate or professional throwers in the United States. As a result, great caution should be exercised in directly extrapolating this clinical data to the overhead throwing athlete.

Potential advantages of biceps tenodesis versus labral repair are multiple. By removing a significant pain generator from the anterior aspect of the shoulder, obviating the need for superior labral healing to the superior glenoid, and eliminating the potential for a repair construct with excess rigidity and capsulo-ligamentous overconstraint, biceps tenodesis is a very attractive treatment alternative. In addition, biceps tenodesis allows for the maintenance of the normal length–tension relation of the biceps, which helps to prevent muscle atrophy and fatigue cramping in comparison to tenotomy (22,37). It is a straightforward procedure that has demonstrated excellent outcomes with a low complication rate. In the clinical series reported by Mazzocca et al. (54), a total of 41 of 50 patients who underwent subpectoral biceps tenodesis were evaluated at a mean of 29 months postoperatively. Thirty-one patients had concomitant rotator cuff repairs with subacromial decompression. There was a statistically significant improvement from baseline to most recent follow-up for all measured clinical outcome scores. Nho et al. (55) reported the number and types of complications after open subpectoral biceps tenodesis over a 3-year period. Among 373 total patients, 8 presented with postoperative complications for an incidence of 0.7% per year. There were two patients (0.2%) with persistent bicipital pain, and two patients (0.2%) with failure of fixation with an associated popeye deformity. There was only one patient (0.1%) with each of the following complication: Wound infection, temporary musculocutaneous neuropathy, complex regional pain syndrome, and proximal humerus fracture (55). In addition, biceps tenodesis allows for a shorter and more predictable postoperative rehabilitation compared to SLAP repair. We typically use a sling for our biceps tenodesis patients for 4 weeks and avoid resisted elbow flexion activities for 8 weeks all while working with physical therapy on regaining and maintaining full shoulder ROM. Following this initial protection period, patients are advanced to throwing at 3 months and are released to unrestricted athletics at 6 months.

Two recent biomechanical studies have advanced our understanding of the complex role that the superior labrum and long head of the biceps play in the glenohumeral joint and have provided additional support for the recommendation to perform a biceps tenodesis as the procedure of choice in the management of type II SLAP lesions. Strauss et al. (56) showed that creation of either an anterior or a posterior type II SLAP lesion in a cadaver model led to significant glenohumeral translations in all directions. Following tenodesis, repair of the posterior SLAP lesions led to restoration of the glenohumeral stability; however, repair of the anterior SLAP lesion did not restore stability. Interestingly, although tenodesis of the long head of biceps did not restore the baseline glenohumeral translations seen in the normal shoulders, there was no significant difference in the glenohumeral translation seen after biceps tenodesis in shoulders with either anterior or posterior SLAP lesions (56). The findings of this study suggest no negative effect biceps tenodesis in the setting of superior labral tear. However, it does bring into question the need for repair of SLAP lesion in conjunction with LHB tenodesis in the throwing shoulder to restore normal biomechanical translation. In addition, it calls into question current techniques for repair of anterior based lesions as in this study, suture anchor repair was unable to restore anterior translation to normal.

In further support for long head of the biceps tenodesis for the treatment of SLAP lesions, Giphart et al. (57) carried out an elegant study examining the in vivo characteristics of the superior labrum and biceps anchor. This study aimed to address the discrepancy in the cadaveric studies showing that the long head of biceps stabilizes the glenohumeral joint, with the clinical findings suggesting that there are no clinically relevant changes in glenohumeral position after either tenodesis or tenotomy of the long head of the biceps. Biplane fluoroscopy and EMG of the biceps was used to determine dynamic three-dimensional glenohumeral positions in five patients who had undergone open subpectoral biceps tenodesis. The motion of the uninjured contralateral shoulder was compared in order to determine normal values for the subject. The findings indicate that in otherwise healthy shoulders, long head of biceps tenodesis does not significantly alter glenohumeral translation during dynamic motions (57). This again supports our assertion that biceps tenodesis should be considered in the treatment of patients with isolated SLAP tears, because no clinically relevant alterations in glenohumeral kinematics have been identified in the literature thus far.

SURGICAL TECHNIQUE

Our preferred treatment for patients with isolated type II SLAP lesions is to perform a mini-open subpectoral biceps tenodesis with interference screw fixation. Controversy exists about the location and method of fixation after a biceps tenodesis. The biceps tenodesis can be performed either proximally, with the tendon maintained within the bicipital groove or just below the groove in a

supra-pectoral position (58), or distally where the tendon is removed from the bicipital groove (37). We agree with the advocates for distal fixation of the biceps tendon, because removing the long head of biceps from the bicipital groove and excising the proximal portion eliminates a potential pain generator from the shoulder, while maintaining the normal length–tension relationship of the biceps. It has been found that the power of the biceps after biceps tenodesis ranged from 90% to 100% of the unaffected contralateral side (37,59,60). Biomechanics studies have shown that the interference screw technique provided the highest ultimate load to failure and the least amount of displacement after cyclic loading when compared to other fixation methods (22,37,61–63).

Our approach to addressing type II SLAP lesions involves a diagnostic arthroscopy in the beach-chair position of both the glenohumeral joint and subacromial space to confirm the diagnosis of SLAP lesion and to assess for any concomitant pathology. After confirming the presence of an isolated type II SLAP lesion we then debride the SLAP lesion and arthroscopically release the long head of the biceps tendon. Currently, there is no consensus regarding if and when the SLAP lesion requires concomitant repair in the setting of LHB tenodesis and we do not routinely repair the labrum. After the release of the long head of the biceps, the operating room table is lowered to 30 degrees from the beach-chair position. We perform a mini-open sub-pectoral biceps tenodesis with interference screw fixation and utilize the technique recently described by members of our group (37,64).

In this technique, the arm is abducted and internally rotated so that the inferior border of the pectoralis tendon becomes palpable. We then make a 3-cm long incision either along the axillary fold or the medial aspect of the arm, and this incision typically begins 1 cm superior to the inferior border of the pectoralis tendon and continues 2 cm distally (Fig. 26-6). Dissection is carried down directly over the humerus and great care is taken to avoid overzealous exposure medially in order to avoid possible injury to the neurovascular structures. After identifying the inferior border of the pectoralis major tendon, the fascia over the coracobrachialis and biceps muscles are incised from proximal to distal. Digital palpation is then used to identify the tendon of the long head of the biceps, which is located in the bicipital groove just medial to the pectoralis major insertion. The long head of the biceps tendon is then pulled out of the wound and clamped at the proximal end of tendon.

A Krakow whip-stitch using a No. 2 nonabsorbable suture is passed from 15 mm proximal to the musculotendinous junction and the remaining 20 mm of tendon proximal to the stitch is excised in order to maintain the anatomic length–tension relationship for the biceps after the tenodesis. Attention is then turned to the humerus, and a periosteal elevator and bovie is used to expose the bone approximately 1 cm proximal to the

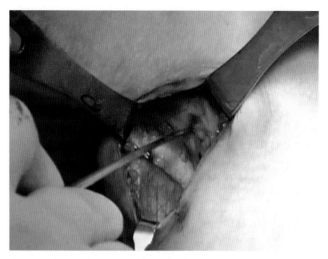

▲ **FIGURE 26-6:** Surgical exposure via sub-pectoral approach. The incision is made just distal to the axilla. The interval between the pectoralis major and short head biceps is opened to expose the long head biceps, located just medial to the pectoralis major tendon.

inferior border of the pectoralis major tendon. A guide-wire in then placed centered in the humerus and a cannulated reamer is used to prepare the humeral tunnel. Typically an 8-mm reamer is utilized though a smaller 7-mm or larger 9-mm tunnel can be considered based on patient and tendon size. An interference screw system with a self-docking driver is then used to complete the tenodesis (Arthrex, Naples, Florida). One end of the Krackow suture is passed through the tenodesis screwdriver and screw, and the other limb of the suture is left out. The screwdriver is then placed into the bone tunnel and care should be taken to ensure that the tendon is fully seated within the tunnel. The interference screw is then advanced until it is flush with the surrounding bone and the two suture limbs are tied together. Positioning of the long head biceps musculotendinous junction 1 cm proximal to the inferior border of the pectoralis major tendon will allow the surgeon to reproduce the

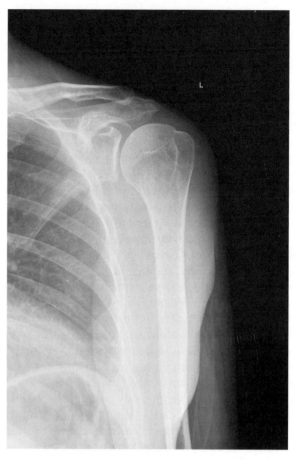

▲ **FIGURE 26-7:** Radiograph of right shoulder following sub-pectoral biceps tenodesis. The tunnel can be visualized in the proximal diaphysis demonstrating level of fixation.

normal length–tension relationship and cosmetic appearance of the muscle (Fig. 26-7). The wound is then irrigated in a standard manner and closed with No. 2-0 absorbable monofilament suture and then Dermabond (Ethicon, Somerville, NJ) is applied and we believe that this helps to reduce the risk of contamination from the axilla.

SUMMARY

While the incidence of symptomatic superior labral tears is relatively low, SLAP lesions can cause significant pain and functional limitation, especially in the overhead athlete. Controversy exists within the sports medicine and shoulder surgery literature as to the ideal management of type II SLAP lesions. While the current standard of care is arthroscopic repair, recent evidence demonstrating less than ideal outcomes following SLAP repair and unpredictable rates of return to athletic activity have led to the search for alternative treatment options. Tenodesis of the long head of the biceps tendon has evolved and presents significant potential advantages over arthroscopic repair in the management of type II injuries. As a straightforward surgical procedure with excellent outcomes, low complication rates, a simplified rehabilitation, and increasing biomechanical data to support its use, we believe that biceps tenodesis represents a preferred treatment option for most patients with improved clinical outcomes and lower rates of complications. However, further clinical study is needed to determine clinical outcomes following long head of the biceps tenodesis in the overhead athlete including ability to return to sport, and to identify which patient groups are best managed with tenodesis alone, primary SLAP repair alone, or a combination of repair plus tenodesis.

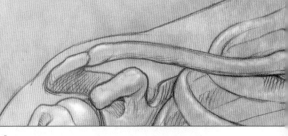

Transfer the Long Head of the Biceps

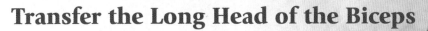

Nicole Sliva / Elizabeth Gausden / Moira M. McCarthy /
Stephen J. O'Brien

INTRODUCTION

Most people do not recognize the clinical implications of the LHBT originating within the glenohumeral joint, and its possibilities as a contributor to intra-articular pain, and its relationship to the glenoid labrum (65). Experience has taught us to view these two structures now as one functional entity, that is, the "biceps–labrum complex". Although the tendon of the long head of the biceps (LHBT) is a common source of shoulder pain, it is often under-diagnosed in the setting of multiple pathologies of the shoulder. In addition, just as there is debate over the biomechanical function of the LHBT, there remains no consensus on management of this clinical problem.

In 1985, Andrews et al. (21) first observed glenoid labrum tears in 73 throwing athletes. Based on the observation that 83% of the labral tears in his study involved the biceps–labrum "junction" intra-articularly, Andrews proposed that the traction of the biceps tendon during the throwing motion in the labrum essentially "pulled it off." One cadaveric study found that the biceps anchor experienced consequential tension and failed at the biceps anchor when in the simulated late cocking phase of throwing as opposed to the deceleration phase (66). The late cocking phase of a throw creates significant stress on the superior labrum. Another cadaveric study confirmed that in the late cocking phase of throwing the arm experiences maximum external rotation, suggesting that in this position, the orientation of the biceps anchor could play a role in the creation of a SLAP lesion (67).

Subsequently, in 1990, Snyder et al. developed the acronym S.L.A.P., for Superior Labral tear Anterior to Posterior, and proposed the classification system widely used today. In type I lesions, the tear consists of fraying at the superior labrum. In type II lesions—the most common—the tear involves fraying at the edge of the labrum and a detached biceps anchor. Type III lesions are the classic bucket-handle tear in the superior labrum. Type IV lesions contain a bucket-handle tear to the superior labrum in conjunction with a tear to the biceps tendon (68).

Based on the experience of the senior author (SJO), we have developed an algorithmic approach to the treatment of biceps–labrum complex lesions, where the decision making involves preoperative clinical evaluation, MRI evaluation, and arthroscopic evaluation.

DEMOGRAPHICS OF PATIENTS AT HIGH RISK FOR BICEPS–LABRUM COMPLEX INJURIES

Sport

Overhead throwing athletes are particularly susceptible to injury due to patterns of chronic repetitive stress overload. However, this also occurs with acute trauma in contact sports (5,16,21,23,67,69–76).

Age

Studies demonstrate that age relates to the likelihood of having a symptomatic biceps–labrum complex lesion. In a large study by Zhang et al., the authors noted an increase in evidence of SLAP repair, particularly in individuals between the ages of 20 to 29 and 40 to 49. The prevalence of SLAP repair recorded in this study increased 105% between 2004 and 2009 (51). In a comparison on professional to amateur baseball pitchers, Gowan et al. found that amateur athletes demand higher biceps activity to accelerate and decelerate the arm than their professional counterparts. The higher demand may put amateurs at a higher risk of injury (71).

DIAGNOSING BICEPS INVOLVEMENT IN BICEPS–LABRUM COMPLEX LESIONS

The "3-Pack Examination" was developed by the senior author (SJO: "3-Pack Examination" for lesions of the biceps labrum complex: A prospective validation study) which involves evaluation of the biceps–labrum complex with regard to the three areas for clinical concern, that is, the bicipital groove (1), the "junction" where the LHBT exits the shoulder (2), and intra-articular portion (3). In two separate, recently completed studies, we have found that the 3-Pack physical examination was more effective than MRI for diagnosing and treating lesions of the biceps–labrum complex. We also found that the intra-observer reliability for the 3-Pack Examination is quite high (77).

The clinical diagnostic evaluation depends upon three components of examination: The tenderness due to palpation of the bicipital groove as compared to the contralateral side (1), a positive "throwing test" in which

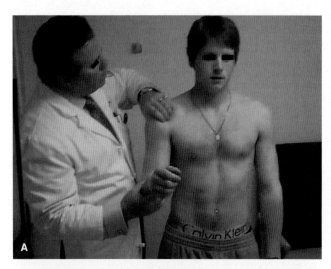

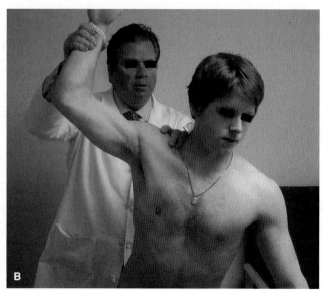

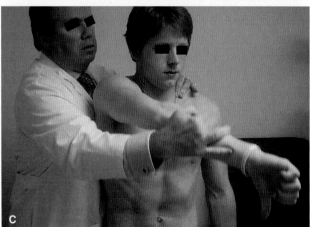

▲ **FIGURE 26-8:** The 3-Pack Examination. **(A)** Palpation of the bicipital groove: The examiner will ask if this is the patient's pain upon palpation, and compare this to the contralateral side. The result of the test is positive only if it replicates the patient's clinical pain. **(B)** The throwing test. The patient replicates the motion of throwing a ball overhead by elevating the arm with maximal external rotation. Then, the patient steps forward with the contralateral leg while the physician resists the forward motion of the throwing arm. The result of the test is positive only if it replicates the patient's clinical pain. **(C)** The active compression test. In this test the patient's arm is forward flexed to 90 degrees and adducted 10 to 15 degrees. The thumb points downward, internally rotating the shoulder. The patient then provides resistance while the physician applies downward force. The patient then repeats the test with the palm of the hand up. A positive active compression test is when the pain present in the thumb down position is relieved in the palm up position. Again, the result of the test is positive only if it replicates the patient's clinical pain. (Reprinted by permission of Steven O'Brien)

the forward motion of the patient's arm is resisted as the individual attempts a simulated overhead throw (2), and a positive active compression test (3) (Fig. 26-8). In each finding of the 3-Pack Examination, the physician compares each finding to the contralateral side and asks the key question, "Is this your pain?"

The algorithm for treatment of biceps–labrum complex lesions depends on the presence or absence of biceps symptoms in the setting of a labrum tear. There are three indications for labrum repair in the setting of painful biceps labrum complex lesions. The first indication is a labral tear with no evidence of biceps involvement, meaning no bicipital groove tenderness, a negative throwing test that rules out a junctional lesion, or a negative Arthroscopic Active compression test (with no incarceration of the LHBT) (1). The second indication is labral tears associated with instability of the inferior glenohumeral ligament complex (IGHLC) (2). Finally, a third indication is labrum tears with biceps involvement that have healthy labrum tissue to repair even after the LHBT

has been removed from the glenohumeral joint (3). The treatment for other labrum tears would be debridement.

In utilizing this algorithm in a group of 300 consecutive patients with symptomatic biceps–labrum complex lesions, 25% of the patients with labral tears underwent labral repair alone and the other 75% underwent biceps transfer with either labral repair or labral debridement (78).

EVOLUTION OF TREATMENT OF BICEPS–LABRUM COMPLEX INJURIES

Conservative Care of SLAP Tears

The literature on conservative management of SLAP tears is scant. In a study of nonoperative treatment for SLAP tears, Edwards et al. showed that 67% of the overhead athletes in his study could not return to sport at their previous level. The authors concluded that the majority of overhead athletes with SLAP tears would ultimately require surgical intervention in order to return to competitive play (15).

Review of the literature did not show any studies on the conservative treatment of SLAP tears with intra-articular corticosteroid injection. However, the senior author (SJO: Personal communication) has noted this to be an effective conservative measure in athletes that allows for at least temporary relief of pain and improvement in return to play in the short term.

CONSERVATIVE CARE OF BICEPS (GROOVE) TENDINITIS

Conservative management for biceps tendonitis commonly consists of ice, rest, anti-inflammatory injection, and corticosteroid injections (79–81). In 80 athletes treated by Jobe et al. with a rehabilitation program involving shoulder strengthening exercises and temporary activity modification, 50% of them returned to the same competitive level of play. Sport-specific subgroup analysis, however, showed that only 25% of swimmers had good results and 34% of throwers had good results. The authors postulated that activity levels for each patient determines how successful conservative management for shoulder pathology will be (73). Shoulder injections into the biceps sheath are an accepted clinical practice, and in a study done by Hashiuchi et al. (82), ultrasound-guided injections proved to be much more accurate than unguided shoulder injections.

SLAP REPAIR

Debridement

Cordasco et al. looked at debridement of unstable SLAP lesion in 27 patients of which 93% were overhead athletes. At 2-year follow-up, the authors found that 63% of these patients experienced excellent pain relief, and 45% were able to return to their preinjury level of activity (83).

Surgical Repair

According to a study done by Katz et al. (84), 32% of patients that have undergone operative treatment experience suboptimal results following an isolated SLAP repair, or a SLAP in conjunction with rotator cuff repair, Bankhart repair, excision of the distal clavicle, or sub-acromial decompression. In a study by Brockmeier et al., type II SLAP repair outcomes were studied in 47 patients with a mean follow-up time of 2.7 years. Thirty-four of these forty-seven patients were athletes. Overall, these patients exhibited significant improvements, with

increases in ASES and L'Insalata scores from 62 and 62 to 97 and 93, respectively, and 74% of athletes returned to this preinjury level. However, the authors noted that a traumatic etiology could lead to a better ability to return to sport, since 92% of athletes with a traumatic etiology returned, but only 64% of athletes with an atraumatic etiology returned. Of the athletes enrolled in the study, 74% were able to return to their preinjury level of competition (14). Most studies show an improvement in functional scores following SLAP Repair, especially in short-term follow-up.

Return to Sport

Cohen et al. (85) reported that only 14 of 29 athletes were able to return to sport and compete at their preinjury level. Further, following arthroscopic repair of 31 SLAP lesions using a trans-rotator cuff approach, only 44% of patients returned to full preinjury activity levels (86). In a 2010 study by Friel et al., they reported on the results of 48 patients that underwent type II SLAP repair after a mean follow-up of 3.4 years. Overall, patients exhibited an increase in the average ASES score from 54.49 to 83.37. However, of the 13 overhead athletes in the study, only 7 returned to their previous level of sport, and 5 of the 6 that did not return claimed the reason to be shoulder pain. Further, of the four patients that required revision surgery, two were overhead athletes (87).

ARGUMENT FOR NEED TO ADDRESS BICEPS AT SAME TIME

A recent study by Provencher et al. (88) showed that approximately 40% of the type II SLAP repairs done in an active military population needed a second procedure to address the biceps tendon to effect complete relief of their pain. After a mean follow-up for 40 months, the authors found that 66 of the 179 patients were considered clinical failures. When the authors amended 50 of the 66 shoulders using a tenodesis revision procedure, they found an improvement in average ASES scores from the mid-60s to mid-80s. Patients with labral tears presenting with biceps pain do well when the physician addresses concomitant biceps pathology. This points to the importance of the "three-pack evaluation" preoperatively to evaluate fully the biceps–labral complex (88).

Boileau recorded the differences in result between 10 patients undergoing SLAP repair and 15 patients undergoing biceps tenodesis. The constant scores both improved, with a higher satisfaction score of 89 for tenodesis and 83 for SLAP repair. Boileau concluded that arthroscopic biceps tenodesis is an effective alternative to repair (30).

BICEPS SURGERY

Tenotomy

Tenotomy of the LHBT, in which the biceps tendon is released from its origin, is a common surgical option for managing biceps tendon pathology. Tenotomy is a relatively simple procedure that demands less rehabilitation, and allows the patient to return back to activity more quickly than tenodesis. In a study performed by Gill et al. in 30 shoulders undergoing tenotomy, the complication rate was 13% after 19 months follow-up (89,90). Gill et al. (90) concluded that 90% of patients could return to their preinjury level of sport, and that 96% did not require further pain medication. Kelly et al. (91) reported on 54 patients that underwent tenotomy and found that 95% had a decrease in biceps tendon pain and 95% decrease of pain in the bicipital groove when palpated. Although these results are good, it was disheartening that a large number of patients under age 60 had fatigue discomfort and cramping, and many younger patients were frustrated with the cosmetic result (Fig. 26-9). Further, 70% of patients exhibited a Popeye sign: 82.7% men and 36.5% women. No significant loss of strength was seen in patients over 60 years of age, but it was prevalent in the younger patients. In a study done by Boileau and Chuinard, the occurrence of the Popeye sign was significantly higher in those that underwent tenotomy instead of tenodesis (61% vs. 3%) (92). Osbahr et al. (93) disclosed a 12% complication rate—indicated by anterior shoulder pain, muscle spasms, or cosmetic deformity—following tenotomy of 80 patients.

Tenodesis

Tenodesis, or reattaching the proximal LHBT stump to a more distal region of the humerus or local soft tissue, is an effective therapeutic modality. Proponents of tenodesis stress that it re-establishes muscle length as well as eliminating fatigue discomfort. It also reduces cosmetic deformity (Popeye sign) (94). Eakin et al. (70) recommended tenodesis for patients that have localized biceps pathology. In the study published by Boileau et al. in 2009, 15 patients that underwent tenodesis did not require another operation after an average 35 months of follow-up. Tenodesis has been described as a suitable procedure for active young patients (30).

While tenodesis leads to a more cosmetically favorable outcome by avoiding the Popeye sign, it is a more complex operation with longer postoperative rehabilitation than tenotomy, and has potential complications. Osbahr et al. (93) disclosed a complication rate of 33% in 80 patients undergoing tenodesis, exhibiting either muscle spasm or anterior shoulder pain following tenodesis. In a study involving 353 patients undergoing tenodesis, 7 experienced complications following surgery: Two had a resulting Popeye deformity, two had persistent bicipital pain, one had neurological complications, one developed a wound infection, and one developed reflex sympathetic nerve dystrophy (55). Another study noted a patient who developed heterotopic ossification following tenodesis, greatly limiting shoulder motion (95).

Transfer

In a biceps transfer, the long head of the biceps tendon is released from the anchor on the superior labrum and transferred into the subdeltoid space. After removing it entirely from the bicipital groove, it is then sutured to the conjoint tendon (Fig. 26-10). The procedure is done with the patient in the beach-chair position (96). Diagnostic arthroscopy allows the physician to examine the full extent of the biceps tendon and other potential pain generators in the shoulder. The procedure is performed using posterior, superolateral, anterolateral, and inferior arthroscopic portals in order to maximize visualization of the LHBT as it is tenotomized and moved to the subdeltoid space. This arthroscopic technique allows for excellent visualization and successful soft tissue healing (80).

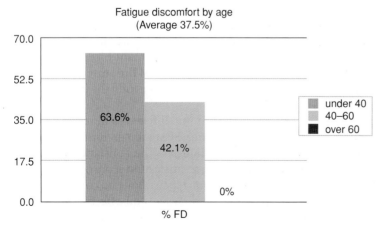

Fatigue discomfort by age
(Average 37.5%)

◀ **FIGURE 26-9:** In "Arthroscopic release of the long head of the biceps tendon: Functional outcome and clinical results" by Kelly et al., there was a clear delineation between patients less than or greater than 60 years of age. These results led the authors to conclude that age 60 is a distinguishing age for which kind of treatment a patient would receive, with patients older than 60 receiving a biceps tenotomy, and patients 60 and below receiving a biceps transfer. (Reprinted by permission of Steven O'Brien)

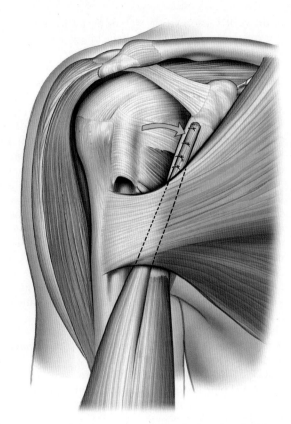

▲ **FIGURE 26-10:** Biceps transfer. The long head of the biceps is removed from the "bicipital tunnel" (groove and overlying hood), and transferred anterior to the lateral edge of conjoint tendon. (Reprinted by permission of Steven O'Brien)

Drakos et al. addresses the importance and success of biceps transfers. The authors of the study examined 40 subjects following transfer of the long head of the biceps with a minimum follow-up of 2 years. Upon weight testing, no patient exhibited a statistically significant change in biceps strength. The authors concluded that a biceps transfers is a trustworthy surgical intervention for patients who are active and suffer from chronic biceps pain (80).

The senior author (SJO) has now successfully performed approximately 500 Biceps Transfers over the last 10 years, and it has proven to be a reliable solution to solving shoulder pain stemming from the biceps tendon that limits cosmetic deformity, alleviates fatigue discomfort, obviates the need for bone tendon healing with its potential complications, and places the LHBT "co-linear" with the conjoint tendon. It also gets the LHBT out of the groove entirely, eliminating concomitant groove pathology as a source of pain. Finally, it appears to heal to the conjoint tendon with regenerative healing, rather than healing with "scar" formation to bone, which can lead to daily pain, and the very troubling complications of Reflex Sympathetic Dystrophy.

Not all patients are appropriate candidates for biceps transfer. In the study done by Kelly et al. (91), the authors suggested that tenotomy is appropriate in patients 60 years and older, as these patients did not exhibit any decrease in strength following a tenotomy procedure, and no patients over 60 years old had a concern over a cosmetic deformity. Of the 210 patients treated arthroscopically in this study, 18% underwent tenotomy of LHBT and exhibited significant improvement in mobility, activity, and pain levels when compared to the nontenotomized patients (74). Other studies have also concluded that tenotomy is the preferred procedure for elderly patients (74,90). Recognizing which kind of patient is going to benefit from tenodesis or transfer, rather than tenotomy or labral repair alone is crucial to ensuring a positive outcome.

Indications for a biceps transfer include biceps symptoms in addition to a labrum tear and/or biceps incarceration (95). Further, Drakos et al. demonstrated Biceps Transfer to be an acceptable procedure for patients that are young, active, and suffering from chronic biceps pain. In this study, 25 shoulders underwent biceps transfer, resulting in improved ASES, L'Insalata, and UCLA scores from 78.72, 75.57, and 27.32 to 84.8, 85.2, and 29.5, respectively (80).

In a 2- to 10-year follow-up study following a biceps transfer by Taylor et al., there has been no strength lost in the shoulder when tested with a 4.54-kg (10-lb) weight. Eighty-eight percent of patients rated their results following the biceps transfer as good to excellent. There was no bicipital groove tenderness in 87.5% of patients with palpation, and 94% had a negative active compression test (78). Thus, for the select group of patients that expresses biceps pathology with a SLAP tear, a biceps procedure that fits the patient's needs and the surgeon's preference and surgical skills will ensure the patient does not have ongoing problems.

CONCLUSION

The 3 Pack Examination provides a dependable, reproducible, and algorithmic approach to determine the involvement of the LHBT in generating shoulder pain in the setting of existing labral pathology and SLAP tears.

References

1. Andrews JR, Broussard TS, Carson WG. Arthroscopy of the shoulder in the management of partial tears of the rotator cuff: A preliminary report. *Arthroscopy.* 1985;1(2):117–122.
2. Snyder SJ, Karzel RP, Del Pizzo W, et al. SLAP lesions of the shoulder. *Arthroscopy.* 1990;6(4):274–279.
3. Maffet MW, Gartsman GM, Moseley B. Superior labrum-biceps tendon complex lesions of the shoulder. *Am J Sports Med.* 1995;23(1):93–98.
4. Mileski RA, Snyder SJ. Superior labral lesions in the shoulder: Pathoanatomy and surgical management. *J Am Acad Orthop Surg.* 1998;6(2):121–131.

5. Knesek M, Skendzel JG, Dines JS, et al. Diagnosis and management of superior labral anterior posterior tears in throwing athletes. *Am J Sports Med.* 2013;41(2); 440–460.

6. Kim TK, Queale WS, Cosgarea AJ, et al. Clinical features of the different types of SLAP lesions: An analysis of one hundred and thirty-nine cases. *J Bone Joint Surg Am.* 2003;85-A:66–71.

7. Cook C, Beaty S, Kissenberth MJ, et al. Diagnostic accuracy of five orthopedic clinical tests for diagnosis of superior labrum anterior posterior (SLAP) lesions. *J Shoulder Elbow Surg.* 2012;21(1):13–22.

8. Bencardino JT, Beltran J, Rosenberg ZS, et al. Superior labrum anterior-posterior lesions: Diagnosis with MR arthrography of the shoulder. *Radiology.* 2000; 214(1):267–271.

9. Michener LA, Doukas WC, Murphy KP, et al. Diagnostic accuracy of history and physical examination of the superior labrum anterior-posterior lesions. *J Athl Train.* 2011;46(4):343–348.

10. Karlsson J. Physical examination tests are not valid for diagnosing SLAP tears: A review. *Clin J Sport Med.* 2010; 20(2):134–135.

11. Nam EK, Snyder SJ. The diagnosis and treatment of superior labrum anterior and posterior (SLAP) lesions. *Am J Sports Med.* 2003;31(5):798–810.

12. Provencher MT, McCormick F, Dewing C, et al. A prospective analysis of 179 type 2 superior labrum anterior and posterior repairs: Outcomes and factors associated with success and failure. *Am J Sports Med.* 2013;41(4):880–886.

13. Youm T, ElAttrache NS, Tibone JE, et al. The effect of the long head of the biceps on glenohumeral kinematics. *J Shoulder Elbow Surg.* 2009;18(1):122–129.

14. Brockmeier SF, Voos JE, Williams RJ 3rd, et al. Outcomes after arthroscopic repair of type-II SLAP lesions. *J Bone Joint Surg Am.* 2009;91(7):1595–1603.

15. Edwards SL, Lee JA, Bell JE, et al. Nonoperative treatment of superior labrum anterior posterior tears: Improvements in pain, function, and quality of life. *Am J Sports Med.* 2010;38(7):1456–1461.

16. Sayde WM, Cohen SB, Ciccotti MG, et al. Return to play after Type II superior labral anterior-posterior lesion repairs in athletes: A systematic review. *Clin Orthop Relat Res.* 2012;470(6):1595–1600.

17. Neuman BJ, Boisvert CB, Reiter B, et al. Results of arthroscopic repair of type II superior labral anterior posterior lesions in overhead athletes: Assessment of return to preinjury playing level and satisfaction. *Am J Sports Med.* 2011;39(9):1883–1888.

18. Neri BR, ElAttrache NS, Owsley KC, et al. Outcome of Type II superior labral anterior posterior repairs in elite overhead athletes: Effect of concomitant partial thickness rotator cuff tears. *Am J Sports Med.* 2011;39(1):114–120.

19. Morgan CD, Burkhart SS, Palmeri M, et al. Type II SLAP lesions: Three subtypes and their relationships to superior shoulder instability and rotator cuff tears. *Arthroscopy.* 1998;14(6):553–565.

20. Rhee YG, Lee DH, Lim CT. Unstable isolated SLAP lesion: Clinical presentation and outcome of arthroscopic fixation. *Arthroscopy.* 2005;21(9);1099.

21. Andrews JR, Carson WG Jr, McLeod WD. Glenoid labrum tears related to the long head of the biceps. *Am J Sports Med.* 1985;13(5):337–341.

22. Barber A, Field LD, Ryu R. Biceps tendon and superior labrum injuries: Decision-marking. *J Bone Joint Surg Am.* 2007;89(8):1844–1855.

23. Snyder SJ, Banas MP, Karzel RP. An analysis of 140 injuries to the superior glenoid labrum. *J Shoulder Elbow Surg.* 1995;4(4):243–248.

24. Patzer T, Kircher J, Lichtenberg S, et al. Is there an association between SLAP lesions and biceps pulley lesions? *Arthroscopy.* 2011;27(5):611–618.

25. Ide J, Maeda S, Takagi K. Sports activity after arthroscopic superior labral repair using suture anchors in overhead-throwing athletes. *Am J Sports Med.* 2005;33(4):507–514.

26. Kim SH, Ha KI, Choi HJ. Results of arthroscopic treatment of superior labral lesions. *J Bone Joint Surg Am.* 2002;84-A(6):981–985.

27. Enad JG, Gaines RJ, White SM, et al. Arthroscopic superior labrum anterior-posterior repair in military patients. *J Shoulder Elbow Surg.* 2007;16(3):300–305.

28. Enad JG, Kurtz CA. Isolated and combined Type II SLAP repairs in a military population. *Knee Surg Sports Traumatol Arthrosc.* 2007;15(11):1382–1389.

29. Yung PS, Fong DT, Kong MF, et al. Arthroscopic repair of isolated type II superior labrum anterior-posterior lesion. *Knee Surg Sports Traumatol Arthrosc.* 2008; 16(12):1151–1157.

30. Boileau P, Parratte S, Chuinard C, et al. Arthroscopic treatment of isolated type II SLAP lesions: Biceps tenodesis as an alternative to reinsertion. *Am J Sports Med.* 2009;37(5):929–936.

31. Neuman BJ, Boisvert CB, Reiter B, et al. Results of arthroscopic repair of type II superior labral anterior posterior lesions in overhead athletes: Assessment of return to preinjury playing level and satisfaction. *Am J Sports Med.* 2011;39(9):1883–1888.

32. Cooper DE, Arnoczky SP, O'Brien SJ, et al. Anatomy, histology, and vascularity of the glenoid labrum. An anatomical study. *J Bone Joint Surg Am.* 1992;74(1):46–52.

33. Bedi A, Allen AA. Superior labral lesions anterior to posterior-evaluation and arthroscopic management. *Clin Sports Med.* 2008;27(4):607–630.

34. Vangsness CT Jr, Jorgenson SS, Watson T, et al. The origin of the long head of the biceps from the scapula and glenoid labrum. An anatomical study of 100 shoulders. *J Bone Joint Surg Br.* 1994;76(6):951–954.

35. Keener JD, Brophy RH. Superior labral tears of the shoulder: pathogenesis, evaluation, and treatment. *J Am Acad Orthop Surg.* 2009;17:627–637.

36. Rao AG, Kim TK, Chronopoulos E, et al. Anatomical variants in the anterosuperior aspect of the glenoid labrum: a statistical analysis of seventy-three cases. *J Bone Joint Surg Am.* 2003;85-A:653–659.

37. Nho SJ, Strauss EJ, Lenart BA, et al. Long head of the biceps tendinopathy: diagnosis and management. *J Am Acad Orthop Surg.* 2010;18:645–656.

38. Rodosky MW, Harner CD, Fu FH. The role of the long head of the biceps muscle and superior glenoid labrum in anterior stability of the shoulder. *Am J Sports Med.* 1994;22:121–130.

39. Elser F, Braun S, Dewing CB, et al. Anatomy, function, injuries, and treatment of the long head of the biceps brachii tendon. *Arthroscopy.* 2011;27:581–592.

40. Pagnani MJ, Deng XH, Warren RF, et al. Effect of lesions of the superior portion of the glenoid labrum on glenohumeral translation. *J Bone Joint Surg Am.* 1995;77:1003–1010.

41. Burkart A, Debski RE, Musahl V, et al. Glenohumeral translations are only partially restored after repair of a simulated type II superior labral lesion. *Am J Sports Med.* 2003;31:56–63.

42. Patzer T, Habermeyer P, Hurschler C, et al. The influence of superior labrum anterior to posterior (SLAP) repair on restoring baseline glenohumeral translation and increased biceps loading after simulated SLAP tear and the effectiveness of SLAP repair after long head of biceps tenotomy. *J Shoulder Elbow Surg.* 2012.

43. Yamaguchi K, Riew KD, Galatz LM, et al. Biceps activity during shoulder motion: an electromyographic analysis. *Clin Orthop Related Res.* 1997:122–129.

44. Glousman R, Jobe F, Tibone J, et al. Dynamic electromyographic analysis of the throwing shoulder with glenohumeral instability. *J Bone Joint Surg Am.* 1988;70:220–226.

45. Kim SH, Ha KI, Ahn JH, et al. Biceps load test II: A clinical test for SLAP lesions of the shoulder. *Arthroscopy.* 2001;17:160–164.

46. Connell DA, Potter HG, Wickiewicz TL, et al. Noncontrast magnetic resonance imaging of superior labral lesions. 102 cases confirmed at arthroscopic surgery. *Am J Sports Med.* 1999;27:208–213.

47. Modarresi S, Motamedi D, Jude CM. Superior labral anteroposterior lesions of the shoulder: part 2, mechanisms and classification. *AJR Am J Roentgenol.* 2011;197:604–611.

48. Modarresi S, Motamedi D, Jude CM. Superior labral anteroposterior lesions of the shoulder: part 1, anatomy and anatomic variants. *AJR Am J Roentgenol.* 2011;197:596–603.

49. Waldt S, Burkart A, Lange P, et al. Diagnostic performance of MR arthrography in the assessment of superior labral anteroposterior lesions of the shoulder. *AJR Am J Roentgenol.* 2004;182:1271–1278.

50. Burkhart SS, Morgan CD. The peel-back mechanism: its role in producing and extending posterior type II SLAP lesions and its effect on SLAP repair rehabilitation. *Arthroscopy.* 1998;14:637–640.

51. Zhang AL, Kreulen C, Ngo SS, et al. Demographic trends in arthroscopic SLAP repair in the United States. *Am J Sports Med.* 2012;40:1144–1147.

52. Gorantla K, Gill C, Wright RW. The outcome of type II SLAP repair: a systematic review. *Arthroscopy.* 2010;26:537–545.

53. Cohen SB, Sheridan S, Coiccotti MG. Return to Sports for Professional baseball players after surgery of the shoulder or elbow. *Sports Health.* 2011;3:105–111.

54. Mazzocca AD, Cote MP, Arciero CL, et al. Clinical outcomes after subpectoral biceps tenodesis with an interference screw. *Am J Sports Med.* 2008;36:1922–1929.

55. Nho SJ, Reiff SN, Verma NN, et al. Complications associated with subpectoral biceps tenodesis: low rates of incidence following surgery. *J Shoulder Elbow Surg.* 2010;19:764–768.

56. Strauss EJ, Salata MJ, Sershon R, et al. The Role of the Superior Labrum Following Biceps Tenodesis in Glenohumeral stability. (Unpublished data) 2012.

57. Giphart JE, Elser F, Dewing CB, et al. The long head of the biceps tendon has minimal effect on in vivo glenohumeral kinematics: a biplane fluoroscopy study. *Am J Sports Med.* 2012;40:202–212.

58. Boileau P, Krishnan SG, Coste JS, et al. Arthroscopic biceps tenodesis: a new technique using bioabsorbable interference screw fixation. *Arthroscopy.* 2002;18:1002–1012.

59. Boileau P, Neyton L. Arthroscopic tenodesis for lesions of the long head of the biceps. *Oper Orthop Traumatol.* 2005;17:601–623.

60. Elkousy HA, Fluhme DJ, O'Connor DP, et al. Arthroscopic biceps tenodesis using the percutaneous, intra-articular trans-tendon technique: preliminary results. *Orthopedics.* 2005;28:1316–1319.

61. Ozalay M, Akpinar S, Karaeminogullari O, et al. Mechanical strength of four different biceps tenodesis techniques. *Arthroscopy.* 2005;21:992–998.

62. Kusma M, Dienst M, Eckert J, et al. Tenodesis of the long head of biceps brachii: cyclic testing of five methods of fixation in a porcine model. *J Shoulder Elbow Surg.* 2008;17:967–973.

63. Mazzocca AD, Bicos J, Santangelo S, et al. The biomechanical evaluation of four fixation techniques for proximal biceps tenodesis. *Arthroscopy.* 2005;21:1296–1306.

64. Mazzocca AD, Rios CG, Romeo AA, et al. Subpectoral biceps tenodesis with interference screw fixation. *Arthroscopy.* 2005;21:896.

65. Tuoheti Y, Itio E, Minagawa H, et al. Attachment types of the long head of the biceps tendon to the glenoid labrum and their relationships with the glenohumeral ligaments. *Arthroscopy.* 2005;21(10):1242–1249.

66. Shepard MF, Dugas JR, Zeng N, et al. Differences in the ultimate strength of the biceps anchor and the generation of type II superior labral anterior posterior lesions in a cadaveric model. *Am J Sports Med.* 2004;32(5):1197–1201.

67. Pradhan RL, Itoi E, Hatakeyama Y, et al. Superior labral strain during the throwing motion. A cadaveric study. *Am J Sports Med.* 2001;29(4):488–492.

68. Snyder SJ, Karzel RP, Del Pizzo W, et al. SLAP lesions of the shoulder. *Arthroscopy.* 1990;6(4):274–279.

69. Copeland S. Throwing injuries of the shoulder. *Br J Sports Med.* 1993;27(4):221–227.

70. Eakin CL, Faber KJ, Hawkins RJ, et al. Biceps tendon disorders in athletes. *J Am Acad Orthop Surg.* 1999;7(5):300–310.

71. Gowan ID, Jobe FW, Tibone JE, et al. A comparative electromyographic analysis of the shoulder during pitching. professional versus amateur pitchers. *Am J Sports Med.* 1987;15(6):586–590.

72. Hawkins RJ, Kennedy JC. Impingement syndrome in athletes. *Am J Sports Med.* 1980;8(3):151–158.

73. Jobe F, Moynes DR. Delineation of diagnostic criteria and a rehabilitation program for rotator cuff injuries. *Am J Sports Med.* 1982;10(6):336–339.

74. Kempf JF, Gleyze P, Bonnomet F, et al. A multicenter study of 210 rotator cuff tears treated by arthroscopic acromioplasty. *Arthroscopy.* 1999;15(1):56–66.

75. Manske R, Prohaska D. Superior labrum anterior to posterior (SLAP) rehabilitation in the overhead athlete. *Phys Ther Sport.* 2010;11(4):110–121.

76. Mihata T, McGarry MH, Tibone JE, et al. Biomechanical assessment of type II superior labral anterior-posterior (SLAP) lesions associated with anterior shoulder capsular laxity as seen in throwers: A cadaveric study. *Am J Sports Med.* 2008;36(8):1604–1610.

77. O'Brien SJ, Dawson CK, Newman AM, et al. "3 pack examination" for lesions of the biceps labrum complex: A prospective validation study. (In Progress.)

78. Taylor S, Baret NJ, Newman AM, et al. Arthroscopic transfer of the long head of the biceps tendon: 2-10 year functional outcome and clinical results. (In Progress.)

79. Churgay CA. Diagnosis and treatment of biceps tendinitis and tendinosis. *Am Fam Physician.* 2009;80(5):470–476.

80. Drakos MC, Verma NN, Gulotta LV, et al. Arthroscopic transfer of the long head of the biceps tendon: Functional outcome and clinical results. *Arthroscopy.* 2008;24(2):217–223.

81. Patton WC., McCluskey GM 3rd. Biceps tendinitis and subluxation. *Clin Sports Med.* 2001;20(3):505–529.

82. Hashiuchi T, Sakurai G, Morimoto M, et al. Accuracy of the biceps tendon sheath injection: Ultrasound-guided or unguided injection? A randomized controlled trial. *J Shoulder Elbow Surg.* 2011;20(7):1069–1073.

83. Cordasco FA, Steinmann S, Flatow EL, et al. Arthroscopic treatment of glenoid labral tears. *Am J Sports Med.* 1993;21(3):425–430; discussion 430–431.

84. Katz LM, Hsu S, Miller SL, et al. Poor outcomes after SLAP repair: Descriptive analysis and prognosis. *Arthroscopy.* 2009;25(8):849–855.

85. Cohen DB, Coleman S, Drakos MC, et al. Outcomes of isolated type II SLAP lesions treated with arthroscopic fixation using a bioabsorbable tack. *Arthroscopy.* 2006;22(2):136–142.

86. O'Brien SJ, Allen AA, Coleman SH, et al. The trans-rotator cuff approach to SLAP lesions: Technical aspects for repair and a clinical follow-up of 31 patients at a minimum of 2 years. *Arthroscopy.* 2002;18(4):372–377.

87. Friel NA, Karas V, Slabaugh MA, et al. Outcomes of type II superior labrum, anterior to posterior (SLAP) repair: Prospective evaluation at a minimum two-year follow-up. *J Shoulder Elbow Surg.* 2010;19(6):859–867.

88. Provencher MT, McCormick F, Dewing CB, et al. Revision rates and outcomes of superior labrum anterior posterior 2 repairs: A prospective analysis of 225 patients. paper #208.

89. Frost A, Zafar MS, Maffulli N. Tenotomy versus tenodesis in the management of pathologic lesions of the tendon of the long head of the biceps brachii. *Am J Sports Med.* 2009;37(4):828–833.

90. Gill TJ, McIrvin E, Mair SD, et al. Results of biceps tenotomy for treatment of pathology of the long head of the biceps brachii. *J Shoulder Elbow Surg.* 2001;10(3):247–249.

91. Kelly AM, Drakos MC, Fealy S, et al. Arthroscopic release of the long head of the biceps tendon: Functional outcome and clinical results. *Am J Sports Med.* 2005;33(2):208–213.

92. Boileau P, Chuinard C. Arthroscopic biceps tenotomy: Technique and results. *Oper Tech Sports Med.* 2006;15(1):35–44.

93. Osbahr DC, Diamond AB, Speer KP. The cosmetic appearance of the biceps muscle after long-head tenotomy versus tenodesis. *Arthroscopy.* 2002;18(5):483–487.

94. Romeo AA, Mazzocca AD, Tauro JC. Arthroscopic biceps tenodesis. *Arthroscopy.* 2004;20(2):206–213.

95. Harris AI, Bush-Joseph CA, Bach BR Jr. Massive heterotopic ossification after biceps tendon rupture and tenodesis. *Clin Orthop Relat Res.* 1990;(255):284–288.

96. Verma NN, Drakos M, O'Brien SJ. Arthroscopic transfer of the long head biceps to the conjoint tendon. *Arthroscopy.* 2005;21(6):764.

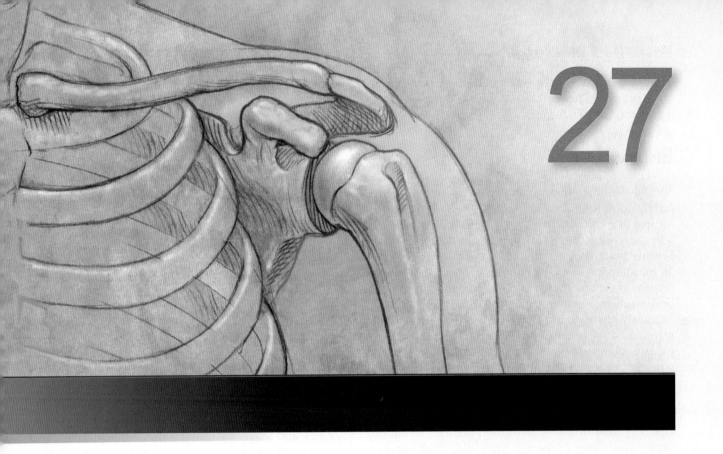

INSTABILITY OF THE SWIMMER'S SHOULDER

Samuel A. Taylor / Moira M. McCarthy /
Joshua S. Dines / David M. Dines

INTRODUCTION

Competitive swimming is an intense, year-round activity. Bak (1) reported that the average elite swimmer puts each shoulder through more than one-half million stroke revolutions during a season. Thus, it comes as no surprise that the shoulder is the most commonly injured joint in this population (1–5). Furthermore, unlike the throwing athlete where there exists an interval of rest between overhead activity, the swimmer repeats the rotational and torque stresses immediately after each stroke cycle. McMaster and Troup (6) reported the prevalence of shoulder pain was 10% and 26% in recreational and elite swimmers, respectively. Other authors have reported even higher numbers (5,7,8).

A number of factors contribute to shoulder vulnerability in this patient population—a selection bias toward those with ligamentous laxity, repetitive overhead motion, and an intense year-round workout routine. Swimmers; therefore, are at risk of developing a unique form of glenohumeral instability stemming from genetic predisposition, microtrauma, and fatigue, respectively. This instability is typically a variant of multidirectional instability (MDI) and not grossly apparent on examination. Rather, instability in the swimmer's shoulder tends to manifest itself clinically as impingement, rotator cuff tendinopathy, and scapular dyskinesia. These athletes pose a unique diagnostic and therapeutic challenge.

EPIDEMIOLOGY

Shoulder injuries among competitive swimmers are relatively commonplace (7). Wolf et al. (5) reviewed the records of 94 NCAA Division I collegiate swimmers over 5 years, to elucidate injury patterns in this population. Seventy percent of women and 73% of men sustained an injury that resulted in a physician visit. The shoulder was the most commonly affected anatomic location in both women (36%) and men (31%). Freshmen had significantly higher injury rates than did their more senior teammates, suggesting an association with the increased yardage demands posed by the transition from high school to college. The elite swimmer trains 2 to 4 hours per day (1) for 5 to 7 days (9) and tallying upward of 100 km each week (10).

In their survey of 432 competitive swimmers, Bak et al. (2) did not find a correlation between swimming stroke and injury frequency. They did; however, note that shoulder injuries occurred more frequently during the butterfly than any other stroke. Another study that looked more specifically at those patients with a chief complaint of shoulder pain, found that the majority of the 36 injured swimmers were women and more than one-third of the cohort reported bilateral shoulder pain (11). Interestingly, patients with bilateral shoulder pain had a significantly longer period of symptoms than the unilateral shoulder pain group—104 weeks compared to 33 weeks. Impingement was nearly ubiquitous. Concomitant pathologic humeral head translation with a positive apprehension sign was seen in 25 of 36 shoulders during examination (anteroinferior most common direction). In a small study of 22 competitive swimmers in Germany, 50% were found to have a positive apprehension sign (8).

EXAMINATION FINDINGS AND PATHOPHYSIOLOGY

"Swimmer's shoulder" is a term used to describe anterior shoulder pain in swimmers. Since its original description (12), it has come to represent a number of disparate pathologies including muscle fatigue, impingement (4), labral tears (13), symptomatic os acromiale (14), and instability (1). In fact, several of these pathologies are interrelated with one leading to the other. For the purpose of this chapter, we will focus on instability and its effects on the glenohumeral joint.

Instability in the swimmer is a variation of the thrower's shoulder with a background of varying degrees of MDI. Because glenohumeral stability is based upon a complex interplay of dynamic and static restraints, disruption or imbalance are rapidly magnified by repetitive use during intensive stroke training and can manifest as pain. For example, the swimmer with baseline laxity relies on other dynamic structures such as the rotator cuff for stability. With the added insult of capsuloligamentous microtrauma, extra stress is imparted on the rotator cuff. Thus, instability will not infrequently manifest as rotator tendinopathy (10).

Many swimmers have some degree of generalized joint laxity represented by a positive sulcus sign. Fifty-one percent of elite swimmers in this cohort had a 1+ sulcus sign and 14% had a 2+ sulcus sign (10). While a wide spectrum of normal glenohumeral mobility exists in the general population, swimmers that ascend to the elite levels may be subject to a biologic selection bias. The same glenohumeral laxity that may lead to superior performance may predispose the athlete to pathologic shoulder processes such as impingement, long head of the biceps tendinitis, rotator cuff tendinitis, and scapulothoracic dyskinesia—a concept that Wilk et al. (15) refers to as the "Thrower's Paradox." Zemek and Magee (16) found that elite swimmers had significantly greater glenohumeral laxity in three of five clinical tests than did recreational swimmers. Sein et al. (10) examined 80 adolescent and young adult elite swimmers with questionnaires, physical examination, and magnetic resonance imaging (MRI). Ninety-one percent of the cohort reported shoulder pain and 84% had clinically reproducible impingement signs. Seventy-one percent had grade 1 (61%) or grade 2 (10%) anterior translation and 38% had grade 1 (33%) or grade 2 (5%) posterior translation. Olivier et al. (17) found anterior–inferior capsuloligamentous laxity in 67% of swimmers.

However, not all studies agree. Jansson et al. (18) evaluated a group of 120 juvenile competitive swimmers for generalized joint laxity and glenohumeral joint laxity. They used the Beighton score and a physical examination that included the drawer test and sulcus test to more specifically assess the shoulder. Male swimmers had a higher degree of general joint laxity compared with the control population, but did not have significant examination findings of glenohumeral instability. Borsa et al. (19) used ultrasound to quantify glenohumeral joint laxity in collegiate level swimmers and an age-matched control population. No significant difference in glenohumeral translation was found among swimmers versus controls, or in swimmers with or without a history of shoulder pain.

These studies highlight an important point—glenohumeral instability in the swimmer's shoulder may present as apprehension but not as overt instability. Instability in the swimmer's shoulder results from repetitive microtrauma incurred by the anterior and inferior capsuloligamentous structures.

Like the throwing athletes, swimmers are not immune to the pathologic effects of glenohumeral internal rotation deficit (GIRD). Torres and Gomes (20) measured GIRD in asymptomatic tennis players, swimmers, and a control group. They found that tennis players had the largest dominant shoulder GIRD (23.9 degrees), followed by swimmers (12 degrees), and then the control population (4.9 degrees). Both tennis players and swimmers had significantly more GIRD than control groups, 27.6 degrees and 17.9 degrees, respectively. Along these same lines, Riemann et al. (21) reported significantly increased external rotation in the dominant upper shoulder among men and women at all levels of competition. Loss of internal rotation was more prominent in college and masters level swimmers than youth or high school swimmers. Olivier et al. (17) found greater asymmetry of external rotation to internal rotation between shoulders in swimmers (ratio 0.52) versus a control population (ratio 0.75). Though it remains controversial, some have suggested that posterior capsular tightness may contribute to anterior instability (22) and the development of Type-II SLAP lesions (23).

In the painful swimmer's shoulder, symptomatic outlet impingement is a commonly reported finding (35% to 91%) (8,11,17,24). Brushoj et al. (4) described arthroscopic findings in 18 competitive swimmers with shoulder pain who failed conservative measures. Labral pathology and subacromial impingement were identified in 61% and 28% of patients, respectively. Arthroscopic subacromial decompression and/or labral debridement resulted in only a modicum of success as only 56% of these patients returned to their preinjury level at an average of 4 months follow-up. Sein et al. (10) found that 69% of swimmers (age 13 to 25 years) had supraspinatus tendinopathy seen on MRI. This supraspinatus tendinopathy is the major cause of shoulder pain in elite swimmers based upon a significant correlation between presence of tendinopathy and training volume (hours and distance).

While it's true prevalence and pathologic implications remain a source of debate, scapular dyskinesia has been implicated in the "swimmer's shoulder" by a number of investigators. Rupp et al. (8) found scapular winging in 5 of 22 swimmers with shoulder pain and scapular protraction in 12 of 22 swimmers. A number of electromyographic studies support altered muscular activation in swimmers with painful versus asymptomatic shoulder (25–27). Madsen et al. (28) reported an 82% cumulative prevalence of scapular dyskinesia which developed during a training workout. In the asymptomatic shoulder, Crotty and Smith (29) did not find a significant difference in scapular positioning based upon DiVeta and Kibler measurements in high school swimmers pre- and post-workout, suggesting no relationship between fatigue and scapular positioning.

Treatment

The mainstay of treatment in swimmers with shoulder pain is conservative. Activity modification along with nonsteroidal anti-inflammatory drugs (NSAIDs) is the critical first intervention. The symptomatic swimmer will be shut down completely until the acute phase has subsided. A sling is not used. Range of motion exercises within midranges are encouraged. Patients should avoid extremes of motion during this initial period of rest. After 10 to 14 days of activity modification and NSAIDs, the patient is reassessed. If they are able to tolerate a pain-free full range of motion, they are progressed to a stretching and strengthening protocol. If the symptoms have not sufficiently ceased, then this initial phase of activity modification is continued for another 2 to 4 weeks.

As the majority of patients with symptomatic glenohumeral instability have a variant of MDI with underlying laxity, the goal of physical therapy should be to strengthen the dynamic stabilizers of the joint. In patients with GIRD, posterior capsular stretching is critical to symptomatic resolution. Core and periscapular strengthening is also a cornerstone of rehabilitation. Whenever possible the patient should be directed to a therapist and/or a trainer who is well versed in proper swim stroke education and stroke technique modification. This is an important, but often overlooked, component of rehabilitation. Duration of rehabilitation is variable and patient specific.

The vast majority of patients respond to the aforementioned protocol, obviating the need for surgical intervention. In the patient with persistent symptoms despite 4 to 6 months of conservative measures or the patient with two or more symptomatic recurrences, one may consider arthroscopic intervention. As swimmers commonly have related and coexisting pathologies, a thorough differential diagnosis and systematic diagnostic arthroscopy is crucial. Other pathologies, such as impingement, rotator cuff tendinopathy, biceps tendinitis, and SLAP lesions may occur concomitantly.

If a true labral tear exists, it may be fixed in the standard fashion. However, it is far more common to find capsular redundancy, which may be anterior and/or posterior. Two important points must be remembered (1): Determine the predominant direction of symptomatic laxity and (2) avoid overtightening the joint. The former is based upon preoperative examination as well as examination under anesthesia. To address the latter, we feel strongly that labral repair or capsular plication should be performed with the shoulder in the 90–90 position; which is 90 degrees abduction and 90 degrees of external rotation. The demands upon the glenohumeral joint for swimmers are very similar to those of the throwing athlete. Overtightening the shoulder is the primary reason for failure in this patient population.

Jones et al. (30) reported on 20 consecutive overhead athletes with recalcitrant symptomatic glenohumeral instability treated with anterior capsular plication. The cohort was of mixed sports (baseball, softball, volleyball, tennis, water polo, and freestyle swimming). At an average follow-up of 3.6 years, 18 of 20 patients had returned to their overhead sport. Seventeen of these 18 patients reported return to preinjury level function. The authors note that the two patients, who were unable to return to overhead sport, had concomitantly repaired rotator cuff tears.

In a more sport-specific outcome series, Montgomery et al. (31) retrospectively reviewed 15 swimmers who underwent arthroscopic capsular plication for symptomatic instability. At an average of 29 months follow-up, 80% of patients had returned to their preinjury level of competition. All reported subjective pain relief and the ASES and L'Insalata scores were 78 and 82, respectively. In this series, 20% of patients did not return to their preinjury performance.

Finally, it is important to recognize the anatomy such as the Buford Complex or sublabral foramen as normal variants and not pathologic entities. Surgical intervention directed at these normally occurring variants will result in excessive tightening and surgical failure. Occasionally; however, unusual pathologies may be encountered. In a small, unreported series by the senior author (David M. Dines) of three elite swimmers with symptomatic instability who were recalcitrant to conservative measures, tear of the anterior capsule was identified emanating from a normally occurring sublabral foramen (Fig. 27-1A,B). The capsular tear was repaired (Fig. 27-1C) and the sublabral foramen left in its naturally occurring state. All three patients returned to sport at a preinjury level.

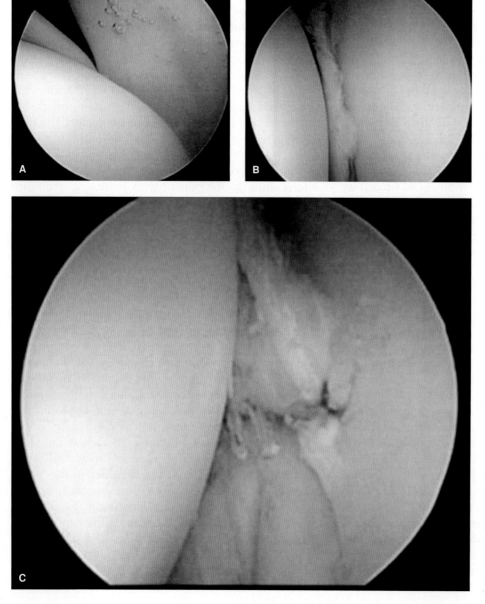

◀ **FIGURE 27-1:** A sublabral foramen is seen at arthroscopy **(A)**. Inferiorly, a tear of the anterior inferior labrum emanating from the apex of the normal sublabral foramen is identified **(B)**. Only the pathologic portion of the labrum is repaired with suture anchors without closure of the normal sublabral foramen **(C)**. Closure of a sublabral foramen can have devastating consequences to shoulder motion in the competitive swimmer.

SUMMARY

The swimmer's shoulder represents a complex diagnostic and therapeutic dilemma. Many different pathologies can coexist with instability including impingement, scapular dyskinesia, biceps tendinitis, GIRD, and rotator cuff pathology. Swimmers, particularly those that compete at the elite levels frequently have some degree of underlying ligamentous laxity. As a result, when instability is present there is typically some component of MDI. As a result of the laxity, swimmers can require significant compensatory use of the dynamic stabilizers of the shoulder including the rotator cuff that can become symptomatic in the setting of training overuse. The mainstay intervention is activity modification, strengthening of the dynamic glenohumeral stabilizers, and improvement of swim stroke mechanics. When extensive efforts at conservative management have failed, represented by persistent symptoms or repeated recurrence, one may consider arthroscopy. If labral repair or capsular plication is indicated, it should be performed in the 90-90 position to avoid overtightening.

References

1. Bak K. Nontraumatic glenohumeral instability and coracoacromial impingement in swimmers. *Scand J Med Sci Sports.* 1996;6(3):132–144.

2. Bak K, Bue P, Olsson G. Injury patterns in Danish competitive swimming. *Ugeskr Laeger.* 1989;151(45): 2982–2984.

3. Bak K. The practical management of swimmer's painful shoulder: Etiology, diagnosis, and treatment. *Clin J Sport Med.* 2010;20(5):386–390.

4. Brushoj C, Bak K, Johannsen HV, et al. Swimmers' painful shoulder arthroscopic findings and return rate to sports. *Scand J Med Sci Sports.* 2007;17(4):373–377.

5. Wolf BR, Ebinger AE, Lawler MP, et al. Injury patterns in division I collegiate swimming. *Am J Sports Med.* 2009; 37(10):2037–2042.

6. McMaster WC, Troup J. A survey of interfering shoulder pain in United States competitive swimmers. *Am J Sports Med.* 1993;21(1):67–70.

7. Richardson AB, Jobe FW, Collins HR. The shoulder in competitive swimming. *Am J Sports Med.* 1980;8(3): 159–163.

8. Rupp S, Berninger K, Hopf T. Shoulder problems in high level swimmers–impingement, anterior instability, muscular imbalance? *Int J Sports Med.* 1995;16(8): 557–562.

9. Tate A, Turner GN, Knab SE, et al. Risk factors associated with shoulder pain and disability across the lifespan of competitive swimmers. *J Athl Train.* 2012;47(2): 149–158.

10. Sein ML, Walton J, Linklater J, et al. Shoulder pain in elite swimmers: Primarily due to swim-volume-induced supraspinatus tendinopathy. *Br J Sports Med.* 2010;44(2):105–113.

11. Bak K, Fauno P. Clinical findings in competitive swimmers with shoulder pain. *Am J Sports Med.* 1997;25(2): 254–260.

12. Kennedy JC, Hawkins R, Krissoff WB. Orthopaedic manifestations of swimming. *Am J Sports Med.* 1978; 6(6):309–322.

13. McMaster WC. Anterior glenoid labrum damage: A painful lesion in swimmers. *Am J Sports Med.* 1986; 14(5):383–387.

14. Bedi A, Rodeo SA. Os acromiale as a cause for shoulder pain in a competitive swimmer: A case report. *Sports Health.* 2009;1(2):121–124.

15. Wilk KE, Meister K, Andrews JR. Current concepts in the rehabilitation of the overhead throwing athlete. *Am J Sports Med.* 2002;30(1):136–151.

16. Zemek MJ, Magee DJ. Comparison of glenohumeral joint laxity in elite and recreational swimmers. *Clin J Sport Med.* 1996;6(1):40–47.

17. Olivier N, Quintin G, Rogez J. The high level swimmer articular shoulder complex. *Ann Readapt Med Phys.* 2008; 51(5):342–347.

18. Jansson A, Saartok T, Werner S, et al. Evaluation of general joint laxity, shoulder laxity and mobility in competitive swimmers during growth and in normal controls. *Scand J Med Sci Sports.* 2005;15(3):169–176.

19. Borsa PA, Scibek JS, Jacobson JA, et al. Sonographic stress measurement of glenohumeral joint laxity in collegiate swimmers and age-matched controls. *Am J Sports Med.* 2005;33(7):1077–1084.

20. Torres RR, Gomes JL. Measurement of glenohumeral internal rotation in asymptomatic tennis players and swimmers. *Am J Sports Med.* 2009;37(5): 1017–1023.

21. Riemann BL, Witt J, Davies GJ. Glenohumeral joint rotation range of motion in competitive swimmers. *J Sports Sci.* 2011;29(11):1191–1199.

22. Burkhart SS, Morgan CD, Kibler WB. The disabled throwing shoulder: Spectrum of pathology part I: Pathoanatomy and biomechanics. *Arthroscopy.* 2003; 19(4):404–420.

23. Grossman MG, Tibone JE, McGarry MH, et al. A cadaveric model of the throwing shoulder: A possible etiology of superior labrum anterior-to-posterior lesions. *J Bone Joint Surg Am.* 2005;87(4):824–831.

24. Bak K, Magnusson SP. Shoulder strength and range of motion in symptomatic and pain-free elite swimmers. *Am J Sports Med.* 1997;25(4):454–459.

25. Scovazzo ML, Browne A, Pink M, et al. The painful shoulder during freestyle swimming. An electromyographic cinematographic analysis of twelve muscles. *Am J Sports Med.* 1991;19(6):577–582.

26. Pink M, Jobe FW, Perry J, et al. The painful shoulder during the butterfly stroke. An electromyographic and

cinematographic analysis of twelve muscles. *Clin Orthop Relat Res.* 1993;(288):60–72.

27. Pink M, Perry J, Browne A, et al. The normal shoulder during freestyle swimming. An electromyographic and cinematographic analysis of twelve muscles. *Am J Sports Med.* 1991;19(6):569–576.

28. Madsen PH, Bak K, Jensen S, et al. Training induces scapular dyskinesis in pain-free competitive swimmers: A reliability and observational study. *Clin J Sport Med.* 2011;21(2):109–113.

29. Crotty NM, Smith J. Alterations in scapular position with fatigue: A study in swimmers. *Clin J Sport Med.* 2000; 10(4):251–258.

30. Jones KJ, Kahlenberg CA, Dodson CC, et al. Arthroscopic capsular plication for microtraumatic anterior shoulder instability in overhead athletes. *Am J Sports Med.* 2012; 40(9):2009–2014.

31. Montgomery SR, Chen NC, Rodeo SA. Arthroscopic capsular plication in the treatment of shoulder pain in competitive swimmers. *HSS J.* 2010;6(2):145–149.

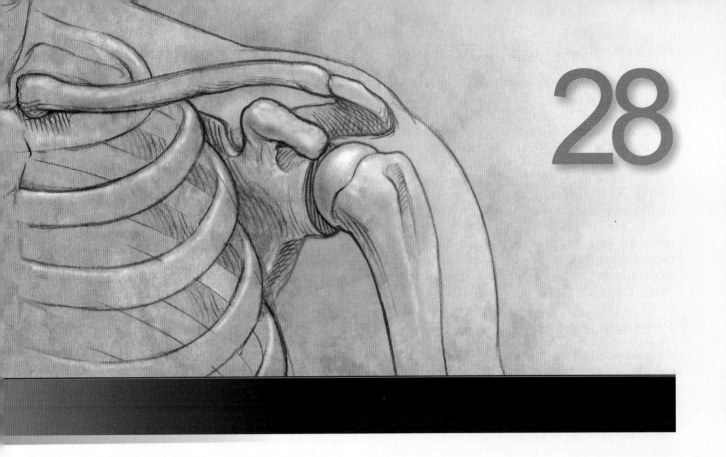

In-season Instability in Contact Athletes

Eddie Y. Lo / Sumant G. Krishnan

Introduction

Glenohumeral instability is a common shoulder injury in athletes, especially those involved in competitive contact sports. While these events more commonly are traumatic and anterior when a full dislocation occurs, subtle subluxations may involve either anterior and/or posterior symptoms. The National Collegiate Athletic Association (NCAA) Injury Surveillance System estimates a rate of glenohumeral instability events of 0.12 per 1,000 exposures (1). The highest rates were associated with contact sports such as football, ice hockey, and wrestling. In these contact sports, the athletes are also at greater risk for recurrent instability episodes simply due to the nature of their sport. Consequently, the management of contact athletes who suffer shoulder instability episodes during the season of play becomes challenging. The principles applied to the management of these contact athletes with regard to "in-season" instability can be applied to all athletes, both noncontact and/or recreational.

History

The appropriate management of a contact athlete with a shoulder instability problem begins with a thorough history (2–10). Although athletes may recall a traumatic injury with the shoulder "coming out of joint," the true presentation of the unstable shoulder can be quite variable. An athlete with complete glenohumeral joint dislocation, defined as dissociation of the articular surfaces, can present with visible deformity of shoulder contour and the sensation of numbness and tingling down the arm. However, other athletes present with chief complaints of "pain," "popping," "shifting," or simply that the "shoulder feels like it pops out." These may or may not be secondary to true glenohumeral instability, so it is important to reconstruct any injury event that may have occurred. Athletes can be extremely accurate in diagnosing their own direction of instability simply through proper questioning.

Reconstructing the Story

The mechanism of injury in the athlete's shoulder is critical to both understanding the pathology present and guiding clinical management (11). Detailed questioning regarding the exact events that preceded the shoulder problem draw a road map leading to the appropriate diagnosis. There are *10 key factors* that must be obtained in the evaluation of the in-season unstable shoulder in order to individualize management:

1. Age
2. Sport played
3. Position played at time of injury
4. Level of participation (recreational, elite nonprofessional, professional, etc.)
5. Arm dominance
6. Arm position at exact moment of injury (if known)
7. Mechanism of trauma (contact, fall, etc.)
8. Degree of trauma (required sideline or hospital reduction, continued playing, etc.)
9. Number of subsequent similar episodes
10. Time of injury relative to "season" of play (beginning, middle, end of season, etc.)

The typical "story" for an athlete with anterior instability is a single traumatic episode with the shoulder relatively abducted and externally rotated at time of contact with the involved arm (i.e., the middle linebacker in American football attempting to tackle a runner going beside him). Conversely, the story for an athlete with posterior instability often involves contact to the injured arm with the shoulder relatively flexed and internally rotated (i.e., the offensive lineman in American football attempting to block an oncoming defender). By recreating the exact events that occurred, accurate diagnosis will follow. This is an important point since often these athletes present with the simple statement that "my shoulder hurts"—rather than a true instability episode.

PHYSICAL EXAMINATION

"Laxity is a sign…instability is a symptom"

The examination of the unstable shoulder has been discussed elsewhere in detail, but a few points require emphasis. Because of the variability of the subjective complaint, physical examination is critically important to confirm the difference between objective shoulder laxity and symptomatic instability. Laxity is a physiologic joint motion that is natural to the patient. Instability is a symptomatic translation of the shoulder joint that reproduces what the patient experiences. Completion of shoulder examination must include signs of generalized ligamentous laxity as described by Wynne-Davies criteria (12). Active motion, passive motion, and strength examinations are helpful in assessing the overall function of the shoulder.

The load and shift test applies anterior and posterior translational forces, while comparison of the inferior sulcus to the contralateral side in neutral and external rotations offers insight into inferior symptoms. Specific provocative tests such as the apprehension, relocation, and "surprise" tests can be helpful in confirming the degree of instability (13–17).

Nearly every athlete with symptomatic instability will present with scapular dyskinesis. This is important to both assess and document, as the degree of scapular dyskinesis can augment the degree of symptomatic instability experienced. Evaluation of range of glenohumeral motion with and without the scapula stabilized ("scapular stabilization maneuver") can provide important additional information regarding the degree of symptoms relative to the shoulder joint itself.

RADIOGRAPHIC EVALUATION

The appropriate radiographic evaluation of the unstable shoulder has been discussed elsewhere, but it should be noted that the evaluating physician must have orthogonal radiographs prior to any advanced imaging (18,19). The missed diagnosis of a locked dislocation (especially in a physically large athlete) can be avoided by attention to this detail. A complete series of plain radiography including true anteroposterior, scapular Y, and axillary lateral views are necessary to document dislocation or concentric reduction of the shoulder.

In the senior author's treatment algorithm, complete radiographic series should be the first-line evaluation for patients with instability. Any sideline or emergency room x-ray films confirming the direction of instability can be helpful. Additional advanced imaging consisting of either computed tomographic or magnetic resonance imaging will be performed to evaluate (1) soft tissue injury and (2) bone injury to the glenoid and/or humeral head.

OTHER FACTORS

One unique factor in the management of the athlete with in-season instability is their social context. In addition to managing the patient's expectations, the treating physician must also interact with family, trainers, coaches, and (if professional) agents who all can be intimately in the care of the respective athlete. Although the final treatment plan must be based on discussion and informed consent from the athlete (or parents if the athlete is a minor), the final management decision is often not reached until all of the aforementioned parties have been consulted by the athlete or (if consent has been granted by the athlete) by the treating physician.

Management of those expectations must involve honest and frank discussion regarding the (1) injury diagnosis, (2) treatment plan, (3) expected time to return to play, and (4) final success of the treatment recommended. In many cases, the expectations of the athlete and his/her social network may not be the same as the expectations of the physician with regard to expected outcome. Managing those expectations can be as critical to the athlete's success as an operative or nonoperative in-season technique.

OPTIONS FOR THE IN-SEASON UNSTABLE SHOULDER

The treatment of the in-season athlete involves only two options: Immediate nonoperative management or immediate operative management. When deciding on what is appropriate for the athlete in question, the physician must balance the risk of recurrent instability (if play is allowed to continue) versus the attendant risks of operative management (including the possibility of failure to return to previous level of play). There are no surgical techniques that provide perfect success with no recurrent instability as well as perfect return to previous level of play. Similarly, there are no nonoperative measures that perfectly prevent recurrence of instability. To further confound the decision, there are no guarantees that either operative or nonoperative management will prevent other noninstability related shoulder disorders, such as dislocation arthropathy or rotator cuff tears. Hence, there is no "right answer" for every in-season athlete.

Physicians and athletes must discuss all options before determining the option that provides the least harm to the longevity of the involved shoulder as well as allows the best chance (if desired) to return to play. Additional instability episodes can further damage

articular surfaces, destabilize the joint, and lower the rate of future successful treatment (20,21). Biomechanical studies suggest that cyclic loading at subfailure levels can stretch the inferior glenohumeral ligament and predispose to chronic instability (22). In the series by Taylor and Arciero (20), all patients with acute traumatic injuries were found to have Bankart lesions without capsular disruption. In contrast, Larrain et al. (23) evaluated patients with recurrent instabilities and found chronic cases to be associated with 95.5% capsuloligamentous elongation and higher rate of bony deficiencies (36% vs. 17.5%). In this series, recurrent instability after surgical repair is also higher in the chronic group (8.3% vs. 5.1%). In Yiannakopoulos' series, chronic instability patients also associated with higher rate of anterior labrolgamentous periosteal sleeve avulsion (ALPSA) lesions, concomitant Hill-Sachs injuries, and capsular laxity (24).

Delaying surgical treatment also carries a potential risk for future arthritis. Buscayret et al. (25) evaluated chronic instability episodes and found that eventual risk of arthritis to be associated with not only the number of instability episodes, but also age of onset, delay of surgery, having associated bony defects, and duration of follow-up. Franceschi et al. (26) identified a separate cohort of recurrent dislocators and found overall recurrence rate of 16.6%, which is higher than treatment of acute dislocators. Ten percent of the patients without preoperative arthritis were found to have degenerative changes at 2 years. Having increased number of dislocations, lower average age, increased length of follow-up, delay of surgery, increased anchor use, and having degenerative labrum predisposed the patients to more degenerative changes.

Rehabilitation

Nonoperative treatment can include immobilization, behavioral changes, and physical therapy. Immobilization therapy can be utilized as the definitive treatment or a temporizing measure. Itoi et al. (27) first proposed using an external rotation brace as the definitive treatment for anterior instability. The principle is to coapt the labrum back to the anteroinferior glenoid. In his cohort, there was a significant reduction in redislocation rate (20% vs. 38%). However, other authors were not able to reproduce these results (28,29). In Itoi's cohort, the patients' age was as high as 90 years old and may be of a different cultural background. This cohort may have a different natural history of instability as compared to young, active athletes.

Alternatively, athletes may be treated with an athletic brace as a temporizing measure until the off-season. As previously discussed, timing of the treatment is as important as the demand of the athlete. Factors including senior season, level of competition (high school, college, professional), contract year, and number of games in season all play a factor in determining the ultimate treatment. In addition, position of the player and the associated demand on his shoulder also influences the success of bracing therapy.

There has been only one study evaluating the adequacy of the athletic brace. Buss et al. (30) treated 30 athletes with acute or recurrent anterior shoulder instability. After the instability episode, immediate physical therapy was performed with range of motion and strengthening exercises. When the athletes had full motion and symmetric strength, they resumed their athletic activities. For contact athletes, a brace was given to statically restrict the abduction and extension motions. In this cohort, only 3 of 30 patients (10%) were unable to return to play. However, when specially questioned, the brace was not able to hold the glenohumeral joint adequately reduced. There were on average 1.4 recurrent episodes in 11 (41%) of the athletes. Four (13.3%) underwent surgery during the season, but 12 (40%) were able to at least delay surgery until the end of the season.

Based on the sparse evidence-based recommendations, best practice for the nonoperative management of the in-season athlete should begin with minimal immobilization until pain resolves (1 to 2 days). Gentle physical therapy exercises involving scapular isometrics and range of motion to tolerance begins during the first week following injury. Aquatic therapy is extremely beneficial at this stage. Early neuromuscular stimulation of the posterior rotator cuff (infraspinatus) and deltoid can aid muscle recovery. Once full range of motion is obtained (whenever that may be), strengthening is progressed from closed chain exercises to open chain strengthening. Return to play is allowed when the shoulder demonstrates objective (goniometric) full range of motion and resisted strength of the cuff musculature symmetric to the contralateral uninjured side. There should also be no symptoms of apprehension in any provocative (anterior or posterior) testing position based on the original instability diagnosis.

"The First Shot is the Best Shot"

When deciding on operative management for the unstable shoulder, success rates are comparable between arthroscopic and open surgical techniques. These have been discussed elsewhere, but a few studies bear repeating. Arciero et al. (2) treated 21 cadets with arthroscopic Bankart repair with 14% recurrence. Bottoni et al. (3) treated 10 military soldiers with arthroscopic tacks and had 11% recurrence rate. Kirkley et al. (4) treated 16 patients with transglenoid suturing and had 19% recurrence rate. Jakobsen et al. (6) treated 37 patients with open anchor repair and had 8% failure rate at 10 years. Robinson et al. (7) treated 84 patients with arthroscopic Bankart repair and had 7% recurrence at 2 years.

Balg and Boileau (18) evaluated 131 consecutive patients with traumatic recurrent anterior instability and identified six risk factors associated with potential failure of arthroscopic Bankart repair. Risk factors included age younger than 20, involvement in competitive sports, shoulder hyperlaxity, presence of Hill-Sachs lesions, and loss of inferior glenoid contour (31,32).

Regardless of operative technique used, the physician and athlete must be aware of the lesions being managed (soft tissue and/or bone) and the postoperative rehabilitation associated with that particular technique. Return to play has not been shown to be expectantly different with either arthroscopic or open surgical techniques, as most contact athletes will not attempt full return to contact sport for a minimum of 6 months after surgery (33).

IN-SEASON MANAGEMENT OF THE UNSTABLE SHOULDER IN CONTACT ATHLETES

The senior author has proposed a practical and stepwise algorithm for managing instability episodes in athletes during season of play (33) (Fig. 28.1). The algorithm is based on a set of three binary questions, once appropriate history (*10 key factors*), physical examination (*laxity vs. instability*), and imaging (*CT arthrography with three-dimensional reconstructions*) have been reviewed:

1. Soft-tissue lesion versus significant bone lesion?
2. First instability episode versus secondary (recurrent) episode?
3. Level of play: Recreational/collegiate versus elite collegiate/professional?

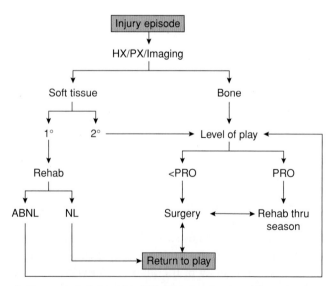

▲ **FIGURE 28-1:** Algorithm for managing instability episodes in athletes during season of play.

Discussion at each step of this algorithm involves the physician, the athlete, and any social circumstances that may affect the final decision (high school senior season, collegiate final playoff or bowl game, contract year for professional athlete, etc.). For those athletes who refuse recommended surgical treatment if the physician recommends such, nonoperative rehabilitation can be pursued—but the risks of recurrence and further glenohumeral damage must be highlighted.

References

1. Owens BD, Agel J, Mountcastle SB, et al. Incidence of glenohumeral instability in collegiate athletics. *Am J Sports Med.* 2009;37(9):1750–1754.
2. Arciero RA, Wheeler JH, Ryan JB, et al. Arthroscopic Bankart repair versus nonoperative treatment for acute, initial anterior shoulder dislocations. *Am J Sports Med.* 1994;22(5):589–594.
3. Bottoni CR, Wilckens JH, DeBerardino TM, et al. A prospective, randomized evaluation of arthroscopic stabilization versus nonoperative treatment in patients with acute, traumatic, first-time shoulder dislocations. *Am J Sports Med.* 2002;30(4):576–580.
4. Kirkley A, Werstine R, Ratjek A, et al. Prospective randomized clinical trial comparing the effectiveness of immediate arthroscopic stabilization versus immobilization and rehabilitation in first traumatic anterior dislocations of the shoulder: Long-term evaluation. *Arthroscopy.* 2005;21(1):55–63.
5. Boileau P, Villalba M, Héry JY, et al. Risk factors for recurrence of shoulder instability after arthroscopic Bankart repair. *J Bone Joint Surg Am.* 2006;88(8):1755–1763.
6. Jakobsen BW, Johannsen HV, Suder P, et al. Primary repair versus conservative treatment of first-time traumatic anterior dislocation of the shoulder: A randomized study with 10-year follow-up. *Arthroscopy.* 2007;23(2):118–123.
7. Robinson CM, Jenkins PJ, White TO, et al. Primary arthroscopic stabilization for a first-time anterior dislocation of the shoulder. A randomized, double-blind trial. *J Bone Joint Surg Am.* 2008;90(4):708–721.
8. Owens BD, DeBerardino TM, Nelson BJ, et al. Long-term follow-up of acute arthroscopic Bankart repair for initial anterior shoulder dislocations in young athletes. *Am J Sports Med.* 2009;37(4):669–673.
9. Hovelius L, Olofsson A, Sandström B, et al. Nonoperative treatment of primary anterior shoulder dislocation in patients forty years of age and younger. A prospective twenty-five-year follow-up. *J Bone Joint Surg Am.* 2008;90(5):945–952.
10. Robinson CM, Howes J, Murdoch H, et al. Functional outcome and risk of recurrent instability after primary traumatic anterior shoulder dislocation in young patients. *J Bone Joint Surg Am.* 2006;88(11):2326–2336.
11. Milano G, Grasso A, Russo A, et al. Analysis of risk factors for glenoid bone defect in anterior shoulder instability. *Am J Sports Med.* 2011;39(9):1870–1876.
12. Wynne-Davies R. Acetabular dysplasia and familial joint laxity: Two etiological factors in congenital dislocation of the hip. A review of 589 patients and their families. *J Bone Joint Surg Br.* 1970;52(4):704–716.
13. Neer CS 2nd, Foster CR. Inferior capsular shift for involuntary inferior and multidirectional instability of the shoulder. A preliminary report. *J Bone Joint Surg Am.* 1980;62(6):897–908.
14. Hawkins RJ, Schutte JP, Janda DH, et al. Translation of the glenohumeral joint with the patient under anesthesia. *J Shoulder Elbow Surg.* 1996;5(4):286–292.
15. Jobe FW, Kvitne RS, Giangarra CE. Shoulder pain in the overhand or throwing athlete. The relationship of anterior instability and rotator cuff impingement. *Orthop Rev.* 1989;18(9):963–975.
16. Lo IK, Nonweiler B, Woolfrey M, et al. An evaluation of the apprehension, relocation, and surprise tests for anterior shoulder instability. *Am J Sports Med.* 2004;32(2):301–307.
17. Krishnan SG, HR, Bokor DJ. Clinical evaluation of shoulder problems. In: Rockwood CA, ed. *The Shoulder.* Philadelphia, PA: WB Saunders; 2004.
18. Balg F, Boileau P. The instability severity index score. A simple pre-operative score to select patients for arthroscopic or open shoulder stabilisation. *J Bone Joint Surg Br.* 2007;89(11):1470–1477.
19. Itoi E, Lee SB, Amrami KK, et al. Quantitative assessment of classic anteroinferior bony Bankart lesions by radiography and computed tomography. *Am J Sports Med.* 2003;31(1):112–118.
20. Taylor DC, Arciero RA. Pathologic changes associated with shoulder dislocations. Arthroscopic and physical examination findings in first-time, traumatic anterior dislocations. *Am J Sports Med.* 1997;25(3):306–311.
21. Chuang TY, Adams CR, Burkhart SS. Use of preoperative three-dimensional computed tomography to quantify glenoid bone loss in shoulder instability. *Arthroscopy.* 2008;24(4):376–382.
22. Pollock RG, Wang VM, Bucchieri JS, et al. Effects of repetitive subfailure strains on the mechanical behavior of the inferior glenohumeral ligament. *J Shoulder Elbow Surg.* 2000;9(5):427–435.
23. Larrain MV, Montenegro HJ, Mauas DM, et al. Arthroscopic management of traumatic anterior shoulder instability in collision athletes: Analysis of 204 cases with a 4- to 9-year follow-up and results with the suture anchor technique. *Arthroscopy.* 2006;22(12):1283–1289.
24. Yiannakopoulos CK, Mataragas E, Antonogiannakis E. A comparison of the spectrum of intra-articular lesions in acute and chronic anterior shoulder instability. *Arthroscopy.* 2007;23(9):985–990.
25. Buscayret F, Edwards TB, Szabo I, et al. Glenohumeral arthrosis in anterior instability before and after surgical treatment: Incidence and contributing factors. *Am J Sports Med.* 2004;32(5):1165–1172.
26. Franceschi F, Papalia R, Del Buono A, et al. Glenohumeral osteoarthritis after arthroscopic Bankart repair for anterior instability. *Am J Sports Med.* 2011;39(8):1653–1659.
27. Itoi E, Hatakeyama Y, Sato T, et al. Immobilization in external rotation after shoulder dislocation reduces the

risk of recurrence. A randomized controlled trial. *J Bone Joint Surg Am.* 2007;89(10):2124–2131.

28. Finestone A, Milgrom C, Radeva-Petrova DR, et al. Bracing in external rotation for traumatic anterior dislocation of the shoulder. *J Bone Joint Surg Br.* 2009;91(7):918–921.

29. Liavaag S, Brox JI, Pripp AH, et al. Immobilization in external rotation after primary shoulder dislocation did not reduce the risk of recurrence: A randomized controlled trial. *J Bone Joint Surg Am.* 2011;93(10):897–904.

30. Buss DD, Lynch GP, Meyer CP, et al. Nonoperative management for in-season athletes with anterior shoulder instability. *Am J Sports Med.* 2004;32(6):1430–1433.

31. Sekiya JK, Jolly J, Debski RE. The effect of a Hill-Sachs defect on glenohumeral translations, in situ capsular forces, and bony contact forces. *Am J Sports Med.* 2012;40(2):388–394.

32. Burkhart SS, De Beer JF. Traumatic glenohumeral bone defects and their relationship to failure of arthroscopic Bankart repairs: Significance of the inverted-pear glenoid and the humeral engaging Hill-Sachs lesion. *Arthroscopy.* 2000;16(7):677–694.

33. Abboud JA, Armstrong AA. Management of anterior shoulder instability: Ask the experts. *J Shoulder Elbow Surg.* 2011;20:173–182.

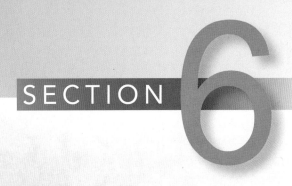

INSTABILITY AFTER ARTHROPLASTY

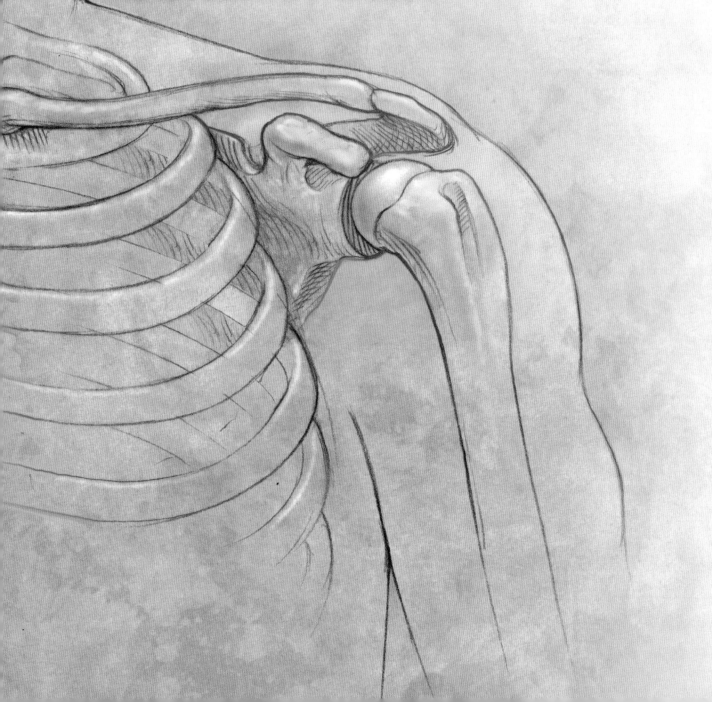

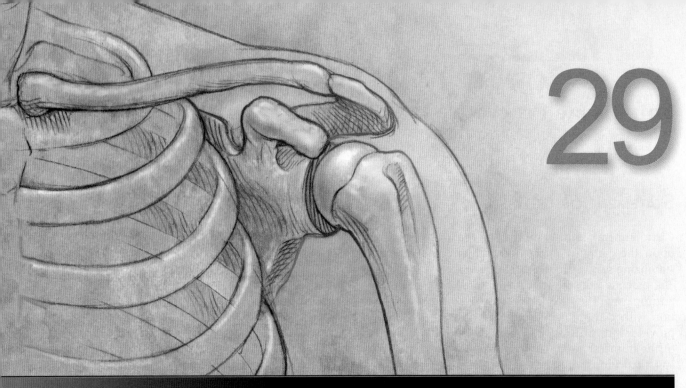

ANTERIOR INSTABILITY AFTER ANATOMIC ARTHROPLASTY

*I*nstability following shoulder arthroplasty can be a devastating complication. It may be the result of poor surgical technique during the index arthroplasty; or can develop secondary to trauma or soft tissue pathology. The appropriate treatment depends on the cause of the instability. There are cases in which soft tissue procedures can be done such as a posterior capsular plication in certain cases of posterior instability. In other cases, component revision is necessary. Expected outcomes of revision surgery for instability following shoulder arthroplasty are directly related to the cause of the instability. The ensuing chapters will review the different ways to treat both anterior and posterior instabilities following shoulder arthroplasty.

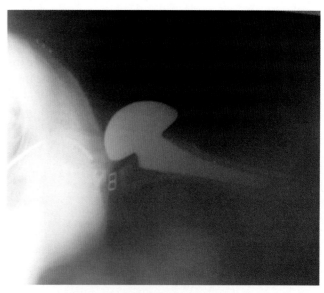

Soft Tissue Procedure Is Sufficient

Kristofer J. Jones / David M. Dines

STATEMENT OF THE ISSUE

Glenohumeral joint stability is primarily dependent upon the complex interaction of static and dynamic stabilizing soft tissue structures given the lack of inherent osseous constraint. Conventional total shoulder arthroplasty (TSA) requires extensive soft tissue dissection with disruption of some of these structures and provides little articular constraint given the conformity of the humeral and glenoid components. For this reason, meticulous repair of soft tissue stabilizers is of paramount importance to ensure the appropriate balance of glenohumeral stability and mobility.

Anterior instability following TSA is one of the most commonly reported complications and while there are a multitude of factors that can contribute to postoperative instability, subscapularis insufficiency is typically the offending cause. While component malposition (excessive anteversion) and/or inappropriate sizing have been recognized as potential factors that play a role in anterior instability, we have found that soft tissue failure is more prevalent. In the case of component-related issues, revision or reverse total shoulder arthroplasty (reverse TSA) are certainly indicated. However, if incompetent soft tissue stabilizers are encountered, we prefer to address the problem with soft tissue reconstruction in order to avoid any complications that are inherent to procedures involving removal of well-fixed implants and concerns regarding implant longevity following reverse TSA, especially in younger patients.

INTRODUCTION

Glenohumeral instability in the setting of shoulder arthroplasty is an unusual, but disabling complication with a reported incidence ranging from 0% to 29%, and an overall average incidence of 2.8% (1,2). Postoperatively, instability is a significant source of pain and dysfunction and revision procedures are often indicated to ameliorate symptoms (3,4). When evaluating a patient with the aforementioned complaints, it is important to have a high index of suspicion for postoperative instability, as soft tissue compromise involving the glenohumeral capsule, rotator cuff, or both is one of the most common reasons for revision procedures (5,6).

Prosthetic instability is generally classified according to the direction of humeral displacement (superior, anterior, posterior, or inferior) as well as the offending etiology (soft tissue failure, component malalignment, or a combination of these factors) (Fig. 29-1). In cases where component positioning is adequate, the most common cause of anterior instability following conventional shoulder arthroplasty is subscapularis insufficiency. Wirth and Rockwood (7,8) reported that excessive humeral anteversion, anterior deltoid dysfunction, and subscapularis insufficiency were the main contributing factors to anterior instability; however, they believed that subscapularis compromise was the requisite factor necessary to cause anterior displacement. The subscapularis muscle provides anterior compressive forces that are required to balance posterior forces as well as static restraint to anterior displacement. In general, subscapularis ruptures can be the result of poor tissue quality secondary to multiple procedures, poor attention to meticulous repair, inappropriate humeral head component sizing resulting in increased lateral offset and tension on the subscapularis repair (i.e., "overstuffing"), and aggressive physical therapy during the early stages of rehabilitation (3,5,6,9,10). In a retrospective review of 41 patients by Miller et al. (6), approximately two-thirds of the experimental cohort demonstrated subscapularis dysfunction following conventional shoulder arthroplasty, as evidenced by a positive lift-off and belly-press examination at a mean follow-up of 1.9 years. It should be noted that the authors observed a trend toward better clinical and functional outcomes when bone tunnels

▲ **FIGURE 29-1:** Axillary radiograph demonstrating anterior instability of the humeral prosthesis.

were utilized to repair the tendon (transosseous repair); however, given the poor results following anatomic soft tissue repair, the authors recommended lesser tuberosity osteotomy to improve subscapularis healing at the site of repair. To date, there have been no prospective randomized studies that demonstrate lesser tuberosity osteotomy techniques reduce subscapularis failure and while the authors' assertion regarding optimal techniques to improve subscapularis healing remains controversial, this study highlights the fact that subscapularis healing and function are critical for the overall success and longevity of TSA.

PATIENT EVALUATION

History

Comprehensive evaluation should always begin with a complete history, as it is important to note that not all patients with shoulder dysfunction resulting from instability will subjectively report subluxation or dislocation. In the overwhelming majority of cases, patients will initially present with pain and weakness localized to the operative shoulder. Miller et al. (10) reported that 100% of patients diagnosed with anterior instability secondary to subscapularis insufficiency initially presented with complaints of debilitating pain, while only 43% noted anterior instability.

A careful history will reveal specific activities or glenohumeral positions that reproduce symptoms, thus providing valuable insight into the direction of instability. For example, a patient with anterior instability will often complain of pain or apprehension with the shoulder in a position of abduction and external rotation. The onset of symptoms should also be carefully elucidated, as anterior instability secondary to component malposition (i.e., excessive anteversion) will often manifest early in the postoperative period. Conversely, humeral component oversizing with excessive lateral offset may lead to gradual attrition of the subscapularis and late instability. Patients with early subscapularis failure will often present in the immediate postoperative period and frequently describe a discrete event such as a "pop or snap" after forced external rotation or extension.

The primary indications for the index procedure and pre-existing conditions can provide important diagnostic clues. For example, patients with rheumatoid arthritis frequently have poor soft tissue quality with associated rotator cuff pathology that may compromise postoperative results (11,12). In addition, previous surgical procedures that violate the integrity of the subscapularis tendon may predispose patients to poor postoperative healing. Miller et al. (10) noted that approximately 43% (3/7) of patients that presented with postoperative instability underwent open surgical stabilization procedures (Putti–Platt) prior to primary TSA. As always, infection must always be considered in any case of failed arthroplasty and may present as overt instability.

Physical Examination

A careful physical examination is mandatory to obtain an accurate diagnosis and guide successful treatment. Obvious signs of infection (erythema, warmth, drainage) and compromised wound healing should be excluded. Inspection of muscular contour should also be performed to detect any signs of atrophy or obvious deformity that may indicate anterior humeral head subluxation or even a fixed dislocation. Both active and passive range of motion should be examined, with particular attention paid to positions of apprehension and the limits of external rotation. Any indication of increased passive external rotation in the operative extremity may represent subscapularis insufficiency. Motor strength testing of all components of the rotator cuff as well as the deltoid and scapular stabilizers should be evaluated. Focused examination of the subscapularis should include the belly-press and lift-off tests, as early diagnosis and repair of subscapularis is paramount to success in the revision setting (10,13,14). Ultimately, chronic subscapularis failures are more challenging to repair and yield less predictable results.

Diagnostic Imaging

Radiologic examination is an important adjunct when attempting to diagnose prosthetic instability. Plain radiographs should always include a true AP view in 45 degrees of internal and external rotations, a scapular Y view, and an axillary view. Evaluation of component position and sizing is important in order to determine the underlying cause of prosthetic failure. In addition, secondary osseous changes in cases of chronic fixed dislocation should be detected to aid in decisions regarding revision surgical procedures. The axillary view is particularly helpful in identifying the direction of instability as well as glenoid version. In some cases, anterior subluxation greater than 5 mm may be indicative of subscapularis insufficiency (15).

Various studies have demonstrated significant variability in the quantification of glenoid version on axillary views and thus, we now utilize computerized tomography (CT) to measure glenoid version and assess glenoid bone stock in the revision setting (16,17). Despite the presence of metal artifact, novel magnetic resonance imaging (MRI) sequences now provide more accurate assessment of surrounding soft tissue structures. With limited pulse-sequence parameter modification, rotator cuff tears can be diagnosed with a reported sensitivity of 91% and specificity of 80% following TSA (18). Given

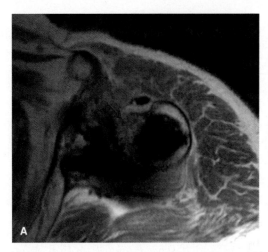
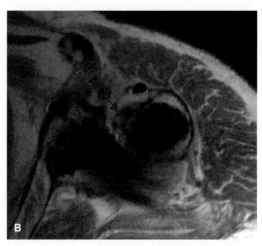

▲ **FIGURE 29-2: A** and **B:** Multiacquisition variable-resonance image combination (MAVRIC) MRI sequence designed to suppress metal artifact. This sequence of axial images demonstrates a chronic subscapularis tear (*arrows*) in a patient that underwent total shoulder arthroplasty.

the detail of these newly acquired sequences, MRI can play a significant role in the evaluation of subscapularis insufficiency when clinically suspected (Fig. 29-2A,B).

TREATMENT

Given the relative rarity of this complication, few studies have reported on long-term outcomes following surgical management of anterior instability in the setting of TSA. Recent literature suggests that prosthetic instability is a challenging problem with less than optimal functional outcomes following revision surgery. Sanchez-Sotelo et al. attempted to define the etiology of instability and the precise risk factors that may lead to an unsatisfactory clinical outcome. According to the authors, the preoperative direction of instability was the only factor that was significantly associated with the final outcome after revision surgery. Interestingly, of the 19 shoulders that failed revision procedures, approximately 74% (14/19) were treated for anterior instability. Once again, the integrity of the subscapularis cannot be emphasized enough, as 79% (15/19) of patients with anterior instability were found to have a disrupted subscapularis (9).

The success of primary subscapularis tendon repair has been reported in a few case series. Moeckel et al. (3) described seven patients diagnosed with anterior instability secondary to subscapularis rupture following TSA. Each patient underwent primary repair and the overall failure rate at a minimum of 2 years was 43% (3/7). Three patients with recurrent instability required static reconstruction of the anterior capsule with Achilles allograft to provide a satisfactory outcome (Fig. 29-3A,B). Alternative options for restoration of a static anterior buttress include iliotibial band graft or even xenograft augmentation (19).

In a study by Miller et al. (10), the authors attempted to treat seven patients with anterior instability secondary to subscapularis insufficiency. While the tendon was primarily repaired in three cases, four patients with poor tendon quality (57%) required transfer of the pectoralis major tendon to serve as an additional anterior buttress and restore balance to the anterior–posterior force couple. Interestingly, 50% (2/4) of these patients required additional procedures because of persistent anterior instability. A recent study by Elhassan and Warner demonstrated similarly poor results, as the authors evaluated three patient cohorts comprised of 10 patient each following

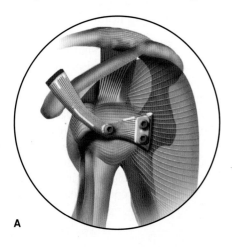
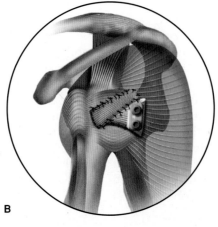

◀ **FIGURE 29-3: A** and **B:** Static reconstruction of the anterior capsule with bone-Achilles tendon allograft. Using this technique, the bone block of the allograft is secured to the glenoid neck with a lag screw and a washer. The tendon is similarly secured to the lesser tuberosity.

A   B

pectoralis major tendon transfer for irreparable tears of the subscapularis. Group I (subscapularis insufficiency following failed instability procedure) and III (subscapularis insufficiency with massive rotator cuff tear) demonstrated better functional outcomes and lower failure rates compared to those patients in group II (subscapularis insufficiency following TSA). The authors noted that preoperative anterior subluxation of the humeral head was a prognostic factor that was predictive of tendon transfer failure.

Endres and Warner recently reported two cases of anterior instability following TSA treated with a modified Latarjet procedure. Though technically challenging, the authors reported successful stabilization at a mean follow-up of 4.5 years (20). In severe cases of instability, salvage with reverse TSA may be the only remaining surgical option to provide adequate restraint.

AUTHOR'S PREFERRED TREATMENT

Clinical results suggest that anterior instability following TSA is a challenging problem and when we consider the available surgical options, several important factors must be considered. We acknowledge that the etiology of anterior instability following TSA can be multifactorial and in these cases, soft tissue imbalance and component malpositioning should be addressed. However, in the setting of appropriately sized and positioned components, we favor soft tissue reconstruction to improve stability.

In our treatment algorithm, we initially consider the timing of the subscapularis rupture and the potential quality of the tissue, as several authors have reported that primary repair is most successful when performed early after traumatic rupture (10,13). In the acute setting, we favor direct tendon-to-tendon repair utilizing bone tunnels if possible (Fig. 29-4A,B). In cases where the subscapularis tissue is thin and tenuous from previous procedures or underlying inflammatory disease, we will consider reinforcing the tendon with xenograft, Achilles, or ITB graft.

Unfortunately, in many cases the diagnosis is delayed and the tendon may not be primarily reparable. In the chronic setting, a primary repair can still be performed utilizing absorbable suture anchors with the

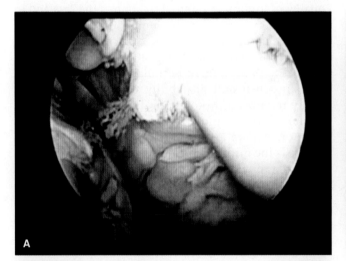
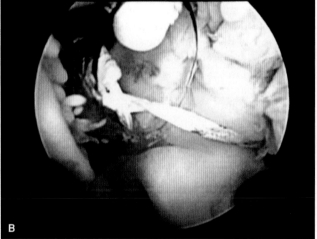
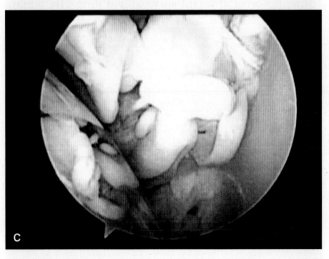

▲ FIGURE 29-4: Primary side-to-side arthroscopic subscapularis repair following acute traumatic rupture.

suture limbs passed through both ends of the tendon if it is still competent and elastic. If there is any uncertainty regarding the quality of fixation, a xenograft, Achilles, or ITB graft may be used to augment the repair. While this approach maintains some dynamic stability, it requires reasonable subscapularis muscle function. Thus, in cases where the muscle quality is in question (i.e., fatty atrophy), we favor a technique previously described by the senior author that utilizes an Achilles tendon–bone allograft to create an anterior static stabilizer between the glenoid neck and the humerus. The patient should be counseled that this procedure will provide adequate stability but may result in range of motion limitations. In addition to primary tendon repair and/or allograft supplementation, other authors have advocated pectoralis tendon transfers either above or under the conjoined tendon to create a dynamic stabilizing force. As previously discussed, results following this procedure have been mixed and we do not typically employ this technique. In the cases performed by the senior author, a subcoracoid transfer is used because we believe it recreates an anatomic vector similar to the subscapularis muscle.

Altogether, the best treatment for prosthetic instability is prevention through careful and considerate surgical techniques. Proper component placement along with durable subscapularis repair during the index procedure should preclude this devastating complication. As previously highlighted, the success of this procedure is largely dependent upon subscapularis function in the postoperative setting so careful attention to proper fixation is paramount to ensure adequate healing. Ultimately, subscapularis repair can be accomplished in a number of ways depending upon the tendon quality, substance, and elasticity. In cases where the tendon quality is compromised or shortened due to previous surgical procedures, we prefer to use a lesser tuberosity osteotomy to achieve bone-to-bone healing. In routine cases with reasonable tendon quality, the senior author prefers to use a transosseous tendon-to-bone or tendon-to-tendon repair (Fig. 29-5). In some younger patients with excellent quality tendon, primary repair will suffice. Following repair, it is important to determine the

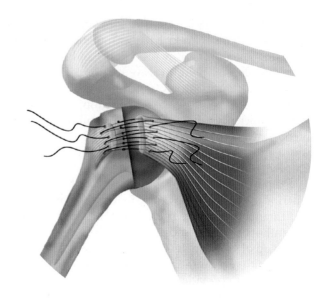

▲ **FIGURE 29-5:** Transosseous tendon to bone repair. Prior to humeral stem insertion, three no. 5 ethibond sutures are inserted through the humerus in a transosseous fashion. The humeral stem is impacted into place and the two suture limbs are subsequently placed through the tenotomized subscapularis in a figure-of-eight fashion. The three suture limbs are then securely tied.

quality of fixation in external rotation at the side and in abduction to determine the limits of range of motion during rehabilitation. In most cases, we tend to limit external rotation to less than 30 degrees for the first 4 weeks to protect the subscapularis repair.

In conclusion, instability after shoulder arthroplasty requires a thorough evaluation of component version and subscapularis integrity. In cases where the components are appropriately placed and soft tissue failure is the primary contributing factor to postoperative instability, we favor soft tissue reconstruction as the ideal surgical alternative. In cases where the tendon is insufficient to accommodate primary repair, graft augmentation can improve clinical results. In the most severe cases, serious consideration should be given to reverse TSA as a potential salvage procedure; however, implant survival and longevity remain a genuine concern.

Revision of Components Is Necessary

Grant Garrigues / Gerald R. Williams, Jr

INTRODUCTION

The rise in the number of anatomic shoulder arthroplasties (ASAs), including TSA and humeral head replacement (HHR), continues with approximately 47,000 ASA[1] per year in the United States in 2008 and projected to rise by 322% by 2015 (21,22). This rise is, in part, driven by the success of ASA for pain relief, functional improvement, and implant survivorship (23). However, the overall complication is as high as 15% in one systematic review (1). Instability makes up for approximately 30% of these complications, affecting approximately 5% of all ASAs, second only to rotator cuff tears in frequency (1,24–26). Eighty percent of all instability cases are anterosuperior, making anterior instability one of the most common complications following ASA (1,25).

The pain and dysfunction patients experience due to an unstable arthroplasty is significant (26). The poor experience reported in the literature of soft tissue reconstructions and an understanding of the pathoanatomy that leads to this instability, suggests that component revision is generally necessary when treating instability of an ASA (3,27–29). Types of component revision include maintaining an anatomic arthroplasty and changing the head size, the humeral stem, or the glenoid versus converting to a reverse TSA.

Neer described his series of 194 total shoulders, with minimum 2-year follow-up, in 1982 (27). This series included anatomic TSA for a variety of indications including cuff-tear arthropathy, glenohumeral joint fusion, neoplasm, and revision cases, in addition to osteoarthritis and inflammatory arthritis. They noted two anterior dislocations within the first 6 weeks after surgery. Both were closed reduced and immobilized before resuming the exercise program. No redislocations occurred; however, one of their unstable arthroplasty patients had recurrent subluxations (27). To the best of our knowledge, there are no known further reports of closed treatment for this condition in the English-speaking medical literature.

In 1993, Moeckel et al. (3) retrospectively reviewed the Hospital for Special Surgery experience with unstable ASA and found seven cases of anterior shoulder instability. Despite their early recognition (average time to revision surgery 8 1/2 weeks) their attempts at subscapularis repair had a high failure rate. Three of seven

cases had recurrent dislocation or subluxation, requiring a second revision. The second revision involved an Achilles allograft to create a static soft tissue restraint between the glenoid and the humerus. With minimum follow-up of 18 months (18 to 36 months), all three shoulders remained stable. Unfortunately, this static stability came at the expense of motion, with an average elevation of 85 degrees (range, 78 to 93) and 5 degrees external rotation (range, 15 to 20) (3).

While this paper is often cited to support soft tissue reconstruction for stabilization, it should be noted that the authors themselves point out that component revision was a frequent part of the treatment strategy: 3/7 patients required glenoid component revision or removal, 1/7 required a custom-made modular head to increase the retroversion, and 4 of the 5 modular humeral prosthesis were revised by downsizing the head (3).

Wirth and Rockwood (27) presented the results of their series of more than 400 arthroplasty cases in 1995. Of their 43 revision cases, 18 were for instability. Three of these had minimum 2-year follow-up and were in the anterior direction. Of these cases, decreased retroversion of the humeral component was present in every case and disruption of the subscapularis was present in two of three. Their approach to this multifactorial problem included revision of the humeral component to restore proper version, coracoacromial ligament reconstruction, and pectoralis major tendon transfer. They note that stability was achieved in all but one shoulder, but given the publication venue as an AAOS abstract, the details of the individual patients are not available (27).

The Mayo clinic experience from 1985 to 1999 was reviewed by Sanchez-Sotelo et al. (9). After reviewing over a 1,000 arthroplasty cases, including those with primary ASA performed at the Mayo clinic and those referred from other physicians, they noted 33 patients with instability, with 14 of these described as anterosuperior instability and 5 described as anterior instability. Glenoid loosening was present in one case, one case had excessive glenoid anteversion, and two cases had excessive humeral anteversion. There were no noted component abnormalities in any of the remaining 15 cases. The soft tissues were more frequently at issue. Fifteen of the nineteen anterior or anterosuperior cases were noted to have a subscapularis tear, with additional cases noted to have anterosuperior rotator cuff thinning or a "stretched" subscapularis. In stark contrast to prior studies, even with a mean time between the index arthroplasty and the treatment of instability of 23 months

---

[1]This number includes an unknown number of reverse TSA.

(range, 28 days to 11 years), they were able to reattach the subscapularis in every case, though one required a dura mater allograft. Despite their impressive ability to achieve a soft tissue repair and their soft tissue rebalancing efforts, the results of soft tissue reconstruction in these skilled hands were marginal. Only 15/19 were "unsatisfactory" on the Neer rating, 11/19 remained unstable, 3/19 required resection arthroplasty. Only 5/19 were stable, with the majority of those still rating their outcome as "unsatisfactory" (9).

Deutsch et al. (28) reviewed a series of 32 patients who underwent glenoid revision surgery after anatomic TSA. Twelve patients had concomitant instability, with the majority, 9/12, having an anterior instability component. They concluded that the eccentric loads on the glenoid imparted by the instability likely predisposed to glenoid component loosening. As noted by prior authors, they found that anterior instability was associated with postoperative subscapularis rupture, anterior soft tissue insufficiency, and malrotation of the humeral component. Of the 5/9 patients with instability only in an anterior direction (not anterosuperior) all 5 had subscapularis tears. Revision of the glenoid was an inclusion criterion for the study, but humeral revision was also almost universally required (8/9 cases). Two of the humeral-sided revisions were for stem loosening, two head revisions for abrasive wear and resizing, three stem revisions for malposition, and one stem revision for exposure. In addition to revising the stem when malpositioned and repairing any repairable rotator cuff tears, the treatment strategy included Achilles allograft reconstruction of the anterior soft tissue envelope in 5/9 cases. Their results in these challenging cases are sobering, with only two patients ultimately achieving a stable joint (one required revision to glenohumeral joint fusion) and some patients made worse by the operation (28).

While all of the above series frequently include both component revision and soft tissue repair in their treatment strategy, this data on treatment of anterior instability in an ASA comes from the era prior to the 2003 FDA approval of the reverse TSA. This implant has improved the functional results of shoulder arthroplasty in the cuff deficient shoulder by substituting increased implant constraint for the absent centering effect of the rotator cuff. For this reason, instead of performing a tendon transfer or allograft soft tissue reconstruction and revising a failed anatomic glenohumeral arthroplasty for the version and glenoid loosening issues that frequently occur with subscapularis insufficiency, the reverse TSA can address many of these problems simultaneously.

With a more current treatment algorithm, Melis et al. (29), looked at 37 anatomic TSA cases with aseptic glenoid loosening. Out of 37, 29 had subscapularis insufficiency, postulated to be the cause of the glenoid loosening, and 13 had instability. Treatment with revision to reverse TSA yielded consistent improvement,

with an average increase in elevation from 68 to 121 degrees and improvement in the average constant score from 25 to 55 points. They noted that reverse shoulder arthroplasty is a reliable option to treat glenohumeral instability, rotator cuff insufficiency, and even glenoid bone loss. In addition they also observed that revision of the prosthetic components provides the best outcomes while soft tissue reconstructions can be expected to yield poorer results (29).

EVALUATION

The causes of anterior instability are numerous, and will be reviewed in detail below. However, the most common cause of anterior instability after ASA is subscapularis insufficiency (25). While the etiology can be a result of either an implant-related issue or a soft tissue deficiency (Table 29-1), there is frequently a combination of a number of contributory factors, so a thorough evaluation is critical (9,27).

Subscapularis Insufficiency

The most common cause of anterior shoulder instability after anatomic arthroplasty is subscapularis insufficiency (25). Failure of the subscapularis can be attributed to surgical technique, poor tissue quality, inappropriately sized or positioned components, a fall or trauma in the early postoperative period, or over exuberant physical therapy (30). The subscapularis has a dual role in anterior instability—acting as the primary anterior compressor to balance the posterior rotator cuff, as well as acting as a static soft tissue restraint (25,30). Miller et al. (6,12) are credited with raising the awareness of this important complication. They reported a rate of reoperation for subscapularis tear after shoulder arthroplasty of 5.8% (10). In fact, it appears that the incidence of subscapularis insufficiency may be even higher, with abnormal lift-off examination in 67.5% and abnormal belly-press in 66.5% of postarthroplasty patients in their initial series (6). Further studies have confirmed the significance of this problem, with rotator cuff tears estimated to be the one of the most

TABLE 29-1 **Causes of Anterior Instability after Anatomic Shoulder Arthroplasty**

Soft tissue	Subscapularis insufficiency
	Anterior deltoid dysfunction
Implant	Humeral component
	Anteversion
	Overstuffing
	Other humeral factors
	Glenoid component
	Anteversion
	Overstuffing
	Other glenoid factors

common complications after shoulder arthroplasty with half of these involving the subscapularis (1).

While clearly not every patient with subscapularis insufficiency has instability, this risk factor is frequently found in published series of anterior shoulder instability after ASA. In the series by Moeckel et al. (3), seven cases of anterior instability, all had subscapularis tears. Wirth and Rockwood (27) reported on 3 cases of anterior instability, and 2/3 were found to have subscapularis tears. Sanchez-Sotelo et al. (9) noted 15 of the 19 anterior or anterosuperior instability cases had a subscapularis tear, and the additional cases were described as having a thinned or stretched subscapularis.

Evaluation

When evaluating a patient with a failed arthroplasty, the search for subscapularis insufficiency starts with a high index of clinical suspicion. The chief complaint may include a history of dislocation or subluxation, but frequently patients complain of pain or loss of function (26). The history should start with the first episode of any shoulder issue—often unrecognized instability was present before the arthroplasty was performed. In addition, a thorough history, including operative reports, of any prior surgical procedures is critical. Specifically, operations that include take down or lengthening of the subscapularis will place the patient at risk for subscapularis rupture (25). These reports may also make comments about the intraoperative stability, tissue quality, and any other balancing procedures performed at the same setting.

The safe zone reported by the index surgeon for motion without repair tension should be noted and compared with the patient's recollection of their postoperative motion. Overaggressive therapy or a fall in the postoperative period can cause subscapularis rupture. Patients may recall a distinct pop when the repair failed with external rotation or extension (10). A history of medical conditions should also be obtained, especially risk factors for rotator cuff rupture or poor subscapularis healing such as inflammatory arthritis, tobacco use, and diabetes. While subscapularis insufficiency may be attritional, it more frequently occurs when the initial repair fails before it is allowed to heal fully. Thus instability usually presents earlier than other failures, at an average of 2.1 years from the index procedure (1). In fact, in Moeckel's series, the patients returned to the operating room an average of 81/2 weeks (3).

Physical examination tests are similar to those of the nonarthroplasty shoulder (Fig. 29-6). The lift-off and belly-press tests are paramount in assessing the integrity of the subscapularis (6,31). Translation can also be tested with load-and-shift testing, while apprehension, especially in abduction and external rotation is also helpful. Active range of motion testing will often show a loss of elevation, as the loss of the anterior force couple challenges forward flexion. Passive range of motion may

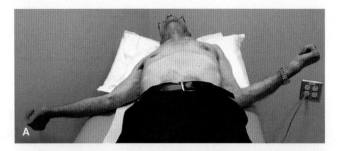
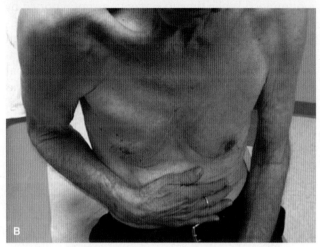

▲ **FIGURE 29-6:** A 75-year-old man presents with right shoulder pain and loss of elevation that has been present since his anatomic arthroplasty 2 years ago. **(A)** Increased passive external rotation and **(B)** an abnormal belly-press test indicate subscapularis insufficiency. (Copyright Grant Garrigues 2013)

show an increase in passive external rotation with subscapularis insufficiency, but this is not always the case. In fact, patients may have a decrease in passive range of motion and thus both stiffness and instability. If the shoulder is not stiff, a positive abdominal compression test is indicative of subscapularis deficiency.

Imaging findings of subscapularis insufficiency include anterior subluxation on the axillary lateral view, with greater than 5 mm being diagnostic (32). This same imaging series may also show glenoid loosening, frequently found with subscapularis insufficiency as the absent anterior cuff leads to anterior–posterior "rocking horse" forces on the glenoid, similar to those described by Franklin et al. (33). CT arthrogram can be helpful to evaluate both the implant as well as the surrounding soft tissues (32). While newer MRI protocols allow the soft tissues to be visualized even in the presence of a metallic implant. Sperling et al. (18) showed 91% sensitivity and 80% specificity for MRI in the diagnosis of rotator cuff tears after arthroplasty. More recently, ultrasound has been validated as a method to assess the subscapularis' integrity after arthroplasty (34).

Treatment and Results

The subscapularis has dual stabilizing functions, both active and passive, and soft tissue reconstruction attempts to restore one or both of these. Early recognition is critical to attempt repair, as the subscapularis will retract and atrophy over time, worsening the prognosis for the results of repair (31). However, as discussed above, even with early recognition and a reparable tendon, the results of soft tissue repairs are unpredictable and often poor. Moeckel et al. (3) recognized the issue early, but still had 3/7 with either recurrent dislocation or subluxation requiring a second revision operation. Stability was finally achieved, but at the expense of a great deal of motion loss. While time to surgery was not reported by Deutsch et al. (28), they had similar difficulties repairing the subscapularis, used a similar reconstruction with 5/9 cases requiring an Achilles allograft capsular reconstruction, and had similar sobering results in this patient population. The average postoperative flexion was 74 degrees, only two patients were stabilized by the revisions, one of these required revision to glenohumeral fusion, and some patients were made worse (28). In Sanchez-Sotelo's series they were impressively always able

to repair the subscapularis, but their results were similarly sobering with 14/19 having persistent instability after their soft tissue repairs and rebalancing (9). While subscapularis insufficiency was present in two of three cases in Wirth's series, requiring pectoralis major transfer (Fig. 29-7), they noted decreased retroversion of the humeral component and revised the humerus in all cases (27,35). This component revision strategy proved more effective than soft tissue repairs alone, though the patient-by-patient results are not available for this abstract.

Given the challenges of repairing the subscapularis after failure in an arthroplasty situation, many surgeons currently find revision to reverse total shoulder a more predictable operation. As discussed above, Melis et al. (29) evaluated this strategy. They concluded that soft tissue reconstructions can be expected to yield poorer results and that reverse shoulder arthroplasty is a reliable option to treat glenohumeral instability, rotator cuff insufficiency, and even glenoid bone loss (Fig. 29-8).

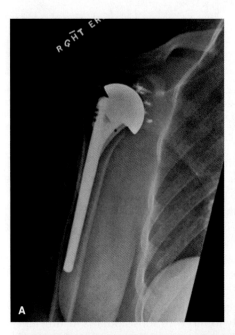
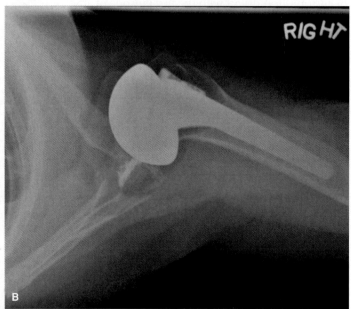
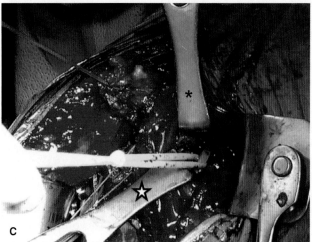

▲ **FIGURE 29-7:** A 35-year-old woman with multiple failed anterior instability operations and a painful, unstable hemiarthroplasty **(A)**. Evaluation revealed anterior subluxation on the axillary lateral view **(B)** and an abnormal belly press. Given her young age, conversion to reverse TSA was not advisable and a pectoralis major transfer was performed. **(C)** The superior Army–Navy retractor (*asterisk*) is retracting the clavicular head of the pectoralis major (tagged with white suture), just medial to the conjoint tendon. This reveals the musculocutaneous nerve (yellow vessel loop). The inferior Army–Navy retractor (*open star*) is retracting the conjoint tendon from the medial side. Even in this case, revision was necessary as the humeral head was removed to allow posterior capsular releases for soft tissue balancing. A smaller humeral head was used to allow repair of the scant remaining anterior soft tissues. (Copyright Grant Garrigues 2013)

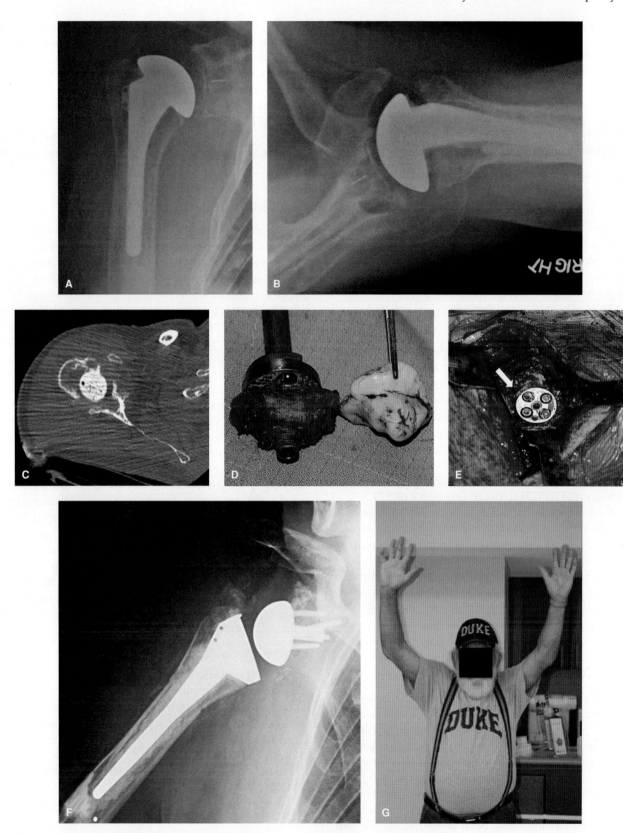

▲ **FIGURE 29-8: (A, B)** A 68-year-old man with a painful, unstable, pseudoparalytic, loose, infected, total shoulder. His belly-press test was abnormal. **(C)** After debridement and antibiotic spacer, a cavitary glenoid defect was present. The metaglene is implanted on the iliac crest, then removed with structural bone graft. **(D)** This graft is fashioned to match a cement imprint made intraoperatively of the cavitary defect. **(E)** The graft is visible *(white arrow)* after the metaglene has been screwed into place. Two-year follow-up shows **(F)** complete graft incorporation, **(G)** good range of motion, no pain, or signs of residual infection. (Copyright Grant Garrigues 2013)

Compromised Anterior Deltoid

A compromised anterior deltoid can result from scarring and nerve stretch injury during a deltopectoral approach or even frank nerve disruption and deltoid dehiscence during a transdeltoid approach. Any of these injuries causes an imbalance where a normal anterior and lateral (middle) heads of the deltoid are not counterbalanced, leading to an anteriorly directed force.

Evaluation

Physical examination to inspect prior surgical scars and evaluate atrophy is the most helpful. Isolating each head of the deltoid individually on examination is generally sufficient, but EMG can provide objective data if the electromyographer is alerted to assess each deltoid head separately. In the case of deltoid dehiscence, a palpable, often painful defect can be felt.

Treatment and Results

While this is a frequent comorbidity with other causes of anterior instability, there is little data on treatment of this complication alone. Deltoid dehiscence can be treated with attempted mobilization and repair, but nerve injury and muscle fibrosis are more problematic scenarios. Groh et al. reviewed Rockwood's referral series of 33 patients with deltoid dehiscence and three patients with axillary nerve injury. All patients were dissatisfied; eight had anterior or anterior–superior instability. This condition was described as an operative disaster, causing irrevocable pain and loss of function (36,37).

Unfortunately, deltoid deficiency not only compromises the result of an ASA, it may also compromise the ability for a successful revision to reverse. Separate biomechanical cadaveric studies by Gulotta et al. (38 and Schwartz et al. 39) indicate that the anterior deltoid is critical for abduction in the scapular plane with an RSA. An intact subscapularis may be able to compensate for a deficient deltoid (38), but, as noted above, the irreparable subscapularis is frequently the reason for revision.

Overstuffing

Overstuffing occurs when the capsule and rotator cuff tissues are under increased tension due to abnormally increased offset between their humeral and scapular attachments. This can occur from a glenoid component that is thick, leading to a lateralized joint line, for example, early metal-backed designs. More commonly, this is seen with an oversized head, an insufficient humeral head cut, or a varus stem position (40). The average lateral humeral offset has been measured at 56 mm (range, 40 to 67) and if this anatomic relationship is not respected, overstuffing or undertensioning of the soft tissues may result (41). Overstuffing leads to stiffness, but also increased tension on the subscapularis repair and thus risk for instability due to subscapularis

insufficiency. This leads to an excessively tight posterior capsule and a deficient anterior structure—a clear setup for anterior instability. Undertensioning leads to lax soft tissues that may cause instability as well, but this problem is less common clinically.

Articular malposition by as little as 4 mm can change the tension on the capsular structures, leading to changes in translation in a cadaveric model. This type of prosthetic positioning can also lead to impingement of any uncovered areas of the proximal humerus, another potential cause of instability (42).

Evaluation

Physical examination of an overstuffed joint may reveal the signs and symptoms of subscapularis insufficiency listed above. In addition, while the joint may have anterior instability, there may also be coexistent stiffness as the tissues that remain intact are under excessive tension. Specifically, passive internal rotation and forward elevation will be limited from a tight posterior and inferior capsule.

Plain film radiographs are extremely helpful for evaluation of this problem. The grashey view in neutral rotation will show the humeral implant in profile and can be helpful to assess for varus stem positioning, an oversized humeral head, or an excessively thick glenoid component. A frequent technical error is under resection of osteophytes and then implanting a humeral head on the basis of the size of the native head plus the crown of osteophytes—the appropriateness of the humeral head size can be judged from plain x-rays. If the contralateral shoulder is not involved, templating off well-arm x-rays can give a sense for the appropriate implant dimensions. On the glenoid side, the poor results seen with early metal-backed designs has been postulated to result at least partially from the increased thickness of these components leading to overstuffing (43,44). Finally, the advanced imaging listed above can be helpful to further evaluate for the frequently coexistent problem of subscapularis insufficiency.

Treatment and Results

In Moeckel's series, they discuss that in 4/5 shoulders with anterior instability and a modular head, they replaced the head with a smaller component (3). It is not clear whether this component revision was necessary to correct a previously overstuffed joint, or if an undersized, nonanatomic head used to allow the subscapularis to be under decreased tension at the time of revision.

Humeral Component Version

The normal, anatomic retroversion of the humeral head varies significantly from 7 to 50 degrees with respect to the axis of elbow flexion, with a mean generally around 30 degrees (30). Many authors have postulated that decreased retroversion of the humeral component is a risk factor for anterior instability (29). In hemiarthroplasty for fracture, increased retroversion has been associated with increased tuberosity failure. This is postulated to occur due to increased tension on the greater tuberosity repair (45). Analogously, it has been proposed that decreased retroversion of the humeral component puts increased tension on the subscapularis repair for a given amount of external rotation, though this intuitive connection has not been studied. In fact, in a cadaveric model, of an anatomic arthroplasty implanted in various degrees of retroversion, the version made no difference as it was essentially "rotating a sphere" with no overall effect on the soft tissue length–tension relationships (46).

Evaluation

The patient may complain of increasing instability with further levels of external rotation, either at the side or in abduction. A humeral head osteotomy with a decreased level of retroversion may leave articular bone intact in the back. While the change in version may not affect the stability directly, this extra bone can lead to overstuffing and therefore, subscapularis insufficiency, so the signs and symptoms of those conditions listed above may be present. To evaluate version, a CT with cuts through the elbow and the shoulder can be used to measure the amount of retroversion (Fig. 29-9).

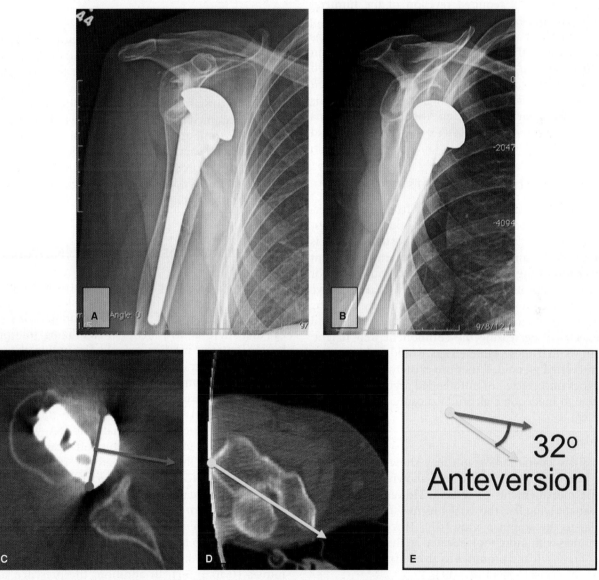

▲ **FIGURE 29-9: (A, B)** Two views of a dislocating total shoulder arthroplasty. The patient suffered dislocations with any external rotation beyond neutral, even with her arm at the side. The belly-press test was intact, but a CT of the entire humerus **(C, D, E)** revealed a significantly anteverted humeral component. We recommend the following practical method for evaluation. Viewing the axial CT cuts, hold a ruler on the screen across the transepicondylar axis. Then, with the ruler held in place, the image is scrolled to humeral head. The angle between the ruler held on the screen and the position of the humeral head can be easily measured using the Cobb angle tool present on most imaging systems. (Copyright Grant Garrigues 2013)

Treatment and Results

Wirth and Rockwood (27) noted decreased retroversion in all three of their cases of anterior instability. Their treatment protocol included restoring the proper version of the humeral component, in addition to addressing coexistent subscapularis and/or glenoid based issues.

Sanchez-Sotelo et al. (9) noted abnormal humeral anteversion in two of their cases with anterosuperior instability. While soft tissue rebalancing and subscapularis repair were the mainstays of their treatment, out of all 33 instability cases (including all directions) 8 required revision of the humeral stem for component malposition and 9 required revision of the humeral stem for glenoid exposure.

Deutsch et al. (28) were reporting on a series were revision of the glenoid was an inclusion criterion for the study, but humeral revision was also required in almost every case (8/9). Two of the humeral-sided revisions were for stem loosening, two head revisions for abrasive wear and resizing, three stem revisions for malposition, and one stem was revised to aid exposure.

Glenoid Component Version

The glenoid face is generally within 10 degrees of perpendicular to plane of the scapular body (16). Excessive retroversion from uncorrected posterior wear is a well-known cause of posterior instability (40) but anteversion of the glenoid can similarly cause anterior instability. Iannotti et al. (40) showed that excessive posterior version causes posterior instability both by creating a posteriorly directed joint reaction force and by effectively decreasing the component wall height. It follows that these same effects would hold true for an anteverted glenoid. Either pre-existent anterior wear that goes uncorrected or unintended asymmetric reaming due to inadequate glenoid exposure can cause this problem.

Evaluation

An axillary lateral radiograph may show this malposition, but axial CT scans have been shown to yield more precise measurements of version. However, even with the patient lying flat, the axial cuts may not be perpendicular to the scapular body (47). Three-dimensional CT models with more sophisticated analyses is a current area of research and promises to give improved accuracy in version measurement (47–49).

A far more common glenoid abnormality seen with anterior instability is a loose glenoid, as noted in the series by Moeckel et al., Sanchez-Sotelo et al., Deutsch et al., and Melis et al. (3,9,28,29). For this reason, a CT arthrogram can be helpful to evaluate both the version of the component, evaluate for loosening,

and to evaluate the rotator cuff integrity with one study (50,51).

Treatment and Results

Wirth reported one case with anterior glenoid wear. Sanchez-Sotelo et al. (9) noted one case of excessive prosthetic glenoid anteversion that experienced anterior instability. This patient remained unstable with an "unsatisfactory" Neer rating. While the experience in the literature of this particular complication is limited, correction of abnormal glenoid version is recommended if this is felt to contribute to the anterior instability.

Other Glenoid Factors

A variety of native and prosthetic glenoid factors influence intrinsic stability of the glenoid. Defects of the native glenoid, such as bony Bankart lesions, can predispose to anterior instability after ASA in the same ways they cause instability in native shoulders. In addition, various parameters such as glenoid width and conformity have some role to play, but wall height seems be the prosthetic parameter with the largest role to play in stability of the prosthetic glenoid (30,52). These factors are critical for glenoid prosthetic design, but are beyond the scope of this chapter.

PREVENTION OF ANTERIOR INSTABILITY

As discussed extensively above, an intact subscapularis is critical in preventing anterior instability. It is the opinion of the authors that the subscapularis is so critical that there is no functional stabilizing role played by the anterior-inferior capsule (including the superior glenohumeral ligament, coracohumeral ligament, middle glenohumeral ligament, and the anterior portion of the inferior glenohumeral ligament complex). We routinely dissect out and remove these capsular structures en bloc on every anatomic TSA (Fig. 29-10). Our confidence in removing this soft tissue stems from the success of the lesser tuberosity osteotomy (31). While no study to date has proven that lesser tuberosity osteotomy decreases the rate of subscapularis insufficiency or anterior instability (53), and fatty infiltration with an intact remains an unsolved problem (54), the results with this technique show healing rates that are improved over subscapularis tenotomy or peel techniques (6,10,31,54). In addition, the presence of the lesser tuberosity fragment allows subscapularis healing to be assessed confidently with routine x-rays (Figs. 29-11 and 29.12). In the case of an acute injury, the integrity of the subscapularis–lesser tuberosity complex can be assessed quickly and, if necessary, allow early repair. The authors have had the opportunity to

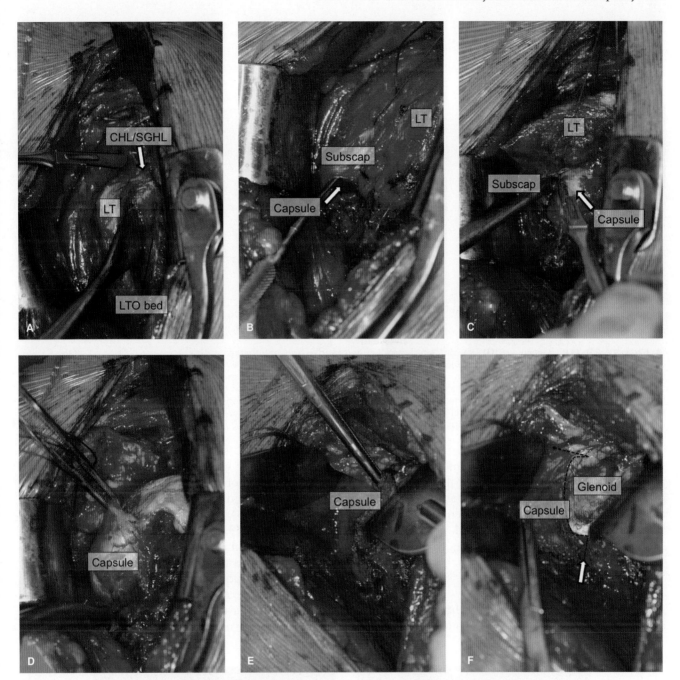

▲ **FIGURE 29-10:**   Lesser tuberosity osteotomy and capsulectomy. **(A)** Removing the lesser tuberosity from the cancellous bed. **(B)** Bluntly dissecting the subscapularis off the underlying capsule medially. **(C)** Sharply dissecting the subscapularis free of the capsule laterally to reveal **(D)** the underlying anterior-inferior capsule. After the axillary nerve is dissected free, the **(E)** external and **(F)** synovial sides of the capsule to be removed are seen. (*continued*)

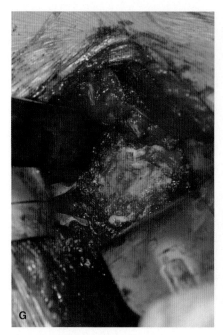
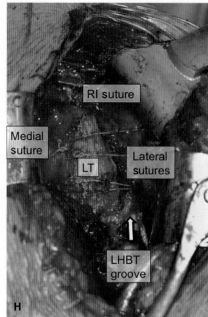
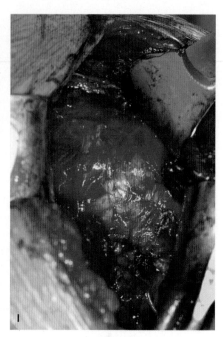

▲ **Figure 29-10:** *(Continued)* **(G)** The contracted capsule is removed as a sheet from the coracoid base around the anterior/inferior glenoid to just posterior of the inferior glenoid pole. **(H)** The lesser tuberosity is repaired to its bony bed with a series of sutures through bone and around the prosthesis. **(I)** External rotation showing the improvement in motion with capsulectomy and the lesser tuberosity moving as a unit with the humerus. CHL/SGHL, coracohumeral ligament/superior glenohumeral ligament; LT, lesser tuberosity; LTO, lesser tuberosity osteotomy, Subscap, subscapularis; RI, rotator interval; LHBT, long head biceps tendon. (Copyright Grant Garrigues 2013)

fix three avulsed lesser tuberosities following shoulder arthroplasty and they have observed that the presence of the lesser tuberosity makes repair easier by providing a clear demarcation of the avulsed tendon and a solid bony structure to pass sutures around.

Conclusions

Anterior instability after an ASA is a challenging clinical scenario. A careful review of the literature clearly shows that even in the era before the reverse total shoulder prosthetic component revision was frequently required to address overstuffing (3), humeral component anteversion (9,27,28), glenoid anteversion (9), or for glenoid exposure (9,28). Attempts at soft tissue reconstruction have an extremely high failure rate (3) with frequent stiffness (3,28), recurrent instability (3,9,28), and a high proportion of dissatisfied patients (9,28). In addition, the rapid retraction and atrophy of the subscapularis, means that even with early recognition, direct repair may not be possible (3,27) and a pectoralis

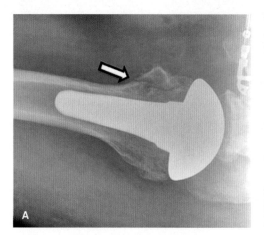
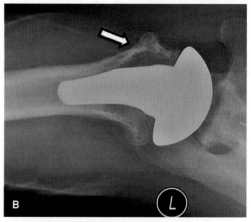

▲ **Figure 29-11:** Axillary lateral x-rays at **(A)** 2 weeks and **(B)** 3 months showing the lesser tuberosity osteotomy and bony, anatomic healing. (Copyright Grant Garrigues 2013)

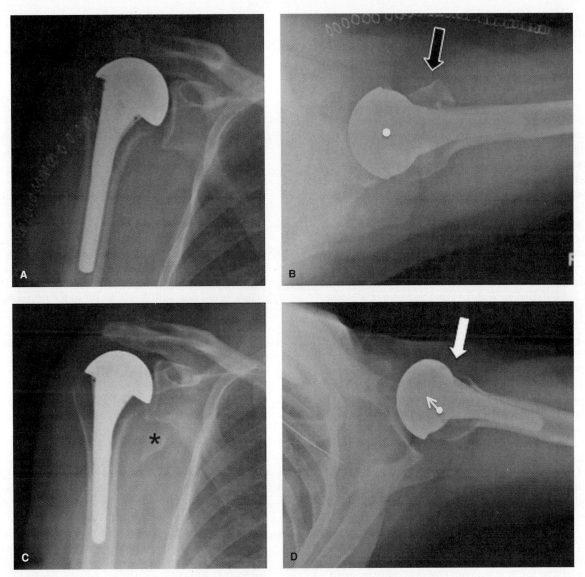

▲ **FIGURE 29-12:** Two-week **(A)** AP and **(B)** axillary lateral x-rays after hemiarthroplasty with an extended coverage head for rotator cuff arthropathy. The lesser tuberosity (*black arrow*) is near its proper position and the humeral head remains centered (*yellow dot*). At 6 weeks, after the patient was involved in an altercation, the **(C)** AP view shows displacement of the lesser tuberosity (*asterisk*) and the **(D)** axillary lateral shows anterior subluxation due to the dethatched subscapularis (*yellow arrow.*) (Copyright Grant Garrigues 2013)

major tendon transfer (35), with or without allograft capsular reconstruction may be the only salvage option (3,28). Moreover, even when soft tissue repair or reconstruction is being performed, it is most often done in combination with humeral head downsizing, humeral stem change in version or height, or glenoid component removal or revision (3,9,27,28). Despite these heroic efforts, the results of soft tissue repair or reconstruction and maintenance of an anatomic arthroplasty are still poor (3,9,27,28). Therefore, in many cases, revision to reverse TSA is the current treatment of choice to treat the soft tissue deficiencies, component loosening or malposition, and loss of function that accompanies an unstable ASA.

References

1. Bohsali KI, Wirth MA, Rockwood CA Jr. Complications of total shoulder arthroplasty. *J Bone Joint Surg Am.* 2006; 88(10):2279–2292.
2. Warren RF, Coleman SH, Dines JS. Instability after arthroplasty: The shoulder. *J Arthroplasty.* 2002;17(4 Suppl 1): 28–31.
3. Moeckel BH, Altchek DW, Warren RF, et al. Instability of the shoulder after arthroplasty. *J Bone Joint Surg Am.* 1993;75:492–497.
4. Godeneche A, Boileau P, Favard L, et al. Prosthetic replacement in the treatment of osteoarthritis of the shoulder: Early results of 268 cases. *J Shoulder Elbow Surg.* 2002;11:11–18.

5. Brems JJ. Complications of shoulder arthroplasty: Infections, instability, and loosening. *Instr Course Lect.* 2002;11:315–321.

6. Miller SL, Hazrati Y, Klepps S, et al. Loss of subscapularis function after total shoulder replacement: A seldom-recognized problem. *J Shoulder Elbow Surg.* 2003;12:29–34.

7. Wirth MA, Rockwood CA Jr. Complications of shoulder arthroplasty. *Clin Orthop.* 1994;307:47–69.

8. Wirth MA, Rockwood CA Jr. Complications of total shoulder-replacement arthroplasty. *J Bone Joint Surg Am.* 1996;78:603–616.

9. Sanchez-Sotelo J, Sperling JW, Rowland CM, et al. Instability after shoulder arthroplasty: Results of surgical treatment. *J Bone Joint Surg Am.* 2003;85(4):622–631.

10. Miller BS, Joseph TA, Noonan TJ, et al. Rupture of the subscapularis tendon after shoulder arthroplasty: Diagnosis, treatment, and outcome. *J Shoulder Elbow Surg.* 2005;14(5):492–496.

11. Stewart MP, Kelly IG. Total shoulder replacement in rheumatoid disease: 7- to 13-year follow-up of 37 joints. *J Bone Joint Surg.* 1997;79:68–72.

12. Trail IA, Nuttall D. The results of shoulder arthroplasty in patients with rheumatoid arthritis. *J Bone Joint Surg Br.* 2002;84:1121–1125.

13. Gerber C, Krushell RJ. Isolated rupture of the tendon of the subscapularis muscle: Clinical features in 16 cases. *J Bone Joint Surg Br.* 1991;73:389–394.

14. Tokish JM, Decker MJ, Ellis HB, et al. The belly-press test for the physical examination of the subscapularis muscle: Electromyographic validation and comparison to the lift-off test. *J Shoulder Elbow Surg.* 2003;12(5):427–430.

15. Gerber A, Warner JJ. Management of glenoid bone loss in shoulder arthroplasty. *Tech Shoulder Elbow Surg.* 2001;2:255–266.

16. Friedman RJ, Hawthorne KB, Genez BM. The use of computerized tomography in the measurement of glenoid version. *J Bone Joint Surg Am.* 1992;74:1032–1037.

17. Nyffeler RW, Jost B, Pfirrmann CW, et al. Measurement of glenoid version: Conventional radiographs versus computed tomography scans. *J Shoulder Elbow Surg.* 2003; 12(5):493–496.

18. Sperling JW, Potter HG, Craig EV, et al. Magnetic resonance imaging of painful shoulder arthroplasty. *J Shoulder Elbow Surg.* 2002;11(4):315–321.

19. Ianotti JP, Antoniou J, Williams GR, et al. Iliotibial band reconstruction for treatment of glenohumeral instability associated with irreparable capsular deficiency. *J Shoulder Elbow Surg.* 2002;11:618–624.

20. Endres NK, Warner JJ. Anterior instability after total shoulder replacement: salvage with modified Latarjet procedure. A report of 2 cases. *J Shoulder Elbow Surg.* 2010;19(2):e1–e5.

21. Kim SH, Wise BL, Zhang Y, et al. Increasing incidence of shoulder arthroplasty in the United States. *J Bone Joint Surg Am.* 2001;93(24):2249–2254.

22. Day JS, Lau E, Ong KL, et al. Prevalence and projections of total shoulder and elbow arthroplasty in the United States to 2015. *J Shoulder Elbow Surg.* 2010;19(8):1115–1120.

23. Deshmukh AV, Koris M, Zurakowski D, et al. Total shoulder arthroplasty: Long-term survivorship, functional outcomes, and quality of life. *J Shoulder Elbow Surg.* 2005;14(5):471–479.

24. Chin PY, Sperling JW, Cofield RH, et al. Complications of total shoulder arthroplasty: Are they fewer or different? *J Shoulder Elbow Surg.* 2006;15:19–22.

25. Cofield RH, Edgerton BC. Total shoulder arthroplasty: Complications and revision surgery. *Instr Course Lect.* 1990;39:449–462.

26. Hasan SS, Leith JM, Campbell B, et al. Characteristics of unsatisfactory shoulder arthroplasties. *J Shoulder Elbow Surg.* 2002;11(5):431–441.

27. Neer, CS, II, Watson, KC, Stanton, FJ. Recent experience with total shoulder replacement. *J Bone Joint Surg Am.* 1982;64:319–337.

28. Deutsch A, Abboud JA, Kelly J, et al. Clinical results of revision shoulder arthroplasty for glenoid component loosening. *J Shoulder Elbow Surg.* 2007;16(6):706–716.

29. Melis B, Bonnevialle N, Neyton L, et al. Glenoid loosening and failure in anatomical total shoulder arthroplasty: Is revision with a reverse shoulder arthroplasty a reliable option? *J Shoulder Elbow Surg.* 2012;21:342–349.

30. Matsen FA III, Clinton J, Rockwood CA Jr, et al. Glenohumeral arthritis and its management. In: Matsen FA III, Rockwood CA Jr, eds. *The Shoulder.* 4th ed. Philadelphia, PA: Saunders; 2009.

31. Gerber C, Pennington SD, Yian EH, et al. Lesser tuberosity osteotomy for total shoulder arthroplasty. *J Bone Joint Surg Am.* 2006;88(Suppl 1 Pt 2):170–177.

32. Gerber A, Ghalambor N, Warner JJ, et al. Instability of shoulder arthroplasty: Balancing mobility and stability. *Orthop Clin North Am.* 2001;32(4):661–670.

33. Franklin JL, Barrett WP, Jackins SE, et al. Glenoid loosening in total shoulder arthroplasty. Association with rotator cuff deficiency. *J Arthroplasty.* 1988;3(1):39–46.

34. Ives EP, Nazarian LN, Parker L, et al. Subscapularis tendon tears: A common sonographic finding in symptomatic postarthroplasty shoulders. *J Clin Ultrasound.* 2013;41(3):129–133.

35. Wirth MA, Rockwood CA Jr. Operative treatment of irreparable rupture of the subscapularis. *J Bone Joint Surg Am.* 1997;79:722–731.

36. Groh G, Simoni M, Rolla P, et al. Loss of the deltoid after shoulder operations: An operative disaster. *J Shoulder Elbow Surg.* 1994;3:243–253.

37. Sher JS, Iannotti JP, Warner JJ, et al. Surgical treatment of postoperative deltoid origin disruption. *Clin Orthop Relat Res.* 1997;(343):93–98.

38. Gulotta LV, Choi D, Marinello P, et al. Anterior deltoid deficiency in reverse total shoulder replacement: A biomechanical study with cadavers. *J Bone Joint Surg Br.* 2012;94(12):1666–1669.

39. Schwartz DG, Kang SH, Lynch TS, et al. The anterior deltoid's importance in reverse shoulder arthroplasty: A cadaveric biomechanical study. *J Shoulder Elbow Surg.* 2013;22(3):357–364.

40. Iannotti JP, Spencer EE, Winter U, et al. Prosthetic positioning in total shoulder arthroplasty. *J Shoulder Elbow Surg.* 2005;14(11):111 S–121 S.

41. Iannotti JP, Gabriel JP, Schneck SL, et al. The normal glenohumeral relationships. An anatomic study of

one hundred and forty shoulders. *J Bone Joint Surg Am.* 1992;74(4):491–500.

42. Williams GR Jr, Wong KL, Pepe MD, et al. The effects of articular malposition after total shoulder arthroplasty on glenohumeral translations, range of motion, and subacromial impingement. *J Shoulder Elbow Surg.* 2001;10(5):399–409.
43. Boileau P, Abidor C, Krishnan SG, et al. Cemented polyethylene versus uncemented metal-backed glenoid components in total shoulder arthroplasty: A prospective, double-blind, randomized study. *J Shoulder Elbow Surg.* 2002;11(4):351–359.
44. Fox TJ, Cil A, Sperling JW, et al. Survival of the glenoid component in shoulder arthroplasty. *J Shoulder Elbow Surg.* 2009;18(6):859–863.
45. Boileau P, Krishnan SG, Tinsi L, et al. Tuberosity malposition and migration: Reasons for poor outcomes after hemiarthroplasty for displaced fractures of the proximal humerus. *J Shoulder Elbow Surg.* 2002;11(5):401–412.
46. Spencer EE Jr, Valdevit A, Kambic H, et al. The effect of humeral component anteversion on shoulder stability with glenoid component retroversion. *J Bone Joint Surg Am.* 2013;87(4):808–814.
47. Hoenecke HR Jr, Hermida JC, Flores-Hernandez C, et al. Accuracy of CT-based measurements of glenoid version for total shoulder arthroplasty. *J Shoulder Elbow Surg.* 2010;19(2):166–171.
48. Ganapathi A, McCarron JA, Chen X, et al. Predicting normal glenoid version from the pathologic scapula: a comparison of methods in 2- and 3-dimensional models. *J Shoulder Elbow Surg.* 2011;20(2):234–244.
49. Iannotti JP, Ricchetti ET, Rodriguez EJ, et al. Development and validation of a new method of 3-dimensional assessment of glenoid and humeral component position after total shoulder arthroplasty. *J Shoulder Elbow Surg Am.* 2013 ; doi:10.1016/j.jse.2013.01.005. [Epub ahead of print]
50. Yian EH, Werner CM, Nyffeler RW, et al. Radiographic and computed tomography analysis of cemented pegged polyethylene glenoid components in total shoulder replacement. *J Bone Joint Surg Am.* 2005;87(9):1928–1936.
51. Badet R, Boileau P, Noel E, et al. Arthrography and computed arthrotomography study of seventy patients with primary glenohumeral osteoarthritis. *Rev Rhum Engl Ed.* 1995;62(9):555–562.
52. Harryman DT II, Sidles JA, Harris SL, et al. The effect of articular conformity and the size of the humeral head component on laxity and motion after glenohumeral arthroplasty. *J Bone Joint Surg Am.* 1995;77:555–563.
53. Lapner LC, Sabri E, Rakhra K, et al. Comparison of lesser tuberosity osteotomy to subscapularis peel in shoulder arthroplasty: a randomized controlled trial. *J Bone Joint Surg Am.* 2012;94(24):2239–2246.
54. Gerber C, Yian EH, Pfirmann CA, et al. Subscapularis muscle function and structure after total shoulder replacement with lesser tuberosity osteotomy and repair. *J Bone Joint Surg Am.* 2005;14(2):128–133.

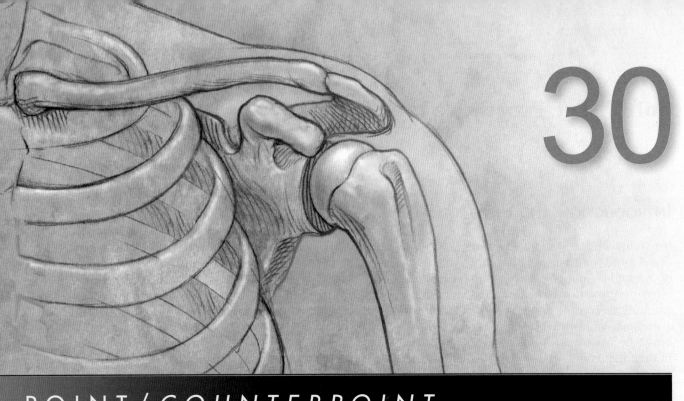

30

POINT/COUNTERPOINT

POSTERIOR INSTABILITY AFTER ANATOMIC ARTHROPLASTY

INTRODUCTION

Instability after arthroplasty is a not-uncommon complication. Approximately 2–3% of complications after Total Shoulder Arthroplasty (TSA) or Humeral Hemiarthroplasty (HHR) involve posterior dislocation or subluxation.

Although in most cases, revision of the component version is necessary, there are rare times when the components are perfectly positioned and the soft tissue envelope is the problem. In these cases, an arthroscopic tendon-capsule plication may restore stability. Occasionally, cruciate graft supplementation may be necessary. One of these soft tissue reconstruction techniques may be considered in instability cases with correct component positioning.

Soft Tissue Procedure Is Sufficient

Felix H. Savoie, III / Michael J. O'Brien

INTRODUCTION AND EPIDEMIOLOGY

Instability after total shoulder arthroplasty (TSA) is one of the more common complications, with an incidence of 2.8% (1). Although more common in the anterior direction, posterior instability may be more disabling and lead to eccentric glenoid wear. In addition, arthritis associated with posterior subluxation may not be corrected by a standard total shoulder replacement (2). In this chapter, we are going to look at the options for correction of posterior instability after TSA.

EVALUATION

In an unstable total shoulder, the first task is to evaluate the positioning of the components. In cases in which the source of the subluxation component is malalignment, soft tissue procedures are contraindicated until component malposition is corrected. Although it has often been recommended that in cases with preoperative glenoid retroversion, the humeral component may be anteverted to compensate for the deformity, it has been shown in literature that this is not really effective (3). Therefore, correct alignment of both the glenoid and humeral components is the most effective way to ensure the absence of instability (4). We have found CT scanning to be the best method of evaluation for component positioning. One simple option is to do a true anterior–posterior scapula view with the forearm stabilized in 20 degrees of external rotation. In this view, one should see the replaced glenohumeral joint as being perfectly aligned.

If the components are in correct position, posterior instability may occur due to soft tissue defects. The most common etiologies of soft tissue only induced instability are infraspinatus thinning and rotator interval laxity.

MANAGEMENT

There is a difference between posterior dislocation and posterior subluxation. A traumatic posterior dislocation may be managed by closed reduction and bracing in external rotation. The injured soft tissues may heal over a 4- to 6-week period of protection. Recurrent dislocation or subluxation will require more treatment.

POSTERIOR SUBLUXATION

In cases in which the components are correctly positioned, soft tissue reconstruction can be effective. Both arthroscopic and open surgical management can lead to satisfactory results. The key is to determine on the initial evaluation if the problem is the posterior soft tissues, the rotator interval, or both. Posterior soft tissue insufficiency (Fig. 30-1) is often more due to laxity in the infraspinatus and capsule combined. More commonly, widening of the rotator interval with concomitant laxity of the superior glenohumeral ligament (SGHL) and coracohumeral ligament (CHL) (Fig. 30-2) allows posterior subluxation to occur with resultant eccentric wear on the glenoid. Although it is more common to have stiffness due to rotator interval contracture, this subluxation can be both functionally disabling and lead to early prosthetic failure.

Posterior soft laxity is best corrected by plication sutures. These sutures are placed through both tendon and capsule, beginning laterally and extending medially until stability is restored. It is important to keep the arm in neutral rotation to prevent over tightening.

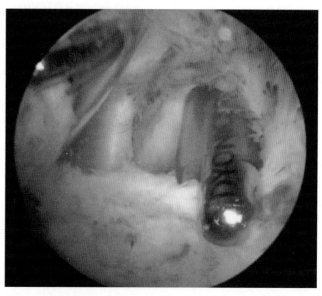

▲ FIGURE 30-1: The arthroscopic view of a posteriorly subluxated humeral head due to posterior soft tissue insufficiency is illustrated. Note the reflection of the glenoid on the prosthetic humeral head.

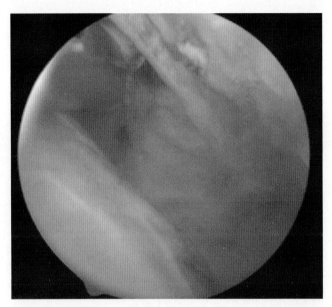

▲ **FIGURE 30-2:** An arthroscopic view of widening of the rotator interval with concomitant laxity of the SGHL and CHL. Note the reflection of the shaver on the humeral head.

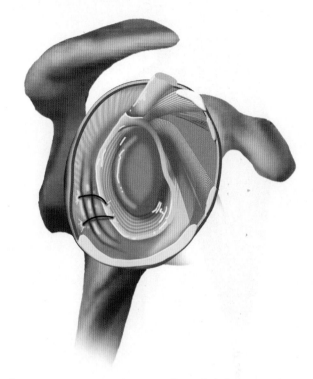

▲ **FIGURE 30-3:** Arthroscopically guided placement of a permanent stitch shuttled via a monofilament suture passer, retrieved, and then tied subacromially.

Technique 1: Arthroscopy

Initially, a diagnostic arthroscopy is performed in routine fashion to determine the amount of glenoid wear and to look for loosening. The arthroscope is then placed in the anterior portal to allow visualization of the posterior soft tissues. A spinal needle is introduced approximately 3 cm distal to the posterolateral corner of the acromion along the posterior edge of the humeral head. A No. 1 PDS (Ethicon, Somerville, NJ) suture is shuttled into the joint and then retrieved retrograde through the posterior cannula which is retracted outside the tendon of the infraspinatus and teres minor. A permanent stitch is shuttled via the PDS suture and then tied subacromially (Fig. 30-3). These steps are repeated moving medially until stability is restored. In most cases of posterior subluxation after arthroplasty, it will require four sutures.

Technique 2: Open

A small incision is made along the posterior acromion in line with the interval between the posterior and middle heads of the deltoid muscle. It is limited to 3 cm distal to the tip of the acromion to avoid injury to the axillary nerve. The two heads of the triceps are split, revealing the posterior rotator cuff musculature. At this point, you have two options. Option A involves simply placing vertical No. 5 Ethibond (Ethicon, Somerville, NJ) sutures through both capsule and tendon without taking down any tissue. These "double bites" allow an accordion effect to the posterior soft tissues similar to the arthroscopic technique, with restoration of stability. Option B involves a "T" split of

the soft tissues, with shifting of the inferior tendon and capsule superiorly and the double breasting of the superior flap over the inferior. This is more effective if there is lateral damage and less effective for general midjoint laxity (Fig. 30-4).

ROTATOR INTERVAL CLOSURE

In cases in which the subluxation is thought to be due to over release or failure of the rotator interval to heal, an interval plication can be performed either arthroscopically or open. The same spinal needle technique bridging supraspinatus to subscapularis as previously described can be performed using a monofilament suture shuttle. It is important in these cases to keep the arm externally rotated 90 degrees to prevent loss of external rotation. This may also be performed open through a small incision at the top of the deltopectoral interval (Fig. 30-5).

POSTERIOR DISLOCATION

In cases of posterior dislocation of the prosthesis, it is most important to evaluate the version of the components (Fig. 30-6). There is no soft tissue reconstruction that will correct for component malposition. However, in a case in which the components are

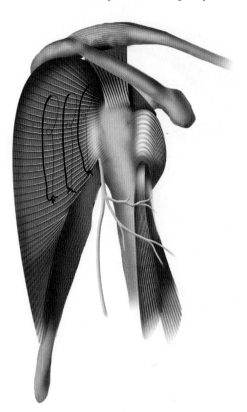

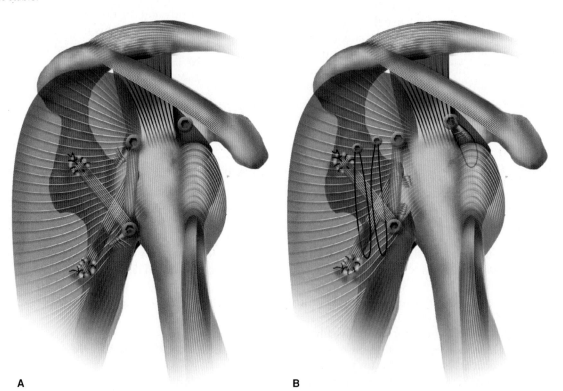

▲ **FIGURE 30-5:** The open approach to rotator interval closure is demonstrated.

▲ **FIGURE 30-4:** The open technique utilizes a mini open posterior–superior approach and then "double vertical passing" of the sutures beginning laterally and progressing medially until the shoulder is stable.

A   B

▲ **FIGURE 30-6:** The posterior graft placement approach is illustrated: The graft is fixated to the inferior glenoid neck using a suture anchor. It is pulled laterally and superiorly and sewn into the conjoined area of the supraspinatus and infraspinatus tendons. The graft is then brought directly inferiorly and sewn into the teres minor tendon. The remaining graft is then brought medially and superiorly and fixated to the superior glenoid neck via another suture anchor.

correctly positioned and there is a dislocation, allograft soft tissue supplementation may lead to creation of a stable joint. The technique for posterior stabilization is a modification of the anterior grafting technique described by Warren et al. (5). A semitendinosis allograft is used via a posterior approach. We favor the posterior deltoid split described above, but one can certainly utilize a more standard approach, provided one is cognizant of the position of the axillary nerve. Once the posterior capsule is exposed, a T-shaped horizontal split with a lateral–vertical incision is used to completely expose the posterior glenohumeral joint. The prosthesis is carefully inspected and correct component positioning confirmed. One end of the graft is then affixed to the glenoid neck at approximately the 7-o'clock posterior-inferior position. This is most easily accomplished by the use of a small double-loaded suture anchor. The graft is then retrieved laterally and superiorly on the humeral head with the arm in neutral rotation and sewn into the conjoined tendon of the posterior supraspinatus and anterior infraspinatus. The graft is then brought inferiorly and sewn into the upper tendon of the teres minor. The free end of the graft is then brought medially and an anchor placed into the upper medial glenoid neck at the 11-o'clock position (Fig. 30-6 A, B). This anchor is used to sew the remaining portion of the graft to the glenoid, creating an X pattern. The inferior limb of the T is then shifted superiorly and can be sewn into the residual infraspinatus tendon. The superior flap is then sewn into the residual teres minor tendon. Additional midmuscle plication stitches can be added as needed.

POSTOPERATIVE COURSE AND REHABILITATION

The patient is usually immobilized in an external rotation brace for 4 weeks for all of the soft tissue reconstructions. During this time frame, therapy is focused on scapular retraction, and hand, forearm, and elbow rehabilitation. At 4 weeks, a slow weaning from the sling along with gentle active-assistive range of motion (ROM) and supine active ROM is initiated, but the patient is asked to continue to sleep in the brace. At 8 weeks postoperative, more aggressive rehabilitation is started and continued until full function is restored.

RESULTS

Very limited results have been reported for this problem. In most cases, the results have been limited to two or three cases with satisfactory results. In our practice, the vast majority of instability cases have been due to component malpositioning and required revision arthroplasty (6).

COMPLICATIONS

The main complication is recurrence of instability. In these cases, there is either an unrecognized component malposition, or insufficient soft tissue or scapular control to maintain stability. Complete prosthetic revision or conversion to the inverse shoulder replacement is the main option for this problem.

Component Revision Is Necessary

Tom Lawrence / John Sperling

INTRODUCTION

Shoulder subluxation or dislocation is a well-recognized complication of anatomic shoulder arthroplasty. Nearly 30% of all complications associated with anatomic TSA relate to glenohumeral instability (7). The overall rate of instability after shoulder arthroplasty is 4.9% of which 20% of cases are posterior (8). As the number of shoulder arthroplasties performed each year is on the rise (9), the shoulder surgeon should have a clear understanding of how to manage the paralleled increased frequency of complications, including that of posterior instability.

ETIOLOGY

In patients with osteoarthritis of the glenohumeral joint, there frequently is contracture and tightening of the anterior capsule and subscapularis tendon, fixed posterior humeral head translation, posterior glenoid erosion, and posterior capsule laxity. Thus from the outset, patients undergoing anatomic TSA are predisposed to posterior instability and these factors need to be addressed to lessen the risk of postoperative posterior instability.

A common mistake during shoulder arthroplasty is not to adequately correct the glenoid retroversion which will promote early loosening via eccentric forces and predispose to posterior instability. Surgical options for preventing glenoid component retroversion and restoring neutral glenoid version include reaming down the high anterior side or structural posterior bone grafting (10). Augmented glenoid components have also been tried although the results have raised concerns regarding the ability to correct instability (11). Previously authors have suggested placing the humeral component in a more anteverted position although more recent biomechanical data has suggested that this does not increase the stability of a shoulder replacement (12).

In addition to correction of glenoid version, tight anterior soft tissues and posterior capsular laxity must be addressed during arthroplasty to provide soft tissue balance and minimize the risk of instability. A careful assessment of the shoulder should be performed at the time of surgery and a general rule is that posterior translation of the humeral head should not exceed 50% of the glenoid diameter. If the head does translate

over 50% and does not reduce spontaneously then this should raise concern and a posterior capsular plication may be performed provided the surgeon is confident that the components have been inserted with the correct version. Despite attempting to correct these factors, there remains a significant risk of posterior instability. In a series of 92 anatomic TSAs performed for patients with primary osteoarthritis and a biconcave glenoid, Walch et al. (13) reported that 5.5% of patients required revision for posterior instability. Hill and Norris (10) reported on 17 patients with abnormal preoperative glenoid version that despite correction of version using glenoid bone grafting and careful soft tissue balancing, 8 of the patients had some form of postoperative instability.

Posterior instability following shoulder arthroplasty may result from excessive humeral retroversion, glenoid retroversion, or failure to balance the soft tissues. Most authors, however, suggest that the etiology for posterior instability is most likely multifactoral in nature. Moeckel et al. (14) reported on three cases of posterior instability and found that retroversion of the glenoid and humeral component in combination with a tight subscapularis were causative factors. Wirth and Rockwood (15) published on seven cases of posterior instability, four of which demonstrated humeral retroversion greater than 80 degrees and four of which had significant posterior glenoid erosion. Sanchez-Sotelo et al. (16) reported on 33 shoulders with anterior (17) or posterior (14) instability. Based upon radiographic, clinical, and intraoperative findings, the authors attributed instability to abnormal soft tissue tension in 21 shoulders, component malpositioning in 1 shoulder, and a combination of factors in 11 cases. Excessive posterior capsular laxity was implicated in 10 of the 14 shoulders with posterior instability, one of which also had excessive anterior capsular tightness.

COMPONENT REVISION OPTIONS AND RESULTS OF TREATMENT

Surgical management of posterior instability after shoulder arthroplasty has traditionally involved improving component position and soft tissue balance including release of tight anterior structures and plication of the lax posterior capsule (15,18). When considering shoulder arthroplasty revision for posterior instability, the surgeon should have a thorough understanding of the factors that predispose to the problem to optimize the chance of a successful outcome. Few studies have reported on the results after revision for posterior instability after shoulder arthroplasty. Furthermore, due to the limited number of patients, these reports have combined anterior and posterior instability cases making the results more difficult to evaluate.

Moeckel et al. (14) reported on seven cases of anterior instability and three cases of posterior instability in a series of 236 TSAs. Revision surgery restored stability in all seven of the anteriorly unstable shoulders whereas of the three with posterior instability, only two were stable at follow-up. The final patient failed two revisions and eventually underwent component removal. In a multicenter study performed by Ahrens et al. (19) consisting of 29 patients with posterior instability, revision surgery was successful in only 53% of cases. In the Mayo clinic (16) series of revision procedures for instability, 8 of the 14 shoulders with posterior instability underwent posterior capsule plication. However, 7 of the 14 patients required additional revision surgery in an attempt to restore stability. The authors concluded that surgical treatment of instability after shoulder instability is associated with a moderately high failure rate.

The results of these studies suggest that the surgical treatment of posterior instability after shoulder arthroplasty with unconstrained anatomic components is associated with a significant failure rate, particularly when soft tissue procedures alone are performed. On this basis, reverse shoulder arthroplasty (RSA) has emerged as an attractive revision alternative. RSA provides increased stability due to greater constraint and conformity enhanced by the increased tension within the deltoid muscle which generates greater compressive forces across the glenohumeral joint. However, whilst a high rate of satisfactory results has been reported in patients with cuff-tear arthropathy, more modest results have been reported in the setting of revision arthroplasty (17).

Melis et al. (20) recently published a retrospective multicenter cohort study of 37 consecutive anatomical TSA revised to RSA with bone grafting for aseptic glenoid loosening or failure. Six (16%) of these patients had evidence of posterior shoulder instability. At a mean follow-up of 47 months, 86% of the total patient group was satisfied or very satisfied. The average Constant score increased from 24 to 55 and active anterior elevation from 68 to 121 degrees. Twenty-two of the 29 (76%) associated bone grafts were incorporated in the glenoid. Eight patients (21%) needed a subsequent reoperation because of recurrent or new complications. The authors concluded that despite high complication and reoperation rates, revision with RSA and bone grafting is a reliable option which provides the benefit both of glenoid bone stock reconstruction and of resolving soft tissue insufficiency and prosthetic instability. Walker et al. (21) performed a retrospective case series of 24 consecutive patients with failed TSA who were treated with conversion to RSA of which 19 were related to instability, 2 having posterior instability. The median total American Shoulder and Elbow Surgeons score improved from 38.5 preoperatively to 67.5, visual analog scale (VAS) pain scores decreased from 5 to 1.5 and function improved from 2 to 6.5. The median Simple Shoulder Test improved from 1 to 5. Fourteen patients rated their outcome as excellent, three as good, three as satisfactory, and two as unsatisfactory. The overall complication rate was 22.7% which included one patient with a postoperative dislocation. The authors concluded that RSA can be an effective treatment for failed TSA by decreasing pain and improving shoulder function although in the revision setting is associated with a higher complication rate.

Abdel et al. (22) recently presented results on 33 unstable anatomic shoulder arthroplasties that were revised to a reverse design of which two patients had posterior instability. Outcomes evaluated included VAS for pain, range of motion, shoulder stability, and Neer rating. The mean age of the patients at the time of revision surgery was 71 years. They were followed for a mean of 42 months (range, 25 to 71 months), or until revision surgery (one patient) or death (death patients). The average time from the index arthroplasty to revision was 26 months. Pain scores improved significantly as did mean active forward elevation from 40 to 97 degrees whereas there was no difference in internal or external rotation. At last follow-up, 31 shoulders (94%) were stable. The remaining two patients experienced dislocations, one at 2.5 weeks postoperatively and the other at 3 months postoperatively. According to the Neer rating system, there were 13 excellent, 10 satisfactory, and 10 unsatisfactory results. The authors concluded that revision to a reverse prosthesis reliably restores shoulder stability with improved pain and active elevation although the overall results are inferior to the outcome with RSA in cuff-tear arthropathy.

Whilst there is currently no literature available directly comparing the results of revision for instability using anatomic versus reverse techniques, these studies suggest that revision to RSA more predictably restores shoulder stability with better clinical outcomes compared to revision using anatomic components. It should be remembered that this is a complex patient group and that complication and revision rates remain high.

OPERATIVE TECHNIQUE

Preoperative Considerations

Prior to revision surgery, the patient must be fully evaluated with a history, clinical examination, and appropriate laboratory tests. In particular, infection should be excluded through the use of erythrocyte sedimentation rate, C-reactive protein, and differential white cell count. If there are any concerns then joint aspiration should be performed. The presence of active infection may necessitate a two-stage rather that one-stage revision procedure.

It is important to know the length of time that the shoulder has been dislocated. Revision for shoulders that have been dislocated for lengthy periods, are more likely to fail if anatomic arthroplasty is performed due to chronic adaptive soft tissue changes.

Previous operative reports should be accessed to confirm the index surgical approach, findings, and type of implant that was used. The surgeon needs to be familiar with the implant that is being revised and have available any necessary instruments to assist removal. A set of revision instruments is crucial to assist implant removal.

Radiographic evaluation should include a true antero-posterior view (Fig. 30-7), scapular Y view, and an axillary view. The degree of posterior subluxation can be determined on the axillary view and allows an initial assessment of the glenoid version (Fig. 30-8). A computed tomography (CT) scan is necessary to more accurately assess glenoid and humeral version, loosening of components, and glenoid bone stock. If

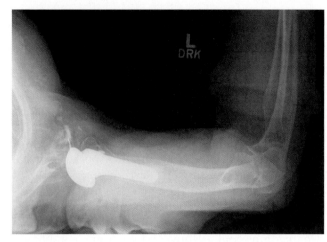

▲ **FIGURE 30-8:** Axillary radiograph of a posteriorly dislocated anatomic TSA. Note the excessively retroverted glenoid component.

abnormal glenoid or humeral version is detected on preoperative imaging studies and the shoulder has not been posteriorly dislocated for an excessive length of time, then the surgeon may consider revision using anatomic components. However, in cases of prolonged and refractory posterior dislocation, particularly where soft tissues and rotator cuff quality are poor or deficient, revision to a reverse arthroplasty is more appropriate (Figs. 30-9 and 30-10). If RSA is planned it is crucial to ensure adequate deltoid function as the RSA

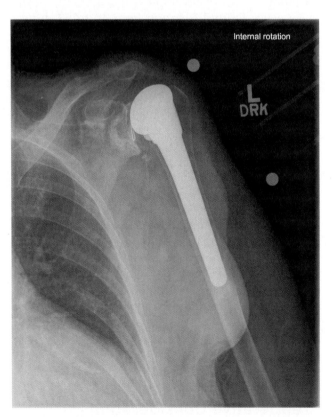

▲ **FIGURE 30-7:** AP radiograph of a posteriorly dislocated anatomic TSA.

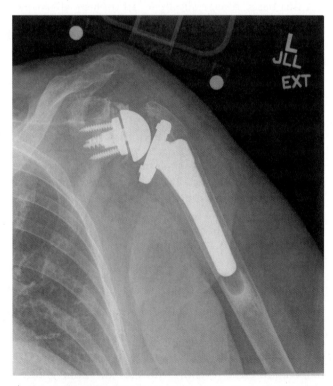

▲ **FIGURE 30-9:** AP radiograph demonstrating revision to RSA.

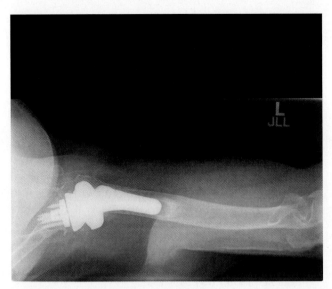

▲ **FIGURE 30-10:** Axillary radiograph demonstrating revision to RSA.

relies on the deltoid for stability and function of the joint.

Operative Technique—Revision to RSA

A deltopectoral approach is used in revision arthroplasty as this is an extensile internervous plane allowing potential access to the humeral shaft to assist with removal of the humeral component. The plane between the deltoid and the underlying humerus and rotator cuff is developed and scar tissue is removed allowing placement of a deltoid retractor to facilitate exposure. The anterior soft tissues are frequently adhered to the conjoint tendon and this interval is carefully developed to protect the axillary nerve. The subscapularis and anterior capsule, which may be deficient in revision cases, are released to allow delivery of the proximal humerus out of the wound.

The humeral component is now addressed having removed surrounding scar tissue and exposed the neck of the prosthesis. In most revision cases to RSA, the humeral component will need to be removed although there are modern platform systems now available that allow conversion of an unstable anatomic shoulder to a reverse without exchange of the humeral component. If the implant is modular, then the head is removed and subsequently the proximal bone-implant or cement-implant interface is disrupted with the use of fine high-speed burrs and narrow osteotomes to facilitate implant removal. A tamp or square-tipped impactor placed under the inferomedial aspect of the neck is struck with a mallet which in most cases will successfully extract the implant. In the situation

where this does not work, a cortical window (23) or osteotomy (24) is required which will later need fixation with cerclage wiring. If present, cement may need to be removed although this process is often difficult and time consuming and, therefore, provided there is no concern regarding infection, it is possible to leave the cement mantle and perform a cement-in-cement revision.

If revision is performed for a posteriorly dislocated anatomic TSA then the glenoid component is removed. For an all polyethylene glenoid that is well fixed, the component is cut into equal segments (typically nine) with a sagittal saw to allow piecemeal removal whilst minimizing damage to the underlying glenoid bone stock. The central peg or keel can then be extracted using a rongeur and the remaining cement mantle can be removed using osteotomes or a high-speed burr. Removal of metal-backed components can be associated with increased glenoid bone loss, so this should be done cautiously in a manner that preserves as much glenoid bone as possible.

Once the glenoid component has been removed, the glenoid should be carefully inspected to assess the location and extent of bone loss. Defects have been previously classified into central, peripheral, and combined which can be mild, moderate, or severe (25). Glenoid bone defects must be addressed to obtain secure fixation of the reverse baseplate and larger defects may require structural bone grafts or may even preclude implantation of a component. The guide pin is positioned in the appropriate location and reaming is kept to a minimum to maintain subchondral bone and allow seating of the baseplate. The baseplate is now secured in place in a standard fashion with a combination of central and peripheral screws. In the situation where bone stock is not deemed sufficient to allow for adequate fixation of the baseplate, bone graft can be placed with a view to performing a second procedure at a later date.

The glenosphere is inserted using the largest available diameter to enhance stability and lessen the chance of dislocation. The humerus is brought back out into the wound taking care not to get caught on the glenosphere in doing so. A trial liner is inserted on the trial humeral component, the shoulder reduced, and the stability and tension are assessed. The trials are now removed and the definitive implants inserted.

Routine closure is performed over a deep drain placed beneath the deltoid. The subscapularis and anterior soft tissue envelope are repaired if possible although frequently, in the revision setting, this is not feasible and the anterior tissues remain detached. The patient is placed in a shoulder immobilizer for up to 6 weeks after surgery and typically only passive motion is allowed during this time.

References

1. Field LD, Dines DM, Zabinski SJ, et al. Hemiarthroplasty of the shoulder for rotator cuff arthropathy. *J Shoulder Elbow Surg.* 1997;6(1):18–23.
2. Gerber C, Costouros JG, Sukthankar A, et al. Static posterior humeral head subluxation and total shoulder arthroplasty. *J Shoulder Elbow Surg.* 2009;18(4): 505–510. doi: 10.1016/j.jse.2009.03.003. Epub 2009 May 29.
3. Spencer EE Jr, Valdevit A, Kambic H, et al. The effect of humeral component anteversion on shoulder stability with glenoid component retroversion. *J Bone Joint Surg Am.* 2005;87(4):808–814.
4. Williams GR Jr, Wong KL, Pepe MD, et al. The effect of articular malposition after total shoulder arthroplasty on glenohumeral translations, range of motion, and subacromial impingement. *J Shoulder Elbow Surg.* 2001;10(5):399–409.
5. Warren RF, Coleman SH, Dines JS. Instability after arthroplasty: The shoulder. *J Arthroplasty.* 2002;17(4 suppl 1): 28–31.
6. Moeckel BH, Altchek DW, Warren RF, et al. Instability of the shoulder after arthroplasty. *J Bone Joint Surg Am.* 1993;75(4):492–497.
7. Chin PY, Spearling JW, Cofield RH, et al. Complications of total shoulder arthroplasty: Are they fewer or different? *J Shoulder Elbow Surgery.* 2006;15(1):19–22.
8. Bohsali KI, Wirth MA, Rockwood CA Jr. Complications of total shoulder arthroplasty. *J Bone Joint Surg Am.* 2006; 88(10):2279–2292.
9. Kim SH, Wise BL, Zhang Y, et al. Increasing incidence of shoulder arthroplasty in the United States. *J Bone Joint Surg Am.* 2011;93(24):2249–2254.
10. Hill JM, Norris TR. Long-term results of total shoulder arthroplasty following bone-grafting of the glenoid. *J Bone Joint Surg Am.* 2001;83-A(6):877–883.
11. Rice RS, Sperling JW, Miletti J, et al. Augmented glenoid component for bone deficiency in shoulder arthroplasty. *Clin Orthop Relat Res.* 2008;466(3):579–583.
12. Spencer EE Jr, Valdevit A, Kambic H, et al. The effect of humeral component anteversion on shoulder stability with glenoid component retroversion. *J Bone Joint Surg Am.* 2005;87(4):808–814.
13. Walch G, Moraga C, Young A, et al. Results of anatomic nonconstrained prosthesis in primary osteoarthritis with biconcave glenoid. *J Shoulder Elbow Surg.* 2012;21(11):1526–1533.
14. Moeckel BH, Altchek DW, Warren RF, et al. Instability of the shoulder after arthroplasty. *J Bone Joint Surg Am.* 1993;75(4):492–497.
15. Wirth MA, Rockwood CA Jr. Complications of total shoulder-replacement arthroplasty. *J Bone Joint Surg Am.* 1996;78(4):603–616.
16. Sanchez-Sotelo J, Sperling JW, Rowland CM, et al. Instability after shoulder arthroplasty: Results of surgical treatment. *J Bone Joint Surg Am.* 2003;85-A(4):622–631.
17. Boileau P, Watkinson DJ, Hatzidakis AM, et al. Grammont reverse prosthesis: Design, rationale, and biomechanics. *J Shoulder Elbow Surg.* 2005;14(1 suppl S):147S–161S.
18. Namba RS, Thornhill TS. Posterior capsulorrhaphy in total shoulder arthroplasty. A case report. *Clin Orthop Relat Res.* 1995;(313):135–139.
19. Ahrens P, Boileau P, Walch G. Posterior instability after unconstrained shoulder arthroplasty. In: Walch G, Boileau P, Molé D, eds. *2000 Shoulder Prostheses: Two to Ten Year Follow Up.* Montpellier, France: Sauramps Medical; 2001: 377–392.
20. Melis B, Bonnevialle N, Neyton L, et al. Glenoid loosening and failure in anatomical total shoulder arthroplasty: Is revision with a reverse shoulder arthroplasty a reliable option? *J Shoulder Elbow Surg.* 2012;21(3):342–349.
21. Walker M, Willis MP, Brooks JP, et al. The use of the reverse shoulder arthroplasty for treatment of failed total shoulder arthroplasty. *J Shoulder Elbow Surg.* 2012;21(4):514–522.
22. Abdel M, Hattrup SJ, Sperling JW, et al. Reverse shoulder arthroplasty for instability after anatomic arthroplasty, presented at AAOS annual meeting, February 16, 2011, San Diego.
23. Sperling JW, Cofield RH. Humeral windows in revision shoulder arthroplasty. *J Shoulder Elbow Surg.* 2005;14(3): 258–263.
24. Johnston PS, Creighton RA, Romeo AA. Humeral component revision arthroplasty: Outcomes of a split osteotomy technique. *J Shoulder Elbow Surg.* 2012;21(4):502–506.
25. Antuna SA, Sperling JW, Cofield RH, et al. Glenoid revision surgery after total shoulder arthroplasty. *J Shoulder Elbow Surg.* 2001;10(3):217–224.

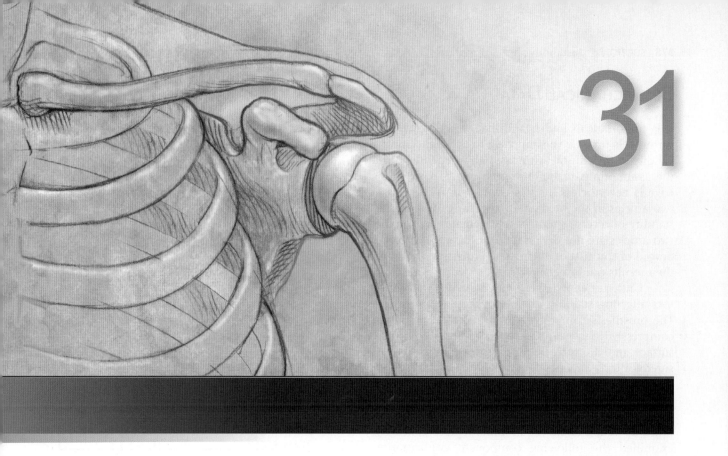

31

Dislocation and Instability in Reverse Shoulder Arthroplasty: Biomechanics, Prevention, Review of the Literature, and Management

Ioannis P. Pappou / Matthew J. Teusink /
Mark A. Frankle

INTRODUCTION

Instability after reverse shoulder arthroplasty (RSA) is reported to happen in 2.4% to 31% of cases (1). It represents the most common complication intrinsic to RSA after the exclusion of hematomas which are nonspecific and occur in up to 21% (2). The purpose of this chapter is to review the biomechanical studies pertinent to the stability of reverse shoulder prostheses, review the literature on instability after reverse shoulder replacement, and finally to discuss its management. Little has been written explicitly about the management of instability after reverse shoulder replacement. The best treatment is prevention and hence a considerable portion of the chapter will be dedicated to the principles surrounding instability prevention. This chapter does not address mechanical component dissociation.

BIOMECHANICAL DATA

It is important to understand that while biomechanical models provide valuable data to the clinician, their validity in the clinical setting is highly dependent upon the assumptions made during testing. A basic knowledge is nevertheless mandatory. Herein we review the two articles in the literature that focus on the intrinsic stability of reverse shoulder replacements. While these two articles are not performed in cadavers and may be devoid of soft tissues, their strength lies in the fact that their results can be generalized.

Gutierrez et al. (3) examined the hierarchy of factors affecting stability of reverse shoulder prostheses. The prosthesis components were mounted in sleds, a compressive load was applied perpendicular to the joint surface and the force required to dislocate was measured for three independent variables: (1) the compressive force, (2) the humerosocket depth (d), and (3) the glenosphere radius (R). This is a well-validated method that has been applied to the study of native shoulder joints as well as anatomic shoulder replacements. They examined the following component configurations: Encore DJO glenosphere 32, 36, 40 mm and Delta III glenosphere 36 mm with standard as well as semiconstrained humerosockets, accounting for eight implant configurations. They also fabricated three pairs of congruent glenospheres and humerosockets out of Delrin to investigate the effect of increasing glenosphere size while keeping the humerosocket depth to socket radius (d/R) stable. The d/R ratio directly expresses the intrinsic articular surface constraint. The results of this study are summarized in Figure 31-1.

The hierarchy of factors was led by compressive force followed by socket depth; glenosphere size played a much lesser role in stability of the RSA device. Similar results were predicted by a mathematical model, suggesting the stability was determined primarily by compressive forces generated by muscles. Measurement of joint resistance to dislocation provides quantitative support to the general concept that RSA devices are much more stable than the normal glenohumeral joint and total shoulder arthroplasty (TSA) devices. The normal glenohumeral joint has a stability force ratio (maximum allowable subluxation force/joint compression force) of approximately 0.5, whereas TSA has less than 1. In contrast, RSA has a stability force ratio greater than 2 and is thus intrinsically more than twice as stable as an anatomic total shoulder.

Favre et al. (4) have investigated the effect of glenoid and humeral component versions on resistance to anterior dislocation of the Delta III reverse prosthesis. They mounted a 36-mm standard prosthesis on specially designed sleds, loaded the joint axially with 40 N and examined the stability force ratio, similar to Gutierrez by

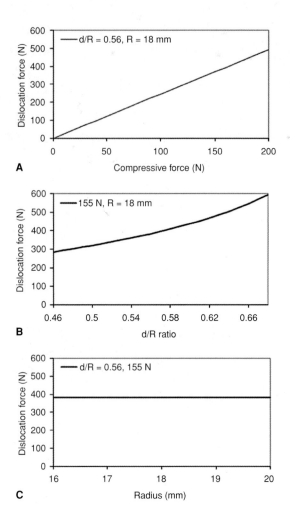

▲ **FIGURE 31-1:** The graphs show the trends present when the analytical model for RSA stability is used to calculate dislocation force. **A:** Force required to dislocate the glenosphere from the humerosocket increases linearly as a function of increasing the compressive load. **B:** Force required to dislocate the glenosphere from the humerosocket increases exponentially as a function of increasing the depth of the humerosocket, represented by the d/R ratio. **C:** Force required to dislocate the glenosphere from the humerosocket remains constant as a function of increasing the radius of the glenosphere. (With kind permission from: Springer Science+Business Media, Clinical Orthopaedics and Related Research and Gutierrez S, Keller TS, Levy JC, et al. Hierarchy of stability factors in reverse shoulder arthroplasty. *Clin Orthop Relat Res.* 2008;466:670–676.)

varying the humeral and glenoid component versions. Two positions were tested; the resting position in 20 degrees of abduction and the abducted position of 60-degree glenohumeral elevation. The latter position was selected to simulate the clinical 90-degree humerothoracic abduction.

In 90 degrees of abduction (i.e., 60 degrees of glenohumeral abduction), no significant influence of the glenosphere version was detected but the effect of humeral component version was highly significant. On average, a change of 10 degrees in humeral component version affected the stability ratio by 21%, whereas an identical alteration in glenoid component version induced a change of the stability ratio of 5%. The standard implant

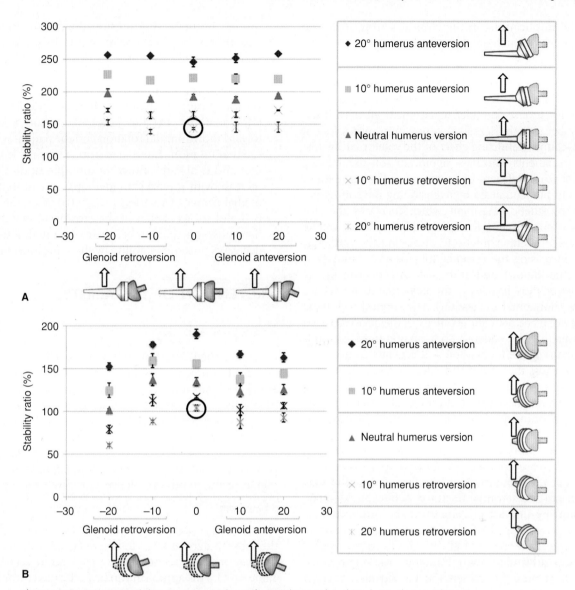

▲ **FIGURE 31-2:** Stability ratios (vertical axis) for **(A)** the simulated 90-degree humerothoracic abduction and **(B)** the resting positions, for the full range of tested glenoid (horizontal axis) and humeral (different points series) component versions. The small drawings represent a cranial view of the testing configuration. Only the dislocating force is drawn (*arrow*). The compressive component is not shown but was present in all cases, pressing the glenoid against the humeral component. The encircled data point represents the standard configuration with the glenoid in neutral version and humeral component in 20-degree retroversion. (Reprinted from: Favre P, Sussmann PS, Gerber C. The effect of component positioning on intrinsic stability of the reverse shoulder arthroplasty. *J Shoulder Elbow Surg.* 2010;19:550–556, with permission from Elsevier.)

configuration yielded the second worst stability ratio of all tested configurations and could only be increased by anteverting the humeral component. The results are summarized in Figure 31-2.

Significant differences in the stability ratio in the resting arm position were also reached for all changes in versions of the humeral component. For the version of the glenosphere, significant differences were reached when the 20-degree glenoid retroversion data were compared to 10-degree retroversion and to neutral glenosphere version. On average, a change of 10 degrees

in humeral or glenoid component version affected the stability ratio by 27% and 15%, respectively. Compared with the standard implant configuration, the stability ratio could only be increased by anteverting the humeral component but could be reduced by retroverting the glenoid component. The stability ratio was higher in the 90-degree abducted position than for the corresponding configurations in the resting position. When both components were in neutral position, the stability ratio was 193% in 90 degrees of arm abduction and 135% for the resting arm position.

The implications in the clinical setting from the basic science research are the following.

1. Compressive forces across the joint are of paramount importance for stability. Patients who suffer from rotator cuff insufficiency and are considered to be candidates for reverse shoulder replacement all have instability because the so called concavity-compression or force-couple stabilizing effect of the rotator cuff is lost (5). In patients who have significant soft tissue laxity (either from deficient or ineffective cuff musculature) this can be neutralized by retensioning the soft tissues with prosthetic placement which increases the distance of the humerus to the scapula. Tensioning can be achieved by either inferiorly displacing the humerus, thus increasing the acromial-tuberosity distance (vertical translation) and/or by laterally displacing the humerus, thus increasing the glenoid tuberosity distance (horizontal translation). The surgical technique of device placement, the geometry of the device selected and altering the patient's bony anatomy are methods of manipulating the tension and generate compressive forces across the reverse shoulder articulation. We will review this in detail in the section on treatment.

   Although Grammont and Baulot (6) advocate overtensioning the deltoid by translating the humerus inferiorly by as much as 3.8 cm (7), this may in fact have deleterious effects. Excessive soft tissue tension may decrease the passive motion, place excessive loads at the bone implant interface and finally may predispose to acromial fractures. Achieving adequate tension by inferior placement of the humerus may predispose to brachial plexus palsy (8) and acromial fractures. Lädermann et al. (9) identified no clinical motion advantage with humeral overlengthening, but shortening the humerus had a detrimental effect on range of motion outcomes.

   The ideal soft tissue to avoid instability and minimize complication from overtensioning is restoration of the natural, anatomic deltoid length. Basic science has long elucidated the deleterious effects of under- or overtensioning a muscle on its force generation potential by moving it out of the optimal range in the Blix curve. The Blix curve describes muscle force generated as a product of pretension and has shown that maximal force developing capacity occurs at the actin–myosin maximal overlap, which is at resting muscle length.

2. Increasing the constraint is an option to increase joint stability—the price paid is decrease in the impingement-free range of motion, although the relationship of constraint and motion may be more complex than in the hip joint (10). Impingement in and by itself may lever the component out of place (11).

3. Increasing the component size does not increase intrinsic joint stability per se. In the clinical scenario

though by increasing tension on the soft tissues it will increase compressive forces on the joint.

4. Manipulation of the component version is an option to increase resistance to anterior dislocation, specifically increasing humeral anteversion. Glenoid retroversion should be avoided. There is price to altering joint anatomy: (a) the range of motion is shifted toward more internal rotation and the patient will lose external rotation. External rotation clinically is important and is already shown in multiple studies not to increase with reverse shoulder replacement that has a medial center of rotation (2,12); (b) by virtue of the ball and socket design of the prosthesis, any component position change that increases anterior stability, decreases posterior stability by the same amount.

PREVENTION OF INSTABILITY

Preoperatively

Optimal patient selection will optimize clinical results or at the very minimum explain to the patient that they are at risk for dislocations if following conditions are noted: Alcoholism, substance abuse, documented noncompliance, severe bone loss compromising secure component fixation and ability to restore soft tissue tension. Assessment of the deltoid function is imperative. Revision surgery is associated with higher dislocation rates in the literature and in our experience which we review below.

Approach

The use of a superolateral approach to avoid violation of the subscapularis appears to be associated with decreased dislocation rates (see review of the literature section and Table 31-1). This approach can be performed through the superior rotator cuff defect thereby minimizing violation of the soft tissue. However, disadvantages include more difficult inferior glenoid exposure, deltoid dehiscence postoperatively, lack of subscapularis tendon excursion, potential for axillary nerve injury, and an increased rate of scapular notching resulting from use of the more difficult inferior exposure (24,48). We use the deltopectoral approach due to its extensile nature, ability to use in revision cases especially when humeral component removal is necessitated through osteotomy, and finally superior visualization of the inferior glenoid enabling us to more accurately place the components. In fracture cases it is not as critical which approach is used, since the subscapularis is left attached to the lesser tuberosity fragment. In summary, the surgeon should use the approach that he is most familiar with, will give him the best visualization with the least amount of morbidity, will allow him to accurately place the components and in case of fracture to manipulate fracture fragments.

(text continues on page 384)

TABLE 31-1 Review of the Literature

	Year	Authors	N	Age (yrs)	f/u (mos)	D/L	SS rep	Subsc+	Subsc−	Approach	Infect	MRCT	CTA	Rev	FS	OA	RA	Fx
1	2012	Hattrup et al. (13)	19	70	37	1	7/19			DP	0/1						19a	
2	2012	Walker et al. (14)	22	68	39.6	1				DP	0/1			22				
3	2012	Willis et al. (15)	16	65	37	0				DP					16			
4	2012	Garrigues et al. (16)	11	80.5	43.2	0				DP								11
5	2012	Clark et al. (17)	120	68.5	13.2	5	65/120	2/65	3/55	DP		32	39	20	7			21
6	2011	Gallo et al. (11)	57	66	18.8	9				DP	4/9		36	18	3			
7	2011	Ekelund and Nyberg (18)	27	68	56	0	0/18			AL prim + DP rev	0/0			9			18	
8	2011	Trappey et al. (19)	212 Pri	66	24	11 Pri	161/284	1/161	14/123	DP 282, AL 2	n/a but 3 rsxn	25	119		25	13	5	16
8	2011	Trappey et al. (19)	72 Rev			6 Rev				DP in all REV				72				
9	2011	Sadoghi et al. (20)	68	66	42	0				DP		68						
10	2011	Nolan et al. (21)	71	74	24	2	70/71			DP			71					
11	2011	Cazeneuve and Cristofari (22)	35	75	86	4				AL								35
12	2011	Austin et al. (23)	28 Pri	72.3	16.4	1				DP 10, SUP 15			23		4			
12	2011	Austin et al. (23)	28 Rev	71.2	20.8	0				DP				28				

(continued on page 382)

TABLE 31-1 Review of the Literature (continued)

	Year	Authors	N	Age (yrs)	f/u (mos)	D/L	SS rep	Subsc+	Subsc−	Approach	Infect	MRCT	CTA	Rev	FS	OA	RA	Fx
13	2011	Naveed et al. (24)	49	81	39	0				DP 38, AL 12			49					
14	2011	Valenti et al. (25)	76	73	44	0				AL		17	56					
15	2011	Young et al. (26)	10	77	22	0				DP							10	
16	2010	Muieri et al. (27)	60	71	52	1				DP		60						
17	2010	Holcomb et al. (28)	21	70.4	36	0				DP							21	
18	2009	Young et al. (29)	49	78.9	38	1				DP 43, SUP 6		2	19	4	8	14	1	
19	2009	Wierks et al. (30)	20	73	9	2				DP			16	4				
20	2009	Holcomb et al. (31)	14	70.6	33	2				DP				14				
21	2009	Edwards et al. (32)	138	68	36	7	62/138	0/62	7/76	DP		10	60	33	21		5	
22	2009	Gallinet et al. (33)	19	74	12.4	0				DP								19
23	2009	Grassi et al. (34)	26	42	42	1				DP = 11, L = 15		2		3	3			
24	2008	Klein et al. (35)	20	74.8	33.2	2				AL								20
25	2008	Cuff et al. (36)	96	72	27.5					DP		96						
26	2007	Wall et al. (12)	191	72.7	39.9	15	137	"No diff"	"No diff"	DP		34	59	45		53	1	2
27	2007	Levy et al. (37)	29	69	"24 min"	5	69/69			DP				29				
28	2007	Gohlke and Rolf (38)	34	68	31.5	3				DP				34				

#	Year	Author	N	Age	Follow-up	D/L				Approach							
29	2007	Levy et al. (39)	19	72	44	0				DP			19				19
30	2007	Bufquin et al. (40)	43	78	22	1				DP 23, AL 20							
31	2006	Frankle et al. (41)	62	71	33	0				DP		62					
32	2006	Boileau et al. (42)	45	72.2	40	3				DP 41, AL 5	21	19	5				
33	2005	Werner et al. (2)	58	68	38	5				DP	19	17	21	1			
34	2004	Vanhove and Beugnies (43)	14	71	31	0				AL	14						
35	2003	Woodruff et al. (44)	13	64	87	0				DP						17	
36	2001	Rittmeister Kerschbaumer (45)	8	60.25	54.3	0				AL 5							8
37	2001	Jacobs et al. (46)	7	72	16	0				AL	7						
38	2001	De Wilde et al. (47)	5	34–73	"23–39"	0				Clavicle ostoetomy			5				
TOTAL			1912			92 4.8%	571/856 66.7%	3/288 1%	24/254 9.5%		400	652	385	88	80	105	124

Patient in Hattrup's series has inflammatory arthritis but not RA.

Patients ultimately were infected and treated with resection arthroplasty.

N, number of shoulders; Pri, primary cases; Rev, revision cases; D/L, dislocations; SS repair, documented repair of the subscapularis; Subscap +, number of dislocations in cases with repaired subscapularis; Subscap −, number of dislocations in cases with unrepaired or irreparable subscapularis.

Approach: DP, deltopectoral; AL, deltoid split; Sup, deltoid split and detachment of anterior deltoid from acromion.

Infect, coexistence of infection in cases of instability.

Indications are broken down into the following categories: MRCT, massive rotator cuff tears; CTA, cuff tear arthropathy; Rev, revision of previous implant; hemi or total to reverse arthroplasty; FS, fracture sequelae; OA, osteoarthritis with large cuff tear; RA, rheumatoid; Fx, acute proximal humerus fracture.

Component Placement to Avoid Impingement

Decreasing impingement may decrease instability rates. Gutierrez et al. (49) have investigated the hierarchy of factors affecting impingement-free abduction range of motion and have found that lateralizing the center-of-rotation offset from 0 to 10 mm to be the most important factor, followed by inferior positioning of the glenoid, inferior glenosphere tilt, humeral neck-shaft angle, and prosthetic size. Some authors recommend inferior placement of Grammont style prostheses with overhang of the metaglene to avoid notching and adduction deficit (50). This may have deleterious effects at the bone implant interface by decreasing the surface area available for ingrowth and concentrating the stresses on a smaller surface. It lengthens the arm by displacing the humerus distally.

In order to avoid an adduction deficit due to inferior impingement, the hierarchy of component placement is somewhat different. The most important is a humeral component that most resembles an anatomic neck-shaft angle (130 degrees as opposed to more valgus neck shaft of 150 degrees), inferior position and inferior tilting of the glenosphere relative to the glenoid bony surface and finally humeral socket depth (49).

Placing the glenosphere component with a 15-degree inferior tilt has been shown to increase compressive forces on the baseplate–bone interface and should thus maximize implant longevity and osseous ingrowth (51,52).

Optimizing Soft Tissue Tension

Compressive forces across the joint are very important for stability. The two basic ways to increase them are to displace the humerus laterally in relation to the scapula and inferiorly in relation to the acromion. We will review in the treatment section how the surgeon can exploit component position, technique, and osseous anatomy to achieve the desired result adjusting it to the situation at hand. Intraoperatively, assuming that the reconstruction has produced optimal soft tissue tension the question begets: How does one assess tension in RSA? The constrained design of the joint obviates the traditional assessment of humeral head translation on the glenoid.

Intraoperative Assessment of Soft Tissue Tension

Several authors have described their technique of achieving optimal soft tissue length and judging joint stability intraoperatively. Boileau et al. (42) has described observing tension on the conjoint tendon—this technique is subjective and requires experience. Lädermann et al. (53) described a radiographic method of determining optimal deltoid tension based on humeral length by determining the length of the contralateral humerus preoperatively on scaled radiographs. Trappey et al. (19) use intraoperative trialing to assess soft tissue tension. They place incrementally sized polyethylene spacers on the humeral component until axial motion between the glenosphere and the humeral component is less than 2 mm with longitudinal traction.

Seitz (54) recommends firm two-thumbs pressure to obtain a reduction followed by a difficult three-finger uncoupling using the thumbs and index and middle finger in opposite directions to obtain uncoupling. This degree of stable coupling should allow a "rubbery tension" on the deltoid. Trial implants with varied thickness spacers should be tested sequentially until a secure, stable reduction is achieved with retentive (semiconstraint) liners to afford greater stability if necessary.

Our technique is tailored to the amount of preoperative bony deformity as reported by Klein et al. (55). Glenosphere selection is based, first, on the presence of a glenoid defect and, second, on the ability of the components to provide stability without restricting motion. In the presence of a glenoid defect, a larger glenosphere was selected for 46% (26/56) of shoulders to adequately cover the defect. In glenoids without bone loss, a smaller size (32 mm [−4-mm offset], which has a 6-mm center of rotation lateral to the glenoid surface, for female patients and 32 mm [neutral offset], which has a 10-mm center of rotation lateral to the glenoid surface, for male patients) is routinely used. We place the glenosphere to match the 135-degree neck cut of the humerus. We then place the humerosocket in such a way to closely mimic the anatomic head cut; that is, the top of the humerosocket to the tuberosity distance is minimal. Much of this process is done visually, as we inspect the native relationship of the lateral offset of the humerus with respect to the glenoid. After examining this, we select a glenosphere and humeral socket size that reproduces this spatial relationship. Because of the semiconstrained nature of the implant, we do not use the usual methods that are employed to assess stability in an anatomic shoulder arthroplasty, such as evaluating the amount of humeral translation. To ensure that there is minimal postoperative stiffness, we assess the ease with which the articulation reduces. It should not take great force or manipulation of the arm to relocate the humerus for trialing.

During trialing, the arm should easily forward elevate overhead without forceful effort or osseous impingement, yet the articulation should be stable on both internal and external rotations without the subscapularis in place. There should be sufficient laxity for the surgeon to slide his/her index finger over the lip of the socket and, by applying a laterally directed force to the socket and extending the humerus, easily dissociate the components. Trialing is used as a second confirmation of our choice to ensure that the joint remains located throughout a range of motion. We feel that the actual soft tissue tension required is variable between individuals and do not typically rely as heavily on this aspect.

REVIEW OF THE LITERATURE

We performed a literature search on PubMed using the terms "reverse shoulder arthroplasty," "reverse shoulder replacement," and "reverse shoulder prosthesis.". Nonclinical articles were discarded. Duplicate series using the same pool of patients were discarded and only the ones with latest follow-up were used. Multicenter studies were excluded if individual surgeons published newer, larger series with their personal results thus avoiding using a common pool of patients. Series with incomplete description of the complications and no clinical outcome were excluded (including the large series by Farshad and Gerber (56), where 11 dislocations out of 341 cases were reported for a 3.1% incidence). Finally by review of each individual article and their reference list we ensured that the literature list was up to date and complete. Grammont and Baulot's (6) seminal article had poor description of his patient population and methods; no dislocations were reported. Their two follow-up articles were unavailable to us after attempts to directly access that journal and interlibrary loan request (57,58). Series exclusively on tumor reconstruction were excluded since this subset of patients has many peculiarities and the series are small.

The results are summarized in Table 31-1. These are all level IV or retrospective series, no meta-analysis is possible, only a systematic review. We identified *1.912 cases* in this review, which is the largest to date and found a cumulative dislocation incidence of *92/1912 or 4.8%.* We specifically sought out to investigate if the specific diagnosis or at least revision versus primary arthroplasty plays a role, what is the effect of subscapularis repair and approach and whether coexistence of infection and dislocation was documented in other series. We also wanted to extract data on the dislocation direction since it is poorly described in clinical series but biomechanical data suggest that RSA may be more prone to lateral dislocations (59). Finally we wanted to investigate the treatment described by other authors.

Meaningful analysis of the dislocation incidence in primary versus revision RSA and among the various indications for RSA was precluded by incomplete reporting by most authors. In series comparing primary to revision cases Trappey et al. (19) documented higher dislocation rates in revision versus primary cases (8.3% vs. 5.2%) without statistical significance; Austin et al. (23) reported low rates in both revision and primary cases (0% and 3.6%); Wall et al. (12) reported significantly higher rates of dislocation in revision (37% vs. 13%). Meaningful analysis of the dislocation rates

comparing various indications was impossible due to incomplete reporting.

The data on the effect of subscapularis repair on postoperative dislocation rates is conflicting with some studies showing a clear benefit (19,32) and others showing no benefit (12,17) in repair, but overall favor repairing the subscapularis (Table 31-1). Our review of the literature revealed a 1% incidence of dislocation in cases with documented subscapularis repair versus 9.5% in cases where the tendon was not repaired or was irreparable. A complete release or tenotomy of the subscapularis and release of the underlying middle and inferior glenohumeral during exposure of the glenoid predisposes the shoulder to anterior instability during deltopectoral approaches and we hence recommend that every effort should be made to repair the subscapularis.

The anterolateral approach seems to be related with low incidence of dislocation in series where it is used explicitly. Incomplete reporting in series where both approaches were used precludes statistical analysis. Moreover, many series use it for fractures, which represent a distinct clinical entity; the subscapularis is attached to the lesser tuberosity and the surgeon works through the fracture line. Hence, in fractures there is no theoretical benefit of the deltopectoral versus anterolateral approach.

Table 31-2 summarizes the data on the timing, etiology, and treatment of dislocations in the literature whenever reported.

MANAGEMENT OF INSTABILITY/ DISLOCATION AFTER RSA

Little has been written about best evidence on management of postoperative instability.

The first step is to ascertain if there is any identifiable cause of dislocation. Examples are patient activity/compliance, implant malposition, bone or soft tissue deficiency, and the result of inadequate surgical technique. The direction of instability is usually anterior-lateral and occurs following extension, adduction, and internal rotation. The surgeon needs to rule out infection by laboratory tests (ESR, CBC, CRP) and if necessary joint aspiration. The treatment strategy in the case of documented infection is geared toward infection eradication. There is no standardized treatment with one or two stage protocols in RSA and in fact, several studies found favorable results with component retainment and one-stage debridement/mobile component exchange in infected RSA (60,61).

If the humeral and glenoid components appear to be well fixed but dissociated, an attempt at closed reduction in the office is often possible without sedation or any anesthesia. Axillary nerve/deltoid dysfunction should be assessed before and after reduction. The shoulder is then taken through a range of motion and stability is assessed.

TABLE 31-2 Summary of Treatment on Dislocations (D/L)

	Year	Authors	D/L	Closed	Stable	OR	OR/pt	Comments on Etiology and Final Outcome
1	2012	Hattrup et al. (13)	1	1/1	1/1	—	—	Stable
2	2012	Walker et al. (14)	1	1/1	1/1	—	—	Early (5 wks), stable
5	2012	Clark et al. (17)	5	5	0	5	n/a	No information on timing, outcome, and what operative treatment
6	2011	Gallo et al. (11)	9	n/a	n/a	9	1.6	All 9 had an abnormal of subscapularis tendon (3 absent, 6 intact or partially torn of moderate or poor quality). Superior metaglene tilt: 2, superior metaglene position: 3, Greater tuberosity compromised in 4/9. All 6 dislocations within 6 mos. 4/9 (44%) had concurrent infection, 3 with *Propionibacterium acnes*. Final outcome: 3 chronic dislocations, 3 explants, 3 stable
8	2011	Trappey et al. (19)	11 Pri	8/11	3/8	3/11	1.2	9/11 within 8 wks. 7 stable, 2 resection arthroplasty, 2 continued instability
8	2011	Trappey et al. (19)	6 Rev	4/6	1/4	2/6	1.4	6/6 within 6 wks. 4 stable, 1 resected, 1 dislocated/infected
10	2011	Nolan et al. (21)	2	2/2	2/2	—	—	One patient dislocated on OR day, reduced stable. Second dislocation at 33 mos, subluxing but patient satisfied, no further treatment
11	2011	Cazeneuve and Cristofari (22)	4	0/4	0/4	4	n/a	3/4 excised portion of greater tuberosity that was impinging, these shoulders were then stable. 1/4 was revised due to excessive humeral component anteversion
12	2011	Austin et al. (23)	1 Pri	—	—	1	—	Stable after surgery
16	2010	Mulieri et al. (27)	1	1/1	1/1	—	—	Stable
18	2009	Young et al. (29)	1	1/1	1/1	—	—	Early post-op after a fall, stable
19	2009	Wierks et al. (30)	2	—	—	—	—	No discussion
20	2009	Holcomb et al. (31)	2	—	—	1	1	Larger glenosphere, stable
21	2009	Edwards et al. (32)	7	2/7	2/2	5	1	All within 2 mos, all stable
23	2009	Grassi et al. (34)	1	1/1	1/1	—	—	Stable
24	2008	Klein et al. (35)	2*	2	1/2	—	—	Same patient had two dislocations on post-op day 9 and 10. Stable after second reduction
25	2008	Cuff et al. (36)	4	4	1/4	2	1	1/4 early, 3 happened at 3, 7 and 27 mos post-op. 3/4 stable ultimately. 1 chronic dislocation, not revised due to health and low function
26	2007	Wall et al. (12)	15	—	—	—		No discussion
27	2007	Levy et al. (37)	5	2/4	0/2	—	—	Very complex patients. 1 dislocation at 25 mos, reduced and stable. One patient had two dislocations, reduced and stable at last follow-up, later diagnosed with dystonia. One dislocation at 8 mos required open reduction. One patient had a postoperative dislocation, stable postreduction and then redislocated after a massive stroke; painless and satisfied hence no treatment. Last patient had multiple previous surgeries; 4 mos after revision RSA had dislocation, rerevised, was unstable and unsatisfied ultimately
28	2007	Gohlke and Rolf (38)	3	—	—	3	1	Stable after surgery
31	2006	Boileau et al. (42)	3	—	—	3	1	Stable after surgery
32	2007	Bufquin et al. (40)	1	—	—	—	—	Atraumatic anterior dislocation at 6 wks. No pain, no intervention
33	2005	Werner et al. (2)	5	—	1	4	1	Three patients stable after lateralization, 1 converted to hemi, 1 closed reduction all stable at final follow-up

Closed, patients where closed treatment was attempted; Stable, successful closed treatment; OR, patients ultimately requiring surgery; OR/pt, average number of procedures per patient of those patients who ultimately required surgery; until stable or final outcome (resection or unstable/infected).

If the shoulder is stable with the arm at the side and can allow hand-to-mouth motion with a reduction performed without anesthesia, closed treatment is initiated. The shoulder is immobilized in an abduction/external rotation sling for a minimum of 6 weeks. Extension, adduction, and internal rotation are avoided. If the reduction in the office fails, a closed reduction in the OR is attempted next. It has been our experience however that closed reductions under anesthesia have not been possible except for one case. The surgeon must therefore be prepared to perform an open reduction and if necessary revision of components if the dislocation is irreducible or unstable.

The guidelines below are also applicable in cases of infection after excisional debridement and mobile or total component exchange.

In the case of an open reduction the surgeon needs to assess soft tissue tension, mechanical impingement (osseous or soft tissue), bony deficiency, and erroneous version of the prosthesis which are amenable to a mechanical solution by appropriate component revision.

In the setting of correctly positioned components and appropriate soft tissue tension it has been our experience that inferior soft tissue impingement is the most likely cause of instability. A critical portion of the open reduction is thus removal of all the soft tissue surrounding the inferior half of glenosphere. Removal of soft tissue from the axillary pouch can be difficult, especially in the revision setting in a patient with scarring and heterotopic bone but is critical and should be performed. The surgeon should be cognizant of the axillary nerve by palpation, exposure, or nerve monitoring.

Finally, if no specific disorder is appreciated or in the case of generalized decoaptation (generalized soft tissue laxity as first described by Grammont), increasing soft tissue tension will lead to increased compres-

sive forces. A more constraint humerosocket may also be used as it provides added stability.

Table 31-3 provides a list of how the surgeon can exploit various techniques to alter soft tissue tension and tailor it to the clinical situation at hand. Figure 31-3

TABLE 31-3   Surgical and Implant Factors That Can Help Restore Soft Tissue Tension

Prosthetic Factors
- Varying glenosphere offset and size
- Different humeral neck-shaft angles (a varus or valgus component)
- Varying thickness of humeral inserts

Surgical Factors
- Altering the level of the humeral osteotomy
- Offsetting placement of the humerosocket
- Changing placement of the glenosphere

Techniques to Restore Soft Tissue Tension by Lengthening the Humerus
- Placement of the glenosphere with inferior translation
- Placement of the glenosphere with inferior tilt
- Using an inferiorly eccentric glenosphere
- Using a larger glenosphere with inferior overhang
- Using a valgus humeral neck-shaft angle
- Humeral augments

Techniques to Restore Soft Tissue Tension Through Compressive Force Across the Glenohumeral Joint
- Placement of glenosphere with lateral offset
- Using a varus humeral component
- Translating humeral component so the intramedullary stem is lateral to socket

With kind permission from: Springer Science+Business Media, Clinical Orthopaedics and Related Research and Walker M, Brooks J, Willis M, et al. How reverse shoulder arthroplasty works. *Clin Orthop Relat Res.* 2011;469:2440–2451.

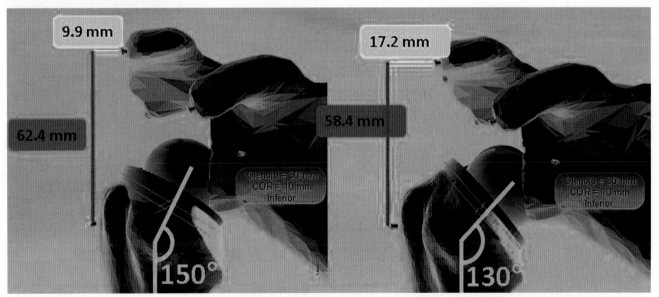

▲ FIGURE 31-3:   Effect of varus and valgus humeral components on vertical and lateral translations.

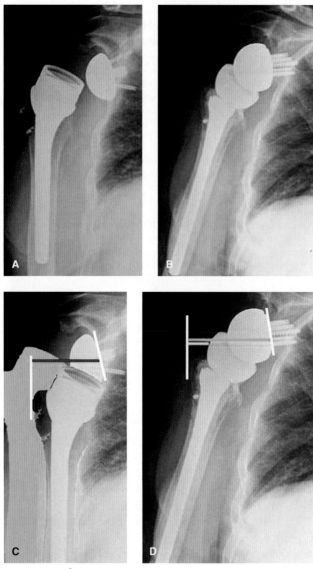

▲ FIGURE 31-4: A: Preoperative radiographs of a patient who presented to us with a dislocated reverse shoulder arthroplasty performed elsewhere and was already revised to a thicker metaphyseal augment, thicker polyethylene and constraint humerosocket. B: Postoperative radiograph. C,D: Illustrating the effect of a prosthesis with a more lateral center of rotation in increasing soft tissue tension without excessive inferior translation and achieving stability.

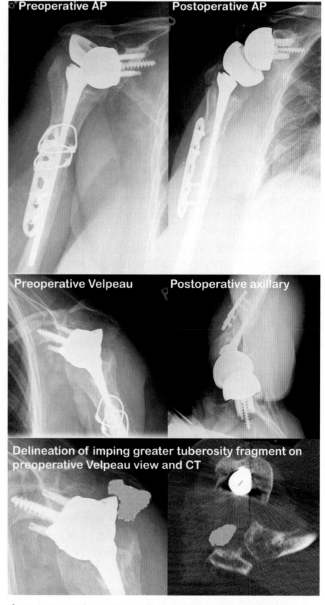

▲ FIGURE 31-5: This patient had a failed hemiarthroplasty with tuberosity mal/nonunion that was revised to a reverse arthroplasty. He then had a postoperative fracture, was treated with ORIF, allograft/cabling and presented to us with instability. On the preoperative AP radiograph the shoulder is dislocated, whereas it is reduced on the Velpeau axillary. The magnified Velpeau view and CT scan delineate the fragment of greater tuberosity adjacent to the AC joint that was mechanically impinging and lead to dislocations. During the revision operation, that fragment was excised (not visible on postoperative radiographs) and the shoulder remained stable and located.

demonstrates for example how with all other factors being equal (glenosphere size, tilt and inferior placement, same polyethylene implant and no metaphyseal augments), the difference in the neck-shaft angle of the implant produces different amount of vertical and horizontal translations. An implant with more valgus produces more inferior translation versus lateral translation and vice versa.

Figure 31-4 shows a case where dislocation of a reverse prosthesis—already revised by another experienced surgeon for instability without success—was managed successfully by increasing soft tissue tension and lateralizing the center of rotation. Figure 31-5 illustrates a case of dislocating reverse prosthesis due to

osseous impingement of a malunited greater tuberosity fragment. Resection of that fragment lead to stability.

OUR EXPERIENCE

We have reviewed our database on reverse total shoulder replacements since 2003 and have identified 31 patients treated for instability. The most common pre-operative diagnoses were osteoarthritis with rotator cuff tear accounting for 12 cases (39%) and failed hemiarthroplasty with 8 cases (26%). Nearly half (48%) of the cases we treated had previous shoulder arthroplasty surgery. The most common glenosphere sizes used in these cases was 32-mm neutral offset in 8 (26%), 32-mm −4 lateral offset in 5 (16%), and 40-mm neutral offset in 4 (13%). Additional procedures including proximal humeral and/or glenoid bone grafting or muscle transfer was performed in conjunction with the index RSA in 11 cases (35%). The average time to first dislocation was 152 days with nearly half (15/31) occurring in the first 90 days.

Treatment

The majority of cases (22/31 or 71%) were initially managed with closed reduction, while 28% (6/31) underwent, directly, revision surgery to a larger glenosphere. In all of these cases the revision consisted of a larger glenosphere and socket of which 44-mm plus 8-mm lateral offset was the most common size (50%). Three patients underwent component removal and placement of an antibiotic cemented hemiarthroplasty for deep infection (one of these patients ultimately underwent second stage reimplantation of an RSA with a 40-mm neutral glenosphere). Of the 22 shoulders initially managed with closed reduction, approximately half (12/22 or 54%) remained stable whereas the rest had continued instability. Those with continued instability were treated with revision to a larger glenosphere and socket in six shoulders (28%). The most common glenosphere used in these cases was 36 mm with neutral offset. All of these patients remained stable at final follow-up. Four shoulders (19%) remained unstable and either declined or were medically unfit to undergo revision surgery. The average final ASES score in patients treated for instability was 67.4.

Infection should be considered in all cases of instability following RSA. In our series nearly 40% (12/31) shoulders had documented or suspected infection following their dislocation episode.

CONCLUSIONS

- Instability is the most common complication after RSA with a cumulative incidence of 4.8% in the literature.
- Achieving optimal soft tissue tension and accurate component placement is the key to decrease its incidence.
- Subscapularis repair appears to lower the risk of dislocation significantly.
- Infection must be ruled out.
- Early dislocations can often be managed with closed treatment.

- In late dislocations closed treatment may be attempted but more often require surgical treatment.
- The surgeon has to assess if there are specific mechanical factors related to the dislocation (i.e., impingement, component malposition) and address them.
- If no specific risk factor is identified, an inferior periglenoid scar removal and component revision or adjustment to increase soft tissue tension with or without a constrained humerosocket should restore stability.
- The techniques to change soft tissue tension as the surgeon desires were presented.

References

1. Cheung E, Willis M, Walker M, et al. Complications in reverse total shoulder arthroplasty. *J Am Acad Orthop Surg.* 2011;19:439–449.
2. Werner CM, Steinmann PA, Gilbart M, et al. Treatment of painful pseudoparesis due to irreparable rotator cuff dysfunction with the Delta III reverse-ball-and-socket total shoulder prosthesis. *J Bone Joint Surg Am.* 2005;87:1476–1486.
3. Gutierrez S, Keller TS, Levy JC, et al. Hierarchy of stability factors in reverse shoulder arthroplasty. *Clin Orthop Relat Res.* 2008;466:670–676.
4. Favre P, Sussmann PS, Gerber C. The effect of component positioning on intrinsic stability of the reverse shoulder arthroplasty. *J Shoulder Elbow Surg.* 2010;19:550–556.
5. Aluisio FV, Osbahr DC, Speer KP. Analysis of rotator cuff muscles in adult human cadaveric specimens. *Am J Orthop (Belle Mead NJ).* 2003;32:124–129.
6. Grammont PM, Baulot E. Delta shoulder prosthesis for rotator cuff rupture. *Orthopedics.* 1993;16:65–68.
7. Jobin CM, Brown GD, Bahu MJ, et al. Reverse total shoulder arthroplasty for cuff tear arthropathy: The clinical effect of deltoid lengthening and center of rotation medialization. *J Shoulder Elbow Surg.* 2012;21:1269–1277.
8. Van Hoof T, Gomes GT, Audenaert E, et al. 3D computerized model for measuring strain and displacement of the brachial plexus following placement of reverse shoulder prosthesis. *Anat Rec (Hoboken).* 2008;291:1173–1185.
9. Lädermann A, Walch G, Lubbeke A, et al. Influence of arm lengthening in reverse shoulder arthroplasty. *J Shoulder Elbow Surg.* 2012;21:336–341.
10. Gutierrez S, Luo ZP, Levy J, et al. Arc of motion and socket depth in reverse shoulder implants. *Clin Biomech (Bristol, Avon).* 2009;24:473–479.
11. Gallo RA, Gamradt SC, Mattern CJ, et al. Instability after reverse total shoulder replacement. *J Shoulder Elbow Surg.* 2011;20:584–590.
12. Wall B, Nove-Josserand L, O'Connor DP, et al. Reverse total shoulder arthroplasty: A review of results according to etiology. *J Bone Joint Surg Am.* 2007;89:1476–1485.
13. Hattrup SJ, Sanchez-Sotelo J, Sperling JW, et al. Reverse shoulder replacement for patients with inflammatory arthritis. *J Hand Surg Am.* 2012;37:1888–1894.
14. Walker M, Willis MP, Brooks JP, et al. The use of the reverse shoulder arthroplasty for treatment of failed total shoulder arthroplasty. *J Shoulder Elbow Surg.* 2012;21:514–522.

15. Willis M, Min W, Brooks JP, et al. Proximal humeral malunion treated with reverse shoulder arthroplasty. *J Shoulder Elbow Surg.* 2012;21:507–513.

16. Garrigues GE, Johnston PS, Pepe MD, et al. Hemiarthroplasty versus reverse total shoulder arthroplasty for acute proximal humerus fractures in elderly patients. *Orthopedics.* 2012;35:e703–e708.

17. Clark JC, Ritchie J, Song FS, et al. Complication rates, dislocation, pain, and postoperative range of motion after reverse shoulder arthroplasty in patients with and without repair of the subscapularis. *J Shoulder Elbow Surg.* 2012;21:36–41.

18. Ekelund A, Nyberg R. Can reverse shoulder arthroplasty be used with few complications in rheumatoid arthritis? *Clin Orthop Relat Res.* 2011;469:2483–2488.

19. Trappey GJ 4th, O'Connor DP, Edwards TB. What are the instability and infection rates after reverse shoulder arthroplasty? *Clin Orthop Relat Res.* 2011;469: 2505–2511.

20. Sadoghi P, Vavken P, Leithner A, et al. Impact of previous rotator cuff repair on the outcome of reverse shoulder arthroplasty. *J Shoulder Elbow Surg.* 2011;20:1138–1146.

21. Nolan BM, Ankerson E, Wiater JM. Reverse total shoulder arthroplasty improves function in cuff tear arthropathy. *Clin Orthop Relat Res.* 2011;469:2476–2482.

22. Cazeneuve JF, Cristofari DJ. Long term functional outcome following reverse shoulder arthroplasty in the elderly. *Orthop Traumatol Surg Res.* 2011;97:583–589.

23. Austin L, Zmistowski B, Chang ES, et al. Is reverse shoulder arthroplasty a reasonable alternative for revision arthroplasty? *Clin Orthop Relat Res.* 2011;469:2531–2537.

24. Naveed MA, Kitson J, Bunker TD. The Delta III reverse shoulder replacement for cuff tear arthropathy: A single-centre study of 50 consecutive procedures. *J Bone Joint Surg Br.* 2011;93:57–61.

25. Valenti P, Sauzieres P, Katz D, et al. Do less medialized reverse shoulder prostheses increase motion and reduce notching? *Clin Orthop Relat Res.* 2011;469:2550–2557.

26. Young AA, Smith MM, Bacle G, et al. Early results of reverse shoulder arthroplasty in patients with rheumatoid arthritis. *J Bone Joint Surg Am.* 2011;93:1915–1923.

27. Mulieri P, Dunning P, Klein S, et al. Reverse shoulder arthroplasty for the treatment of irreparable rotator cuff tear without glenohumeral arthritis. *J Bone Joint Surg Am.* 2010;92:2544–2556.

28. Holcomb JO, Hebert DJ, Mighell MA, et al. Reverse shoulder arthroplasty in patients with rheumatoid arthritis. *J Shoulder Elbow Surg.* 2010;19:1076–1084.

29. Young SW, Everts NM, Ball CM, et al. The SMR reverse shoulder prosthesis in the treatment of cuff-deficient shoulder conditions. *J Shoulder Elbow Surg.* 2009;18:622–626.

30. Wierks C, Skolasky RL, Ji JH, et al. Reverse total shoulder replacement: Intraoperative and early postoperative complications. *Clin Orthop Relat Res.* 2009;467:225–234.

31. Holcomb JO, Cuff D, Petersen SA, et al. Revision reverse shoulder arthroplasty for glenoid baseplate failure after primary reverse shoulder arthroplasty. *J Shoulder Elbow Surg.* 2009;18:717–723.

32. Edwards TB, Williams MD, Labriola JE, et al. Subscapularis insufficiency and the risk of shoulder dislocation after reverse shoulder arthroplasty. *J Shoulder Elbow Surg.* 2009;18:892–896.

33. Gallinet D, Clappaz P, Garbuio P, et al. Three or four parts complex proximal humerus fractures: Hemiarthroplasty versus reverse prosthesis: A comparative study of 40 cases. *Orthop Traumatol Surg Res.* 2009;95:48–55.

34. Grassi FA, Murena L, Valli F, et al. Six-year experience with the Delta III reverse shoulder prosthesis. *J Orthop Surg (Hong Kong).* 2009;17:151–156.

35. Klein M, Juschka M, Hinkenjann B, et al. Treatment of comminuted fractures of the proximal humerus in elderly patients with the Delta III reverse shoulder prosthesis. *J Orthop Trauma.* 2008;22:698–704.

36. Cuff D, Pupello D, Virani N, et al. Reverse shoulder arthroplasty for the treatment of rotator cuff deficiency. *J Bone Joint Surg Am.* 2008;90:1244–1251.

37. Levy J, Frankle M, Mighell M, et al. The use of the reverse shoulder prosthesis for the treatment of failed hemiarthroplasty for proximal humeral fracture. *J Bone Joint Surg Am.* 2007;89:292–300.

38. Gohlke F, Rolf O. [Revision of failed fracture hemiarthroplasties to reverse total shoulder prosthesis through the transhumeral: Method incorporating a pectoralis-major-pedicled bone window]. *Oper Orthop Traumatol.* 2007;19:185–208.

39. Levy JC, Virani N, Pupello D, et al. Use of the reverse shoulder prosthesis for the treatment of failed hemiarthroplasty in patients with glenohumeral arthritis and rotator cuff deficiency. *J Bone Joint Surg Br.* 2007;89:189–195.

40. Bufquin T, Hersan A, Hubert L, et al. Reverse shoulder arthroplasty for the treatment of three- and four-part fractures of the proximal humerus in the elderly: A prospective review of 43 cases with a short-term follow-up. *J Bone Joint Surg Br.* 2007;89:516–520.

41. Frankle M, Levy JC, Pupello D, et al. The reverse shoulder prosthesis for glenohumeral arthritis associated with severe rotator cuff deficiency. A minimum two-year follow-up study of sixty patients surgical technique. *J Bone Joint Surg Am.* 2006;88(suppl 1 pt 2): 178–190.

42. Boileau P, Watkinson D, Hatzidakis AM, et al. Neer Award 2005: The Grammont reverse shoulder prosthesis: Results in cuff tear arthritis, fracture sequelae, and revision arthroplasty. *J Shoulder Elbow Surg.* 2006;15:527–540.

43. Vanhove B, Beugnies A. Grammont's reverse shoulder prosthesis for rotator cuff arthropathy. A retrospective study of 32 cases. *Acta Orthop Belg.* 2004;70:219–225.

44. Woodruff MJ, Cohen AP, Bradley JG. Arthroplasty of the shoulder in rheumatoid arthritis with rotator cuff dysfunction. *Int Orthop.* 2003;27:7–10.

45. Rittmeister M, Kerschbaumer F. Grammont reverse total shoulder arthroplasty in patients with rheumatoid arthritis and nonreconstructible rotator cuff lesions. *J Shoulder Elbow Surg.* 2001;10:17–22.

46. Jacobs R, Debeer P, De Smet L. Treatment of rotator cuff arthropathy with a reversed Delta shoulder prosthesis. *Acta Orthop Belg.* 2001;67:344–347.

47. De Wilde L, Mombert M, Van Petegem P, et al. Revision of shoulder replacement with a reversed shoulder prosthesis (Delta III): Report of five cases. *Acta Orthop Belg.* 2001;67:348–353.

48. Simovitch RW, Zumstein MA, Lohri E, et al. Predictors of scapular notching in patients managed with the Delta III reverse total shoulder replacement. *J Bone Joint Surg Am.* 2007;89:588–600.

49. Gutierrez S, Comiskey CA 4th, Luo ZP, et al. Range of impingement-free abduction and adduction deficit after reverse shoulder arthroplasty. Hierarchy of surgical and implant-design-related factors. *J Bone Joint Surg Am.* 2008;90:2606–2615.

50. de Wilde LF, Poncet D, Middernacht B, et al. Prosthetic overhang is the most effective way to prevent scapular conflict in a reverse total shoulder prosthesis. *Acta Orthop.* 2010;81:719–726.

51. Gutierrez S, Greiwe RM, Frankle MA, et al. Biomechanical comparison of component position and hardware failure in the reverse shoulder prosthesis. *J Shoulder Elbow Surg.* 2007;16:S9–S12.

52. Gutierrez S, Walker M, Willis M, et al. Effects of tilt and glenosphere eccentricity on baseplate/bone interface forces in a computational model, validated by a mechanical model, of reverse shoulder arthroplasty. *J Shoulder Elbow Surg.* 2011;20:732–739.

53. Lädermann A, Williams MD, Melis B, et al. Objective evaluation of lengthening in reverse shoulder arthroplasty. *J Shoulder Elbow Surg.* 2009;18:588–595.

54. Seitz WH. Instability after reverse total shoulder arthroplasty: A balancing act. *Seminars in Arthroplasty* 2009;20:104–114.

55. Klein SM, Dunning P, Mulieri P, et al. Effects of acquired glenoid bone defects on surgical technique and clinical outcomes in reverse shoulder arthroplasty. *J Bone Joint Surg Am.* 2010;92:1144–1154.

56. Farshad M, Gerber C. Reverse total shoulder arthroplasty-from the most to the least common complication. *Int Orthop.* 2010;34:1075–1082.

57. Baulot E, Chabernaud D, Grammont PM. [Results of Grammont's inverted prosthesis in omarthritis associated with major cuff destruction. Apropos of 16 cases]. *Acta Orthop Belg.* 1995;61(suppl 1):112–119.

58. Baulot E, Garron E, Grammont PM. [Grammont prosthesis in humeral head osteonecrosis. Indications–results]. *Acta Orthop Belg.* 1999;65(suppl 1):109–115.

59. Henninger HB, Barg A, Anderson AE, et al. Effect of lateral offset center of rotation in reverse total shoulder arthroplasty: A biomechanical study. *J Shoulder Elbow Surg.* 2012;21:1128–1135.

60. Beekman PD, Katusic D, Berghs BM, et al. One-stage revision for patients with a chronically infected reverse total shoulder replacement. *J Bone Joint Surg Br.* 2010;92:817–822.

61. Zavala JA, Clark JC, Kissenberth MJ, et al. Management of deep infection after reverse total shoulder arthroplasty: A case series. *J Shoulder Elbow Surg.* 2012;21:1310–1315.

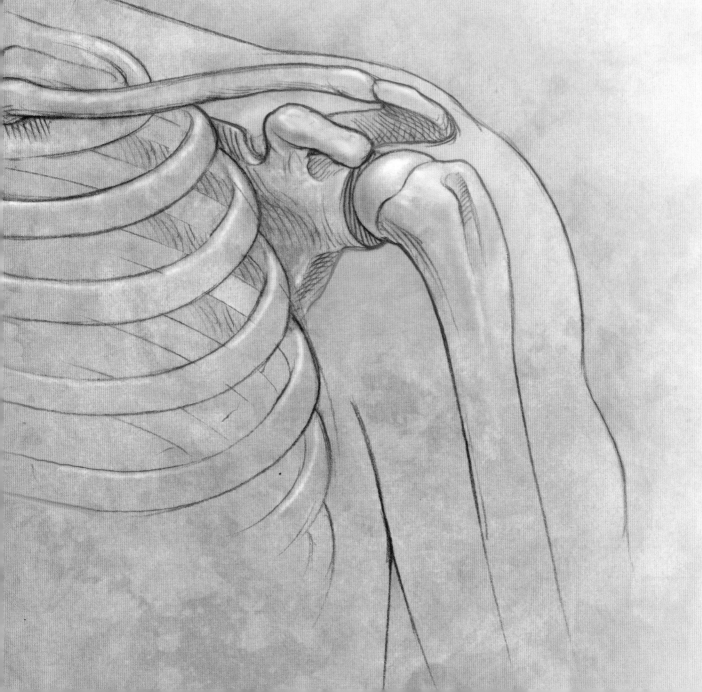

SPECIAL CONSIDERATIONS

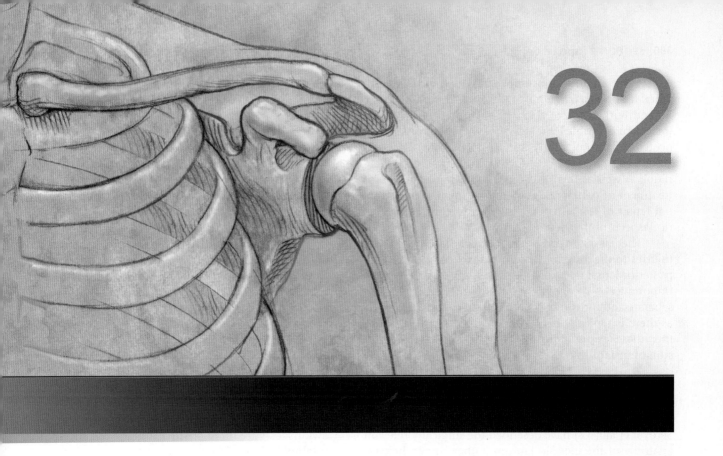

ARTHROSCOPIC TREATMENT OF PANLABRAL TEARS

Rachel M. Frank / Frank McCormick / John McNeil /
CDR Matthew T. Provencher

INTRODUCTION

Glenohumeral instability is a commonly encountered diagnosis in the young, athletic patient population. Instability is most often due to lesions of the glenoid labrum and/or surrounding joint capsule, and is typically characterized by location. Anterior shoulder instability accounts for the vast majority of cases, and is usually due to a traumatic lesion of the anterior glenoid labrum, commonly known as the Bankart lesion (1–5). While less common, posterior shoulder instability is a well-described clinical entity, and is often due to posterior labrum disruptions (6–8). Finally, superior labrum lesions are also found in this patient population, often in overhead-throwing athletes. First recognized by Andrews et al. (9) and later described by Snyder et al. (10) as SLAP (superior labrum, anterior, and posterior) lesions; the description, classification, and treatment of these lesions have continued to evolve over the past decade (11–22). Superior labral detachment tears provide the potential for progressive microinstability and subsequent secondary instability with involvement of other areas of the labrum.

Advances in arthroscopic techniques and surgeon awareness have thus increased our ability to recognize more complex lesions involving multiple areas around the labrum. In 2004, Powell et al. (23) first characterized the appearance of a "circumferential" detachment of the entire labrum from the glenoid. Powell classified this combined anterior, posterior, inferior, and superior labral lesion as a panlabral SLAP type-IX lesion. In 2005, Lo and Burkhart (24) also described their arthroscopic treatment of "triple labral lesions" with anterior labrum, posterior labrum, and SLAP type-II lesions. Recently, Tokish et al. (25,26) described both their surgical technique as well as their outcomes following arthroscopic treatment of panlabral lesions requiring a circumferential repair of the anterior, posterior, inferior, and superior aspects of the glenoid labrum.

There is a growing body of evidence to suggest that injuries to the anterior labrum may extend to extensive posterior labral tears and vice-versa (23–31). Of utmost importance is recognizing that these lesions are likely separate and indistinct from multidirectional instability as there is typically no baseline collagen disorder. Further, these lesions are considered the end-stage progression of instability.

RELEVANT ANATOMY

Seroyer et al. (32) have described the surgically relevant anatomy of the glenoid labrum. Other comprehensive reviews of common labral anatomy as well as anatomical variants have also been published (33,34). It is important to understand that while the rotator cuff is clearly a critical component of dynamic shoulder stability (35,36), the glenohumeral capsulolabral structures are important static restraints contributing to overall shoulder stability (35,37–39). The labrum itself acts as a static stabilizer by increasing the concavity-compression mechanism of the humeral head in the glenoid socket, and increasing the depth of the humeral articulation (40–42). The joint capsule and glenohumeral ligaments (inferior, middle, superior) play substantial roles in stabilization depending on the position of the shoulder.

Patients presenting with panlabral lesions typically describe a traumatic onset of symptoms. The majority of patients will have experienced an initial anterior instability event and then experience subsequent episodes of recurrent instability or dislocations that cause an increase in extent of tear as well as glenohumeral cartilage and bone damage. These patients will describe their inciting injury as having occurred with their arm in the classic position of abduction and external rotation. Other patients will present with posterior instability episodes and in these cases will report a traumatic event with the arm in the position of forward flexion, adduction, and internal rotation. Patients will often complain of progressive pain and ease of instability. Often patients will have had progressive symptoms for two or more years prior to presentation, and they may also have undergone previous surgical procedures (25,26,28). They will usually not complain of weakness. Different from isolated Bankart or SLAP lesions, patients

with panlabral lesions will usually have positive symptoms and apprehension in all planes of motion.

PHYSICAL EXAMINATION

Physical examination should incorporate a complete assessment of both shoulders. This is important in order to assess for other possible etiologies of their complaints, including generalized laxity or multidirectional instability. The comprehensive examination should include assessment of muscle tone and appearance, range of motion, strength, and provocative maneuvers. Specific signs for panlabral lesions are rare and are difficult to elucidate. More common is significant guarding with numerous positive provocative maneuvers. Specifically, patients may experience pain-induced limitation of strength testing during an active compression test (43). Most patients will also have a positive apprehension test. Patients will also usually have a positive push–pull test for posterior laxity (43). Impingement maneuvers including the Neer and Hawkins tests are often positive, but are not specific for panlabral lesions (25).

DIAGNOSTIC IMAGING

All patients presenting with shoulder pain and a clinical concern for panlabral pathology should have plain radiographs. While x-rays do not show the labrum itself, they can be helpful in evaluating the contour of the glenoid rim and humeral head, which can change treatment choices depending on the extent of disease. A standard shoulder series including an anterior–posterior view of shoulder in the plane of the scapula, scapular-Y view, and axillary view should be performed. Other specialized views can be obtained as indicated, including a Stryker notch view and/or West Point view to assess for Hill-Sachs lesions and/or glenoid bone loss, respectively.

If bone loss is suspected, computed tomography (CT), and specifically three-dimensional CT can be used to further define the osseous morphology of the glenohumeral joint. As noted in multiple recent studies, both glenoid bone loss (i.e., bony Bankart) and humeral head lesions (i.e., Hill-Sachs defects) are associated with recurrent glenohumeral instability (44–47). Patients with circumferential labral lesions may thus have concomitant bony defects on either the glenoid surface and/or the humeral head. Depending on the location and size of such defects, treatment to address not only the labrum but also the bone loss may be warranted.

Magnetic resonance imaging (MRI) and magnetic resonance arthrography (MRA) are the diagnostic studies of choice in the noninvasive evaluation of patients

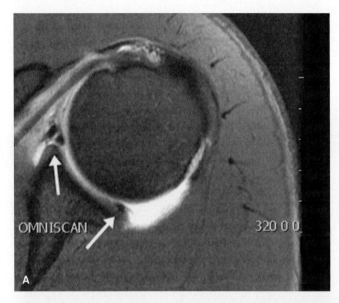
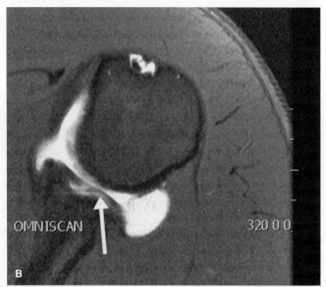
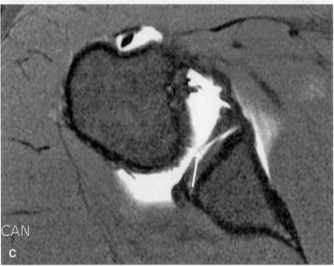
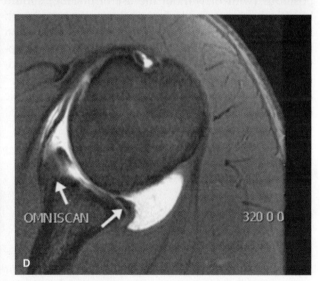

▲ FIGURE 32-1: **A:** Axial magnetic resonance arthrogram of anterior and posterior labral tear (*white arrows*). **B:** Axial magnetic resonance arthrogram of tear with inferior extension, in a tear that is total of 300 degrees of the glenoid labrum. **C:** Axial magnetic resonance arthrogram of the inferior most portion of the tear. **D:** Same series in the midportion of glenoid with anterior and posterior tears.

with suspected panlabral lesions (Fig. 32-1). It should be noted that even with contrast enhancement, imaging is notoriously unreliable. In the recent case series presented by Ricchetti et al. (28), labral pathology was found in 91% of patients with noncontrast MRI studies, compared with 100% of patients undergoing MRA. However, tears in more than one area of the labrum were only found in 27% and 72% of patients undergoing MRI and MRA, respectively. Furthermore, 13% of all studies (combined MRI and MRA) accurately reported combined anterior, posterior, and superior labrum lesions. Tokish et al. (25), who reported an overall accuracy of 77% shoulders undergoing MRA, reported similar numbers. Overall, despite MRA findings, in the setting of instability with pain, and positive provocative tests, the surgeon should be prepared for the arthroscopic diagnosis of panlabral tears.

INDICATIONS AND CONTRAINDICATIONS

Given the relatively low prevalence of panlabral lesions, it is difficult to describe absolute indications and contraindications for surgical fixation. Proposed indications and contraindications are described in Table 32-1.

NONOPERATIVE TREATMENT

Nonoperative treatment of panlabral lesions is rare, as patients typically present with long-standing pain, instability, and debilitation. As such, most patients have exhausted nonoperative treatment by the time they present with circumferential labral pathology. If a patient is not deemed suitable for operative fixation, or is unwilling

TABLE 32-1 **Indications and Contraindications for Surgery**

Indications	• Recurrent instability • Pain despite conservative treatment
Contraindications	• Significant glenoid bone loss of 20% or more • Additional procedures required before, or in addition to, panlabral repair • Extensive glenohumeral arthritis • Unwilling to comply with rehabilitation • Multiple medical comorbidities that preclude surgical candidacy

to comply with the required postoperative rehabilitation protocol, several modalities can be attempted. Activity modification and avoidance of provocative shoulder positions (with or without the use of bracing) should be attempted. A formal physical therapy program with a focus on appropriate strengthening, proprioception training, and scapulothoracic coordination may be helpful (48,49). Other modalities for pain control including oral anti-inflammatory medications (NSAIDs) and cryotherapy may be helpful with regard to symptomatic relief; however, such measures will not be useful for improving the actual underlying instability.

SURGICAL TREATMENT

Authors' Preferred Technique

Our preferred surgical position is in the lateral position (26). Given the potential for a long anesthetic time, we ensure to pad all bony prominences with low weights for arm traction. We are sure to perform detailed marking of anatomic landmarks for portal placement, anticipating soft tissue swelling (Fig. 32-2). A detailed examination under anesthesia (EUA) provides valuable information for surgical planning. Much of our decision making is based on the quantification of anterior and posterior laxity via ASES classification (50).

The surgical stepwise progression is listed in Table 32-2. We begin with a comprehensive diagnostic arthroscopy from the modified (slightly lateral) posterior portal. We refrain from placing an anterior portal until our surgical assessment and plan is completed. Next,

TABLE 32-2 **The Surgical Stepwise Progression**

Diagnostic arthroscopy
Posterior capsulolabral preparation
Anterior capsulolabral preparation
Posterior and inferior capsulolabral repair
Anterior capsulolabral repair
SLAP preparation and repair

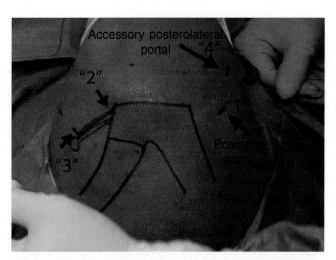

▲ **FIGURE 32-2:** Arthroscopic portal setup with a patient in the lateral decubitus position. The primary portals are **(1)** standard posterior portal; **(2)** anterosuperior portal (off the anterolateral edge of the acromion which comes into the joint high in the rotator interval); **(3)** midglenoid portal (just lateral to the coracoid process which comes in just above the subscapularis); **(4)** posterolateral 7-o'clock portal (4 cm directly lateral to the posterolateral corner of the acromion, which comes in at the 7-o'clock position of the inferior glenoid).

we create an anterosuperior portal using "outside-in" technique under direct visualization, just anterior to the biceps, followed by a 7-mm cannula (Arthrex, Naples, FL). We then create a midglenoid (anteroinferior) working portal, with entry into joint just superior to subscapularis and lateral to allow placement of anchor into glenoid, using an 8.25-mm cannula (Arthrex, Naples, FL). Finally, an accessory posterolateral portal may be placed percutaneously or cannulated depending on the extent of labral tear (Fig. 32-3).

It is our general preference to repair the posterior labrum first in the anticipation of significant swelling making this more difficult later in the case. Our highest priority is completing the anterior and posterior segments prior to the superior repairs do to maneuverability constraints developing with the progressive stabilization and swelling. We perform most of our soft tissue and bony preparation work using the anterosuperior portal as this allows the inferior–anterior portal to serve as a working portal for anterior and posterior labrum preparation and the posterior portal to aid in posterior labrum and glenoid preparation. While preparing the posterior glenoid and labrum, we determine if the posterolateral portal warrants a cannulated portal. This decision is based on the need for a posterior-inferior labral repair with anchor placement at the 6-o'clock to 8-o'clock position. A Beath pin from an ACL kit (or an anchor-inserter drill-sleeve) is placed with spinal needle removal, and enables numerous anchors to be placed using the same percutaneous incision if one does not wish to cannulate.

Anchor placement is done first through the posterolateral portal. Our surgical goal is to repair the posterior IGHL, anterior IGHL, MGHL, and reduce capsular laxity. Therefore, we often place 4 to 6 anchors at

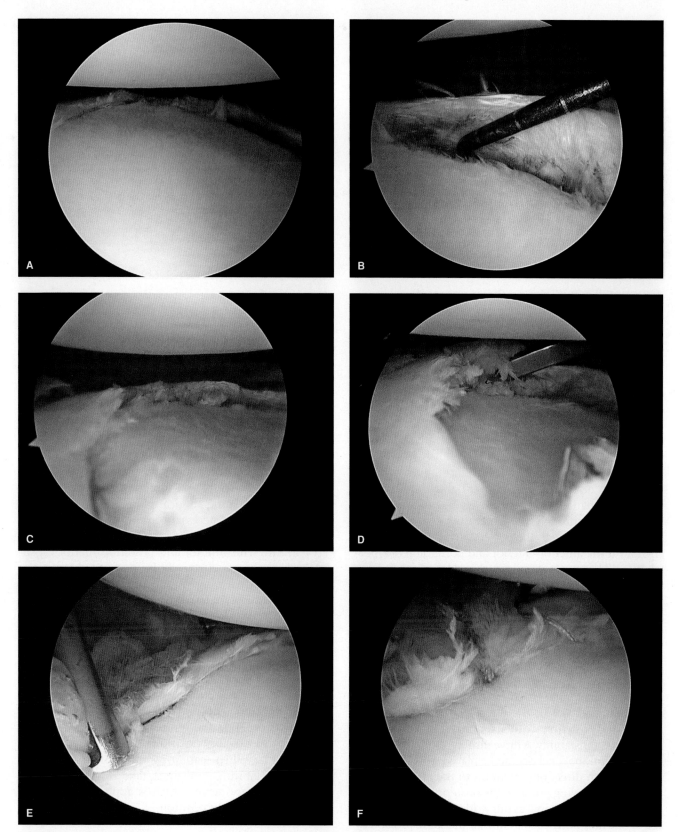

▲ FIGURE 32-3: **A:** Arthroscopic image as viewed from the anterosuperior portal of an anterior, inferior, and posterior labral tear (overall a panlabral tear configuration). **B:** Anterior component of the tear. **C:** Posterior component of the tear. **D:** Arthroscopic preparation for tear capsulolabral repair. **E:** Starting first with posterior repair, an anchor inserter is brought in from the posterolateral (7-o'clock) portal. **F:** The posterior and inferior repair is finalized and posteriorly repaired and inferiorly repaired. (*continued*)

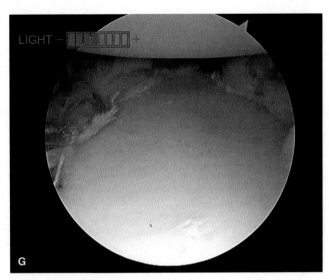

▲ **FIGURE 32-3:** (*Continued*) **G:** Final repair of anterior, inferior, and posterior labral tear.

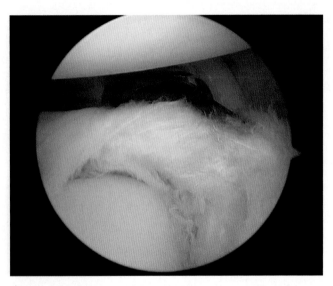

▲ **FIGURE 32-4:** Arthroscopic image as viewed from posterior of a SLAP II tear in a patient with a panlabral tear.

the inferior glenoid with anterior and posterior extension predicated on findings at EUA and intra-articular assessment. As much, the degree of capsular plication, coupled with labral repair, is based on the degree of directional instability. We typically perform capsular tuck of 5 to 10 mm, however, if there is a skybox view of the glenoid, we will perform a larger capsular plication with the labral repair. Our goal is to finish with a balanced and centered humeral head after surgical completion, but to not risk localized over-tightening that will threaten the patient's postoperative range of motion.

Viewing through the anterosuperior portal, we begin working through the posterolateral portal to place anchors at the anterior–inferior and posteroinferior portal. We will begin our capsular tuck and labral repair here, without tying the sutures, but docking the sutures in the posterior portal or outside of the posterolateral portal cannula. Next we will place an anchor anterior through the anterior–inferior portal to capture the MGHL and anterior labrum. The sutures are placed outside of the working cannula once the soft tissue is captured. Finally, we will place a posterior anchor through the posterior portal. We then progressively tie all knots starting inferior and working our way up the glenoid, alternating between anterior and posterior. We then repeat our EUA and assess for persistent instability. A drive thru sign should be eliminated. Additional anchors can be placed where needed.

We then direct our attention to the SLAP tear. We transfer our viewing portal to the posterior portal. Using the anterosuperior portal as our working portal, we begin soft tissue and bony preparation in the same previously described manner (Fig. 32-4). We focus our bony preparation at the 10:30 to 12:30 position. In some cases, the labral-biceps complex is so unstable, that the glenoid morphology is our clue to soft tissue reapproximation. The anchor is placed via a percutaneous anterolateral portal (located just off the anterolateral corner of the

acromion 3 to 4 mm) through the rotator interval, or rotator cuff muscle belly. We prefer one anchor placed posterior to the biceps. We feel this approach is more efficient intraoperatively, biomechanically equivalent to more anchors, with less risk of stiffness by incorporating the SGHL in the repair. If another anchor is warranted posteriorly, we will place through the posterior cannula. We place a single-loaded suture in a simple configuration, with the knot away from the glenoid.

PEARL: Perform a complete diagnostic arthroscopy before initiating surgical plan. Prioritize the posterior repair where necessary in anticipation of future swelling.

PEARL: The anterior and posterior inferior capsulolabral repair can effectively be performed using the anterosuperior viewing portal and the posterolateral working portal.

PEARL: We find efficient glenoid preparation is obtained using a 3.5-mm resector blade set on forward-shaver function and used as a fine burr (Smith and Nephew Endoscopy, Andover, MA).

Placing the burr through the posterior portal enables fine-tuning of the glenoid preparation.

Spend sufficient time with preparation, and make sure to incorporate the entire posterior labrum from 6-o'clock to 12-o'clock position.

PEARL: When capturing the inferior capsular pouch and labrum, one must take care inferiorly to avoid the axillary nerve, which is approximately 2 cm from the 5:30 to 6:30 position.

REHABILITATION

We place the patient in a neutral rotation sling to be worn at all times. Rehabilitation following panlabral repair is typically performed in phases. Our preferred

TABLE 32-3   Outcomes

Author	Year, Journal	N	Follow-up	Technique	Outcomes	Complications
Ricchetti et al.	2012, AJSM	44	42 mos (16–78)	Arthroscopic panlabral repair, mean anchors n = 8	ASES: 90 ± 18 Penn: 90 ± 15	30% (n = 13) • 7% revision surgery • 11% recurrent instability event
Mazzocca et al.	2011, AJSM	20	28 mos (14–47)	Arthroscopic 270-degree labral repair (anterior, inferior, posterior) No SLAP repair	ASES: 93 SANE: 91 SST: 11 Constant: 95	• 15% failure rate (n = 3) with recurrent instability • 10% stiffness (n = 2)
Tokish et al.	2009, JBJS	39	32 mos (24–53)	Arthroscopic panlabral repair, mean anchors n = 7	ASES: 90 SF12: 90 SANE: 89 All returned to preop activity levels for at least one season	15% (n = 6) • Recurrent instability (n = 2) • Stiffness (n = 2) • Recalcitrant biceps tendinitis (n = 2)

protocol involves three specific phases as follows: Phase 1 (0 to 6 weeks), sling with abduction pillow (UltraSling; DonJoy, Vista, CA), daily pendulums and ROM of elbow, wrist, and hand with passive ROM in the scapular plane at 2 weeks with formalized physical therapy; Phase 2 (6–24), discontinue use of sling and abduction pillow at 6 weeks, begin structured program to achieve full active and passive shoulder range of motion by 12 weeks, begin strengthening of deltoid, rotator cuff, and scapular stabilizers after full, painless, active ROM is restored; Phase 3, progressive sport-specific return to activity as strength permits, with return to sports at approximately 6 to 9 months postoperatively.

OUTCOMES

A summary of available studies is presented in Table 32-3 (23–31, 51). In the largest series, Tokish et al. (25) reported reliable reduction in pain, instability, and achievement of primarily good to excellent outcomes in 41 shoulders undergoing arthroscopic repair of circumferential glenoid labrum lesions using the technique described above. In particular, all high level athletes in this study returned to their activity for at least one season; however, the overall rate of failure was 15%, with two cases each of

recurrent instability, stiffness, or persistent SLAP lesions. Ricchetti et al. (28) presented comparable outcomes in 44 patients at an average 42 months following surgery, with a mean postoperative ASES score of 90 ± 18.

Complications

Complications following arthroscopic panlabral repair are rare, and are similar to those reported for arthroscopic anterior instability, posterior instability, and SLAP repair. Ricchetti et al. (28) reported several complications (n = 13, or 30%) in their cohort of 44 patients, including portal drainage (n = 1), stiffness (n = 6) with one patient requiring repeat surgery for arthroscopic release, progression to glenohumeral arthritis requiring total shoulder arthroplasty 4 years after panlabral repair (n = 1), and recurrent instability (n = 5) with one patient requiring repeat stabilization surgery. Tokish et al. (25) reported several complications as well, including recurrent dislocation (n = 2) with both patients experiencing dislocation following one competitive football season after initial repair and both requiring revision stabilization, stiffness (n = 2) with both patients requiring repeat surgery for arthroscopic release, and persistent SLAP lesions with recalcitrant biceps tendinitis (n = 2) with both patients requiring biceps tenodesis.

SUMMARY

Patients presenting with circumferential labral lesions will often have vague, nonspecific complaints, and diagnosis can thus be challenging. A high index of suspicion in patients with persistent pain and instability following an original instability event is necessary. Appropriate diagnostic workup with MRI/MRA is useful; however, the diagnosis is often made during the diagnostic arthroscopy. Arthroscopic stabilization of panlabral lesions is technically complicated but when performed in the appropriate patient, can be very effective.

References

1. Bankart ASB. The pathology and treatment of recurrent dislocation of the shoulder joint. *Br J Surg.* 1938;26:23–29.

2. Bottoni CR, Wilckens JH, DeBerardino TM, et al. A prospective, randomized evaluation of arthroscopic stabilization versus nonoperative treatment in patients with acute, traumatic, first-time shoulder dislocations. *Am J Sports Med.* 2002;30:576–580.

3. DeBerardino TM, Arciero RA, Taylor DC, et al. Prospective evaluation of arthroscopic stabilization of acute, initial anterior shoulder dislocations in young athletes. Two- to five-year follow-up. *Am J Sports Med.* 2001;29:586–592.

4. Kim SH, Ha KI, Cho YB, et al. Arthroscopic anterior stabilization of the shoulder: Two to six-year follow-up. *J Bone Joint Surg Am.* 2003;85-A:1511–1518.

5. Taylor DC, Arciero RA. Pathologic changes associated with shoulder dislocations. Arthroscopic and physical examination findings in first-time, traumatic anterior dislocations. *Am J Sports Med.* 1997;25:306–311.

6. Provencher MT, LeClere LE, King S, et al. Posterior instability of the shoulder: Diagnosis and management. *Am J Sports Med.* 2011;39:874–886.

7. Bigliani LU, Pollock RG, McIlveen SJ, et al. Shift of the posteroinferior aspect of the capsule for recurrent posterior glenohumeral instability. *J Bone Joint Surg Am.* 1995;77:1011–1020.

8. Kim SH, Ha KI, Park JH, et al. Arthroscopic posterior labral repair and capsular shift for traumatic unidirectional recurrent posterior subluxation of the shoulder. *J Bone Joint Surg Am.* 2003;85-A:1479–1487.

9. Andrews JR, Carson WG Jr, McLeod WD. Glenoid labrum tears related to the long head of the biceps. *Am J Sports Med.* 1985;13:337–341.

10. Snyder SJ, Karzel RP, Del Pizzo W, et al. SLAP lesions of the shoulder. *Arthroscopy.* 1990;6:274–279.

11. Sayde WM, Cohen SB, Ciccotti MG, et al. Return to play after type II superior labral anterior-posterior lesion repairs in athletes: A systematic review. *Clin Orthop Relat Res.* 2012;470:1595–1600.

12. Neuman BJ, Boisvert CB, Reiter B, et al. Results of arthroscopic repair of type II superior labral anterior posterior lesions in overhead athletes: Assessment of return to preinjury playing level and satisfaction. *Am J Sports Med.* 2011;39:1883–1888.

13. Modarresi S, Motamedi D, Jude CM. Superior labral anteroposterior lesions of the shoulder: Part 1, anatomy and anatomic variants. *AJR Am J Roentgenol.* 2011;197:596–603.

14. Modarresi S, Motamedi D, Jude CM. Superior labral anteroposterior lesions of the shoulder: Part 2, mechanisms and classification. *AJR Am J Roentgenol.* 2011;197:604–611.

15. Jia X, Yokota A, McCarty EC, et al. Reproducibility and reliability of the Snyder classification of superior labral anterior posterior lesions among shoulder surgeons. *Am J Sports Med.* 2011;39:986–991.

16. Friel NA, Karas V, Slabaugh MA, et al. Outcomes of type II superior labrum, anterior to posterior (SLAP) repair: Prospective evaluation at a minimum two-year follow-up. *J Shoulder Elbow Surg.* 2010;19:859–867.

17. Abrams GD, Safran MR. Diagnosis and management of superior labrum anterior posterior lesions in overhead athletes. *Br J Sports Med.* 2010;44:311–318.

18. Brockmeier SF, Voos JE, Williams RJ 3rd, et al. Outcomes after arthroscopic repair of type-II SLAP lesions. *J Bone Joint Surg Am.* 2009;91:1595–1603.

19. Yung PS, Fong DT, Kong MF, et al. Arthroscopic repair of isolated type II superior labrum anterior-posterior lesion. *Knee Surg Sports Traumatol Arthrosc.* 2008;16:1151–1157.

20. Seroyer S, Tejwani SG, Bradley JP. Arthroscopic capsulolabral reconstruction of the type VIII superior labrum anterior posterior lesion: Mean 2-year follow-up on 13 shoulders. *Am J Sports Med.* 2007;35:1477–1483.

21. Funk L, Snow M. SLAP tears of the glenoid labrum in contact athletes. *Clin J Sport Med.* 2007;17:1–4.

22. Enad JG, Gaines RJ, White SM, et al. Arthroscopic superior labrum anterior-posterior repair in military patients. *J Shoulder Elbow Surg.* 2007;16:300–305.

23. Powell SE, Nord KD, Ryu RK. The diagnosis, classification, and treatment of SLAP lesions. *Op Tech Sports Med.* 2004;12:99–110.

24. Lo IK, Burkhart SS. Triple labral lesions: Pathology and surgical repair technique-report of seven cases. *Arthroscopy.* 2005;21:186–193.

25. Tokish JM, McBratney CM, Solomon DJ, et al. Arthroscopic repair of circumferential lesions of the glenoid labrum. *J Bone Joint Surg Am.* 2009;91:2795–2802.

26. Tokish JM, McBratney CM, Solomon DJ, et al. Arthroscopic repair of circumferential lesions of the glenoid labrum: Surgical technique. *J Bone Joint Surg Am.* 2010;92(suppl 1 pt 2):130–144.

27. Lindauer KR, Major NM, Rougier-Chapman DP, et al. MR imaging appearance of 180–360 degrees labral tears of the shoulder. *Skeletal Radiol.* 2005;34:74–79.

28. Ricchetti ET, Ciccotti MC, O'Brien DF, et al. Outcomes of arthroscopic repair of panlabral tears of the glenohumeral joint. *Am J Sports Med.* 2012;40:2561–2568.

29. Dickens JF, Kilcoyne KG, Haniuk E, et al. Combined lesions of the glenoid labrum. *Phys Sportsmed.* 2012;40:102–108.

30. Dickens JF, Kilcoyne KG, Giuliani J, et al. Circumferential labral tears resulting from a single anterior glenohumeral instability event: A report of 3 cases in young athletes. *Am J Sports Med.* 2012;40:213–217.

31. Warner JJ, Kann S, Marks P. Arthroscopic repair of combined Bankart and superior labral detachment anterior and posterior lesions: Technique and preliminary results. *Arthroscopy.* 1994;10:383–391.

32. Seroyer ST, Nho SJ, Provencher MT, et al. Four-quadrant approach to capsulolabral repair: An arthroscopic road map to the glenoid. *Arthroscopy.* 2010;26:555–562.

33. Dunham KS, Bencardino JT, Rokito AS. Anatomic variants and pitfalls of the labrum, glenoid cartilage, and glenohumeral ligaments. *Magn Reson Imaging Clin N Am.* 2012;20:213–228.

34. Tischer T, Vogt S, Kreuz PC, et al. Arthroscopic anatomy, variants, and pathologic findings in shoulder instability. *Arthroscopy.* 2011;27:1434–1443.

35. Turkel SJ, Panio MW, Marshall JL, et al. Stabilizing mechanisms preventing anterior dislocation of the glenohumeral joint. *J Bone Joint Surg Am.* 1981;63:1208–1217.

36. Debski RE, Sakone M, Woo SL, et al. Contribution of the passive properties of the rotator cuff to glenohumeral stability during anterior-posterior loading. *J Shoulder Elbow Surg.* 1999;8:324–329.

37. Lintner S, Levy A, Kenter K, et al. Glenohumeral translation in the asymptomatic athlete's shoulder and its relationship to other clinically measurable anthropometric variables. *Am J Sports Med.* 1996;24:716–720.

38. Ovesen J, Nielsen S. Stability of the shoulder joint. Cadaver study of stabilizing structures. *Acta Orthop Scand.* 1985; 56:149–151.

39. O'Connell PW, Nuber GW, Mileski RA, et al. The contribution of the glenohumeral ligaments to anterior stability of the shoulder joint. *Am J Sports Med.* 1990;18:579–584.

40. Lippitt S, Matsen F. Mechanisms of glenohumeral joint stability. *Clin Orthop Relat Res.* 1993;(291):20–28.

41. Matsen FA 3rd, Chebli C, Lippitt S. Principles for the evaluation and management of shoulder instability. *J Bone Joint Surg.* 2006;88:648–659.

42. Lazarus MD, Sidles JA, Harryman DT 2nd, et al. Effect of a chondral-labral defect on glenoid concavity and glenohumeral stability. A cadaveric model. *J Bone Joint Surg.* 1996;78:94–102.

43. Tokish JM, Krishnan SG, Hawkins RJ. Clinical examination of the overhead athlete: The "differential-directed" approach. In: Krishnan SG, Hawkins RJ, Warren RF, eds. *The Shoulder and the Overhead Athlete. A Holistic Approach.* Philadelphia, PA: Lippincott Williams & Wilkins; 2004:23–49.

44. Provencher MT, Frank RM, Leclere LE, et al. The Hill-Sachs lesion: Diagnosis, classification, and management. *J Am Acad Orthop Surg.* 2012;20:242–252.

45. Piasecki DP, Verma NN, Romeo AA, et al. Glenoid bone deficiency in recurrent anterior shoulder instability: Diagnosis and management. *J Am Acad Orthop Surg.* 2009;17: 482–493.

46. Bhatia S, Ghodadra NS, Romeo AA, et al. The importance of the recognition and treatment of glenoid bone loss in an athletic population. *Sports Health.* 2011;3:435–440.

47. Provencher MT, Bhatia S, Ghodadra NS, et al. Recurrent shoulder instability: Current concepts for evaluation and management of glenoid bone loss. *J Bone Joint Surg Am.* 2010;92(suppl 2):133–151.

48. Lodha S, Mazloom S, Resler A, et al. Shoulder instability treatment and rehabilitation. In: Brotzman SB, Manske RC, eds. *Clinical Orthopaedic Rehabilitation.* Philadelphia, PA: Elsevier; 2011:106–111.

49. Burkhead WZ Jr, Rockwood CA Jr. Treatment of instability of the shoulder with an exercise program. *J Bone Joint Surg Am.* 1992;74:890–896.

50. Hawkins RJ, Schutte JP, Janda DH, et al. Translation of the glenohumeral joint with the patient under anesthesia. *J Shoulder Elbow Surg.* 1996;5:286–292.

51. Mazzocca AD, Cote MP, Solovyova O, et al. Traumatic shoulder instability involving anterior, inferior, and posterior labral injury: A prospective clinical evaluation of arthroscopic repair of 270 degrees labral tears. *Am J Sports Med.* 2011;39:1687–1696.

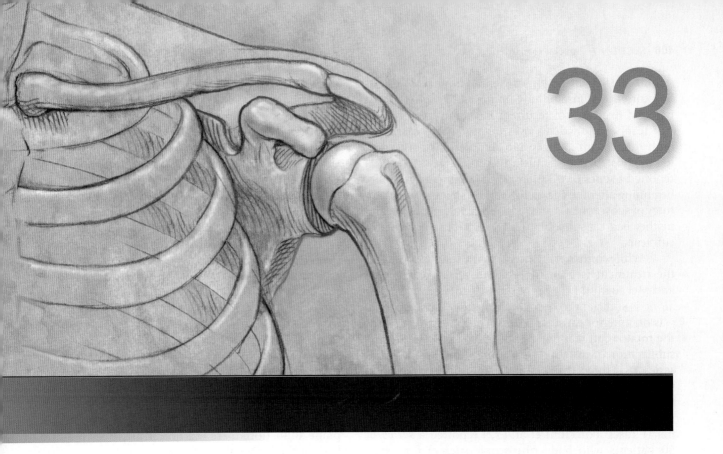

33

Recurrent Anterior Instability of the Shoulder Associated with Full-thickness Rotator Cuff Tear

Gilles Walch / Xinning Li /
Christopher J. Smithers / Patric Raiss

INTRODUCTION

Full-thickness rotator cuff tears associated with anterior glenohumeral instability are rare in patients younger than 40 years. This is in contrast to patients over 40 years, where cuff tears secondary to traumatic anterior dislocation occur in 34% to 100% of cases (1–4). Recurrent instability, however, is uncommon in this age group, observed in 0% to 33% of cases (0% Simonet and Cofield (5), 4% Pevny et al. (6), 4% Hawkins et al. (1), 14% Rowe (7), 22% Gumina and Postacchini (8), and 33% Neviaser et al. (9)). Because of this uncommon combination, very little research has been devoted to recurrent instability associated with full-thickness rotator cuff tears. Craig (10) reported three such cases in patients over 60 years, emphasizing the "posterior mechanism" initially described by McLaughlin (11), which describes recurrent instability in this age as related to the loss of dynamic stabilizers (rotator cuff tear) as opposed to the "anterior mechanism" in younger patients, where failure of static stabilizers (Bankart lesion or glenoid bone loss) results in recurrence of instability. Gumina and Postacchini (8) reported five cases of recurrent instability with rotator cuff tears in individuals over 60 years: Five cases had both rotator cuff and capsulolabral lesions contradicting the posterior mechanism theory. Neviaser et al. (2) reported a series of 11 patients with recurrent instability beginning after the age of 40 years: All had isolated ruptures of subscapularis and glenohumeral ligaments, and neither had capsulolabral lesions nor posterior rotator cuff tears.

While controversy exists as to the lesions observed, the treatment is even more controversial. Craig (10) and McLaughlin (11) proposed that rotator cuff repair alone is sufficient to treat the instability, because there was no anterior capsular lesion. Thus, the treatment of the rotator cuff tear will be sufficient to prevent future subluxation or instability. In Gumina and Postacchini's series (8), three cases had a stabilization associated with rotator cuff repair and two cases had isolated rotator cuff repair. For Neviaser et al. (9) subscapularis repair to the lesser tuberosity was enough to stabilize his 11 cases. Porcellini et al. (12) reported a series of 50 patients who had arthroscopic surgery for recurrent anterior instability associated with a full-thickness rotator cuff tear: All patients underwent arthroscopic anterior capsulolabral and rotator cuff repair. Hawkins et al. (1) reported two cases in which he did not repair the rotator cuff; Araghi et al. (13) reported two cases treated similarly. In 1987, we reported Trillat's experience of 24 cases of recurrent instability in patients over 40 years with rotator cuff tears and upward migration of the humeral head highly suggestive of massive rotator cuff tear: The treatment of instability without cuff repair achieved satisfactory results in 85% of these patients (14). Full-thickness rotator cuff tears with instability therefore pose several problems or questions: That of the anatomy of lesions to explain the recurrence and the treatment. Should the surgeon perform (1) a cuff repair, (2) anterior stabilization, or (3) both at the same time?

The aim of this chapter is to provide some answers to the above question from a review of the literature, retrospective series of surgically treated patients and the senior author's personal experience in managing this particular patient population.

BIOMECHANICAL EFFECTS OF ROTATOR CUFF TEAR AND INSTABILITY

Several authors have evaluated the contribution of rotator cuff to shoulder stability. Su et al. (15) found that transection of the anterosuperior rotator cuff tendon resulted in increased anterior and anterosuperior translations of the humeral head under higher loading conditions. This is especially true when the tear involves the anterior insertion of the rotator cuff cable, which is a thickened area of the rotator cuff originally described with Burkhart. However, with isolated small sectioning of the supraspinatus tear, there was no increase in glenohumeral translation even with higher loads. Parsons et al. (16) also found significant increases in both the magnitude and the direction of the joint reactive forces when the supraspinatus tendon was in combination with either the anterior (subscapularis tendon) or the posterior cuff (infraspinatus or teres minor tendon). In contrast, isolated supraspinatus tendon tear, either partial or full thickness, did not alter the joint reactive forces. Hsu et al. (17) also support the above findings in a biomechanical study of 12 cadavers. The authors found the tears' size and location (anterior tears) had the most influence on shoulder stability. Patients with rotator cuff tears also have altered in vivo glenohumeral and scapula thoracic kinematics. Paletta et al. (18) utilized a two-plane x-ray method to analyze 15 patients with rotator cuff tears and found that with scapular plane abduction, there was abnormal superior translation of the humeral head compared to normal shoulders. This abnormal translation was restored in 86% of 14/15 patients 2 years after the rotator cuff repair. Yamaguchi et al. (19) also reported similar alteration to the glenohumeral translation in patients with rotator cuff tears. Evidence from the literature does suggest that rotator cuff provides an essential function in shoulder stability and glenohumeral kinematics.

SENIOR AUTHOR'S (G. W.) EXPERIENCE IN MANAGING ROTATOR CUFF TEAR AND INSTABILITY

Patient Demographics

Between January 1988 and December 2002, 1,450 patients with recurrent anterior instability were treated surgically by the senior author (G. W.). Among this population, we found 28 shoulders in 27 patients with an associated rotator cuff tear confirmed with arthro-CT or arthro-MRI preoperatively. There were 22 men and 5 women, with mean age 53.1 years (25 to 71), and the dominant side was involved in 66% of the cases. The initial dislocations were all traumatic, with 50% skiing related. The mean number of dislocations was 2.6 (0 to 20), and four patients presented with recurrent subluxations. One patient presented with a complete sensorimotor deficit of the axillary nerve after the first dislocation, with complete recovery after 7 months. The average time between the first dislocation and surgery was 6.1 years (1 to 23 years).

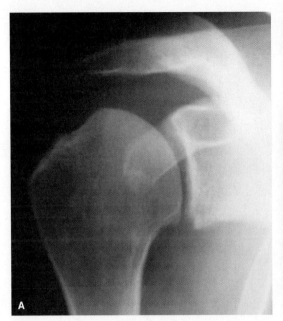 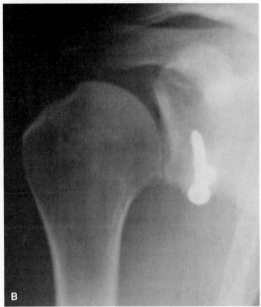

▲ **FIGURE 33-1:** (BOS) First dislocation by skiing, then recurrent dislocation (>10 episodes). **A:** Glenoid fracture—Hill-Sachs lesion, arthritis stage 1. Supraspinatus tear. **B:** Latarjet procedure + supraspinatus repair 25 years old. 10-year follow-up, 35 years old, stable. Constant score at 89 points, arthritis stage 2.

Patient Presentation and Radiographic Findings

Presentations included recurrent instability and apprehension in 14 cases (50%), chronic nocturnal pain following traumatic instability in 10 cases (36%), and a combination of these two for the remaining 4 cases (14%). Preoperatively, all patients underwent a complete clinical examination, including range of motion measurement, testing rotator cuff integrity, signs of instability, and Constant score (15). The average Constant score was 64.3 (49 to 83). X-rays included fluoroscopically controlled AP shoulder views in internal, external, and neutral humeral rotation, and a Bernageau view. These demonstrated (Tables 33-1 and 33-2) a Hill-Sachs lesion in 27 out of 28 humeral heads and an osseous Bankart lesion in 15 cases, ranging from a small inferior glenoid cortical fragment (Fig. 33-1) to a large anteroinferior glenoid fragment involving approximately a quarter of the glenoid face (Fig. 33-2). Osteoarthritis was present in 10 cases (35.7%), characterized by stage 1 inferior osteophytes (as defined by Parsons et al. (16)) in 7 cases (Fig. 33-3) and stage 2 in 3 cases. All but one patient (who had a massive three-tendon rotator cuff tear and would not consider repair) had additional imaging: 22 cases underwent CT arthrography and 5 cases an MRI (Tables 33-1 and 33-2). A full-thickness isolated supraspinatus tear was present in 12 cases, a combined supra- and infraspinatus tear in 10 cases, a combined supraspinatus and subscapularis tear once and finally, and 5 cases had a

massive tear involving all the three tendons. The long head of biceps tendon was ruptured in five cases, subluxated in six, and dislocated in one. Fatty infiltration of the rotator cuff muscles (17) was present in 18 cases and absent in 10 cases: Supraspinatus was involved in 13, infraspinatus in 15, and subscapularis in 6. (Please see Tables 33-1 and 33-2.)

Surgical Treatment

Two types of procedures were performed: Either an open stabilization of Trillat (20) with a biceps tendon tenodesis (if present) in 19 cases or a Latarjet coracoid transfer associated with a rotator cuff repair in 9 cases. The choice between these two techniques was based on the reparability of the rotator cuff and motivation of the patient. When the cuff was deemed irreparable (subacromial space less than 7 mm on the AP view in neutral rotation and/or Goutallier fatty infiltration of cuff muscle greater than stage 2) or when the patient was not willing to consider cuff repair (age or motivation), Trillat's stabilization (which had previously proved effective in this situation) was proposed.

The Trillat stabilization was performed using the original technique: Following a transdeltoid approach, the joint was entered via the upper edge of subscapularis and explored to look for bony lesions. Fractures of the anterior–inferior glenoid were found in nine cases, and Bankart lesions were found in nine cases. In each case, a rasp was used to fresh the anterior glenoid. The coracoid

(text continues on page 412)

TABLE 33-1 Epidemiologic Data of the Patients Operated on with a Latarjet Procedure and Cuff Repair

Name	Sex	Age, First Dislocation	Circumstances, First Dislocation	Type of Instability	Age at Operation	Hill-Sachs	Glenoid Lesion	Rotator Cuff Tear	FI Muscles	Preoperative Arthritis (Samilson)	Procedure	
											Rotator Cuff	LHB
ANG	M	42	Soccer	Recurrent subluxation	46	+	0	SSp	0	Stage 1	TOR	Tenodesis
BOS	M	18	Ski	Recurrent dislocation	25	+	Fc	SSp	0	Stage 1	TOR	
DES	M	53	Ski	Recurrent dislocation	54	+	Fc	SSp + ISp	0	0	TOR	Tenodesis
GAB	M	48	Ski	Recurrent dislocation	48	+	Bankart	SSp	0	0	2 anchors	Tenodesis
MAR	M	23	Moto	Recurrent dislocation	40	Non	Bankart	SSp + ISp	FI st. 1 ISp	0	TOR	Tenodesis
PAI	M	45	Ski	Recurrent dislocation	49	+	Fc	SSp	0	Stage 1	TOR	Tenodesis
PIC	M	16	Rugby	Recurrent dislocation	39	+	Fc	SSp	0	0	2 anchors	
RAN	M	27	Soccer	Recurrent dislocation	32	+	Fc	SSp + sub-luxation LHB	0	0	2 anchors	Tenodesis
ROM	M	26	Soccer	Recurrent subluxation	28	+	Fc	SSp	0	0	1 anchor	

Fc, fracture; SSp, supraspinatus; ISp, infraspinatus; LHB, long head of biceps; FI, fatty infiltration; TOR, transosseous repair.

TABLE 33-2   Epidemiologic Data of the Patients Operated on with a Trillat Procedure

Name	Gender	Age, First Dislocation	Circumstances	Type of Instability	Age at Operation	Hill-Sachs	Glenoid Lesion	Rotator Cuff Tear	Muscles FI	Preoperative Arthritis (Samilson)	Other
BOE	M	52	Fall	Recurrent dislocation	62	+	Bankart	SSp + ISp	St. 2 SSp, St. 3 ISp	0	
BOR	M	51	Ski	Recurrent dislocation	52	+	Fc	SE + SOE + SScap + ruptured LHB	St. 3 SSp, ISp, SScap	0	
CHA	M	40	Fall	Recurrent dislocation	46	+	Fc	SE + SOE + SScap + luxation LHB	St. 2 SScap, St. 4 ISp	St. 2	Coracoid fracture
COR	F	65	Fall	Recurrent dislocation	70	+	Fc	SSp + ISp	St. 3 SSp, St. 2 ISp	0	
DIS gche	F	57	Fight	Recurrent subluxation	71	+	Fc	SSp + ISp	St. 2 SSp, St. 2 ISp	0	
DIS dte	F	65	Fall	Recurrent dislocation	71	+	Fc	SSp + ISp + subluxation LHB	St. 3 SSp, St. 3 ISp	0	
GUI	M	44	Ski	Recurrent dislocation	57	+	Fc	SSp	0	0	
JAC	F	51	Ski	Recurrent dislocation	61	+	Bankart	SSp + ISp	St. 3 SSp, St. 2 ISp	0	
JAN	M	28	Soccer	Recurrent dislocation	47	+	Bankart	SSp + ISp + SScap	St. 4 ISp	St. 1	
JEA	M	45	Ski	Recurrent dislocation	49	+	Fc	SSp + SScap + ruptured LHB	St. 3 SSp, SScap	St. 2	Coracoid fracture
LAU	M	61	Fall	Recurrent dislocation	63	+	Bankart	SSp + ISp + SScap + ruptured LHB	St. 3 ISp, St. 4 SScap	0	
MAZ	M	58	Ski	Recurrent dislocation	62	+	Fc	SSp	St. 1 ISp	St. 1	

(continued on page 410)

TABLE 33-2 Epidemiologic Data of the Patients Operated on with a Trillat Procedure (continued)

Name	Gender	Age, First Dislocation	Circumstances	Type of Instability	Age at Operation	Hill-Sachs	Glenoid Lesion	Rotator Cuff Tear	Muscles FI	Preoperative Arthritis (Samilson)	Other
MET	M	50	Ski	Recurrent dislocation	61	+	Bankart	SSp + ISp + SScap + ruptured LHB	St. 3 ISp, St. 1 SSp, SScap	St. 1	
MOR	M	54	Ski	Recurrent subluxation	55	+	Bankart	SSp + ruptured LHB	St. 1 ISp	0	
NAY	M	55	Fall	Recurrent dislocation	56	+	Bankart	SSp + ISp + subluxation LHB	St. 3 SE, ISp	0	
NIV	F	58	Fall	Recurrent dislocation	59	+	0	SSp + subluxation LHB	St. 3 SSp, St. 1 SScap	0	
PAN	M	57	Ski	Recurrent dislocation	60	+	Bankart	SSp	0	St. 1	
PYA	M	63	Ski	Recurrent dislocation	64	+	Fc	SSp + ISp + subluxation LHB	St. 3 SSp, St. 2 ISp	St. 2	
RAV	F	59	Fall	Recurrent dislocation	61	+	Bankart	SSp + ISp + subluxation LHB	St. 4 SSp, St. 3 ISp	0	

Fc, fracture; SSp, supraspinatus; ISp, infraspinatus; Sscap, subscapularis; LHB, long head of biceps; FI, fatty infiltration.

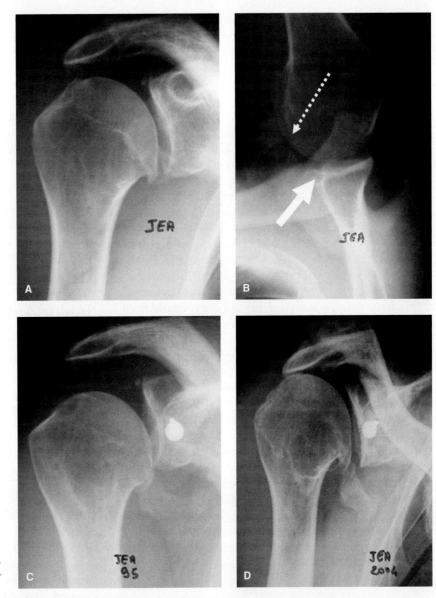

▶ **FIGURE 33-2:** (JEA) First dislocation by skiing, 45 years old, then recurrent subluxation and dislocation (four episodes). Ruptured SSp + SScap, FI st. 3 Ssp – st. 4 SScap. **A,B:** Arthritis stage 1, glenoid rim fracture, nonunion of the coracoid. **C:** Trillat procedure + tenodesis of LHB when 49 years old. **D:** Follow-up 9 years. Constant score 77 points. Very satisfied, stable. Arthritis stage 3.

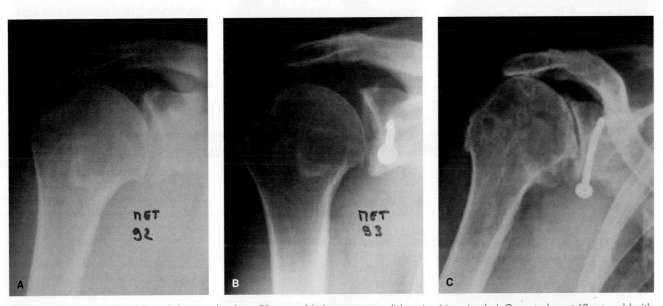

▲ **FIGURE 33-3:** (MET) First dislocation by skiing 50 years old, then recurrent dislocation (six episodes). Operated on at 60 years old with rupture of SSp + ISp + SScap + LHB. **A:** ISp fatty infiltration stage 3 and stage 1, Ssp and Sscap arthritis stage 1. **B:** Trillat procedure + tenodesis of LHB (61 years old). **C:** Follow-up 13 years (73 years old), stable, Constant score 77 points, very satisfied despite an arthritis stage 4.

was then osteotomized at its base, and carefully lowered and medialized so that its tip did not extend lateral to the glenohumeral joint. The fixation was by a Hahn nail in 14 cases and by a malleolar screw in 5 cases. In cases where the biceps had not already ruptured, tenodesis was performed by either suturing to the subscapularis or by resorbable interference screw (21). Postoperatively, a simple sling was worn for 15 days with early passive rehabilitation commenced immediately. Use of the shoulder for activities of daily living was allowed gradually from the fifteenth day and sporting activity from 3 months.

The other nine patients underwent stabilization with a modified Latarjet–Patte stabilization (subscapularis split in the line of its fibers) (22–24) associated with rotator cuff repair. The deltopectoral approach was used, but the skin incision was extended proximally and laterally to allow for a deltoid split used for the cuff repair. Firstly, the coracoid transposition was performed through the deltopectoral interval and the coracoid fixed by two malleolar screws. Small fragments of the anterior edge of the glenoid were resected and isolated Bankart lesions, found twice, were decorticated. One case had no anterior–inferior glenoid lesion identified at the time of operation. A separate anterolateral deltoid split was then made, an acromioplasty performed and the cuff repaired by a transosseous double-U technique (25). Six patients required a tenodesis of the long head of the biceps by a resorbable interference screw. Patients were placed in a 20-degree abduction splint for 1 month, then a simple sling for the second month. Passive rehabilitation was commenced immediately postoperatively to preserve passive range of motion. Stretching was commenced from the second month and continued until the end of the sixth month, at which time the resumption of sports activities was allowed. No weights training exercises were allowed prior to the end of the sixth month.

Review of Patients

There were no patients lost to follow-up. The authors reviewed 22 and 6 were reviewed by phone interview with physical examination performed by their local doctor or orthopedic surgeon. Data collected included range of motion, rotator cuff strength, the Constant score, and the Duplay score for instability (14). The subjective outcome was assessed by asking the patients if they were very satisfied, satisfied, uncertain, or disappointed with the outcome of their surgery. A radiologic assessment included fluoroscopically controlled AP shoulder views in internal, external, and neutral humeral rotation, and a Bernageau view.

Statistics

To compare qualitative variables, the exact Fisher test or the chi-square test were used. For quantitative variables, analysis of variance (Anova) and the Bonferroni test for multiple comparisons were used. The level of significance was set at $p < 0.05$.

Senior Author's Results (G. W.)

Overall Results

The 28 shoulders in 27 patients were reviewed at a mean of 73.5 months (24 to 178), and the mean age at the time of follow-up was 59.1 years (30 to 74). Subjectively, 26 patients were satisfied or very satisfied (96%) and 1 patient was disappointed. The Constant score had increased from 64.3 to 78.1 ($p < 0.05$), with details of the different components listed in Table 33-3. The Duplay score at the time of review was 88/100.

Complications and Revisions

Three patients who underwent the Trillat procedure had recurrent instability. In one case, the patient suffered a single dislocation following a fall while ice skating 7 years postoperatively that required a reduction under general anesthesia. At 5 years of follow-up after the dislocation, aged 73 years, the patient had no further dislocations and was "very satisfied." In the other two cases, multiple recurrent dislocations occurred after the initial procedure. In one patient, the first episode of instability occurred 6 months postoperatively and required revision to convert the Trillat procedure to a Latarjet–Patte. At

TABLE 33-3 Pre- and Postoperative Constant Score

Constant Score	Preoperative	Postoperative	p
Pain (/15)	7.5	13.1	$p < 0.05$
Activity (/20)	11.6	17.6	$p < 0.05$
Mobility (/40)	37.8	36.4	NS
Strength (kg × 2) (/25)	7.4	11	$p < 0.05$
Constant score (/100)	64.3	78.1	$p < 0.05$

NS, not significant.

TABLE 33-4 Comparison of the Results Between Trillat Procedure and Latarjet + Cuff Repair

	Trillat	Latarjet + Cuff Repair
n	19 cases	9 cases
Age at follow-up	65.5 yrs	45.8 yrs
Follow-up	75.3 mos	69.6 mos
Results Duplay score/100	82.9 points	98.8 points
Recurrence of instability	3 cases	0 case
Constant score (100 points)	72.4	90.7
Adjusted Constant score (%)	86.3	95.2
Strength (kg × 2)	8.4	16.4
Subjective results	Very satisfied: 14 cases Satisfied: 4 cases Disappointed: 1 case	Very satisfied: 7 cases Satisfied: 2 cases
External rotation at 0-degree abduction	47.3 degrees	56 degrees
External rotation at 90-degree abduction	82 degrees	77 degrees

the final follow-up 11 years later, the shoulder is stable and the patient "very satisfied." The last patient had two recurrences 6 and 7 years after the initial operation; aged 70 years old, he refused revision surgery and was disappointed with his result. Four other complications were observed: One adhesive capsulitis, one superficial wound infection that resolved with antibiotic treatment, and two nail migrations following Trillat procedures that requiring reoperation for simple removal.

Radiographic Findings

The radiographs showed progressive osteoarthritis, with the prevalence increasing from 35.7% to 64.3%. Based on the Walch et al. (14) staging, seven patients had stage 1 osteoarthritis, seven patients stage 2, two patients stage 3, and four patients stage 4 characterized by severe joint space narrowing with or without osteophyte formation.

Results Based on the Operative Procedure

The Trillat and Latarjet–Patte procedures were performed on very different populations: The average age of patients treated using the Trillat technique was 20 years higher than that of the Latarjet–Patte. Cuff lesions (Tables 33-1 and 33-2) were also very different between these two populations. Comparison of the functional and subjective results of the two operations is therefore not worthwhile. The recurrence rate after Latarjet with cuff repair is zero in this short series, compared with 16% after stabilization by the Trillat technique without

cuff repair (Table 33-4). The rate of revision after the Trillat procedure (two recurrences and two nail removals) was 10.5%, while there were no revisions following the Latarjet–Patte procedure. The rate of postoperative arthritis was 44% after Latarjet–Patte and 84% after Trillat, but again age prevents any meaningful comparison.

Statistical Correlations

We correlated the sex of patients, the affected side, the age at first dislocation, the type of instability, the number of dislocations and age at surgery with glenoid lesions (fracture or not), Hill-Sachs lesions, preoperative osteoarthritis, tendon ruptures, fatty infiltration, and clinical and radiographic results. Age at first dislocation, preoperative delay, and age at operation are significantly associated with the number of ruptured tendons and fatty infiltration of the rotator cuff muscles ($p < 0.05$). The average age of patients without postoperative osteoarthritis was 50.4 years, whereas it was 62.7 years for patients with osteoarthritis ($p < 0.05$). We did not find any significant difference in age between the different stages of osteoarthritis. The preoperative delay between the first dislocation and the surgery and the number of dislocations did not correlate with the occurrence of osteoarthritis ($p > 0.1$). We did not find any correlation with sex, the affected side, preoperative osteoarthritis, osseous Bankart lesions, Hills-Sachs lesions, and the number of dislocations. Furthermore, we did not find any correlation between the initial complaint of patients (pain or instability) and subjective or objective outcomes.

Literature Review and Discussion

The results reported in this book chapter should be interpreted in reference to the two different patient groups: The first consists of five patients under 40 years who had a full-thickness cuff tear associated with recurrent dislocations, and the second consists of 23 patients over 40 years who have recurrent dislocations associated with a cuff tear. Hawkins et al. (26) described five cases of full-thickness cuff tear following anterior traumatic dislocation in patients under 40 years, Throckmorton and Albright (27) reported an 18-year-old patient with anterior instability and both a Bankart lesion and a rotator cuff tear that was surgically repaired, and two cases of isolated rotator cuff tears in the setting of posterior dislocation have also been reported in patients younger than 40 years (28,29). Our five patients were all men who suffered their first dislocation secondary to a sports accident. Weakness and/or the presence of nocturnal pain associated with recurrent instability may help identify this complication and lead to additional preoperative imaging.

Recurrent dislocations in patients whose first episode occurred beyond 40 years have been reported in 0% to 33% of cases (2,4,6–9). The association with a cuff tear seems curiously rare. Araghi et al. (13) reported on a series of 11 patients treated surgically for recurrent instability that are over 40 years, and 9 showed no tear. Similarly, Hawkins et al. (1) described eight similar cases, with only two demonstrating a cuff tear. However, Gumina and Postacchini (8) described eight cases operated on for recurrent instability that began after the age of 60, and only three did not have a rotator cuff tear. We believe that in adults over 40 years, an anterior dislocation can cause a rotator cuff tear, but there is no evidence to demonstrate that the rotator cuff tear is the primary etiology of the recurrence. This is in contrast to the proposed "posterior mechanism" (10,11), which suggests that recurrent dislocations in this age group are secondary to the cuff rupture. Neviaser et al. (9) suggested that subscapularis has an important role in recurrence at this age: They reported 11 cases of recurrent anterior instability that had an isolated avulsion of the subscapularis at the lesser tuberosity without a Bankart lesion. We have found no case in our series corresponding to this description. On the contrary, all our patients had bone lesions and typical capsuloligamentous instability: A Hill-Sachs lesion was present in 96.5%, an anteroinferior bony Bankart in 53.5%, and a soft tissue Bankart injury in 39.3%. In only two patients (7.1%) there was no capsuloligamentous injury, however, these two patients had a Hill-Sachs lesion. Similarly, none of our patients had isolated subscapularis rupture. In this series of 28 cases of recurrent dislocation associated with a cuff tear, the "anterior mechanism" therefore seems to be the predominant, if not exclusive cause for recurrence, as in younger patients. In regard to cuff tears, with the exception of isolated subscapularis tears,

we found all the typical patterns. No data in our series indicate whether the cuff tear was a consequence of the first traumatic dislocation or a recurrence.

The treatment of anterior instability associated with rotator cuff tears is controversial. It is important to note that in the literature, the vast majority of articles relate to single episodes of instability associated with rotator cuff tears in patients over 40 years. In recurrent instability, Neviaser et al. (9) proposed repairing isolated subscapularis tears. All the patients in their series were stable, pain free, and had recovery of full mobility. Gumina and Postacchini (8) reported five surgically treated cases: The three patients who had a rotator cuff repair associated with anterior stabilization obtained a satisfactory result; however, the two cases that had only cuff repairs had further instability. Hawkins et al. (1) reported the outcomes of two cases of recurrent anterior instability in patients over 40 years of age with repair of the rotator cuff (one patient also had Magnuson–Stack repair). Postoperatively, both patients had poor functional outcome; however, recurrence of instability was eliminated. Pevny et al. (6) retrospectively reviewed 52 patients over the age of 40 years with traumatic anterior shoulder dislocation. Full-thickness rotator cuff tears were identified in 18 patients (35%); however, only 12 patients (23%) had isolated cuff tears. Of these, six patients had nonoperative treatment and six had rotator cuff repair. In the six patients that had a rotator cuff repair, five (84%) had excellent or good results with no recurrent instability at greater than 2 years of follow-up. Only 50% of the patients with isolated rotator cuff tears (3/6) achieved excellent or good results with nonoperative treatment. Recurrent instability was seen only in two patients (4%) in their series with all treatment methods (nonoperative and operative).

In the series of patients we published in 1987, 24 patients with recurrent dislocation after 40 years treated surgically by Albert Trillat had direct or indirect radiologic evidence of rotator cuff tears. With a mean follow-up of 10.8 years, 63% had a good result according to the criteria of Rowe, and 88% were satisfied. Stability was normal in 75% of the cases, four patients (17%) were apprehension test positive, one patient (4%) had recurrent subluxations, and only one patient (4%) had further dislocations and had to be revised. We learned from this series that the Trillat stabilization procedure was satisfactory even in this age group, if the patients had a significant cuff tear recognized on preoperative radiographs by upward migration of the humeral head. Therefore, we continued with this procedure when the cuff was considered irreparable: In cases of subacromial narrowing, severe fatty infiltration of supraspinatus or infraspinatus, in the elderly or in cases where the patient was not motivated to undergo appropriate rehabilitation. In addition to these good historical results, the rationale for Trillat stabilization compared to the Latarjet procedure was based upon respecting the subscapularis muscle/tendon, which, instead of being split, was retensioned and lowered by the transferred coracoid (14). Of the 19 patients in this new series with the Trillat procedure, we can confirm that none have lost active mobility, 94% are satisfied or very satisfied, despite a 16% recurrence rate. This recurrence rate is comparable to the 14.5% recurrence that we observed after Trillat stabilization of anterior instability in younger patients (14).

However, when a decision was made to repair the rotator cuff, we performed a Latarjet–Patte stabilization with an open repair. We did not observe any recurrence of instability, 100% of the patients were satisfied or very satisfied, and the mean Constant score was 90.7 points. However, we have not performed imaging to assess the anatomical result of the rotator cuff repair. The rate of pre- and postoperative arthritis in this patient population is particularly important because we have observed 37.5% of osteoarthritis preoperatively and 64.3% postoperatively. There was no significant difference in age between patients who did or did not show preoperative osteoarthritis (51 vs. 54 years). In contrast, the age of postoperative patients with osteoarthritis was statistically higher than the age in those without osteoarthritis (62.6 vs. 50.4 years, $p < 0.05$), which implies that instability surgery may contribute to osteoarthritis progression in people over 40 years. In the large series of 570 cases of recurrent anterior instability presented at the SOFCOT symposium in 1999 (30), Buscayret et al. (31) presented a preoperative osteoarthritis rate of 9.5% with a mean age of 32 years. At the median postoperative follow-up of 6.5 years, the rate rose to 29%, which was the same irrespective of procedure, Bankart or Latarjet–Patte. There is more than 20 years difference in average age between this series and the patients presented in this chapter, so a comparison is impossible. Similarly, we cannot compare the rates of osteoarthritis after Latarjet–Patte or after Trillat procedure, since the average ages at review were 45.8 and 65.5, respectively. Therefore, we cannot conclude on the influence of repair of the rotator cuff on the prognosis of osteoarthritis in our series. We have found no comparable series of Bankart repairs which would allow us assess the role of stabilization procedures in the progression of arthritis, but we have seen in the SOFCOT symposium series that the rate of osteoarthritis was the same after Bankart repair and coracoid transfer (30). Neviaser et al. (2) did not report the radiologic findings of his series of 11 cases of stabilization by repair of isolated subscapularis tears.

Besides the small series reported in the literature, Porcellini et al. (12) reported a surprisingly large series of 50 anterior dislocations associated with a full-thickness tear of the rotator cuff. All patients in their series underwent arthroscopic surgery over a 2-year period: All patients had anterior capsulolabral lesions, and the series included five cases that presented with an isolated rupture of the subscapularis. Every patient in the study had an arthroscopic cuff repair and capsulo-ligamentous repair. There were no irreparable cuff tears (patients with a subacromial space less than 5 mm were excluded from the study), and two cases (4%) had recurrence of instability and required a Latarjet stabilization. No pre- or postoperative imaging is reported, preventing any analysis of the incidence of osteoarthritis. In regard to case numbers, this series is similar in size to the entire literature and all were treated in an extremely short period, but it does address the more recent issue about the role of arthroscopy in the treatment of these combined lesions. If reliable in the longer term, this is indeed the ideal solution because it allows treatment of both lesions in a much less invasive manner. However, arthroscopic repair can only be safely proposed when there is no severe muscle fatty infiltration and when bone lesions of the anterior margin of the glenoid permit anchor placement (32). According to these criteria, only four of our cases (14%) were appropriate candidates for arthroscopic treatment and all other patients had either a massive irreparable cuff tears preventing cuff repair or severe bony Bankart lesion.

Another treatment option is isolated arthroscopic or open rotator cuff repair, based on the rationale that return of active humeral head stabilizers will be sufficient to maintain stability. Araghi et al. (13), Craig (10), and Hawkins et al. (1) used this treatment approach, but they did not report their results; however, Gumina and Postacchini (8) reported two failures. We believe that recurrent instability is dependent upon bony and capsuloligamentous lesions of the anteroinferior glenoid rim (present in 93% of cases in our series), and this treatment option runs the risk of recurrence with possible rupture of repaired tendons.

CONCLUSION

In conclusion, recurrent instability associated with a full-thickness cuff tear is a rare entity representing only 2% of recurrent anterior instability cases. The typical lesions of anterior–inferior instability are present in 93% of the cases and rotator cuff tears observed have similar characteristics to those typically observed in this age group. The indication for surgery is based on instability or pain secondary to the rotator cuff tear. The choice of surgical technique depends on the reparability of the rotator cuff, which requires assessment of the size and retraction of the tear along with cuff muscle fatty infiltration with a systematic preoperative CT arthrography. When the cuff is considered reparable, the Latarjet–Patte coracoid transfer associated with open cuff repair resulted in stability in 100% of the cases in our series. Arthroscopy does seem an ideal and elegant solution, but its results need to be further evaluated. Isolated stabilization by Trillat procedure restored stability in 86% of our cases with irreparable cuff tears. This type of surgery does however pay a heavy price, with a 64% rate of osteoarthritis.

It will be very interesting to see whether arthroscopic solutions will reduce this frequency despite the age of this population. Furthermore, there is not enough evidence in the literature to conclude that isolated repair of the rotator cuff without addressing the anteroinferior capsulolabral structures (Trillat or Latarjet procedure) will suffice to prevent recurrent subluxations or dislocations. In our series of patients with instability and rotator cuff tears, we fell that the "anterior mechanism" was the primary contributor to stability. Thus, we recommend addressing the anterior lesion as the essential aspect of the management plan and also to repair the rotator cuff if the muscle is of good quality with either an open or an arthroscopic technique.

References

1. Hawkins RJ, Bell RH, Hawkins RH, et al. Anterior dislocation of the shoulder in the older patient. *Clin Orthop Relat Res.* 1986;(206):192–195.
2. Neviaser RJ, Neviaser TJ, Neviaser JS. Anterior dislocation of the shoulder and rotator cuff rupture. *Clin Orthop Relat Res.* 1993;(291):103–106.
3. Ribbans WJ, Mitchell R, Taylor GJ. Computerised arthrotomography of primary anterior dislocation of the shoulder. *J Bone Joint Surg Br.* 1990;72(2):181–185.
4. Toolanen G, Hildingsson C, Hedlund T, et al. Early complications after anterior dislocation of the shoulder in patients over 40 years. An ultrasonographic and electromyographic study. *Acta Orthop Scand.* 1993;64(5):549–552.
5. Simonet WT, Cofield RH. Prognosis in anterior shoulder dislocation. *Am J Sports Med.* 1984;12:19–24.
6. Pevny T, Hunter RE, Freeman JR. Primary traumatic anterior shoulder dislocation in patients 40 years of age and older. *Arthroscopy.* 1998;14(3):289–294.
7. Rowe CR. Prognosis in dislocations of the shoulder. *J Bone Joint Surg Am.* 1956;38-A(5):957–977.
8. Gumina S, Postacchini F. Anterior dislocation of the shoulder in the elderly patient. *J Bone Joint Surg Am.* 1997;79:540–543.
9. Neviaser RJ, Neviaser TJ, Neviaser JS. Concurrent rupture of the rotator cuff and anterior dislocation of the shoulder in the older patient. *J Bone Joint Surg Am.* 1988;70(9):1308–1311.
10. Craig EV. The posterior mechanism of acute anterior shoulder dislocations. *Clin Orthop Relat Res.* 1984; (190):212–216.
11. McLaughlin H. Injuries of the shoulder and arm. In: Mc Laughlin H, Harrisson L, eds. *Trauma.* Philadelphia, PA: WB Saunders; 1959.
12. Porcellini G, Paladini P, Campi F, et al. Shoulder instability and related rotator cuff tears: Arthroscopic findings and treatment in patients aged 40 to 60 years. *Arthroscopy.* 2006;22(3):270–276.
13. Araghi A, Prasarn M, St Clair S, et al. Recurrent anterior glenohumeral instability with onset after forty years of age: The role of the anterior mechanism. *Bull Hosp Jt Dis.* 2005;62(3–4):99–101.
14. Walch G, Neyret P, Charret P, et al. L'opération de Trillat pour luxation récidivante antérieure de l'épaule. Résultats à long terme de 250 cas avec un recul moyen de 11,3 ans. *Lyon Chir.* 1989;85:25–31.
15. Su WR, Budoff JE, Luo ZP. The effect of anterosuperior rotator cuff tears on glenohumeral translation. *Arthroscopy.* 2009; 25(3):282-9.
16. Parsons IM, Apreleva M, Fu FH, et al. The effect of rotator cuff tears on reaction forces at the glenohumeral joint. *J Orthop Res.* 2002;20(3):439–446.
17. Hsu HC, Luo ZP, Cofield RH, et al. Influence of rotator cuff tearing on glenohumeral stability. *J Shoulder Elbow Surg.* 1997;6(5):413–422.
18. Paletta GA Jr, Warner JJ, Warren RF, et al. Shoulder kinematics with two-plane x-ray evaluation in patients with anterior instability or rotator cuff tearing. *J Shoulder Elbow Surg.* 1997;6(6):516–527.
19. Yamaguchi K, Sher JS, Andersen WK, et al. Glenohumeral motion in patients with rotator cuff tears: A comparison of asymptomatic and symptomatic shoulders. *J Shoulder Elbow Surg.* 2000;9(1):6–11.
20. Trillat A, LeClerc-Chalvet F. *Luxation récidivante de l'épaule.* In: Trillat A, Chalvet F, eds. Paris: Masson; 1973.
21. Edwards TB, Walch G. Biceps tenodesis: Indications and techniques. *Op Tech Sports Med.* 2002;10:99–104.
22. Latarjet M. A propos du traitement des lésions récidivantes de l'épaule. *Lyon Chir.* 1954;49: 994–1003.
23. Patte D, Bernageau J, Trodineau J, et al. Epaules douloureuses et instables. *Rev Chir Orthop.* 1980;66:157–166.
24. Walch G, Boileau P. Latarjet–Bristow procedure for recurrent anterior instability. *Tech Shoulder Elbow Surg.* 2000;3:136–141.
25. Walch G, Edwards TB. Double U suturing technique for repair of the rotator cuff. *Tech Shoulder Elbow Surg.* 2002;3:136–141.
26. Hawkins RJ, Morin WD, Bonutti PM. Surgical treatment of full-thickness rotator cuff tears in patients 40 years of age or younger. *J Shoulder Elbow Surg.* 1999;8(3):259–265.
27. Throckmorton T, Albright J. Case report: Concurrent anterior shoulder dislocation and rotator cuff tear in a young athlete. *Iowa Orthop J.* 2001;21:76–79.
28. Schoenfeld AJ, Lippitt SB. Rotator cuff tear associated with a posterior dislocation of the shoulder in a young adult: A case report and literature review. *J Orthop Trauma.* 2007;21(2):150–152.
29. Steinitz DK, Harvey EJ, Lenczner EM. Traumatic posterior dislocation of the shoulder associated with a massive rotator cuff tear: A case report. *Am J Sports Med.* 2003;31(6):1010–1012.
30. Coudane H, Walch G. Instabilité antérieure de l'épaule. *Rev Chir Orthop.* 2000;86:91–149.
31. Buscayret F, Edwards TB, Szabo I, et al. Glenohumeral arthrosis in anterior instability before and after surgical treatment. Incidence and contributing factors. *Am J Sports Med.* 2004;32:1165–1172.
32. Boileau P, Brassart N, Watkinson DJ, et al. Arthroscopic repair of full-thickness tears of the supraspinatus: Does the tendon really heal? *J Bone Joint Surg Am.* 2005; 87(6):1229–1240.

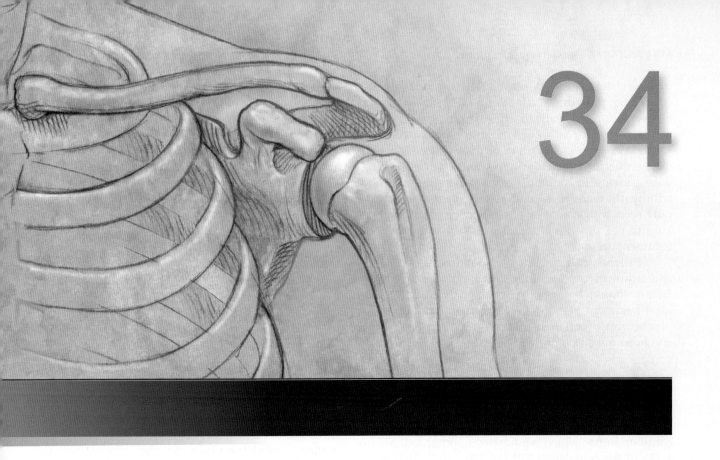

34

COMBINED ANTERIOR INSTABILITY AND GLENOHUMERAL ARTHRITIS

Bryan J. Loeffler / Joseph A. Abboud

INTRODUCTION

Patients with combined anterior instability and glenohumeral arthritis represent a challenging set of clinical scenarios and the management of these patients should be tailored on the basis of a careful review of the patient's symptoms, physical examination findings, prior surgical history, and imaging. Combined instability and glenohumeral arthritis has been referred to as "arthritis of recurrent dislocation" (1), "arthritis of instability" (2), or "dislocation arthropathy" (3), and it may occur with instability previously treated operatively or nonoperatively. The term "capsulorrhaphy-induced arthropathy" (4) specifically refers to arthritis that develops following instability surgery. Arthritis from intra-articular anchor placement, hardware migration, or chondrolysis following instability surgery (5,6) represents yet another subset of patients with combined instability and glenohumeral arthritis.

Most commonly, these patients present with decreased, painful range of motion, and a history of glenohumeral instability (7). In particular, postcapsulorrhaphy patients may have marked internal rotation contractures. The associated posterior humeral head subluxation and posterior glenoid wear can be more severe than is seen with primary osteoarthritis (OA) (1,8). Stabilization procedures for anterior instability which place excessive tension on the anterior soft tissues can contribute

417

to these changes (1,9). While many of the nonanatomic stabilizing procedures historically described are no longer performed, patients who had these operations in the past are predisposed to arthritis at a relatively young age. An understanding of these procedures and their sequelae is therefore important when evaluating these patients. In addition, because postcapsulorrhaphy arthropathy tends to occur at a younger age than is typically seen with osteo- or inflammatory glenohumeral arthritis (1), this can further increase the complexity of treatment options.

Patients with combined glenohumeral instability and arthritis require a thoughtful approach, and many factors should be considered when determining the ideal treatment plan. Surgical treatment may be complex because of soft tissue contractures, altered anatomy, and bone or soft tissue deficiencies.

Anterior Glenohumeral Instability

Anteroinferior glenohumeral dislocation is a relatively common injury, which is estimated to occur in 0.5% to 1.7% of the population (10,11). The cartilage damage and bone injury which occur with traumatic shoulder dislocation are thought to predispose patients to degenerative changes in the glenohumeral joint (12). In addition, surgically induced factors have been identified which can contribute to the development of articular cartilage degeneration.

Although the development of glenohumeral arthrosis is a known potential sequela of both operative and nonoperative management of shoulder instability, the reported prevalence varies widely. Across the literature, the quoted incidence of arthritis from instability typically refers to the percentage of patients who develop any radiographic changes of arthritis. However, the rates of severe radiographic arthritis, symptomatic arthritis, and arthritis requiring shoulder arthroplasty are significantly lower than those with merely radiographic changes.

Treatment

The management of anterior instability can be categorized into nonoperative and operative treatment. Nonoperative treatment includes a rehabilitation program aimed at strengthening the rotator cuff, deltoid, and scapular stabilizers. The exact incidence and severity of arthritis following nonoperative anterior instability is unknown. In a series of 245 patients treated nonoperatively for an anterior dislocation, Hovelius et al. (13) reported a 20% incidence of radiographic degenerative changes at 10 years. Mild radiographic changes were seen in 11% and moderate to severe changes were observed in 9%. Arthroplasty for dislocation arthropathy had not been performed in any of the patients at the

10-year follow-up. The authors also reported no correlation between the number of dislocations and the development of arthritis (13). The strongest risk factors for developing arthritis after nonoperative management of an instability event appear to be age at the time of dislocation and the presence of bony lesions (14).

Operative Treatment

Arthritis has been reported to develop in a range of 12% to 69% of shoulders following surgery for anterior instability (15–19). Surgical factors such as intra-articular placement of anchors or other hardware which can cause articular impingement (5), lateral overhang of the transferred coracoid (20), and excessive tightening of the anterior soft tissues (9) have been identified as contributors to the development and/or progression of glenohumeral arthritis.

Operative management of anterior instability may be divided into anatomic and nonanatomic procedures. Discussion of the indications and techniques of each of these procedures is beyond the scope of this chapter, but a familiarity of these procedures is imperative for the surgeon considering revision surgery after a prior anterior stabilization.

Anatomic Procedures

Arthroscopic Bankart Repair with or without Capsular Shift

Little data on glenohumeral arthropathy following arthroscopic Bankart repair exists (14,17,21). Although the exact incidence of arthrosis in this patient population is unknown, Buscayret et al. (14) reported an 8.7% incidence of arthropathy at a mean of 3.3 years follow-up, while Franceschi et al. (21) observed a 22% incidence after an average follow-up of 8 years. Older age at the time of first dislocation, increased time between the first instability episode to surgery, increased number of anchors, and a more degenerative labrum are reported risk factors for developing arthritic change (21).

Open Bankart

Longer follow-up exists for patients treated by an open Bankart procedure (22,23) with or without capsular shift (24). Glenohumeral arthritis increased from 4% incidence preoperatively to 17% at a mean of 40 months postoperatively (25) with open Bankart repair and superoinferior capsular shift as described by Neer and Foster (24). Although Buscayret et al. (14) reported a 54% incidence of arthrosis at a mean of 17 years postoperatively, Hovelius et al. (26) found that only 1 of 88 shoulders (1.1%) with a prior Bankart repair went on to shoulder arthroplasty for arthritis at a mean follow-up of 17 years.

Anatomic Glenoid Reconstruction with Osteochondral Bone Graft

Numerous methods of glenoid reconstruction for glenoid bone defects associated with anterior instability have been described including iliac crest autograft (27), distal tibia allograft (28), and glenoid allograft (29). The development of arthrosis following these procedures has not yet been reported.

Rotator Cuff Repair

Rotator cuff repair is performed for instability associated with acute glenohumeral dislocation and rotator cuff tear. This typically occurs in patients greater than or equal to 40 years of age. Buscayret et al. (14) reported that rotator cuff tear at the time of instability event was associated with an increased risk of developing arthritis. Treatment options for patients who have undergone previous rotator cuff repair associated with glenohumeral instability are based upon the current status of the rotator cuff and glenohumeral articular cartilage.

NONANATOMIC PROCEDURES

Coracoid Transfer Procedures

In general, instability procedures utilizing coracoid transfer involve a transfer of the tip of the coracoid with the attached conjoined tendon to the anteroinferior rim of the glenoid where it is secured by screw fixation. Many modifications have developed since the original descriptions of these procedures, including variations of the split in the subscapularis and orientation of the transferred coracoid fragment (30–33). In the original Bristow procedure, the cancellous portion of the coracoid fragment is transferred through a vertical spilt in the subscapularis at its musculotendinous junction to the neck of the glenoid (32). Latarjet (31) described a similar procedure, but he transferred the coracoid fragment through a horizontal split in the subscapularis. In addition, the coracoid was placed flat so that its undersurface laid against the prepared surface of the glenoid neck. Buscayret et al. (14) reported that arthritis develops in 45% of patients following a coracoid transfer at a mean of 12 years postoperatively, and excessive lateralization of the coracoid graft has been reported as a contributor to the development of arthritis (4,20).

Historic Procedures

The Magnuson-Stack (34), Putti-Platt (9,22), Du Toit stapling (35), Max Lange (36), and Eden-Hybinette (37) procedures are some of the more common nonanatomic procedures which have previously been described for the treatment of anterior instability. Procedures which excessively tighten the anterior structures, such as a Putti-Platt, cause loss of external rotation which increases the risk for developing arthritis by altering biomechanics and contact pressures of the joint.

SEQUELAE OF ANTERIOR INSTABILITY

Marx et al. (38) performed a case-control study of patients who underwent shoulder arthroplasty which demonstrated a 10 times greater risk for developing severe arthrosis in patients with a history of nonoperatively treated instability compared to patients with no history of instability. When including patients who had prior instability surgery, a 19 times greater risk of developing severe glenohumeral arthritis was observed.

Increased age at time of first dislocation (21,39), interval from first instability episode to surgery (14,21), increased number of anchors, and poor labral tissue quality are reported risk factors for development of dislocation arthropathy (21). However, there is no consensus as to whether recurrent instability episodes increase the risk for developing degenerative changes in the shoulder. The data from Cameron et al. (39) and Hovelius et al. (13) suggests that the number of instability episodes is not a risk factor for arthritic change. Conversely, Franceschi et al. (21) reported that patients with a higher number of dislocation episodes preoperatively were more likely to develop radiographic arthropathy, and the number of dislocation episodes in patients with stage IV arthritis was higher than in patients with milder arthritis.

It is unclear how anterior stabilization influences the development of arthritis after dislocation. No study has demonstrated that shoulder stabilization prevents the development or progression of degenerative changes; however, no case-control studies comparing cohorts of operatively and nonoperatively treated patients have been reported. Furthermore, postoperative recurrence of instability has not been shown to be a risk for factor for development of arthritis (21).

While some patient characteristics and surgical methods have been identified as risk factors for developing arthritis, overall the reported incidence of 47% to 69% has been similar regardless of the procedure for studies with greater than 10 years follow-up (13–15,18,19,36,40–42). There are a wide array of surgical options for the patient with combined anterior instability and glenohumeral arthritis, and the surgery performed must be individualized based on the patient's complaints, clinical findings, and imaging studies.

EVALUATION

As part of a standard, thorough medical history and physical examination particular attention should be paid to the following pertinent findings.

History

It is important to determine the pattern of instability and specifics of prior instability surgery. The treating surgeon may find it very helpful to obtain prior operative notes before considering revision surgery. The chief complaint should be clarified to help guide the recommended treatment. This may be pain, weakness, ongoing instability, and/or stiffness. The severity of each of these symptoms helps to determine if surgical intervention is warranted and should also influence the decision to perform an instability or arthroplasty procedure. It is also important to assess the patient's functional demands and expectations when determining the treatment plan.

Physical Examination Findings

Inspecting prior incisions can provide clues as to what prior surgery has been performed and whether these incisions may be used in the revision surgery. Active and passive range of motion is checked for both of the patient's shoulders, and the presence of an internal rotation contracture is assessed by testing passive external rotation with the arm at the side. The status of rotator cuff function is very important in this patient population. The subscapularis may be weakened or insufficient in patients with anterior instability and/or prior instability surgery, so its function should be assessed by performing belly press and lift-off tests (43). In addition, older patients who have sustained a glenohumeral dislocation are much more likely to have a rotator cuff tear. It is therefore important to perform Jobe's test (44) and test for the presence of weakness in resisted external rotation and/or lag signs. Ideally, the presence of ongoing instability should be assessed by performing a supine modified load and shift as well as testing for a sulcus sign (24), but patients with painful arthrosis may not tolerate this. In the setting of previous surgery, it is important to consider whether the treating surgeon fully appreciated the proper diagnosis. In particular, multidirectional instability (MDI) may be under recognized. Incomplete surgical treatment of instability may result in combined arthritis and ongoing instability. A peripheral nerve examination with particular attention to the axillary nerve and deltoid function is performed assessing for muscular atrophy as well as function. Electromyography and nerve conduction studies may also be obtained to evaluate nerve function preoperatively if dysfunction is suspected on the basis of physical examination findings.

Imaging

Standard anteroposterior (AP) radiographs in internal and external rotation as well as axillary radiographs are routinely obtained. Computed tomography (CT) or magnetic resonance imaging (MRI) scanning should be performed for any patients with suggestion of glenoid or bony deficiency on standard radiographs. CT is preferred over MRI to evaluate for Hill-Sachs lesions in the humeral head as well as glenoid bone loss. Three-dimensional (3-D) CT has been shown to more accurately characterize glenoid morphology over standard two-dimensional (2-D) CT (45,46), and 3-D reconstruction with humeral subtraction is especially useful in evaluating the glenoid. Anteroinferior glenoid bone wear is most commonly encountered in patients with recurrent or chronic instability, while posterior glenoid wear may be seen in postcapsulorrhaphy patients with anterior soft tissue contractures. In cases where the integrity of the rotator cuff is questioned, MRI is preferred to better evaluate the status of the rotator cuff. Particular attention should be paid to evaluating the subscapularis whenever viewing these studies, as significant fatty infiltration may indicate that subscapularis tissue quality is poor. Poor subscapularis tissue may require soft tissue augmentation or pectoralis transfer.

Laboratory Studies

Infection must always be in the differential when evaluating patients with symptoms of pain after prior surgery. When there is suspicion of infection, these patients should be considered for an infection workup. This is typically initiated by obtaining a white blood cell count with differential, erythrocyte sedimentation rate (ESR), and a C-reactive protein (CRP). If these laboratory values are elevated, then a glenohumeral aspiration should be performed. Bone scan and tagged white blood cell scan may also be performed if clinical suspicion remains following completion of these tests.

TREATMENT

Nonoperative management is preferred for patients with low functional demands and only mild discomfort who may not wish to undergo operative management. Surgical treatment options may also be limited for patients who refuse or are unable to cooperate with postoperative restrictions and rehabilitation. Prosthetic replacement is contraindicated in the setting of active infection. As with any preoperative evaluation, the patient's overall medical condition must be considered prior to recommendation of surgery.

Patients with higher functional demands and significant symptoms which are insufficiently improved with conservative measures are candidates for surgical intervention. The type of operative treatment recommended to patients with arthritis and recurrent or chronic instability is based on the following:

1. Age of the patient
2. Instability pattern
3. Prior instability surgery
4. Presence and amount of humeral bone loss (i.e., size of humeral head defect)
5. Amount and pattern of glenoid bone loss
6. Severity of articular degenerative changes
7. Status of dynamic stabilizers (i.e., the rotator cuff)

Regardless of whether the patient was treated nonoperatively or with some type of stabilization procedure, the following conditions may develop:

1. Stable glenohumeral joint with moderate to severe arthritis
2. Recurrent instability with mild arthritis
3. Recurrent instability with moderate to severe arthritis
4. Chronic dislocation that represents a distinct entity (discussed in detail in Chapter 13)

Preoperative Surgical Plan

Several important factors should be considered when planning for surgery in this patient population. In cases where subscapularis deficiency is present and anatomic total shoulder replacement is planned, the surgeon should request Achilles tendon allograft or plan to perform a pectoralis transfer. When bone grafting is planned for severe glenoid deficiency, potential options include iliac crest autograft, humeral head autograft, distal tibia allograft, or glenoid allograft.

The surgeon may also consider whether to perform glenoid bone grafting at the time of glenoid implantation or in a staged fashion. A concern with bone grafting in one stage is graft resorption and glenoid loosening (47). Single stage structural bone graft and glenoid implantation resulted in 8 out of 17 patients with postoperative instability and 5 patients with glenoid loosening (47). A staged procedure with structural bone grafting to the glenoid and hemiarthroplasty is recommended for younger patients. Theoretically, without placing a glenoid component, the glenoid graft is offloaded, which may allow improved incorporation of the graft. If graft incorporation is observed on follow-up imaging, a glenoid component may be placed as soon as 6 months following the index procedure. Failure of graft incorporation is of particular concern in older patients, who may have decreased healing capability. Therefore, a reverse total shoulder arthroplasty (TSA) may be considered for this population.

In cases where the surgical plan is dependent on intraoperative findings, equipment for multiple surgical options and, when relevant, multiple arthroplasty systems should be available. In addition, we routinely plan for continuous intraoperative nerve monitoring of the brachial plexus due to the risk of nerve injury associated with surgical treatment. This risk may be particularly elevated in revision cases where distorted anatomy and contractures exist (48). Intraoperative nerve monitoring may be considered to improve prevention of neurologic injury (49).

SURGICAL MANAGEMENT

Regardless of prior treatment, patients with combined anterior instability and arthritis can be grouped according to the pattern of their symptoms, examination findings, and images. The recommended surgical treatment is based on these factors.

Stable Shoulder with Symptomatic Arthritis

This scenario may occur in patients previously treated nonoperatively or in those who underwent an anterior stabilization procedure. Matsoukis et al. (4) found that the mean delay from the first instability episode and arthroplasty was 19 years for those treated nonoperatively and 24 years for those undergoing a previous stabilization procedure. Patients who had surgery to tighten anterior soft tissues typically present with significant loss of external rotation and may also have associated posterior glenoid wear (Fig. 34-1).

TSA is preferred over hemiarthroplasty with or without soft tissue interposition because of consistent reports demonstrating superior pain relief and function with TSA (4,50–52). Hemiarthroplasty with glenoid reaming alone is another treatment option which has been advocated (53). Hemiarthroplasty and concomitant biologic glenoid resurfacing has been advocated for young patients with severe arthritis based on encouraging results in some studies (54,55), while others have experienced high rates of early failure with disappointing results using this technique (56).

When mild glenoid bone loss is present, asymmetric reaming of the glenoid is recommended (Fig. 34-1). An augmented glenoid component or more aggressive eccentric reaming can be performed for moderate glenoid wear, while severe glenoid wear should be treated with bone grafting.

Recurrent Instability with Mild Arthritis

Patient age and chief complaint (i.e., arthritic-type pain vs. instability) are the most important factors to consider when determining whether to perform an instability procedure in the setting of degenerative glenohumeral

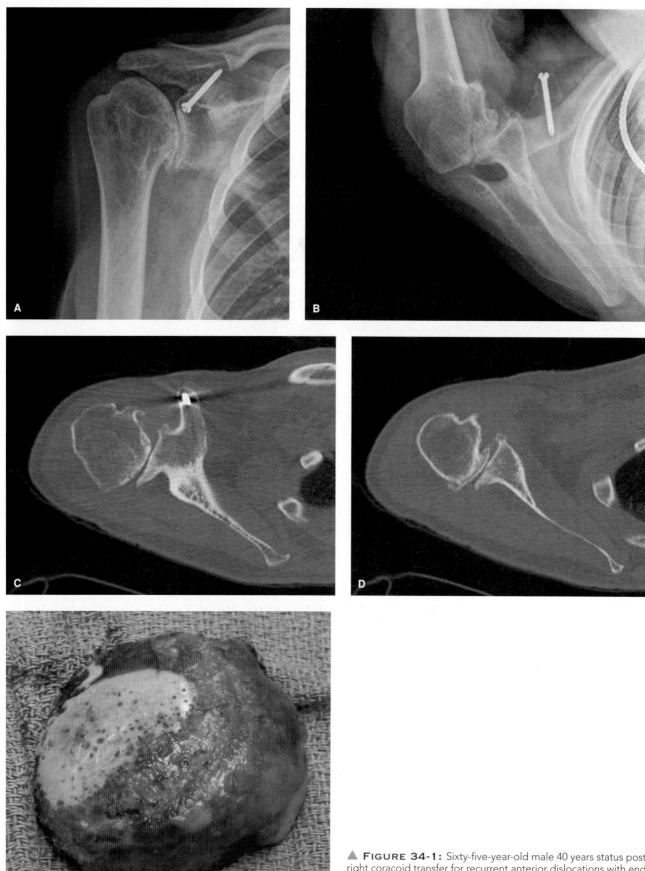

▲ FIGURE 34-1: Sixty-five-year-old male 40 years status post right coracoid transfer for recurrent anterior dislocations with end stage arthritis, posterior humeral head subluxation and posterior glenoid wear **(A,B)**. CT scan demonstrated a biconcave glenoid with 2 to 3 mm of posterior glenoid wear **(C,D)**. The humeral head was severely flattened and worn at the time of surgery **(E)**.

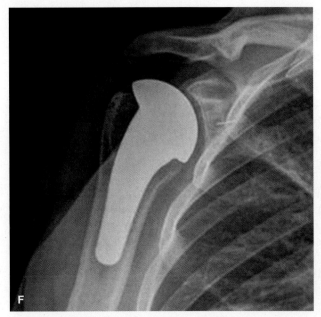

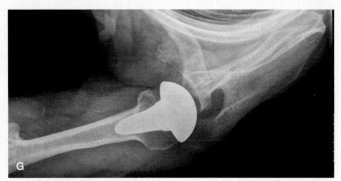

▲ **Figure 34-1:** (*Continued*) One year postoperative x-rays demonstrate correction of glenoid version and humeral head subluxation following total shoulder arthroplasty with asymmetric reaming of the anterior glenoid and screw removal **(F,G)**. Clinically, the patient is pain free with no instability and excellent range of motion.

changes. For younger patients with instability as the primary symptom, a stabilization procedure should be performed. The surgeon should also counsel the patient regarding preexisting degenerative changes in the glenohumeral joint which may require future treatment. Conversely, older patients who primarily describe pain symptoms as opposed to instability symptoms are better candidates for shoulder arthroplasty.

Recurrent Instability with Moderate to Severe Arthritis

In general, TSA is preferred for younger patients with this complex set of findings. Anterior soft tissue reconstruction plus total shoulder replacement may be considered for young patients with subscapularis deficiency. Mild to moderate glenoid wear is managed as described above. When severe glenoid deficiency is present in younger patients, hemiarthroplasty with concomitant glenoid grafting may be necessary. In this setting, glenoid implantation may need to be performed in a staged fashion after graft incorporation.

Elderly patients with instability, arthritis, and glenoid bone deficiency are candidates for reverse shoulder arthroplasty. Bone graft from the resected humeral head may be performed concomitantly if the glenoid is deficient. Reverse shoulder arthroplasty is also favored in the setting of rotator cuff dysfunction, including subscapularis deficiency, in elderly patients.

Salvage procedures may also be considered in some cases. Glenohumeral arthrodesis may be performed for patients unwilling to accept activity restrictions following reverse shoulder replacement or in the setting

of axillary nerve and/or deltoid dysfunction. Resection arthroplasty is another salvage procedure which may be recommended in the presence of chronic infection or severely deficient bone stock which prohibits prosthetic arthroplasty or arthrodesis.

SPECIFIC CONSIDERATIONS FOR REVISION SURGERY FOLLOWING PRIOR INSTABILITY SURGERY

The nature of the previous instability surgery affects the anatomy the surgeon will encounter when performing revision surgery. Obtaining previous operative records and reviewing specifics of the prior procedure(s) can aid the surgeon in preoperative planning. A description of prior instability surgeries with specific considerations follows.

Coracoid Transfer

Young and Rockwood (7) described the challenges associated with revision surgery following a failed Bristow procedure. The authors noted that surgery following a failed Bristow procedure was very complex. Patients presented with painful, recurrent anterior instability, damage to cartilage, and/or coracoid nonunion. Identification and protection of the axillary and musculocutaneous nerves was described as particularly difficult in these cases. The authors advised that the superior and inferior portions of the subscapularis may need to be mobilized separately when the subscapularis has been previously divided horizontally for coracoid transfer to the glenoid. If the transferred coracoid fragment is nonunited, it may either be repaired back to the coracoid or excised with repair of the conjoined tendon to the residual coracoid. Subscapularis deficiency also required augmentation with pectoralis minor and/or major transfer in some cases.

Putti-Platt

In patients who have undergone a Putti-Platt procedure, the subscapularis has been divided approximately 2 cm medial to its insertion. The lateral portion of the subscapularis has been attached to the glenoid or capsulolabral complex, and the medial subscapularis muscle or tendon stump has been repaired lateral to the bicipital groove in a "pants over vest" fashion. When performing shoulder arthroplasty on these patients, the subscapularis should be released off of the humerus and anterior glenoid rim. The subscapularis should be mobilized as is possible, although it is typically scarred in and contracted. In these cases, a z-lengthening or soft tissue graft may be required to restore appropriate subscapularis length and tension (57).

Patients with subscapularis insufficiency may require soft tissue reconstruction with Achilles allograft (58), pectoralis major transfer (7,59,60), or constrained (reverse) arthroplasty. Prior instability procedures, especially where the subscapularis has been released and repaired, may result in poor subscapularis quality leaving it vulnerable to rupture (61). The quality of subscapularis muscle can be evaluated by assessing fatty infiltration on preoperative CT or MRI studies.

For younger patients in whom a pectoralis major transfer is planned, it is recommended that a subcoracoid transfer to the lesser tuberosity be performed as this better replicates the subscapularis force vector compared to transfers superficial to the coracoid (60). Nonetheless, pectoralis major transfer as treatment for irreparable subscapularis tear following TSA has resulted in a high risk of failure, potential for musculocutaneous nerve injury, and oftentimes limited clinical improvements (61,62). Due to these high failure rates, a reverse shoulder arthroplasty is recommended for older patients with significant subscapularis deficiency.

Magnuson-Stack

In the Magnuson-Stack procedure, the subscapularis insertion has been transferred laterally and therefore is less difficult to manage since the subscapularis and anterior structures have not been shortened (8). In these cases, a subscapularis peel should be performed more laterally at the altered insertion site on the greater tuberosity. At the conclusion of the operation, the subscapularis is repaired back to its native insertion site on the lesser tuberosity with transosseous sutures. Performing a tenotomy or releasing the subscapularis directly off of the lesser tuberosity in this situation can leave the surgeon with inadequate subscapularis for repair at the conclusion of the operation.

Max Lange

The Max Lange procedure consists of an anterior capsulorrhaphy with the subscapularis insertion being lateralized. A bone block is also placed at the anteroinferior aspect of the glenoid. Approach to the subscapularis is the same as with the Magnuson-Stack. The bone block is typically left in place unless it causes articular impingement.

Du Toit Open Staple Capsulorrhaphy

Patients who have undergone a prior Du Toit open staple capsulorrhaphy have had their torn anterior capsule and/or labrum reattached to the anterior glenoid rim by staples through a horizontal split in the subscapularis. In cases where the staples loosen or migrate they should be removed; if they are stable and do not interfere with placement of the glenoid component they may be left in place (Fig. 34-2).

TECHNIQUES FOR TREATMENT OF COMBINED ANTERIOR INSTABILITY AND ARTHRITIS WITH ARTHROPLASTY

Arthroplasty for this patient population is often more technically challenging than for a standard primary arthroplasty because of distorted anatomy, anterior soft tissue contractures, and asymmetric glenoid bone loss. The surgical technique described is an anatomic TSA; however, much of the information is applicable for hemiarthroplasty or reverse arthroplasty if that is planned.

Setup

Shoulder arthroplasty is performed in the beach chair position. An examination under anesthesia is performed to determine passive external rotation with the arm at the side. A load and shift test is performed to assess for current instability patterns. Nerve monitoring leads are placed during routine sterile preparation and draping (48,49).

Approach

A deltopectoral approach is utilized, incorporating prior incisions when possible. However, a separate deltopectoral incision is made if the prior incisions will compromise the approach. In revision cases, the cephalic vein may have been previously ligated and may not be apparent. If the vein is present, it is left with the deltoid laterally. The deltopectoral interval may be developed just inferior to the clavicular origins of the pectoralis major and anterior deltoid. Alternatively, the interval may be defined by starting just lateral and distal to the tip of the

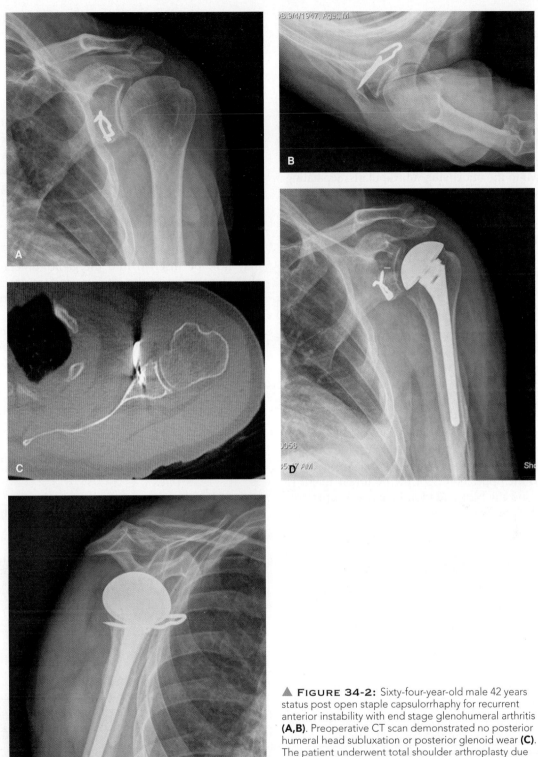

▲ **FIGURE 34-2:** Sixty-four-year-old male 42 years status post open staple capsulorrhaphy for recurrent anterior instability with end stage glenohumeral arthritis **(A,B)**. Preoperative CT scan demonstrated no posterior humeral head subluxation or posterior glenoid wear **(C)**. The patient underwent total shoulder arthroplasty due to severe pain symptoms with inadequate response to nonoperative treatments **(D,E)**. The staples were found to be lodged in the glenoid and did not interfere with the procedure so they were left in place.

coracoid and working distally to the humeral insertions of the deltoid and pectoralis major. While the coracoid is typically used as a reference to guide this approach, the anatomy is greatly altered in the case of prior coracoid transfer making the coracoid a less helpful landmark in this setting. Great care must be taken to stay lateral to the neurovascular structures present medial to the base of the coracoid.

The deltoid and pectoralis major are then mobilized from their clavicular origins down to their humeral insertions. This is often more difficult when prior surgery has been performed due to adhesions and loss of native tissue planes, but it is imperative that these muscles be completely mobilized to optimize exposure. A self-retaining retractor is then placed in the deltopectoral interval, and the clavipectoral fascia is incised longitudinally just lateral to the proximal aspect of the conjoined tendon. The arm is externally rotated to improve exposure deep to the conjoined tendon.

In revision cases, the conjoined tendon is often scarred down to the underlying subscapularis. Separating this layer facilitates exposure and mobilization of the subscapularis, but the surgeon must exercise extreme caution when developing this tissue plane. The axillary nerve and anterior humeral circumflex vessels exist along the anterior–inferior aspect of the subscapularis, and dissection through this plane may put these structures at risk. The axillary nerve is palpated before moving the self-retaining retractor under the conjoined tendon. The musculocutaneous nerve is sometimes palpable running under the conjoined tendon. The three anterior humeral circumflex vessels are identified running transversely along the inferior border of the subscapularis and are cauterized. The arm is then returned to a neutral or slightly internally rotated position to address the subscapularis attachment.

If present, the long head of the biceps tendon provides a landmark to the lesser tuberosity. The biceps tendon sheath is incised up through the rotator interval and to its origin on the supraglenoid tubercle. A soft tissue tenodesis to the upper border of the pectoralis major is performed, and the biceps tendon is released superiorly and excised along with its sheath just proximal to the tenodesis.

Subscapularis Management

The glenohumeral joint may be accessed with a subscapularis peel, tenotomy, or lesser tuberosity osteotomy (LTO). A peel is performed by releasing the subscapularis directly off of its bony attachment to the lesser tuberosity, while a tenotomy is performed 1 cm medial to its insertion.

If the subscapularis remains tethered from prior coracoid transfer, it is recommended to release the tissue passing through it to mobilize the subscapularis. In the absence of a specific reason to manage the subscapularis with a soft tissue release, we prefer an LTO (2) due to the risk of subscapularis failure with other techniques (61,63). A wide curved osteotome is centered on the highest point of the lesser tuberosity with the goal of creating a lesser tuberosity fragment approximately 2 cm long, 1 cm wide, and 5 to 10 mm thick. The superior glenohumeral ligament is released to mobilize the superior soft tissue attachments to the subscapularis. Traction sutures are placed around the lesser tuberosity fragment, which can later be used for transosseous repair.

The inferior subscapularis muscle fibers can be incised horizontally down to the capsule, and an elevator followed by a scalpel is used to separate the subscapularis from the underlying capsule.

Humeral Preparation

The humeral head is now exposed, and the anteroinferior capsule is released off of the surgical neck to access the glenohumeral joint. While the capsule is typically excised in cases of primary arthroplasty without instability, it may be preserved and repaired along with the subscapularis in cases of anterior instability. If an internal rotation contracture is present, an anterior capsulectomy is performed during glenoid exposure. If the surgical plan is dependent on the status of glenoid, a Fukuda may now be inserted into the glenohumeral joint to allow inspection of the articular surface. In cases with soft tissue contractures, this step may be performed after the humeral head cut is performed.

Humeral retractors are placed, and the humeral head is then dislocated by an extension and external rotation maneuver with the arm adducted (Fig. 34-3). In cases of chronic anterior dislocation, the humerus is internally (rather than externally) rotated and a laterally directed force is applied to disengage it from the glenoid rim. Osteophytes are removed around the humeral head to expose the anatomic neck (Fig. 34-4). The rotator cuff is visualized to assess for tearing. If a small tear is noted, this may be

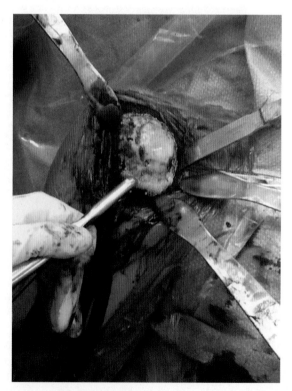

▲ **FIGURE 34-3:** The humeral head is delivered, exposing large peripheral osteophytes.

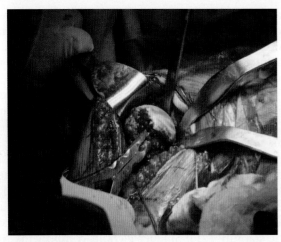

▲ **FIGURE 34-4:** The osteophytes are removed by using a large rongeur to expose the anatomic neck.

repaired during the procedure. Larger or irreparable tears may dictate the need for reverse shoulder arthroplasty.

The humeral head cut is made in the patient's native version along the anatomic neck. Previous recommendations to place the humeral component in excessive anteversion to compensate for glenoid retroversion (64,65) have not been substantiated by recent studies which suggest that this technique does not result in improved stability (66,67). Therefore, a cut along the anatomic neck is recommended to replicate the patient's native version (Fig. 34-5). The rotator cuff must be protected during this cut.

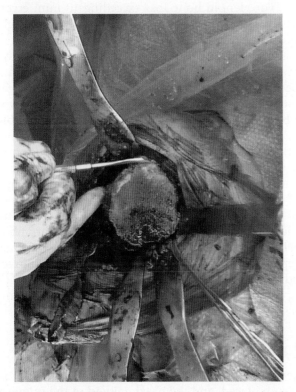

▲ **FIGURE 34-5:** The humeral head has been resected at the level of the anatomic neck.

The humeral canal is then sequentially prepared, paying careful attention to avoid varus preparation. A trial stem is then placed and left in the canal to protect the humerus while the glenoid is addressed.

Glenoid Exposure

Retractors are then removed, and the arm is abducted and externally rotated for glenoid exposure. The operating table may now be slightly tilted away from the surgeon to improve glenoid visualization.

Glenoid exposure may be challenging in revision cases. Care should be taken to optimize exposure while minimizing retraction of the brachial plexus and/or peripheral nerves. These nerves are typically scarred in when prior surgery has been performed, especially in shoulders with chronically limited motion. This adherence to the surrounding soft tissues may tether the nerves, therefore making them more susceptible to stretch injuries. Intraoperative nerve monitoring can be useful to identify nerves at risk of being injured, particularly during glenoid exposure (48).

If a prior coracoid or bone block transfer has been performed, so long as it does not cause articular impingement it is recommended to leave the transfer in place to reduce risk to the axillary and musculocutaneous nerves. A Fukuda retractor or humeral retractor of choice is placed to posteriorly displace the proximal humerus. If external rotation is limited preoperatively, the anterior capsule (Fig. 34-6) is then excised off of the glenoid neck. If anterior instability is present, the anterior capsule is spared and incorporated into the subscapularis repair.

Glenoid Preparation

Reverse retractors are placed around the glenoid to facilitate exposure of the entire labrum. A circumferential labrectomy is performed (Fig. 34-7), and the face of the glenoid is exposed (Fig. 34-8A). The subscapularis muscle is mobilized off of the anterior glenoid neck and subscapularis fossa of the scapula. The presence of glenoid bone loss is quantified by preoperative CT or MRI scan and visually inspected at the time of surgery. Postcapsulorrhaphy arthritis often results in excessively tight anterior soft tissues and subsequent posterior wear, while chronic anterior instability may be accompanied by anterior glenoid bone loss.

The goal for ideal glenoid preparation is to achieve neutral version. Inadequate correction may predispose to early glenoid wear and instability (68,69).

In cases of mild asymmetric anterior or posterior wear, the "high side" may be reamed eccentrically to recreate a more neutral glenoid version and recenter the humeral head (70). For mild wear, we recommend asymmetric reaming up to 3 mm on the high side. Use of a cannulated reaming system allows placement of a

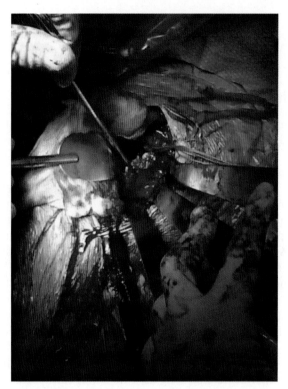

▲ **FIGURE 34-6:** The anterior capsule is isolated, and a Kocher clamp is used to put tension on the capsule (center of image). The anterior capsule is typically excised, but may be retained and incorporated into the subscapularis repair in cases of ongoing anterior instability.

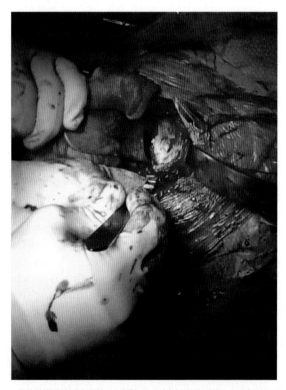

▲ **FIGURE 34-7:** A circumferential labrectomy is performed prior to glenoid reaming.

guide pin to plan version correction and allows for more precise eccentric reaming. The wire is placed in neutral version relative to the axis of the scapula and is aimed at the center of the glenoid vault. A built up reamer is used to ream down the high side.

When instability has led to moderate glenoid bone loss (approximately 3 to 10 mm), eccentric reaming may still be performed; however, there are no clear limits regarding the amount of bone that can safely be reamed with this approach. Alternatively, the use of an augmented glenoid component has been recently recommended (70) to preserve bone stock as compared to eccentric reaming. This also allows for the implantation of a larger glenoid component, which improves prosthetic stability (71). Smaller glenoid components predispose to instability because less translation is required to dislocate the humeral head. In addition, greater bone stock with improved bony support allows for complete seating of the glenoid component. This reduces the risk of glenoid vault perforation with the pegs or keel of the glenoid component. An augmented glenoid component designed with posterior buildup can also be used to treat anterior bone loss by selecting a component designed for the contralateral side and flipping it.

The glenoid component is placed in neutral tilt, which is vertical in the coronal plane. Components placed in excessive superior or inferior tilt (also referred to as inclination), may cause rotator cuff impingement and dysfunction along with edge loading, which predisposes the glenoid component to early wear.

For glenoid bone loss exceeding 10 mm, eccentric reaming may result in inadequate bone for glenoid implantation. Therefore, we recommend structural bone grafting for this severe degree of bone loss (65,70,72). The resected humeral head is typically adequate for this purpose, but in cases where the head is severely flattened, has a large defect, or is otherwise of poor quality an alternate graft should be available. The surgeon should aim the screws to fix the graft such that they do not interfere with the glenoid component pegs or keel. Glenoid bone grafting may be performed at the time of glenoid implantation or in a staged fashion.

Following glenoid preparation (Fig. 34-8B), the holes for the glenoid pegs are suctioned and a thrombin-soaked sponge is placed in the holes while the cement is prepared. The sponge is then removed, cement is injected and pressurized, and the component is implanted and impacted. The component is held in place with thumb pressure until the cement hardens (Fig. 34-8C).

Humeral Head Trial

Glenoid retractors are then removed, humeral retractors are placed, and the proximal end of the humerus is delivered from the wound for humeral trialing.

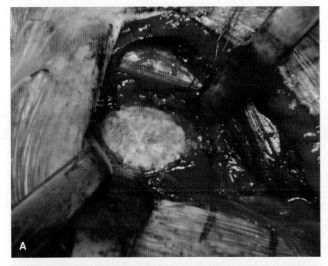

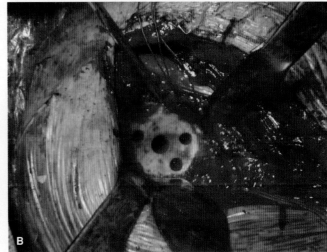

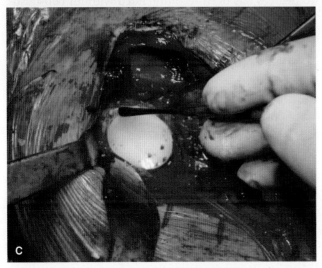

▲ **FIGURE 34-8:** The glenoid is exposed **(A)**, and prepared **(B)** to allow for glenoid component implantation **(C)**.

A concentric or eccentric head should be placed to restore proper humeral head height at 5 to 8 mm above the greater tuberosity. Superior placement of the head can result in increased stress to the superior rotator cuff and edge loading of the glenoid component, which could lead to early wear and failure. In addition, it may result in stiffness due to excessive tension on the inferior ligaments, and weakness of the infraspinatus and subscapularis muscles by raising the center of rotation of the joint and reducing their moment arms (73). Low humeral head position results in greater tuberosity impingement on the acromion, and may result in impaired deltoid function due to inadequate deltoid tensioning. Posterior stability is assessed by applying a posteriorly directed stress with the arm at the side in neutral rotation. Posterior subluxation of approximately 50% or less is desired with this maneuver. In addition, the humeral head should spontaneously recenter in the glenoid component following this maneuver (58). Anterior stability may be assessed by external rotation with the

arm adducted. Even with the subscapularis not yet repaired, the arm should be able to externally rotate to at least 30 degrees without observing anterior subluxation. If instability is noted with trial reduction a slightly thicker humeral head component may be used to increase stability; however, a humeral head that is too large may cause rotator cuff attenuation, pain, decreased motion, and may result in glenoid loosening. Residual posterior instability may be treated by performing a posterior capsulorrhaphy. The posterior capsule may be imbricated with or without the use of percutaneously placed suture anchors in the posterior glenoid rim. Poor soft tissue balancing may result in instability and/or postoperative stiffness.

The final humeral implant and head are then placed. A heavy nonabsorbable suture is placed around the head–neck junction prior to fully seating the component; this is later used to augment the lesser tuberosity repair. After the humeral stem is placed, stability may be reassessed with a trial head prior to final humeral head implantation.

Lesser Tuberosity Repair and Closure

Subscapularis healing is very important for shoulder function and stability following total shoulder replacement. The subscapularis is mobilized as needed to achieve appropriate length and tension for proper soft tissue balancing of the shoulder. If retained, the capsular layer is incorporated into the subscapularis repair. The lateral aspect of the rotator interval is closed with one or two figure of eight nonabsorbable sutures to improve lesser tuberosity stability. More medial placement of these sutures will further limit external rotation, which is often undesirable in this patient population. We perform a transosseous double row repair of the LTO with high-tensile-strength nonabsorbable sutures which are passed around the lesser tuberosity as well as the humeral component. In rare cases when the subscapularis cannot be reduced to the lesser tuberosity following mobilization, subscapularis lengthening procedures or a medialized repair may be considered (74). Subscapularis z-lengthening procedures should be performed judiciously, since lengthening procedures have been associated with an increased risk of subscapularis rupture (61). Following subscapularis repair, gentle external rotation with the arm at the side is performed to guide the postoperative therapy. If the arm externally rotates to 40 degrees, this is the limit allowed in therapy. If less than 40 degrees has been achieved, therapy is restricted accordingly.

A surgical drain is placed. The deltopectoral interval may be reapproximated. Routine closure is performed, and the arm is placed in a sling postoperatively.

REVERSE TOTAL SHOULDER ARTHROPLASTY

Patients indicated for reverse shoulder arthroplasty are approached in a similar manner to those undergoing anatomic TSA. An overview of pertinent technical considerations specific to reverse shoulder arthroplasty is discussed below.

Subscapularis Management

The importance of subscapularis integrity in maintaining stability following reverse shoulder arthroplasty is controversial. While Clark et al. (75) found no detectable effect on stability, range of motion, pain relief, or overall complication rates with repair or no repair of the subscapularis, Edwards et al. (76) reported that an irreparable subscapularis results in an increased risk of postoperative dislocation. Although the subscapularis contribution to stability in reverse shoulder arthroplasty is controversial, when repairable, we handle the subscapularis in essentially the same manner for reverse shoulder arthroplasty as is described above for anatomic TSA. An exception is that in the rare cases where soft tissue grafting or pectoralis major transfer is necessary for subscapularis insufficiency when performing anatomic shoulder arthroplasty, these procedures are not performed in cases of reverse shoulder arthroplasty with subscapularis deficiency.

Humeral Cut

If present, the supraspinatus is excised. The amount of humeral head resected may vary for reverse shoulder arthroplasty, but in general it should be performed above the lesser tuberosity. Retroversion between 0 and 20 degrees has been recommended without consensus; we, therefore, aim for 10 degrees of retroversion with the use of an intramedullary guide rod. Theoretically, a retroverted plane of resection may be recommended if more external rotation is desired postoperatively, while a more anteverted cut would be performed if increased internal rotation is desired.

Glenoid Implantation

The inferior aspect of the baseplate is placed at or slightly lower than the inferior aspect of the glenoid to avoid inferior scapular notching (77). Neutral tilt is preferred since recent data has demonstrated no decrease in scapular notching with inferior tilt (78). Screw fixation is used for the baseplate as opposed to cement used in anatomic TSA. The glenoid sphere component is impacted onto the baseplate.

Stability Assessment

The spacer is placed to restore soft tissue tension with the goal of optimizing stability and deltoid function. While stability is of paramount importance, excessive tension is avoided to reduce the risk of acromion or scapular spine stress fractures.

POSTOPERATIVE PROTOCOLS

For anatomic TSA, range of motion is initiated on postoperative day zero. The limits for range of motion are dependent upon the glenohumeral stability and integrity of the subscapularis after the final components are implanted and the subscapularis repair is performed. For stable shoulders with adequate subscapularis repair, we generally allow 140 degrees of passive forward elevation and 40 degrees of passive external rotation. In the rare cases where a posterior capsular plication has been performed or some residual posterior instability exists, the shoulder may be temporarily immobilized in external rotation. After 6 weeks, subscapularis function is assessed by a belly press test and gentle passive external rotation. Subscapularis failure may present with internal rotation weakness, increased external rotation, and may also be accompanied by ongoing pain. If an LTO has been performed, radiographic signs of healing are assessed as well. If the subscapularis is functional, progressive active shoulder motion followed by strengthening is initiated. In the setting of subscapularis dysfunction, the integrity of the subscapularis repair may be evaluated by ultrasound if a tenotomy has been performed, although the accuracy of this study is operator dependent. If a strong suspicion of subscapularis failure exists, exploration with repair and/or augmentation should be performed.

Patients undergoing reverse shoulder arthroplasty do not perform range of motion exercises postoperatively. Rather, they remain in an abduction pillow for approximately 2 weeks and are then allowed to use the shoulder for light activities below shoulder level. At 6 weeks patients are allowed to perform overhead activities.

RESULTS FOR ANATOMIC ARTHROPLASTY FOR COMBINED ANTERIOR INSTABILITY AND ARTHRITIS

The results following treatment of combined anterior instability and arthritis are fairly limited as this is a relatively uncommon condition. In general, the results are good, but not as good as the results after arthroplasty for primary osteoarthritis. Overall, pain relief is very good in this population and appears to be the most predictable outcome. Improvements in range of motion and function also occur for the majority of patients, but as a whole not to the extent seen with shoulder arthroplasty for primary OA. In addition, higher rates of complications such as instability, loosening, stiffness, and need for revision surgery have been reported after shoulder replacement for arthritis of instability (4,8,79,80). The concern for this increased complication rate is magnified because this patient population tends to be younger than primary OA cohorts.

The first report on this patient population was provided by Neer et al. (1), who found 17 out of 18 patients had excellent or satisfactory results at least 2 years after shoulder arthroplasty for "arthritis of recurrent dislocation." Subsequently, Young and Rockwood (7) reported relief of pain and functional range of motion in all four patients undergoing total shoulder replacement for arthritis after a Bristow procedure. Bigliani et al. (8) reported 13 out of 17 patients (77%) achieved satisfactory results following shoulder replacement after prior instability surgery at a mean of 3 years postoperatively. Pain improved in 94% of patients, and significant increases in range of motion were also reported. Three out of the 17 patients (18%) went on to revision surgery. Green and Norris (79) found improvements in 16 out of 17 patients, with three of these patients (18%) going on to revision surgery. Sperling et al. (81) noted significant pain relief and increased range of motion in 31 patients undergoing shoulder arthroplasty for postcapsulorrhaphy arthritis; however, 11 of these patients (35%) required revision surgery.

Matsoukis et al.'s (4) report on 55 shoulders undergoing arthroplasty with a prior anterior dislocation is the largest series currently published. Significant improvements in Constant score and range of motion were reported at 45 months postoperatively. There were 50 good or excellent results; older age at the time of initial dislocation and presence of a rotator cuff tear were associated with poorer outcomes. A similar rise in Constant score (from 49 to 81 points) at a mean of 44 months postoperatively was reported by Lehmann et al. (80). These authors reported a 40% complication rate with 20% of cases requiring revision surgery out of 45 patients who underwent shoulder arthroplasty for dislocation arthropathy (80). Interestingly, both Matsoukis et al. and Samilson and Prieto (4,3) reported no difference in results when comparing patients with postcapsulorrhaphy arthritis and patients with anterior instability who were previously treated nonoperatively.

S U M M A R Y

The clinical presentation of arthritis occurring after anterior shoulder dislocation and/or surgical stabilization occurs over a wide spectrum. Treatment must be tailored to the patient's symptoms, prior surgical history, and deficiencies of bone and/or soft tissues. Patients are often younger and arthroplasty can be more challenging because of altered anatomy, soft tissue contractures, and asymmetric glenoid wear. Outcomes of arthroplasty for combined instability and arthritis, though limited, have shown inferior results with higher complication rates compared to arthroplasty for primary glenohumeral osteoarthritis. Attention to preoperative evaluation, planning, and intraoperative technique is necessary for optimizing results.

References

1. Neer CS, Watson KC, Stanton FJ. Recent experience in total shoulder replacement. *J Bone Joint Surg Am.* 1982;64(3):319–337.
2. Gerber C, Yian EH, Pfirrmann CA, et al. Subscapularis muscle function and structure after total shoulder replacement with lesser tuberosity osteotomy and repair. *J Bone Joint Surg Am.* 2005;87(8):1739–1745.
3. Samilson RL, Prieto V. Dislocation arthropathy of the shoulder. *J Bone Joint Surg Am.* 1983;65(4):456–460.
4. Matsoukis J, Tabib W, Guiffault P, et al. Shoulder arthroplasty in patients with a prior anterior shoulder dislocation. Results of a multicenter study. *J Bone Joint Surg Am.* 2003;85-A(8):1417–1424.
5. Zuckerman JD, Matsen FA III. Complications about the glenohumeral joint related to the use of screws and staples. *J Bone Joint Surg Am.* 1984;66(2):175–180.
6. Lyons FA, Rockwood CA Jr. Migration of pins used in operations on the shoulder. *J Bone Joint Surg Am.* 1990;72(8):1262–1267.
7. Young DC, Rockwood CA Jr. Complications of a failed Bristow procedure and their management. *J Bone Joint Surg Am.* 1991;73(7):969–981.
8. Bigliani LU, Weinstein DM, Glasgow MT, et al. Glenohumeral arthroplasty for arthritis after instability surgery. *J Shoulder Elbow Surg.* 1995;4(2):87–94.
9. Hawkins RJ, Angelo RL. Glenohumeral osteoarthrosis. A late complication of the Putti-Platt repair. *J Bone Joint Surg Am.* 1990;72(8):1193–1197.
10. Hovelius L. Incidence of shoulder dislocation in Sweden. *Clin Orthop Relat Res.* 1982;(166):127–131.
11. Milgrom C, Mann G, Finestone A. A prevalence study of recurrent shoulder dislocations in young adults. *J Shoulder Elbow Surg.* 1998;7(6):621–624.
12. Taylor DC, Arciero RA. Pathologic changes associated with shoulder dislocations. Arthroscopic and physical examination findings in first-time, traumatic anterior dislocations. *Am J Sports Med.* 1997;25(3):306–311.
13. Hovelius L, Augustini BG, Fredin H, et al. Primary anterior dislocation of the shoulder in young patients. A ten-year prospective study. *J Bone Joint Surg Am.* 1996;78(11):1677–1684.
14. Buscayret F, Edwards TB, Szabo I, et al. Glenohumeral arthrosis in anterior instability before and after surgical treatment: Incidence and contributing factors. *Am J Sports Med.* 2004;32(5):1165–1172.
15. Allain J, Goutallier D, Glorion C. Long-term results of the Latarjet procedure for the treatment of anterior instability of the shoulder. *J Bone Joint Surg Am.* 1998;80(6):841–852.
16. Chapnikoff D, Besson A, Chantelot C, et al. [Bankart procedure: Clinical and radiological long-term outcome]. *Rev Chir Orthop Reparatrice Appar Mot.* 2000;86(6):558–565.
17. O'Neill DB. Arthroscopic Bankart repair of anterior detachments of the glenoid labrum. A prospective study. *J Bone Joint Surg Am.* 1999;81(10):1357–1366.
18. Rosenberg BN, Richmond JC, Levine WN. Long-term followup of Bankart reconstruction. Incidence of late degenerative glenohumeral arthrosis. *Am J Sports Med.* 1995;23(5):538–544.
19. Fabre T, Abi-Chahla ML, Billaud A, et al. Long-term results with Bankart procedure: A 26-year follow-up study of 50 cases. *J Shoulder Elbow Surg.* 2010;19(2):318–323.
20. Hawkins RH, Hawkins RJ. Failed anterior reconstruction for shoulder instability. *J Bone Joint Surg Br.* 1985;67(5):709–714.
21. Franceschi F, Papalia R, Del BA, et al. Glenohumeral osteoarthritis after arthroscopic Bankart repair for anterior instability. *Am J Sports Med.* 2011;39(8):1653–1659.
22. Hovelius L, Thorling J, Fredin H. Recurrent anterior dislocation of the shoulder. Results after the Bankart and Putti-Platt operations. *J Bone Joint Surg Am.* 1979;61(4):566–569.
23. Rowe CR, Patel D, Southmayd WW. The Bankart procedure: A long-term end-result study. *J Bone Joint Surg Am.* 1978;60(1):1–16.
24. Neer CS, Foster CR. Inferior capsular shift for involuntary inferior and multidirectional instability of the shoulder. A preliminary report. *J Bone Joint Surg Am.* 1980;62(6):897–908.
25. Boileau P, Fourati E, Bicknell R. Neer modification of open Bankart procedure: What are the rates of recurrent instability, functional outcome, and arthritis? *Clin Orthop Relat Res.* 2012;470(9):2554–2560.
26. Hovelius L, Vikerfors O, Olofsson A, et al. Bristow-Latarjet and Bankart: A comparative study of shoulder stabilization in 185 shoulders during a seventeen-year follow-up. *J Shoulder Elbow Surg.* 2011;20(7):1095–1101.
27. Warner JJ, Gill TJ, O'hollerhan JD, et al. Anatomical glenoid reconstruction for recurrent anterior glenohumeral instability with glenoid deficiency using an autogenous tricortical iliac crest bone graft. *Am J Sports Med.* 2006;34(2):205–212.
28. Provencher MT, Ghodadra N, LeClere L, et al. Anatomic osteochondral glenoid reconstruction for recurrent glenohumeral instability with glenoid deficiency using a distal tibia allograft. *Arthroscopy.* 2009;25(4):446–452.
29. Tjoumakaris FP, Sekiya JK. Combined glenoid and humeral head allograft reconstruction for recurrent anterior glenohumeral instability. *Orthopedics.* 2008;31(5):497.
30. Gerber C, Terrier F, Ganz R. The Trillat procedure for recurrent anterior instability of the shoulder. *J Bone Joint Surg Br.* 1988;70(1):130–134.
31. Latarjet M. A propos du traitement des luxations recidivantes de l'epaule. *Lyon Chir.* 1954;49(8):994–997.
32. Helfet AJ. Coracoid transplantation for recurring dislocation of the shoulder. *J Bone Joint Surg Br.* 1958;40-B(2):198–202.
33. Patte D, Bernageau J, Rodineau J, et al. [Unstable painful shoulders (author's transl)]. *Rev Chir Orthop Reparatrice Appar Mot.* 1980;66(3):157–165.
34. Magnuson PB, Stack JK. Recurrent dislocation of the shoulder. 1943. *Clin Orthop Relat Res.* 1991;(269):4–8.
35. Du Toit GT, Roux D. Recurrent dislocation of the shoulder; a twenty-four year study of the Johannesburg

stapling operation. *J Bone Joint Surg Am.* 1956;38-A(1): 1–12.

36. Wurnig C, Helwig U, Kabon B, et al. Osteoarthrosis after the Max Lange procedure for unstable shoulders. *Int Orthop.* 1997;21(4):213–216.

37. Hindmarsh J, Lindberg A. Eden-Hybbinette's operation for recurrent dislocation of the humero-scapular joint. *Acta Orthop Scand.* 1967;38(4):459–478.

38. Marx RG, McCarty EC, Montemurno TD, et al. Development of arthrosis following dislocation of the shoulder: A case-control study. *J Shoulder Elbow Surg.* 2002;11(1):1–5.

39. Cameron ML, Kocher MS, Briggs KK, et al. The prevalence of glenohumeral osteoarthrosis in unstable shoulders. *Am J Sports Med.* 2003;31(1):53–55.

40. Hovelius LK, Sandstrom BC, Rosmark DL, et al. Long-term results with the Bankart and Bristow-Latarjet procedures: Recurrent shoulder instability and arthropathy. *J Shoulder Elbow Surg.* 2001;10(5):445–452.

41. Konig DP, Rutt J, Treml O, et al. Osteoarthrosis following the Putti-Platt operation. *Arch Orthop Trauma Surg.* 1996;115(3-4):231–232.

42. van der Zwaag HM, Brand R, Obermann WR, et al. Glenohumeral osteoarthrosis after Putti-Platt repair. *J Shoulder Elbow Surg.* 1999;8(3):252–258.

43. Gerber C, Hersche O, Farron A. Isolated rupture of the subscapularis tendon. *J Bone Joint Surg Am.* 1996;78(7): 1015–1023.

44. Jobe FW, Jobe CM. Painful athletic injuries of the shoulder. *Clin Orthop Relat Res.* 1983;(173):117–124.

45. Scalise JJ, Codsi MJ, Bryan J, et al. The influence of three-dimensional computed tomography images of the shoulder in preoperative planning for total shoulder arthroplasty. *J Bone Joint Surg Am.* 2008;90(11): 2438–2445.

46. Scalise JJ, Bryan J, Polster J, et al. Quantitative analysis of glenoid bone loss in osteoarthritis using three-dimensional computed tomography scans. *J Shoulder Elbow Surg.* 2008;17(2):328–335.

47. Hill JM, Norris TR. Long-term results of total shoulder arthroplasty following bone-grafting of the glenoid. *J Bone Joint Surg Am.* 2001;83-A(6):877–883.

48. Nagda SH, Rogers KJ, Sestokas AK, et al. Neer Award 2005: Peripheral nerve function during shoulder arthroplasty using intraoperative nerve monitoring. *J Shoulder Elbow Surg.* 2007;16(3 suppl):S2–S8.

49. Warrender WJ, Oppenheimer S, Abboud JA. Nerve monitoring during proximal humeral fracture fixation: What have we learned? *Clin Orthop Relat Res.* 2011;469(9): 2631–2637.

50. Bishop JY, Flatow EL. Humeral head replacement versus total shoulder arthroplasty: Clinical outcomes–a review. *J Shoulder Elbow Surg.* 2005;14(1 suppl S):141S–146S.

51. Bryant D, Litchfield R, Sandow M, et al. A comparison of pain, strength, range of motion, and functional outcomes after hemiarthroplasty and total shoulder arthroplasty in patients with osteoarthritis of the shoulder. A systematic review and meta-analysis. *J Bone Joint Surg Am.* 2005;87(9):1947–1956.

52. Gartsman GM, Roddey TS, Hammerman SM. Shoulder arthroplasty with or without resurfacing of the glenoid in patients who have osteoarthritis. *J Bone Joint Surg Am.* 2000;82(1):26–34.

53. Weldon EJ III, Boorman RS, Smith KL, et al. Optimizing the glenoid contribution to the stability of a humeral hemiarthroplasty without a prosthetic glenoid. *J Bone Joint Surg Am.* 2004;86-A(9):2022–2029.

54. Nicholson GP, Goldstein JL, Romeo AA, et al. Lateral meniscus allograft biologic glenoid arthroplasty in total shoulder arthroplasty for young shoulders with degenerative joint disease. *J Shoulder Elbow Surg.* 2007;16(5 suppl): S261–S266.

55. Krishnan SG, Nowinski RJ, Harrison D, et al. Humeral hemiarthroplasty with biologic resurfacing of the glenoid for glenohumeral arthritis. Two to fifteen-year outcomes. *J Bone Joint Surg Am.* 2007;89(4):727–734.

56. Elhassan B, Ozbaydar M, Diller D, et al. Soft-tissue resurfacing of the glenoid in the treatment of glenohumeral arthritis in active patients less than fifty years old. *J Bone Joint Surg Am.* 2009;91(2):419–424.

57. Nicholson GP, Twigg S, Blatz B, et al. Subscapularis lengthening in shoulder arthroplasty. *J Shoulder Elbow Surg.* 2010;19(3):427–433.

58. Moeckel BH, Altchek DW, Warren RF, et al. Instability of the shoulder after arthroplasty. *J Bone Joint Surg Am.* 1993;75(4):492–497.

59. Wirth MA, Rockwood CA Jr. Operative treatment of irreparable rupture of the subscapularis. *J Bone Joint Surg Am.* 1997;79(5):722–731.

60. Galatz LM, Connor PM, Calfee RP, et al. Pectoralis major transfer for anterior-superior subluxation in massive rotator cuff insufficiency. *J Shoulder Elbow Surg.* 2003;12(1):1–5.

61. Miller BS, Joseph TA, Noonan TJ, et al. Rupture of the subscapularis tendon after shoulder arthroplasty: Diagnosis, treatment, and outcome. *J Shoulder Elbow Surg.* 2005;14(5):492–496.

62. Elhassan B, Ozbaydar M, Massimini D, et al. Transfer of pectoralis major for the treatment of irreparable tears of subscapularis: Does it work? *J Bone Joint Surg Br.* 2008;90(8):1059–1065.

63. Miller SL, Hazrati Y, Klepps S, et al. Loss of subscapularis function after total shoulder replacement: A seldom recognized problem. *J Shoulder Elbow Surg.* 2003;12(1):29–34.

64. Wirth MA, Rockwood CA Jr. Complications of total shoulder-replacement arthroplasty. *J Bone Joint Surg Am.* 1996;78(4):603–616.

65. Neer CS, Morrison DS. Glenoid bone-grafting in total shoulder arthroplasty. *J Bone Joint Surg Am.* 1988;70(8): 1154–1162.

66. Iannotti JP, Spencer EE, Winter U, et al. Prosthetic positioning in total shoulder arthroplasty. *J Shoulder Elbow Surg.* 2005;14(1 suppl S):111S–121S.

67. Spencer EE Jr, Valdevit A, Kambic H, et al. The effect of humeral component anteversion on shoulder stability with glenoid component retroversion. *J Bone Joint Surg Am.* 2005;87(4):808–814.

68. Farron A, Terrier A, Buchler P. Risks of loosening of a prosthetic glenoid implanted in retroversion. *J Shoulder Elbow Surg.* 2006;15(4):521–526.

69. Nyffeler RW, Sheikh R, Atkinson TS, et al. Effects of glenoid component version on humeral head displacement and joint reaction forces: An experimental study. *J Shoulder Elbow Surg.* 2006;15(5):625–629.

70. Sears BW, Johnston PS, Ramsey ML, et al. Glenoid bone loss in primary total shoulder arthroplasty: Evaluation and management. *J Am Acad Orthop Surg.* 2012;20(9):604–613.

71. Tammachote N, Sperling JW, Berglund LJ, et al. The effect of glenoid component size on the stability of total shoulder arthroplasty. *J Shoulder Elbow Surg.* 2007;16(3 suppl): S102–S106.

72. Steinmann SP, Cofield RH. Bone grafting for glenoid deficiency in total shoulder replacement. *J Shoulder Elbow Surg.* 2000;9(5):361–367.

73. Nyffeler RW, Sheikh R, Jacob HA, et al. Influence of humeral prosthesis height on biomechanics of glenohumeral abduction. An in vitro study. *J Bone Joint Surg Am.* 2004;86-A(3):575–580.

74. Wirth MA, Rockwood CA Jr. Complications of shoulder arthroplasty. *Clin Orthop Relat Res.* 1994;(307):47–69.

75. Clark JC, Ritchie J, Song FS, et al. Complication rates, dislocation, pain, and postoperative range of motion after reverse shoulder arthroplasty in patients with and without repair of the subscapularis. *J Shoulder Elbow Surg.* 2012;21(1):36–41.

76. Edwards TB, Williams MD, Labriola JE, et al. Subscapularis insufficiency and the risk of shoulder dislocation after reverse shoulder arthroplasty. *J Shoulder Elbow Surg.* 2009;18(6):892–896.

77. Simovitch RW, Zumstein MA, Lohri E, et al. Predictors of scapular notching in patients managed with the Delta III reverse total shoulder replacement. *J Bone Joint Surg Am.* 2007;89(3):588–600.

78. Edwards TB, Trappey GJ, Riley C, et al. Inferior tilt of the glenoid component does not decrease scapular notching in reverse shoulder arthroplasty: Results of a prospective randomized study. *J Shoulder Elbow Surg.* 2012;21(5):641–646.

79. Green A, Norris TR. Shoulder arthroplasty for advanced glenohumeral arthritis after anterior instability repair. *J Shoulder Elbow Surg.* 2001;10(6):539–545.

80. Lehmann L, Magosch P, Mauermann E, et al. Total shoulder arthroplasty in dislocation arthropathy. *Int Orthop.* 2010;34(8):1219–1225.

81. Sperling JW, Antuna SA, Sanchez-Sotelo J, et al. Shoulder arthroplasty for arthritis after instability surgery. *J Bone Joint Surg Am.* 2002;84-A(10):1775–1781.

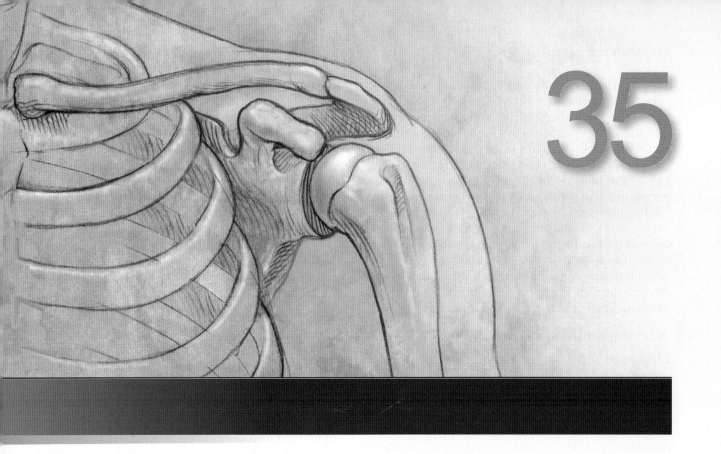

35

RECURRENT GLENOHUMERAL INSTABILITY IN THE EPILEPTIC PATIENT

Patric Raiss / Patrick J. Denard / Gilles Walch

EPIDEMIOLOGY

Epilepsy is a neurologic pathology that can lead to electrical discharges in the brain resulting in a seizure (1). The prevalence of epilepsy is 0.5% whereas the total number of patients who have seizures also related to other pathologies is around 5% (1). Other causes leading to seizures can be different metabolic diseases, traumas, tumors, or drugs. It has been reported that the incidence of shoulder dislocations during seizures is around 0.6%, but this may be underestimated since many dislocations cannot be detected afterward (1–3).

Causes and Pathomechanism of Shoulder Dislocation

There are two possibilities for how a seizure-related shoulder dislocation can occur. First, dislocation can be related due to a fall after the seizure begins. Second, dislocation can also occur due to the extremely powerful and uncoordinated muscle contractures during a seizure (4). Oftentimes the true cause is unknown, as the patient has no memory afterward.

In seizure-related dislocations the humeral head either dislocates anteriorly or posteriorly. Goudie et al. (1) recently described the pathomechanism for both directions of dislocations. For a posterior dislocation the arm is adducted, internally rotated, and forward flexed (5). During a seizure, contractions of the internal rotators of the humeral head (subscapularis, teres major, pectoralis major, and latissimus dorsi) are more powerful than those of the external rotators (infraspinatus and teres minor), leading to superior–posterior displacement of the head against the glenoid and the acromion which may result in a posterior dislocation (1,5,6). For anterior dislocations, the mechanism is abduction and external rotation as has been described comparably in traumatic cases (1).

Accompanied Lesions after Dislocation

Once the humeral head is dislocated the uncoordinated and heavy muscle contractions will fix and press the head against the glenoid bone as long as the seizure occurs. Therefore, large osseous lesions have been described in epileptics with shoulder dislocations on the humeral and the glenoid sides (1,4,7,8).

For anterior dislocations, fractures of the anterior glenoid rim (bony Bankart lesions) varying in size can frequently be detected (1,4,7). In cadaveric studies, it has been demonstrated that instability increases as the size of the glenoid rim fracture enlarges (9–11). Moreover, the size of posterolateral humeral head impression fractures or Hill-Sachs lesions (12) has been shown to be larger in postseizure cases compared to other instability pathology (8). These lesions may be so large that they engage and result in instability during simple activities of daily living.

Posterior shoulder dislocations lead to rim fractures of the posteroinferior glenoid (reverse bony Bankart lesions), also varying in size. A reverse Hill-Sachs lesion can oftentimes be detected at the level of the anatomical neck due to compression to the glenoid. A relationship between the size of the posterior glenoid fracture and the rate of recurrence has been described (13).

Associated injuries that can occur include brachial plexus injuries, coracoid process fractures, tuberosity fractures, and rotator cuff tears (14,15).

Anterior as well as posterior shoulder dislocations can become locked when they are not reduced or misdiagnosed (1). Treatment of these patients can be very challenging.

Causes for Recurrent Dislocations

The main cause for recurrent instability in seizure patients is another seizure (1,8). Although different conservative and operative treatment options have been reported, recurrent dislocations are very frequent and often independent from the stabilization procedure that was chosen (7,8). This can partially be related to patient activity level as recurrent dislocations are more frequent in the younger population (8). Lifestyle changes were discussed as one explanation why seizure-related dislocations are less frequent in older patients (8). In addition, the previously mentioned osseous and soft tissue lesions support the recurrence of instability. Goudie et al. (1) and Steinmann (16) also noted how failure to take antiseizure medications can lead to recurrent seizures. Other disorders like metabolic diseases, diabetes mellitus, or intracerebral pathologies can contribute to recurrent seizures and may need to be excluded by the physician(s) managing the seizure disorder.

CLINICAL ASSESSMENT OF SHOULDER INSTABILITY

A detailed history must be done by the surgeon taking into account patient symptoms, age, practice, sports, number of dislocations, and seizures.

The neurologist or other physician treating the seizures should be contacted to ensure that anticonvulsive therapy is optimized to avoid any further seizures after surgery. It is crucial that the patient, especially a young patient, understand the therapeutic scheme of anticonvulsive medication, and that medication compliance is crucial to reach a stable situation of the shoulder. Without a sufficient antiepileptic medication and in cases of noncompliance, no shoulder stabilization surgery should be performed (8).

The clinical assessment of anterior and posterior shoulder instability in epileptics is comparable to the assessment of unstable shoulder in other patients. Chronic dislocations can usually be detected by severely limited range of motion in elevation and especially in rotation.

For anterior shoulder instability several tests should be performed. The apprehension sign is tested with the patient in front of the examiner. One hand takes the arm of the patient and raises it into 90 degrees of abduction and 90 degrees of external rotation. The other hand is placed on the shoulder with the thumb on the backside and two to three fingers on the front. By increasing external rotation, posterior extension, and pushing the humeral head anteriorly, the patient may become fearful of a recurrent dislocation, oftentimes making it impossible to complete the maneuver. The examiner must be careful not to dislocate the humeral head, and keeps it in place by pressing the finger in front of the shoulder posteriorly.

The relocation test (17) is performed with the patient in a lying position. The affected arm is placed in the position of apprehension. The examiner then provides stability by pushing the humeral head posteriorly back into the glenoid. A decrease in patient apprehension indicates a positive relocation maneuver.

The anterior and posterior drawer signs according to Rockwood (18) are performed by seating the patient in front of the examiner with the shoulders relaxed and the forearms resting on the thighs (19). The examiner uses one hand to stabilize the clavicle and scapula and the other hand is placed around the humeral head. The examiner then pushes the head anteriorly and posteriorly. In a stable shoulder there is only limited mobility. The ability to manually dislocate the humeral head over the glenoid rim or an audible clunk during anterior/posterior translation or reduction suggests a tear of the labrum. Often these patients are apprehensive or have pain during this maneuver. Painless increased glenohumeral mobility, however, can be found in patients with hyperlaxity.

Constitutional laxity of the patient should be examined. We define hyperlaxity as external rotation of 90 degrees or more with the elbow at side. Laxity of the inferior capsule and the inferior glenohumeral ligament should be analyzed using two tests. The sulcus sign is performed with downward traction of the arm resting at the side and a sulcus may occur under the acromion in cases of laxity. The Gagey test (20) is performed on both shoulders with the patient in a sitting position. The scapula is fixed with one hand and with the other hand the patient's arm is maximally abducted. A difference in abduction of 20 degrees or more is defined as laxity of the inferior capsule and ligament.

RADIOGRAPHIC ASSESSMENT OF SHOULDER INSTABILITY

True anteroposterior (AP) radiographs showing the glenoid in profile should be performed in internal, external, and neutral rotations in order to show osseous lesions of the glenoid and especially of the humeral head (Fig. 35-1). Very large Hill-Sachs lesions can frequently be found in these patients. Using three different rotations of the humerus, the surgeon better understands the size and location of the lesion. In AP views, only osseous lesions of the inferior border of the glenoid can be detected.

The comparative profile view of the glenoid according to Bernageau et al. (21) is an excellent method to detect osseous lesions of the anterior glenoid (Fig. 35-2). The above mentioned four radiographs can be enough to make the indication for shoulder-stabilizing surgery. However, to get more detailed information about the size and location of the lesions a computed tomography (CT) scan (with or without contrast agent) has to be performed (1). Three-dimensional reconstructions allow an exact calculation of the amount of bone loss.

We limit the use of magnetic resonance imaging (MRI) in epileptics to those without bone loss where this study is valuable in detecting and classifying soft tissue lesions. However, most epileptics have large bone lesions, which make preoperative MRI unnecessary.

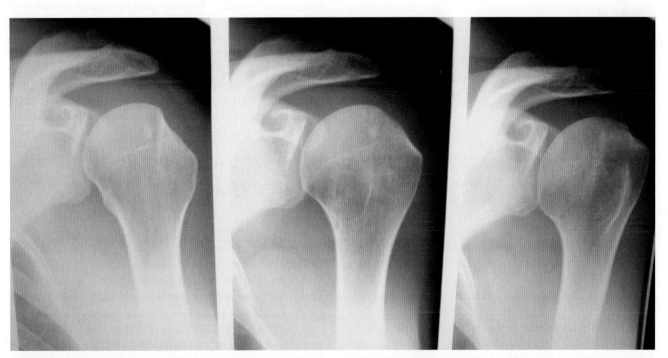

▲ **FIGURE 35-1:** AP view of a left shoulder of a 27-year-old man after multiple recurrent dislocations. In internal rotation **(far left)** a large Hill-Sachs lesion is clearly visible.

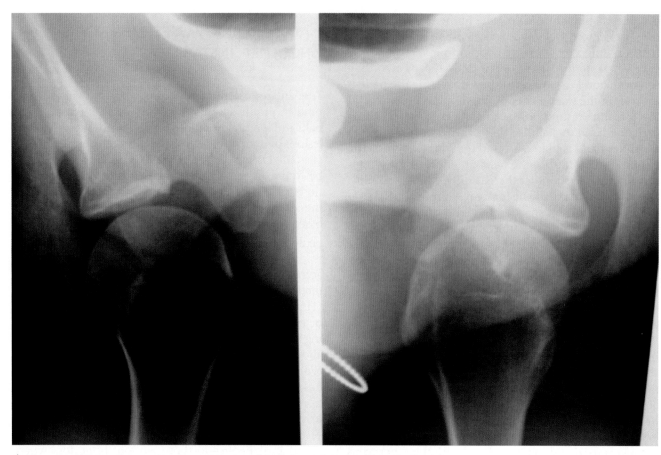

▲ **FIGURE 35-2:** Comparative Bernageau view of the left and right shoulders. On the right image (left shoulder) a fracture of the anterior border of the glenoid with bone loss is visible.

TREATMENT

As previously mentioned, treatment of epileptic patients requires a multidisciplinary approach including the shoulder surgeon, neurologist, physiotherapist, and in some cases the psychiatrist in order to assess the patient's compliance.

Conservative Treatment

As in nonseizure cases, conservative treatment is one option to treat a first-time dislocated shoulder in epileptic patients. In the nonepileptic population, there is currently debate regarding whether the arm should be immobilized in internal or external rotation (22,23). However, there is no consensus or information on which position the arm should be immobilized in after reduction in epileptics.

Bühler and Gerber (7) published a series of epileptic patients with shoulder dislocations in which four (one anterior and three posterior) were treated conservatively and no redislocation occurred. However, no details about the amount of osseous deficiency were reported in this study. In general, large bony lesions of the glenoid and the humerus can be found in this special cohort (8). Therefore, it seems logical that the risk for redislocation is higher compared to nonepileptic patients. A conservative treatment can be effective in a well-controlled epileptic who sustains a traumatic dislocation without large osseous defects (7). In cases with large Hill-Sachs lesions and large glenoid bone deficiency, however, a stabilization procedure should be the treatment of choice in well-controlled patients.

Soft Tissue Procedures for Anterior Dislocation

Goudie et al. (1) stated that an anterior soft tissue stabilization in epileptics may be sufficient in cases with less than 20% bone defect on the glenoid side. This has to be questioned as some authors reported high failure and redislocation rates in epileptics with recurrent seizures even when bone block procedures were chosen for reconstruction of the anterior glenoid (7,8). Bühler and Gerber (7) found that soft tissue stabilization was associated with high redislocation rates due to osseous lesions and recommended against these procedures in the epileptic population.

Bone Buttress Operations for Anterior Dislocations

The anterior aspect of the glenoid can be reconstructed with a bone block from the iliac crest (Eden–Hybinette procedure) (24) or with an allograft. Results of bone buttress operations for epileptic patients with glenoid defects were described in 1995 by Hutchinson et al. (4). Thirteen patients (15 shoulders) with a mean age of 29 years were analyzed at a mean 2.7 years following surgery. Ten dislocations resulted from a seizure, three were traumatic, and two did not have a clear cause. A bone buttress autograft (iliac crest) or allograft (femoral head) was used to reconstruct the anterior glenoid rim. Excellent clinical results and no redislocations were observed, although eight patients continued to have seizures. Moreover, no arthritic changes of the shoulder joint were detected radiographically. These results are unique in literature for anterior shoulder dislocations in epileptic patients.

High redislocation rates after bone block procedures for anterior shoulder dislocations were reported by Bühler and Gerber (7). Next to 17 posterior cases they described 17 cases of anterior dislocations in patients with seizures at a mean follow-up of 10 years. Seven patients treated with an Eden–Lange–Hybinette procedure redislocated afterward. Three of them underwent a reoperation with a bone block procedure while the remaining four were treated conservatively after reduction. None of the shoulders redislocated again. The overall recurrence rate (n = 17) was 47% in this study with five out of eight recurrent dislocations caused by new seizures.

The Latarjet Procedure

The Latarjet procedure has been well described for recurrent anterior instability of the shoulder joint (25). The procedure has three effects which stabilize the humeral head: (I) The sling mechanism of the conjoined tendon that pushes the lower part of the subscapularis muscle and the anteroinferior capsule against the joint, (II) the bone augmentation effect which allows the restoration of the anterior glenoid rim, and (III) the repair of the capsule which is performed using the stump of the resected coracoacromial ligament (25).

Recently, Raiss et al. (8) analyzed the results of the Latarjet procedure in epileptic patients with recurrent anterior shoulder dislocations. Fourteen shoulders in 12 patients with a mean age of 31 years and a mean of 10 dislocations were treated by the same surgeon and had an identical rehab protocol. A slight decrease in external rotation and an increase of osteoarthritic radiographic changes were found after a mean follow-up of 8 years. Six shoulders had a redislocation , all of which were caused by a new seizure in this study (Fig. 35-3). Five patients underwent revision surgery with a very

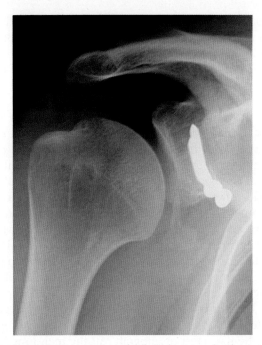

▲ **FIGURE 35-3:** AP view of a shoulder treated with a Latarjet procedure after redislocation. The 4.5-mm malleolar screws are bent and a fracture of the bone block is visible.

large bone buttress from the iliac crest and in two cases redislocation occurred after a new seizure.

The authors concluded that an effective anticonvulsive treatment is essential to avoid further seizures and therefore, further redislocations. Based on this data we feel that shoulder stabilization surgery should be preserved for the well-controlled patient who sustains anterior dislocations during activities of daily living.

The Problem of the Hill-Sachs Lesion

The previously mentioned surgical treatment options for anterior dislocations primarily focus on the restoration of the anterior glenoid rim and only indirectly treat osseous lesions of the humeral head by extension of the glenoid arc (4,7,8). However, as high failure rates have been reported for restoration of the anterior glenoid, and Hill-Sachs lesions can be enormous in epileptics, treatment of these lesions may need to be considered. Humeral head defects can be filled with autograft, allograft, or soft tissues (7,26,27). The remplissage procedure was described as an effective treatment option in combination with a Bankart repair (28,29). To our knowledge, augmentation of the humeral head defect with bone or the remplissage procedure has not been reported in epileptic patients.

Surgical Treatment of Posterior Shoulder Dislocations

The results of surgical treatment after posterior shoulder dislocations in epileptic patients are more satisfactory compared to anterior instability. Moreover, locked posterior dislocations can frequently be observed (7). Bühler and Gerber (7) reported that 15 of 17 posterior dislocations were locked. The number and amount of bone lesions of glenoid were less frequent compared to anterior dislocations in this study and therefore, the main focus was on the repair of the engaging "reverse Hill-Sachs lesion" rather than to restore the glenoid only. Overall two redislocations occurred (12%). In cases where the humeral head defect was augmented with an allo- or autograft, no redislocation was observed after a mean follow-up of 7 years. For small acute defects it is also possible to disimpact and elevate the impressed fracture and to fill the defect with autologous bone (30). Another option to treat the reverse Hill-Sachs lesion is the McLaughlin procedure (31) in which an osteotomy of the lesser tuberosity is performed and then fixed into the defect.

The posterior aspect of the glenoid can be reconstructed by bone buttress procedures with autograft from the iliac crest or allograft. All the mentioned surgeries can be combined with soft tissue procedures like capsular shifts, Bankart repairs, etc. The evidence of all the mentioned surgeries and techniques is limited as only few studies exist dealing with this topic.

Shoulder Arthroplasty for Anterior and Posterior Dislocations

Shoulder arthroplasty is a well-established treatment option for degenerative pathologies of the shoulder joint. Acceptable functional outcomes but high complication rates have been published for nonconstrained shoulder arthroplasty after postinstability arthritis in nonepileptic patients (32–35). Two studies reported on the results of shoulder replacement after fixed anterior glenohumeral dislocations (36,37). One reported about the results of conventional hemi- and total shoulder arthroplasty (37) and the other on the results of cementless surface replacement arthroplasty of the humeral head (36). Redislocations were observed in both studies. Reverse shoulder arthroplasty could potentially reduce the risk of redislocation by lowering and medializing the center of rotation and retensioning the deltoid. However, no studies are available on reverse shoulder replacement surgery in epileptic patients.

CONCLUSION

Shoulder instability in epileptic patients is a special entity that should be distinguished from other instability seen in other populations. Most important is the use of an appropriate anticonvulsive regimen to avoid recurrent seizures as most redislocations result from

a repeat seizure. No operation should be performed in noncompliant patients or patients with ineffective medical treatment. The surgical treatment of recurrent anterior dislocations in the epileptic patient continues to be a challenging problem, and the results after bone block procedures seem to be superior compared to soft tissue operations. However, even bone block procedures should be reserved for the well-controlled epileptic patient who sustains recurrent shoulder dislocations during activities of daily living.

References

1. Goudie EB, Murray IR, Robinson CM. Instability of the shoulder following seizures. *J Bone Joint Surg Br.* 2012; 94:721–728.
2. DeToledo JC, Lowe MR. Seizures, lateral decubitus, aspiration, and shoulder dislocation: Time to change the guidelines? *Neurology.* 2001;56:290–291.
3. Schulz TJ, Jacobs B, Patterson RL Jr. Unrecognized dislocations of the shoulder. *J Trauma.* 1969;9:1009–1023.
4. Hutchinson JW, Neumann L, Wallace WA. Bone buttress operation for recurrent anterior shoulder dislocation in epilepsy. *J Bone Joint Surg Br.* 1995;77:928–932.
5. Shaw JL. Bilateral posterior fracture-dislocation of the shoulder and other trauma caused by convulsive seizures. *J Bone Joint Surg Am.* 1971;53:1437–1440.
6. McLaughlin HL. Posterior dislocation of the shoulder. *J Bone Joint Surg Am.* 1952;24-A-3:584–590.
7. Bühler M, Gerber C. Shoulder instability related to epileptic seizures. *J Shoulder Elbow Surg.* 2002;11:339–344.
8. Raiss P, Lin A, Mizuno N, et al. Results of the Latarjet procedure for recurrent anterior dislocation of the shoulder in patients with epilepsy. *J Bone Joint Surg Br.* 2012;94:1260–1264.
9. Yamamoto N, Itoi E, Abe H, et al. Contact between the glenoid and the humeral head in abduction, external rotation, and horizontal extension: A new concept of glenoid track. *J Shoulder Elbow Surg.* 2007;16:649–656.
10. Yamamoto N, Itoi E, Abe H, et al. Effect of an anterior glenoid defect on anterior shoulder stability: A cadaveric study. *Am J Sports Med.* 2009;37:949–954.
11. Itoi E, Lee SB, Berglund LJ, et al. The effect of a glenoid defect on anteroinferior stability of the shoulder after Bankart repair: A cadaveric study. *J Bone Joint Surg Am.* 2000;82:35–46.
12. Hill HA, Sachs MD. The grooved defect of humeral head. A frequently unrecognized complication of dislocations of the shoulder joint. *Radiology.* 1940;35:690–700.
13. Weishaupt D, Zanetti M, Nyffeler RW, et al. Posterior glenoid rim deficiency in recurrent (atraumatic) posterior shoulder instability. *Skeletal Radiol.* 2000;29:204–210.
14. Robinson CM, Al-Hourani K, Malley TS, et al. Anterior shoulder instability associated with coracoid nonunion in patients with a seizure disorder. *J Bone Joint Surg Am.* 2012;94:e40.
15. Robinson CM, Shur N, Sharpe T, et al. Injuries associated with traumatic anterior glenohumeral dislocations. *J Bone Joint Surg Am.* 2012;94:18–26.

16. Steinmann SP. Posterior shoulder instability. *Arthroscopy.* 2003;19(suppl 1):102–105.

17. Jobe FW, Tibone JE, Jobe CM, et al. The shoulder in sports. In: Rockwood CA, Matsen FA, eds. *The Shoulder.* Philadelphia, PA: Saunders Company; 1990:961–990.

18. Rockwood CA. Subluxations and dislocations about the shoulder. In: Rockwood CA, Green DP, eds. *Fractures in Adults.* 2nd ed. Philadelphia, PA: Lipincott; 2012: 722–950.

19. Gerber C, Ganz R. Clinical assessment of instability of the shoulder. With special reference to anterior and posterior drawer tests. *J Bone Joint Surg Br.* 1984;66:551–556.

20. Gagey OJ, Gagey N. The hyperabduction test. *J Bone Joint Surg Br.* 2001;83:69–74.

21. Bernageau J, Patte D, Debeyre J, et al. [Value of the glenoid profil in recurrent luxations of the shoulder]. *Rev Chir Orthop Reparatrice Appar Mot.* 1976;62:142–147.

22. Liavaag S, Brox JI, Pripp AH, et al. Immobilization in external rotation after primary shoulder dislocation did not reduce the risk of recurrence: A randomized controlled trial. *J Bone Joint Surg Am.* 2011;93:897–904.

23. Itoi E, Hatakeyama Y, Sato T, et al. Immobilization in external rotation after shoulder dislocation reduces the risk of recurrence. A randomized controlled trial. *J Bone Joint Surg Am.* 2007;89:2124–2131.

24. Eden R. Zur Operation der habituellen Schulterluxation unter Mitteilung eines neuen Verfahrens bei Abriss am inneren Pfannenrande. *Dstch Ztschr Chir.* 1918;144:269.

25. Young AA, Maia R, Berhouet J, et al. Open Latarjet procedure for management of bone loss in anterior instability of the glenohumeral joint. *J Shoulder Elbow Surg.* 2011;20:S61–S69.

26. Elkinson I, Giles JW, Faber KJ, et al. The effect of the remplissage procedure on shoulder stability and range of motion: An in vitro biomechanical assessment. *J Bone Joint Surg Am.* 2012;94:1003–1012.

27. Giles JW, Elkinson I, Ferreira LM, et al. Moderate to large engaging Hill-Sachs defects: An in vitro biomechanical comparison of the remplissage procedure, allograft humeral head reconstruction, and partial resurfacing arthroplasty. *J Shoulder Elbow Surg.* 2012;21:1142–1151.

28. Purchase RJ, Wolf EM, Hobgood ER, et al. Hill-sachs "remplissage": An arthroscopic solution for the engaging hill-sachs lesion. *Arthroscopy.* 2008;24:723–726.

29. Boileau P, O'Shea K, Vargas P, et al. Anatomical and functional results after arthroscopic Hill-Sachs remplissage. *J Bone Joint Surg Am.* 2012;94:618–626.

30. Gerber C. Chronic, locked anterior and posterior dislocations. In: Warner JJP, Iannotti JP, Gerber C, eds. *Complex and Revision Problems in Shoulder Surgery.* Philadelphia, PA: Lippincott-Raven; 1997;99–116.

31. Finkelstein JA, Waddell JP, O'Driscoll SW, et al. Acute posterior fracture dislocations of the shoulder treated with the Neer modification of the McLaughlin procedure. *J Orthop Trauma.* 1995;9:190–193.

32. Sperling JW, Antuna SA, Sanchez-Sotelo J, et al. Shoulder arthroplasty for arthritis after instability surgery. *J Bone Joint Surg Am.* 2002;84-A:1775–1781.

33. Lehmann L, Magosch P, Mauermann E, et al. Total shoulder arthroplasty in dislocation arthropathy. *Int Orthop.* 2010;34:1219–1225.

34. Matsoukis J, Tabib W, Guiffault P, et al. Shoulder arthroplasty in patients with a prior anterior shoulder dislocation. Results of a multicenter study. *J Bone Joint Surg Am.* 2003;85-A:1417–1424.

35. Green A, Norris TR. Shoulder arthroplasty for advanced glenohumeral arthritis after anterior instability repair. *J Shoulder Elbow Surg.* 2001;10:539–545.

36. Raiss P, Aldinger PR, Kasten P, et al. Humeral head resurfacing for fixed anterior glenohumeral dislocation. *Int Orthop.* 2009;33:451–456.

37. Matsoukis J, Tabib W, Guiffault P, et al. Primary unconstrained shoulder arthroplasty in patients with a fixed anterior glenohumeral dislocation. *J Bone Joint Surg Am.* 2006;88:547–552.

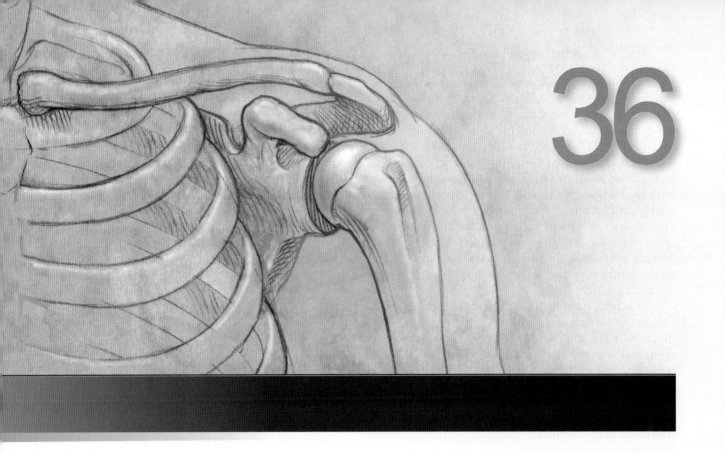

36

INSTABILITY IN PEDIATRIC PATIENTS (OPEN GROWTH PLATES)

Itai Gans / Lawrence Wells

INTRODUCTION

Skeletally immature patients with shoulder instability are a unique subset of patients. Their open growth plates add a level of complexity to the diagnosis and management of their shoulder complaints. Modern child athletes play at higher intensities and at younger ages than ever seen before. By high school, many adolescent athletes concentrate on one sport and play year round, often in multiple leagues. Unfortunately, this also means a decrease in cross-training , increasing their risk of injury. As a result, there has been a dramatic increase in overuse and training-related injuries in children (1). Prompt recognition and treatment of such injuries are critical in preventing long-term functional disability and deformity (2).

Some have argued that young females are disproportionally affected by shoulder instability. Shoulder instability cannot be described as a condition that differentially affects girls, but it is more common in young athletes who are competitive swimmers and gymnasts, both sports in which girls participate more frequently than young boys. While it is true that children with open growth plates are more likely to have a physeal fracture than a dislocation, dislocation is still a common musculoskeletal problem seen by physicians in emergency rooms, family practice offices, and orthopedics practices (3).

Traditionally, children rarely required shoulder surgeries; however, now, many pitchers coming out of high school and joining the major leagues have undergone a surgical procedure for shoulder injuries (1). Management of the in-season athlete can be a challenge in this era of increased desire to obtain scholarship for secondary education and to compete at higher levels in both high school and college. It used to be easier to take young athletes out of sports and let their injuries heal. The modern child and the adolescent athlete face the same kinds of performance pressures as professional athletes with scouts for both professional and collegiate sports teams attending youth sporting events, even at the middle school level (1).

It is important for any physician who treats young patients to be familiar with the differences in skeletal maturity, injury rates, and injury patterns between children and adults. Many graduating family medicine residents treating musculoskeletal conditions show low levels of confidence in treating these injuries (4). As such, if any questions should arise in the treatment of musculoskeletal injuries in skeletally immature patients, consultation to a pediatric orthopedic specialist should be strongly considered.

CLASSIFICATION

The classification of shoulder dislocations in the pediatric population as traumatic or atraumatic is of great importance as the etiology of shoulder instability plays a large role in the choice of treatment.

Atraumatic

There are multiple causes of atraumatic shoulder instability in the pediatric patient including generalized ligamentous laxity, Ehlers-Danlos syndrome, Marfan syndrome, and other ill-defined hyperlaxity conditions (Fig. 36-1). Most commonly these patients will present with generalized ligamentous laxity, which affects about 5% of the population, or ligamentous laxity that has developed slowly secondary to repetitive microtrauma, particularly from sports such as swimming, baseball, or volleyball (5). Atraumatic instability may also occur in individuals who possess congenital or syndromic conditions such as Ehlers-Danlos syndrome and Marfan syndrome. These rare hereditary connective tissue disorders may result in increased joint laxity and poor soft tissue healing. Patients with connective tissue disorders benefit less, and have relatively higher surgical complication rates, than patients without connective tissue disorders, and as such, nonsurgical treatment is highly advised in this patient population (6).

Although rare, voluntary subluxation of the shoulder is another consideration in the treatment of atrau-

matic shoulder instability. Voluntary subluxation of the shoulder tends to occur in the posterior direction (Fig. 36-2). Voluntary subluxators generally benefit from psychological evaluation and support as the voluntary subluxation is often an attention getting behavior. Over time, an involuntary instability can develop as the ligamentous structures of the glenohumeral joint stretch and becomes progressively deficient. The most common pathologic lesion causing pain in those who can voluntarily dislocate the shoulder is excessive capsular laxity rather than the frank labral tears seen in many traumatic dislocations (5).

Traumatic

Trauma to the pediatric shoulder can result in dislocation of the humeral head. Dislocations are commonly seen in adolescents and young adults, with 40% of first episodes occurring before the third decade of life. Associated bony glenoid injuries are more commonly seen in the near skeletally mature adolescent population (7). Most traumatic shoulder dislocations in the pediatric patient however are not associated with a bony injury.

Injury from trauma to the shoulder is not only determined by the mechanism of injury and offending activity, but also dramatically influenced by the extent of skeletal maturity of the injured child. In children, most injuries occur at the chondroosseous junctions of the physes and apophyses rather than the soft tissues. These transition sites between cartilage and bone are at greatest risk during adolescence, when there is a rapid increase in muscle strength and physeal thickening secondary to the teenage growth spurt (8).

The skeletally immature shoulder is also at risk for dislocation in pediatric patients during the birth process. In addition, despite advances in modern obstetric care, traction injury to the brachial plexus sustained during the birth process can result in impairment of upper extremity neuromuscular function. Most commonly, these injuries result in motor weakness of external rotation at the shoulder, causing internal rotation contractures, and subsequent deformity of the skeletally immature glenohumeral joint which can cause severe, recurrent shoulder dislocation (9).

SKELETAL MATURATION

Developmentally in the shoulder and about the scapula, the coracoid area is the first to fuse at about 11 years of age, followed by the glenoid surface and remaining physes, with the medial clavicle fusing last by the age of 25 to 27 (10). The closure of the physis of the medial clavicle, in addition to being the latest physeal closure about the shoulder and upper limb, also shows the greatest variation in maturation (10–12). While there

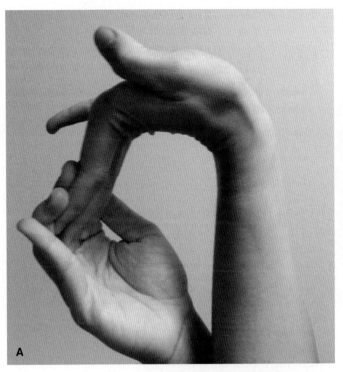

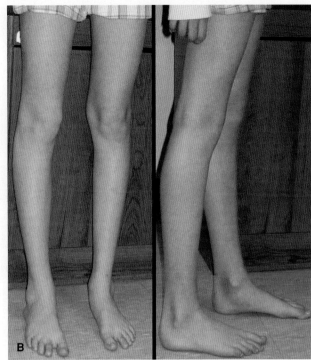

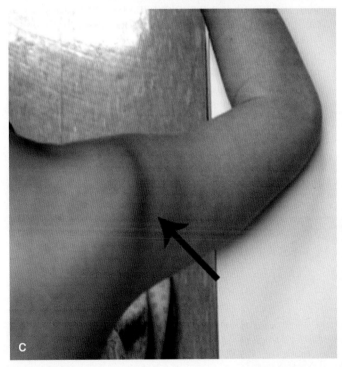

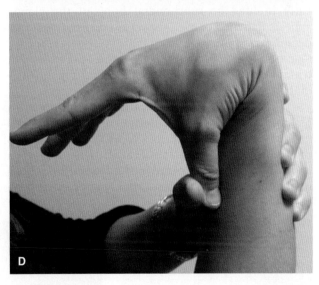

▲ FIGURE 36-1: Physical examination findings in patients with ligamentous laxity. **A:** Hyperextensible metacarpal joints. **B:** Knee hyperextension. **C:** Accentuated sulcus sign. **D:** Thumb to wrist apposition.

is a sex difference in maturation of the skeleton of the upper limb, with females showing an advance relative to males of about 2 years, sex differences in maturation are less noticeable in the scapular girdle. Limited data; however, does show that the female scapular girdle matures slightly ahead of males (10). Table 36-1 shows the timing of physeal closure of the main physes about the shoulder.

It is important to keep in mind that the diagnosis of mature clavicles is overestimated by radiography and computed tomography when compared to direct visual inspection, either in postmortem studies or intraoperatively (14).

For a comparison of normal shoulder radiographs in skeletally immature and mature patients, see Figures 36-3 to 36-5.

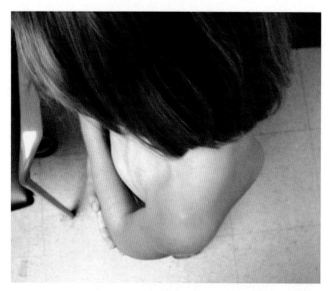

▲ **FIGURE 36-2:** A young patient exhibiting voluntary posterior subluxation of the left shoulder.

TABLE 36-1 **Age of Physeal Closure about the Shoulder**

Physis	Age of Physeal Closure (yrs)	
	Females	Males
Proximal Humerus	14–16	15–17
Base of Coracoid	14–15	15–16
Glenoid Apophysis	15–17	15–17
Distal Clavicle	No Consistent Data[a]	

[a]We were not able to find any data that specifically discussed the closure of the glenoid apophysis or physis of the distal clavicle; however, it is our impression that the maturation parallels that of the coracoid and proximal humerus.

From: Cardoso HF. Age estimation of adolescent and young adult male and female skeletons II, epiphyseal union at the upper limb and scapular girdle in a modern Portuguese skeletal sample. *Am J Phys Anthropol.* 2008;137:97–105 and Ogden JA. *Skeletal Injury in the Child.* 3rd ed. New York, NY: Springer-Verlag; 2000.

Glenoid

Early in life, the subchondral bone of the glenoid appears flattened or even convex on conventional radiography. Despite this radiographic appearance, the cartilaginous glenoid already appears on MRI to have its typical concave configuration and conforms to the shape of the humeral head (15).

The bony glenoid develops from the fusion of two ossification centers. The first center appears at approximately 10 years of age in close proximity to the base of the coracoid. The second ossification center appears at approximately 15 years of age and has a horseshoe configuration (16,17). These ossification centers fuse, undergo

transformation to fatty marrow, and subsequently fuse with the subchondral bone plate. As in adults, the articular surface of the glenoid remains cartilaginous and can be readily identified as a smooth rim of high signal intensity on MRI fluid-sensitive sequences whereas the fibrocartilaginous labrum is of homogenous low signal intensity on all MRI pulse sequences (15). Occasionally, a focal, well-marginated defect in the articular cartilage known as the bare spot of the glenoid can be seen in the center of the glenoid fossa on MRI. This focal thinning is less commonly seen in children than in adults (18).

During skeletal maturation there is a change in the glenoid version, the orientation of the glenoid relative to the angle of the scapula. The glenoid version in children

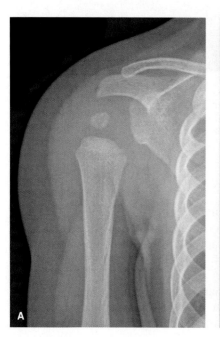
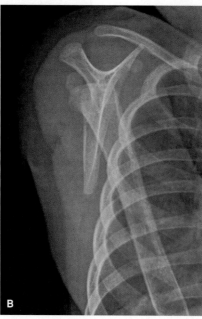

◄ **FIGURE 36-3:** AP **(A)** and trans-scapular Y **(B)** radiographs of a normally located shoulder in a skeletally immature 6-month-old.

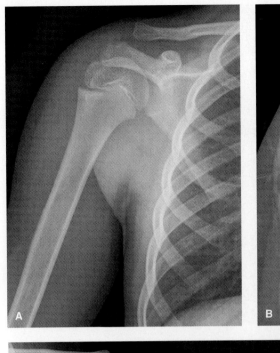
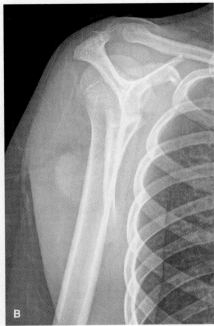
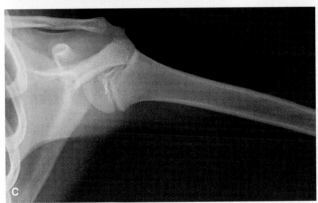

▲ **FIGURE 36-4:**   AP **(A)**, trans-scapular Y **(B)**, and axillary **(C)** radiographs of a normally located shoulder in a skeletally immature 12-year-old.

must be viewed as dynamic. In children younger than 2 years, the mean glenoid version is −6° (or 6 degrees of retroversion). This value steadily increases throughout childhood, reaching adult standards of −1° by the end of the child's first decade of life. However, the normal values of glenoid version have great variability. Approximately 68% of children have slightly retroverted glenoids while the remaining 32% demonstrate mild anteversion (glenoid version > 0°) (19).

Developmentally, reaching adult version may relate to the appearance of the upper ossification center of the glenoid as well as to the appearance of an ossification center at the base of the coracoid which contributes to glenoid formation. The appearance and development of these ossification centers coincide with the end of the first decade of life when adult glenoid version is reached. Children with a hindrance in the normal sequence of progression of glenoid version will clinically have excessive retroversion that may predispose to posterior shoulder instability (19).

Proximal Humerus

The proximal humerus is composed of the proximal humeral physis, which is responsible for the vast majority of the growth of the humerus, and the proximal humeral apophyses, the greater and lesser tuberosities, which are responsible for the expansion of the humeral head and are the attachment points for the rotator cuff tendons. Distally there is a distal humeral physis, consisting of the capitellum and trochlea, and two apophyses, which include the medial and lateral epicondyles. Closure of the proximal humeral physis occurs at approximately 14 to 16 years of age in girls and 15 to 17 years of age in boys (10,16).

Acromion

Three distinct ossification centers merge to form the acromion: The pre-acromion, located more anteriorly; the meso-acromion, which is located in the middle portion; and the meta-acromion, which is more posterior

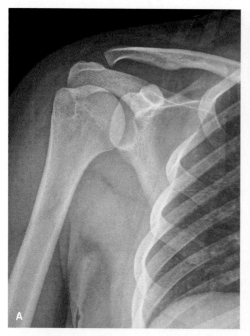

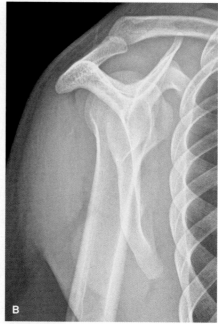

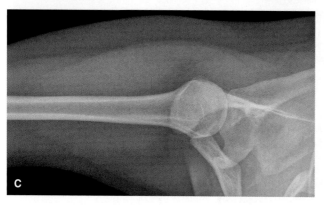

▲ **FIGURE 36-5:** AP **(A)**, trans-scapular
Y **(B)**, and axillary **(C)** radiographs of a normally located shoulder in a skeletally mature
17-year-old.

and forms the acromial angle. These ossification centers form during adolescence and fuse between 17 and
22 years of age (20–22).

NATURAL HISTORY

Conventionally, unidirectional or multidirectional
instability of the shoulder is uncommon in the young
skeletally immature athlete (23–27). In classic studies,
the risk of sustaining a traumatic anterior dislocation
of the shoulder has been estimated to be between 1%
and 2% over one's lifetime, with the risk being highest in childhood and decreasing with age (28–30).
Glenohumeral dislocations in patients 12 years of age
and younger comprise about 1.6% to 4.7% of all glenohumeral dislocations (3,26,27,31). We appreciate
and respect the extensive research that has been done in
determining the rate of shoulder dislocation, led in part
by Hovelius in Sweden; however, in our opinion, these
papers underestimate the rate of shoulder dislocations
in the pediatric patient. This is particularly true in the

subset population of sports injured athletes, commonly
including wrestlers, basketball, and football players.

Bilateral shoulder instability occurs at a rate of
16% in patients from 12 to 22 years of age in contrast to
a rate of only 3% in patients from 30 to 40 years of age
(23). Some studies have even reported a rate for bilateral anterior shoulder instability for patients aged 1 to
20 years of age as high as 24% (32).

Redislocation

Recurrent dislocation is the most common complication
after traumatic anterior shoulder dislocation in young
patients (33). Redislocation in pediatrics, depending on
the patient's age, is the rule, rather than the exception.
This may partially be due to pediatric patients resuming
full activity with a higher frequency than adults, thus
subjecting themselves to stresses that can result in repeat
injury. A shoulder joint with disturbed or attenuated
soft tissue restraints (often the anterior inferior glenohumeral ligament complex) from a first dislocation is
thus at high risk.

Skeletally immature children who resume sports activities soon after shoulder dislocation have the highest recurrence rate (34). Eighty-two percent of young athletes experience redislocation compared to 30% of young nonathletes. Athletes restricted from resuming sports for 6 weeks or more have significantly reduced rates of redislocation and decreased symptomatic instability (35).

Age is the most important denominator for predicting the recurrence of traumatic anterior shoulder dislocation in adolescents (36). Redislocation rates have been reported to be as high as 64% to 95% in patients younger than the age of 20 (25,27,30,37–39), most commonly occurring between 14 and 17 years of age (40). Rates of shoulder dislocations drop to 79% between the ages of 21 and 30 (41) and nearly 0% after the age of 40 (35).

In a classic multicenter study conducted by Hovelius et al. (23) in which patients between 12 and 40 years of age with primary anterior shoulder dislocations were followed prospectively for 10 years, operative treatment was required in 23% of patients experiencing recurrent dislocations. Of patients that went on to surgery, 34% were 12 to 22 years old, 28% were 23 to 29 years of age, and only 9% were between 30 and 40 years of age. Deitch et al. (33) have shown persistent instability necessitating a shoulder stabilization procedure in up to 50% of patients from 11 to 18 years of age.

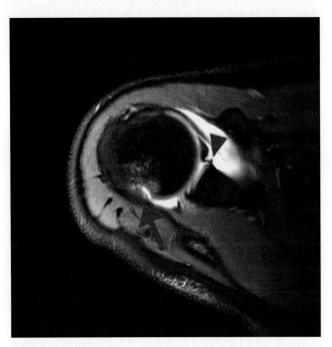

▲ **FIGURE 36-6:** Sequelae due to chronic recurrent shoulder dislocations. *Red arrow*—Hill-Sachs lesion. *Red arrowhead*—Bankart lesion.

ADDITIONAL INJURIES ASSOCIATED WITH DISLOCATION

The main stabilizers of the shoulder joint are the ligaments and the capsule complex. Multiple ligaments are present, but the inferior glenohumeral ligament complex is the most important factor in maintaining shoulder stability. The anterior inferior glenohumeral ligament is most commonly injured during an anterior shoulder dislocation. Detachment of the inferior glenohumeral ligament–labrum complex from the glenoid, the Bankart lesion, is found in 94% to 97% of shoulders after an initial dislocation (42–44).

Recurrent shoulder instability increases the risk of extensive soft tissue and bony injuries with each repeated dislocation (45). In addition to glenohumeral ligament injury, first-time dislocation and recurrent episodes are associated with injuries to the glenoid labrum and muscles of the rotator cuff (46). Figure 36-6 shows the sequelae of chronic recurrent shoulder dislocations on MRI.

As in adult patients, pediatric patients are not immune to possible nerve injury secondary to shoulder dislocations due to the proximity of the brachial plexus, with the greatest risk being to the axillary nerve. Recurrent instability increases the chances of nerve injury.

There does appear to be a modest increased risk of osteoarthritis in young patients with shoulder instability, with worse clinical and radiographic sequelae in instability that tends to occur at a younger age (47).

EVALUATION

History

The mechanisms of injury in traumatic shoulder dislocations in skeletally immature individuals are similar to those of the skeletally mature individuals (48). Patients will often complain of difficulties with activities of daily living, especially overhead activities. Despite this similarity, it is quite important to get a careful and thorough history in pediatric patients with shoulder instability, specifically, its etiology. Determining whether shoulder instability is of traumatic or atraumatic etiology often has significant weight in deciding the course of treatment (49).

Once the etiology of shoulder instability is gleaned, the frequency of shoulder dislocation and prior treatments should be determined. A patient's age is especially important in determining therapy as 92% of patients between 14 and 17 years of age may experience redislocation (40). It is especially important to note any prior attempts or failures at surgical fixation or conservative rehabilitation.

Physical Examination

When physically assessing the pediatric shoulder with instability, it is important to begin with inspection of the appearance of the patient and the arm. One can gather a great deal of information by noticing the way the patient's arm is positioned relative to their body. It is important to perform inspection with the patient's shoulder exposed so that the patient's clothing does not obstruct vision of any obvious deformities. Next, the patient can be lead through passive and active ranges of motion bilaterally to determine if there are any discrepancies between the affected and unaffected sides. Limited range of motion may indicate current dislocation. Patients may also refuse to move shoulders that are dislocated at the time of examination. Note should be made of any crepitance or abnormal scapular patterning through flexion and abduction which may be a sign of long thoracic nerve injury.

Palpation of the shoulder should be performed to determine any point tenderness and a full neurovascular assessment should be completed to determine if there is any neuropraxia, specifically in the distribution of the axillary nerve. Specific tests that may be helpful include the anterior apprehension test which may be positive in those with recurrent shoulder instability. In patients with a positive anterior apprehension test, a relocation test should be performed to ensure that apprehension is resolved with posterior pressure over the humeral head.

A sulcus sign, a soft tissue indentation just below the acromion with downward traction being placed on a relaxed arm at the patients side (Fig. 36-7), is a hallmark of multidirectional instability and is particularly accentuated in patients with ligamentous laxity. The load-and-shift test, which is most reliably done under anesthesia, can also be performed to determine how much laxity and translation the humeral head has within the glenoid. The more translation that can occur, the more instability exists within the shoulder.

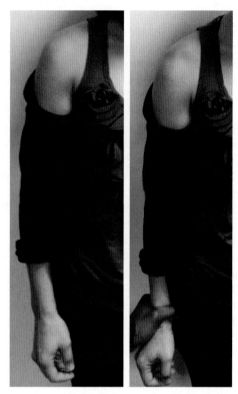

▲ FIGURE 36-7: **(Left)**—normal appearing shoulder. **(Right)**— Sulcus sign upon application of downward traction on the arm.

Imaging

Typically, tangential AP of the scapula, trans-scapular lateral (Y), and axillary radiographs are good studies to obtain in initial evaluation of the unstable shoulder. Figures 36-8 to 36-10 show normal located and abnormal dislocated radiographic images of the shoulder for

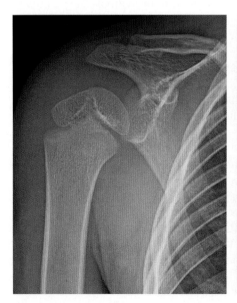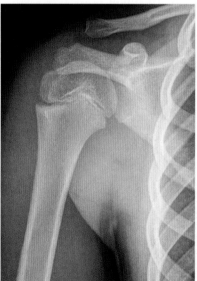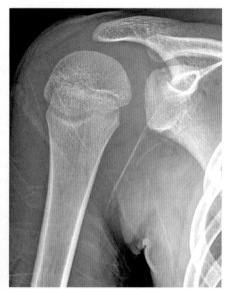

▲ FIGURE 36-8: AP radiographs of the shoulder depicting anterior dislocation **(left)**, normal location **(middle)**, and posterior dislocation **(right)** in skeletally immature patients. The appearance of the humeral head on AP radiograph in posterior dislocation is often referred to as the "light bulb sign."

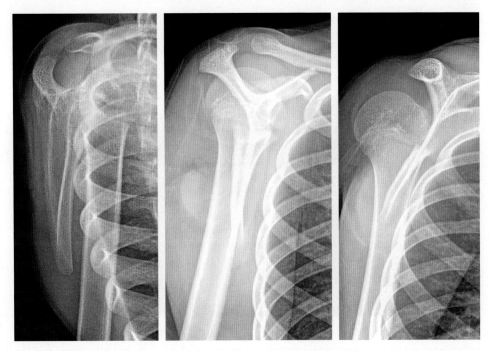

▶ **FIGURE 36-9:** Trans-scapular Y radiographs of the shoulder depicting anterior dislocation **(left)**, normal location **(middle)**, and posterior dislocation **(right)** in skeletally immature patients.

comparison. If radiographic studies are not sufficient to make a full assessment, MRI imaging is often the next step in radiographic evaluation. In the acute setting, such as in traumatic dislocation, MRI might be sufficient to evaluate for further injury. In a patient with recurrent or chronic instability, MRI arthrogram enhances the ability to view injuries to the soft tissue envelope. Injuries to the glenoid labrum are best characterized by intra-articular contrast on MRI (46).

It is important to remember that, despite advances in imaging technology and resolution, studies underestimate the true extent of labral and soft tissue injuries secondary to shoulder dislocations and shoulder instability in adolescent patients. This is especially true in tears of the glenoid labrum, which often extend far beyond the margins identified on MRI when explored arthroscopically (50).

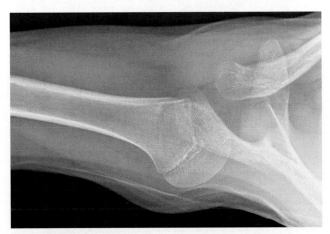

▲ **FIGURE 36-10:** Axillary radiograph of the shoulder depicting posterior dislocation.

TREATMENT

The management of skeletally immature patients with shoulder instability is very similar to the treatment of adult patients, albeit particularly challenging. As in adults, a variety of instability patterns can exist. While historically, treatment has generally been quite conservative, emerging data supports stabilization surgery for first-time traumatic anterior dislocations in active adolescent patients (36). With rehabilitation and exercise without surgery, patients with traumatic subluxation only have a 16% chance of good or excellent results whereas 80% of patients with atraumatic shoulder instability have good or excellent results without surgery (49). Traumatic anterior dislocations often result in Bankart lesions and unacceptably high rates of recurrence without surgical treatment which may include labral repair or capsulolabral plication. Atraumatic shoulder instability may be even more challenging to treat than traumatic shoulder dislocations in the skeletally immature patient. Extended courses of immobilization and rehabilitation may be quite useful although recalcitrant cases may require capsulorrhaphy (51).

If surgical treatment is used, the postoperative course is long and intensive. Physical therapy to restore range of motion and muscle strength is the rule. For athletes, return to sports is allowed only after achievement of complete range of motion, normalized strength, and completion of a progressive functional rehabilitation program (51).

It is important to be aware of the developmental centers of the pediatric bones about the shoulder when

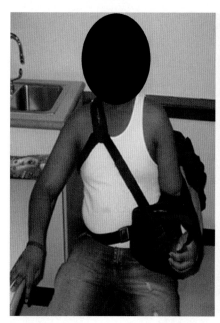
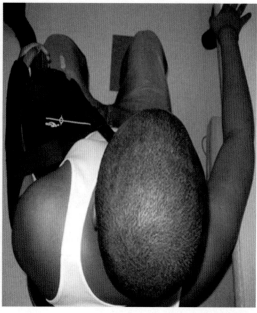

◀ **FIGURE 36-11:** Shoulder immobilization in external rotation.

managing skeletally immature patients with shoulder instability. Identification of Salter-Harris fractures about the physes and avoidance of growth disturbances with operative treatments are essential. Surgical treatment in young athletes has been shown to be both effective and safe (52). Growth impairment due to surgery about open growth plates at the glenoid has not been documented in the literature (53). We agree that surgical stabilization of the shoulder is a safe method of treatment in the pediatric patient and have not observed any clinically apparent growth disturbance with current surgical treatments circa 2013.

Treatment goals include returning to normal or near-normal function, limiting further injury to the shoulder, preventing neurapraxia, and eliminating the risk of redislocation which is quite high in the pediatric patient with shoulder instability (40).

Atraumatic Dislocations

All patients with atraumatic shoulder instability should undergo a course of immobilization as preliminary therapy. Surgery in these patients is usually a last resort used in those who did not respond to immobilization, activity modification, and rehabilitation or physical therapy. In terms of initial immobilization, all types and durations of immobilization have an equal effect on preventing redislocation and decreasing chances of progression to surgery (23).

The position of the shoulder in immobilization is; however, critically important. Reduction of Bankart lesions, which are extremely common in anterior shoulder dislocations, is better with the arm in external rotation than it is with the arm in internal rotation (54) (Figs. 36-11 and 36-12). There is a significant reduction

in redislocation rate of patients treated with immobilization in external rotation as compared to those treated with immobilization in internal rotation. It is important to remember that young patients treated with immobilization in external rotation will have difficulties with sitting at a desk and entering and exiting cars due to the position of their arm. While the reduction in redislocation rates is significant across all age groups, in patients younger than 30 years of age, immobilization in external

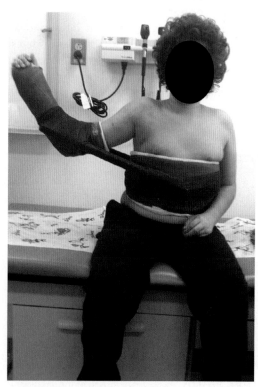

▲ **FIGURE 36-12:** Shoulder spica cast in external rotation.

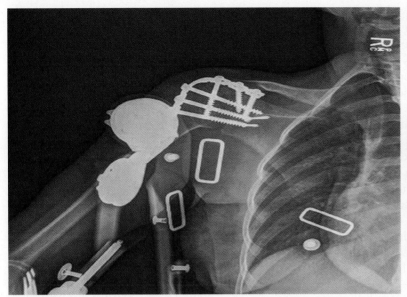
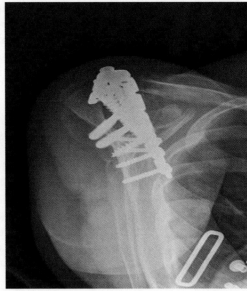

▲ **FIGURE 36-13:** AP **(right)** and trans-scapular lateral **(left)** radiographs of the shoulder status post arthrodesis with scapulohumeral plate in place. *Courtesy of Charles Getz, MD.*

rotation is particularly beneficial with a relative risk reduction of 46.1% (55).

A rigid rehabilitation program is extremely important for proper healing and the highest likelihood of a full return to activity without recurrent dislocation. Physical therapy should include restrengthening, emphasizing the muscles of internal rotation and adduction, range of motion stretches, isotonic and isokinetic exercises, and strict restrictions of activities until all goals of the rehabilitation program have been satisfied (56).

While extreme, in cases of recurrent instability that cannot be managed otherwise, shoulder arthrodesis has been used as a successful treatment. Patients recover with restricted range of motion; however, arthrodesis decreases pain rating and eliminates risk of dislocation due to joint fusion (57) (Figs. 36-13 and 36-14).

Traumatic Dislocations

Almost all pediatric patients with traumatic shoulder dislocations should be treated operatively. One exception is the mid-season athlete with traumatic dislocation, particularly if he or she wants to finish playing the season. Management of the in-season athlete can be quite difficult (1). These patients may benefit from physical therapy and bracing in the interim until the season

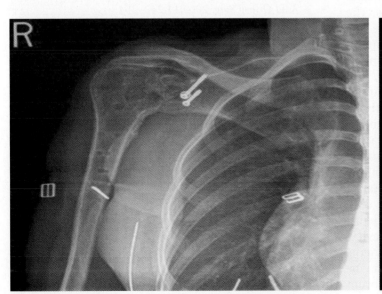
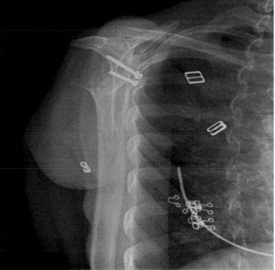

▲ **FIGURE 36-14:** AP **(right)** and trans-scapular lateral **(left)** radiographs of the shoulder status post arthrodesis after plate removal. *Courtesy of Charles Getz, MD.*

is over at which time they can consider surgical treatment. This delay of treatment excludes patients whose sports require overhead activity such as gymnasts, rock climbers, kayakers, and tennis players. This subset of athletes should not be allowed to return to sports until after treatment has been completed due to the high risk of redislocation and further injury (58).

Traumatic dislocations should be treated operatively because surgery dramatically reduces redislocation rates and other sequelae of shoulder dislocation (59). Arthroscopically treated patients with traumatic shoulder dislocation have recurrent instability rates of only 11% to 14%, drastically lower than patients treated nonoperatively who have redislocation rates of 75% to 80% (52,60). Patients with traumatic shoulder dislocations treated nonoperatively also tend to have a small, but clinically meaningful, decrease in quality of life compared to those treated operatively (58).

The surgery of choice in traumatic shoulder dislocations in children before the closure of growth plates is arthroscopic stabilization. Arthroscopic labral refixation for post-traumatic shoulder instability can be carried out using the same surgical procedures as in adults. No evidence of growth disturbance or biodegradation-associated problems has been observed in children and adolescents undergoing labral refixation, and as such, delay until adulthood is not indicated (53). In skeletally immature patients, primary arthroscopic Bankart repair is an effective treatment of traumatic shoulder instability and significantly reduces the rate of recurrent shoulder instability (45,60).

CONCLUSION

Shoulder instability in the pediatric patient can have multiple precipitating factors and presentations. The patient, age, and the mechanism of injury are key factors to consider as treatment options are contemplated. Traumatic instability is likely to have an underlying soft tissue injury which, if left untreated, will likely result in recurrent instability and injury. Atraumatic instability is often associated with an underlying or heritable soft tissue laxity condition that is often best addressed with nonoperative treatment and activity modification. Most traumatic instability occurs in the athletic adolescent and surgical treatment options tend to result in better outcomes than nonoperative treatments. Surgical techniques similar to those used in adult patients can be used in adolescent patients. The authors' observations and experience, and a review of the current literature, have not revealed any patients with clinically apparent growth disturbance with current instability repair techniques anchoring the labrum and glenohumeral ligament complex back to the glenoid.

ACKNOWLEDGMENTS

Nancy Chauvin, MD—Department of Radiology, The Children's Hospital of Philadelphia

Charles Getz, MD—Department of Orthopaedic Surgery, Thomas Jefferson University Hospital

Victor Ho, MD—Department of Radiology, The Children's Hospital of Philadelphia

References

1. McKee J. The changing landscape of youth sports injuries. *AAOS Now.* Nov. 2009.
2. Soprano JV. Musculoskeletal injuries in the pediatric and adolescent athlete. *Curr Sports Med Rep.* 2005;4: 329–334.
3. Wright JM, Paletta GA Jr, Altchek DW, et al. Surgical management of posterior shoulder instability in a ten-year-old boy: A case report and literature review. *Am J Orthop (Belle Mead NJ).* 2000;29:633–637.
4. Matheny JM, Brinker MR, Elliott MN, et al. Confidence of graduating family practice residents in their management of musculoskeletal conditions. *Am J Orthop (Belle Mead, NJ).* 2000;29:945–952.
5. Devgan LL, Gill HS, Faustin C, et al. Posterior dislocation in a voluntary subluxator: A case report. *Med Sci Sports Exerc.* 2006;38:613–617.
6. Weinberg J, Doering C, McFarland EG. Joint surgery in Ehlers-Danlos patients: Results of a survey. *Am J Orthop (Belle Mead NJ).* 1999;28:406–409.
7. Cleeman E, Flatow EL. Shoulder dislocations in the young patient. *Orthop Clin North Am.* 2000;31:217–229.
8. Jaramillo D, Shapiro F. Musculoskeletal trauma in children. *Magn Reson Imaging Clin N Am.* 1998;6: 521–536.
9. Pearl ML. Shoulder problems in children with brachial plexus birth palsy: Evaluation and management. *J Am Acad Orthop Surg.* 2009;17:242–254.
10. Cardoso HF. Age estimation of adolescent and young adult male and female skeletons II, epiphyseal union at the upper limb and scapular girdle in a modern Portuguese skeletal sample. *Am J Phys Anthropol.* 2008;137:97–105.
11. Schmeling A, Schulz R, Reisinger W, et al. Studies on the time frame for ossification of the medial clavicular epiphyseal cartilage in conventional radiography. *Int J Legal Med.* 2004;118:5–8.
12. Webb PA, Suchey JM. Epiphyseal union of the anterior iliac crest and medial clavicle in a modern multiracial sample of American males and females. *Am J Phys Anthropol.* 1985;68:457–466.
13. Ogden JA. *Skeletal Injury in the Child.* 3rd ed. New York, NY: Springer-Verlag; 2000.
14. Meijerman L, Maat GJ, Schulz R, et al. Variables affecting the probability of complete fusion of the medial clavicular epiphysis. *Int J Legal Med.* 2007;121: 463–468.
15. Chauvin NA, Jaimes C, Laor T, et al. Magnetic resonance imaging of the pediatric shoulder. *Magn Reson Imaging Clin N Am.* 2012;20:327–347, xi.

16. Rockwood CA Jr, Matsen FA III. *The Shoulder.* 4th ed. Philadelphia, PA: Saunders/Elsevier; 2009.
17. Ogden JA, Phillips SB. Radiology of postnatal skeletal development. VII. The scapula. *Skeletal Radiol.* 1983;9:157–169.
18. Kim HK, Emery KH, Salisbury SR. Bare spot of the glenoid fossa in children: Incidence and MRI features. *Pediatr Radiol.* 2010;40:1190–1196.
19. Mintzer CM, Waters PM, Brown DJ. Glenoid version in children. *J Pediatr Orthop.* 1996;16:563–566.
20. Macalister A. Notes on the acromion. *J Anat Physiol.* 1893;27:245–251.
21. Sahajpal D, Strauss EJ, Ishak C, et al. Surgical management of os acromiale: A case report and review of the literature. *Bull NYU Hosp Jt Dis.* 2007;65:312–316.
22. Sammarco VJ. Os acromiale: Frequency, anatomy, and clinical implications. *J Bone Joint Surg Am.* 2000;82:394–400.
23. Hovelius L, Augustini BG, Fredin H, et al. Primary anterior dislocation of the shoulder in young patients. A ten-year prospective study. *J Bone Joint Surg Am.* 1996;78:1677–1684.
24. Heck CC. Anterior dislocation of the glenohumeral joint in a child. *J Trauma.* 1981;21:174–175.
25. Hoelen MA, Burgers AM, Rozing PM. Prognosis of primary anterior shoulder dislocation in young adults. *Arch Orthop Trauma Surg.* 1990;110:51–54.
26. Rowe CR. Anterior dislocations of the shoulder: Prognosis and treatment. *Surg Clin North Am.* 1963;43:1609–1614.
27. Rowe CR. Prognosis in dislocations of the shoulder. *J Bone Joint Surg Am.* 1956;38-A:957–977.
28. Hovelius L. Incidence of shoulder dislocation in Sweden. *Clin Orthop Relat Res.* 1982:127–131.
29. Sprangers MA, Aaronson NK. The role of health care providers and significant others in evaluating the quality of life of patients with chronic disease: A review. *J Clin Epidemiol.* 1992;45:743–760.
30. Simonet WT, Melton LJ 3rd, Cofield RH, et al. Incidence of anterior shoulder dislocation in Olmsted County, Minnesota. *Clin Orthop Relat Res.* 1984:186–191.
31. Wagner KT Jr, Lyne ED. Adolescent traumatic dislocations of the shoulder with open epiphyses. *J Pediatr Orthop.* 1983;3:61–62.
32. O'Driscoll SW, Evans DC. Contralateral shoulder instability following anterior repair. An epidemiological investigation. *J Bone Joint Surg Br.* 1991;73:941–946.
33. Deitch J, Mehlman CT, Foad SL, et al. Traumatic anterior shoulder dislocation in adolescents. *Am J Sports Med.* 2003;31:758–763.
34. Marans HJ, Angel KR, Schemitsch EH, et al. The fate of traumatic anterior dislocation of the shoulder in children. *J Bone Joint Surg Am.* 1992;74:1242–1244.
35. Simonet WT, Cofield RH. Prognosis in anterior shoulder dislocation. *Am J Sports Med.* 1984;12:19–24.
36. Cil A, Kocher MS. Treatment of pediatric shoulder instability. *J Pediatr Orthop.* 2010;30:S3–S6.
37. Rowe CR, Sakellarides HT. Factors related to recurrences of anterior dislocations of the shoulder. *Clin Orthop.* 1961;20:40–48.
38. Vermeiren J, Handelberg F, Casteleyn PP, et al. The rate of recurrence of traumatic anterior dislocation of the shoulder.

A study of 154 cases and a review of the literature. *Int Orthop.* 1993;17:337–341.
39. McLaughlin HL, MacLellan DI. Recurrent anterior dislocation of the shoulder. II. A comparative study. *J Trauma.* 1967;7:191–201.
40. Postacchini F, Gumina S, Cinotti G. Anterior shoulder dislocation in adolescents. *J Shoulder Elbow Surg.* 2000;9:470–404.
41. Rowe CR. Acute and recurrent anterior dislocations of the shoulder. *Orthop Clin North Am.* 1980;11:253–270.
42. Rowe CR, Patel D, Southmayd WW. The Bankart procedure: A long-term end-result study. *J Bone Joint Surg Am.* 1978;60:1–16.
43. Taylor DC, Arciero RA. Pathologic changes associated with shoulder dislocations. Arthroscopic and physical examination findings in first-time, traumatic anterior dislocations. *Am J Sports Med.* 1997;25:306–311.
44. Thomas SC, Matsen FA 3rd. An approach to the repair of avulsion of the glenohumeral ligaments in the management of traumatic anterior glenohumeral instability. *J Bone Joint Surg Am.* 1989;71:506–513.
45. Jones KJ, Wiesel B, Ganley TJ, et al. Functional outcomes of early arthroscopic Bankart repair in adolescents aged 11 to 18 years. [Erratum appears in *J Pediatr Orthop.* 2007;27(4):483]. *J Pediatr Orthop.* 2007;27:209–213.
46. MacKenzie JD. MR arthrography made simple: Indications and techniques. *Pediatr Radiol.* 2008;38:S240–S242.
47. Brophy RH, Marx RG. Osteoarthritis following shoulder instability. *Clin Sports Med.* 2005;24:47–56.
48. Sarwark JF, King EC, Janicki JA. Glenohumeral subluxation and dislocation. In: JHK Beaty Jr, ed. *Rockwood and Wilkins' Fractures in Children.* 7th ed. Philadelphia, PA: Lippincott, Williams & Wilkins; 2009:634–644.
49. Burkhead WZ Jr, Rockwood CA Jr. Treatment of instability of the shoulder with an exercise program. *J Bone Joint Surg Am.* 1992;74:890–896.
50. Eisner EA, Roocroft JH, Edmonds EW. Underestimation of labral pathology in adolescents with anterior shoulder instability. *J Pediatr Orthop.* 2012;32:42–47.
51. Geier CD Jr, Paletta GA Jr. Shoulder instability in the skeletally immature athlete. *Oper Tech Sports Med.* 2006;14:159–164.
52. Bottoni CR, Wilckens JH, DeBerardino TM, et al. A prospective, randomized evaluation of arthroscopic stabilization versus nonoperative treatment in patients with acute, traumatic, first-time shoulder dislocations. *Am J Sports Med.* 2002;30:576–580.
53. Kraus R, Pavlidis T, Dongowski N, et al. Children and adolescents with posttraumatic shoulder instability benefit from arthroscopic stabilization. *Eur J Pediatr Surg.* 2010;20:253–256.
54. Itoi E, Sashi R, Minagawa H, et al. Position of immobilization after dislocation of the glenohumeral joint. A study with use of magnetic resonance imaging. *J Bone Joint Surg Am.* 2001;83-A:661–667.
55. Itoi E, Hatakeyama Y, Sato T, et al. Immobilization in external rotation after shoulder dislocation reduces the risk of recurrence. A randomized controlled trial. *J Bone Joint Surg Am.* 2007;89:2124–2131.
56. Aronen JG, Regan K. Decreasing the incidence of recurrence of first time anterior shoulder dislocations

with rehabilitation. *Am J Sports Med.* 1984;12: 283–291.

57. Diaz JA, Cohen SB, Warren RF, et al. Arthrodesis as a salvage procedure for recurrent instability of the shoulder. *J Shoulder Elbow Surg.* 2003;12:237–241.

58. Kirkley A, Werstine R, Ratjek A, et al. Prospective randomized clinical trial comparing the effectiveness of immediate arthroscopic stabilization versus immobilization and rehabilitation in first traumatic anterior disloca-tions of the shoulder: Long-term evaluation. *Arthroscopy.* 2005;21:55–63.

59. Lawton RL, Choudhury S, Mansat P, et al. Pediatric shoulder instability: Presentation, findings, treatment, and outcomes. *J Pediatr Orthop.* 2002;22:52–61.

60. Arciero RA, Wheeler JH, Ryan JB, et al. Arthroscopic Bankart repair versus nonoperative treatment for acute, initial anterior shoulder dislocations. *Am J Sports Med.* 1994;22:589–594.

Index

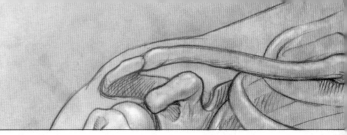

Page numbers followed by *f* indicate figures; those followed by *t* indicate tables.